U0311184

蒙古文手抄普济杂方

Mongolian Manuscripts of Cure-all Prescriptions

中国蒙医药古籍影印珍本

Rare Photocopy of Chinese Mongolian Medicine Ancient Book

民族文字出版专项资金资助项目

图书在版编目（CIP）数据

蒙古文手抄普济杂方：蒙古文 / 辽宁省阜新蒙医药研究所，内蒙古民族大学编. —沈阳：辽宁民族出版社，2018.7（2021.1重印）
（中国蒙医药古籍影印珍本）
ISBN 978-7-5497-1858-0

Ⅰ. ①蒙… Ⅱ. ①辽… ②内… Ⅲ. ①蒙医—药方—汇编—蒙古语（中国少数民族语言）Ⅳ. ①R291.2

中国版本图书馆CIP数据核字（2018）第166850号

蒙古文手抄普济杂方
MENGGUWENSHOUCHAOPUJIZAFANG

出版发行者：辽宁民族出版社
地　　址：沈阳市和平区十一纬路25号　邮编：110003
印　刷　者：辽宁新华印务有限公司
幅 面 尺 寸：210mm×285mm
印　　张：42
字　　数：850千字
出 版 时 间：2018年7月第1版
印 刷 时 间：2021年1月第2次印刷
责 任 编 辑：白兰英
封 面 设 计：杜　江
责 任 印 制：杨　雪
责 任 校 对：代智敏

标准书号：ISBN 978-7-5497-1858-0
定　　价：480.00元

网　　址：www.lnmzcbs.com　　邮购热线：024-23284335
淘宝网店：http://lnmz2013.taobao.com
如有印装质量问题，请与出版社联系调换　联系电话：024-23284340

ᠶᠠᠭᠤ ᠪᠠᠷ ᠰᠠᠶᠢᠨ ᠰᠠᠶᠢᠬᠠᠨ ᠪᠣᠯ ᠤᠯᠠᠮᠵᠢᠯᠠᠯᠲᠤ ᠮᠣᠩᠭᠣᠯ ᠰᠣᠶᠣᠯ ᠤᠨ ᠬᠡᠯᠡᠯᠴᠡᠭᠡᠨ ᠦ ᠭᠣᠣᠯ ᠬᠡᠰᠡᠭ ᠦᠨ ᠨᠢᠭᠡ ᠪᠣᠯᠤᠨ᠎ᠠ ᠃

ᠡᠷᠬᠢᠯᠡᠭᠴᠢ : (ᠵᠠᠰᠠᠭ ᠤᠨ ᠭᠠᠵᠠᠷ ᠤᠨ ᠰᠣᠶᠣᠯ ᠤᠨ ᠣᠷᠤᠨ ᠦ ᠬᠠᠮᠲᠤ ᠡᠮᠬᠢᠳᠬᠡᠯ)

ᠳᠡᠳ ᠡᠮᠬᠢᠳᠬᠡᠭᠴᠢ : ᠪᠠᠶᠠᠷ ᠮᠣᠩᠭᠣᠯ ᠰᠠᠷᠠᠨ ᠭᠡᠷᠡᠯ ᠰᠠᠶᠢᠨ ᠪᠢᠯᠢᠭ

ᠡᠮᠬᠢᠳᠬᠡᠭᠴᠢ : ᠪᠠᠶᠠᠷ ᠵᠣᠷᠢᠭᠲᠤ ᠭᠡᠷᠡᠯ

«ᠤᠯᠠᠮᠵᠢᠯᠠᠯᠲᠤ ᠰᠣᠶᠣᠯ ᠤᠨ ᠥᠪ ᠢ ᠬᠠᠮᠠᠭᠠᠯᠠᠬᠤ ᠶᠢᠨ ᠲᠡᠭᠦᠯ ᠦ ᠰᠤᠷᠭᠠᠯᠢ ᠮᠡᠳᠡᠯᠭᠡ ᠪᠢᠴᠢᠭ ᠤᠨ ᠴᠤᠪᠤᠷᠠᠯ» ᠤᠨ ᠨᠠᠶᠢᠷᠠᠭᠤᠯᠬᠤ ᠡᠷᠬᠢᠯᠡᠭᠴᠢ ᠶᠢᠨ ᠬᠣᠷᠢᠶ᠎ᠠ

ᠡᠷᠬᠢᠯᠡᠭᠴᠢ : ᠮᠥ ᠵᠢᠩ ᠰᠠᠨ ᠯᠢᠶᠣ ᠬᠤᠸᠠ ᠬᠦᠢ ᠲᠤᠩ ᠭᠤᠸᠠ ᠬᠦᠢ ᠰᠤᠸᠸᠸᠸ ᠪᠠᠲᠤᠪᠣᠯᠣᠳ

ᠳᠡᠳ ᠡᠮᠬᠢᠳᠬᠡᠭᠴᠢ : ᠪᠠᠶᠠᠷᠮᠢᠲ᠋ ᠸᠠᠩ ᠴᠢᠨ ᠵᠢᠶᠠᠨ

ᠡᠮᠬᠢᠳᠬᠡᠭᠴᠢ : ᠪᠣᠣ ᠴᠢᠨ ᠬᠠᠯᠠ ᠮᠦ ᠯᠢ ᠯᠢᠩ

«ᠤᠯᠠᠮᠵᠢᠯᠠᠯᠲᠤ ᠰᠣᠶᠣᠯ ᠤᠨ ᠥᠪ ᠢ ᠬᠠᠮᠠᠭᠠᠯᠠᠬᠤ ᠶᠢᠨ ᠲᠡᠭᠦᠯ ᠦ ᠰᠤᠷᠭᠠᠯᠢ ᠮᠡᠳᠡᠯᠭᠡ ᠪᠢᠴᠢᠭ ᠤᠨ ᠴᠤᠪᠤᠷᠠᠯ» ᠤᠨ ᠡᠮᠬᠢᠳᠬᠡᠯ ᠦᠨ ᠬᠣᠷᠢᠶ᠎ᠠ

ᠡᠷᠬᠢᠯᠡᠭᠴᠢ : ᠮᠥᠩᠬᠡᠪᠠᠶᠠᠷ ᠮᠥ ᠰᠠᠷᠠᠨ ᠭᠡᠷᠡᠯ ᠵᠢᠨ ᠯᠢᠩ ᠬᠠᠯᠠ ᠪᠠᠶᠠᠷ ᠮᠥᠩᠬᠡᠪᠠᠶᠠᠷ ᠪᠣᠷᠵᠢᠭᠢᠨ ᠪᠠᠶᠠᠷ ᠮᠣᠩᠭᠣᠯ ᠴᠣᠭᠲᠤ ᠪᠢᠯᠢᠭ ᠬᠠᠯᠠ ᠪᠠᠶᠠᠷ

ᠳᠡᠳ ᠬᠠᠷᠢᠭᠤᠴᠠᠭᠴᠢ ᠶᠢᠨ ᠳᠠᠷᠤᠭ᠎ᠠ : ᠰᠠᠷᠠᠨ ᠭᠡᠷᠡᠯ ᠮᠥ · ᠮᠣᠩᠭᠣᠯ ᠪᠠᠶᠠᠷ ᠮᠣᠩᠭᠣᠯ ᠵᠢᠯ

ᠬᠠᠷᠢᠭᠤᠴᠠᠭᠴᠢ ᠶᠢᠨ ᠳᠠᠷᠤᠭ᠎ᠠ : ᠵᠣᠷᠢᠭᠲᠤ ᠭᠡᠷᠡᠯ ᠮᠣᠩᠭᠣᠯ ᠰᠠᠷᠠᠨ ᠵᠢᠯ

«ᠤᠯᠠᠮᠵᠢᠯᠠᠯᠲᠤ ᠰᠣᠶᠣᠯ ᠤᠨ ᠥᠪ ᠢ ᠬᠠᠮᠠᠭᠠᠯᠠᠬᠤ ᠶᠢᠨ ᠲᠡᠭᠦᠯ ᠦ ᠰᠤᠷᠭᠠᠯᠢ ᠮᠡᠳᠡᠯᠭᠡ ᠪᠢᠴᠢᠭ ᠤᠨ ᠴᠤᠪᠤᠷᠠᠯ» ᠤᠨ ᠲᠥᠰᠥᠯ ᠬᠠᠷᠢᠭᠤᠴᠠᠭᠴᠢ

《中国蒙医药古籍影印珍本》领导小组

《中国蒙医药古籍影印珍本》顾问委员会

《中国蒙医药古籍影印珍本》编辑委员会

ᠡᠮᠦᠨᠡᠬᠢ ᠦᠭᠡ

ᠵᠠᠭᠤᠨ ᠤ 16 ᠳᠤᠭᠠᠷ [illegible] ᠮᠣᠩᠭᠣᠯ [illegible] ᠤᠨ [illegible] ᠪᠣᠯᠵᠤ ᠪᠠᠢᠨ᠎ᠠ ᠃
[illegible] ᠃ [illegible] ᠃ [illegible] ᠃ [illegible]
[illegible] 《 [illegible] 》 [illegible]
[illegible] ᠃
[illegible] ᠃ [illegible]
[illegible] 《 [illegible] 》 ᠪᠤᠶᠤ 《 [illegible] 》 [illegible]
[illegible]
[illegible] ᠃ [illegible]
[illegible] （ [illegible] ） [illegible]
[illegible]
[illegible] ᠃

[illegible] ᠃ [illegible] ᠃
[illegible]
[illegible]
[illegible] ᠃ [illegible]
[illegible]
[illegible]
[illegible] ᠃ [illegible]
[illegible]

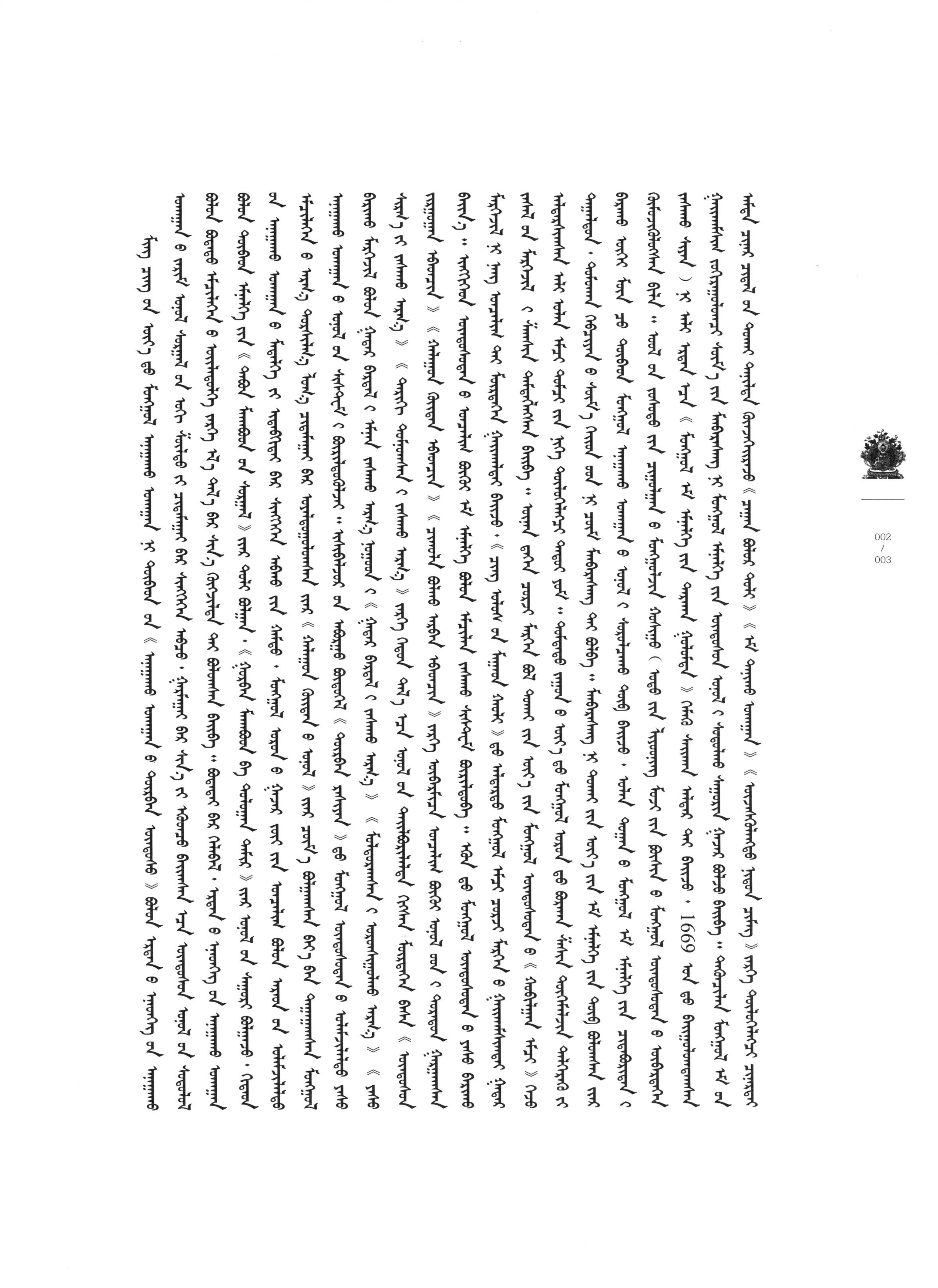

ᠮᠣᠩᠭᠣᠯ ᠬᠡᠯᠡ ᠪᠢᠴᠢᠭ ᠢ ᠮᠣᠩᠭᠣᠯ ᠰᠤᠷᠭᠠᠭᠤᠯᠢ ᠶᠢᠨ ᠰᠤᠷᠭᠠᠨ ᠬᠦᠮᠦᠵᠢᠯ ᠦᠨ ᠬᠡᠷᠡᠭᠰᠡᠯ ᠳᠦ ᠬᠦᠷᠭᠡᠵᠦ ᠪᠠᠢᠨ᠎ᠠ ᠂ ᠲᠡᠷᠡ ᠴᠢ ᠪᠡᠷ ᠰᠤᠷᠭᠠᠭᠤᠯᠢ ᠶᠢᠨ ᠰᠤᠷᠭᠠᠨ ᠳᠦ ᠳᠤᠰᠬᠤ ᠶᠢᠨ ᠬᠠᠮᠲᠤ ᠪᠡᠷ ᠰᠤᠷᠤᠯᠴᠠᠭᠴᠢᠳ ᠤᠨ ᠬᠢᠴᠢᠶᠡᠯ ᠳᠦ ᠪᠠᠷᠢᠮᠲᠠ ᠪᠤᠯᠤᠨ ᠪᠠᠢᠨ᠎ᠠ ᠃

ᠪᠤᠰᠤ ᠂ ᠰᠤᠷᠭᠠᠨ ᠤ ᠪᠠᠢᠭᠤᠯᠤᠯᠭ᠎ᠠ ᠶᠢᠨ ᠬᠠᠮᠲᠤᠷᠠᠯᠴᠠᠭ᠎ᠠ ᠶᠢᠨ ᠂ ᠰᠤᠷᠭᠠᠭᠤᠯᠢ ᠂ ᠰᠤᠷᠭᠠᠭᠤᠯᠢ ᠂ ᠰᠤᠷᠭᠠᠭᠤᠯᠢ ᠰᠤᠷᠭᠠᠭᠤᠯᠢ ᠂ ᠮᠣᠩᠭᠣᠯ ᠰᠤᠷᠭᠠᠭᠤᠯᠢ ᠂ ᠪᠠᠭ᠎ᠠ ᠰᠤᠷᠭᠠᠭᠤᠯᠢ ᠳᠤᠮᠳᠠ ᠬᠡᠯᠡ ᠮᠣᠩᠭᠣᠯ ᠬᠡᠯᠡ ᠪᠢᠴᠢᠭ ᠦᠨ ᠰᠤᠷᠭᠠᠨ ᠢ ᠬᠡᠷᠡᠭᠵᠢᠭᠦᠯᠬᠦ ᠳᠦ ᠰᠤᠷᠭᠠᠨ ᠬᠦᠮᠦᠵᠢᠯ ᠦᠨ ᠰᠢᠨᠡᠴᠢᠯᠡᠯ ᠢ ᠬᠦᠢᠴᠡᠳᠬᠡᠬᠦ ᠳᠦ ᠬᠠᠮᠢᠶ᠎ᠠ ᠲᠠᠢ ᠂ ᠮᠣᠩᠭᠣᠯ ᠬᠡᠯᠡ ᠪᠢᠴᠢᠭ ᠦᠨ ᠰᠤᠷᠭᠠᠨ ᠢ ᠪᠠᠶᠠᠵᠢᠭᠤᠯᠬᠤ ᠳᠤ ᠴᠢᠬᠤᠯᠠ ᠠᠴᠠ ᠪᠠᠷ ᠬᠠᠮᠢᠶᠠᠷᠤᠯᠵᠤ ᠪᠠᠢᠨ᠎ᠠ ᠃ ᠰᠦᠯᠵᠢᠶ᠎ᠡ ᠰᠤᠷᠭᠠᠨ ᠰᠤᠷᠭᠠᠯᠲᠠ ᠶᠢᠨ ᠬᠡᠷᠡᠭᠯᠡᠭᠡ ᠶᠢᠨ 2016 ᠣᠨ ᠤ 《 ᠮᠣᠩᠭᠣᠯ ᠬᠡᠯᠡ ᠪᠢᠴᠢᠭ ᠦᠨ ᠰᠤᠷᠭᠠᠨ ᠬᠦᠮᠦᠵᠢᠯ ᠦᠨ ... 2000 ᠣᠨ ᠤ ... 1980 ᠣᠨ ᠤ ... ᠮᠣᠩᠭᠣᠯ ᠬᠡᠯᠡ ᠪᠢᠴᠢᠭ ᠦᠨ ᠰᠤᠷᠭᠠᠨ ... ᠂ 1987 ᠣᠨ ᠤ ... 1958 ᠣᠨ ᠤ ... ᠮᠣᠩᠭᠣᠯ ᠬᠡᠯᠡ ᠪᠢᠴᠢᠭ ᠦᠨ ... ᠃

ᠡᠳᠡᠭᠡᠷ ᠮᠣᠩᠭᠣᠯ ᠬᠡᠯᠡ ᠪᠢᠴᠢᠭ ᠦᠨ ᠰᠤᠷᠭᠠᠨ ᠬᠦᠮᠦᠵᠢᠯ ᠦᠨ ... ᠃

... 《 ... ᠮᠣᠩᠭᠣᠯ ᠬᠡᠯᠡ ᠪᠢᠴᠢᠭ ᠦᠨ ... 3000 ... 《 ... 》 ... ᠃

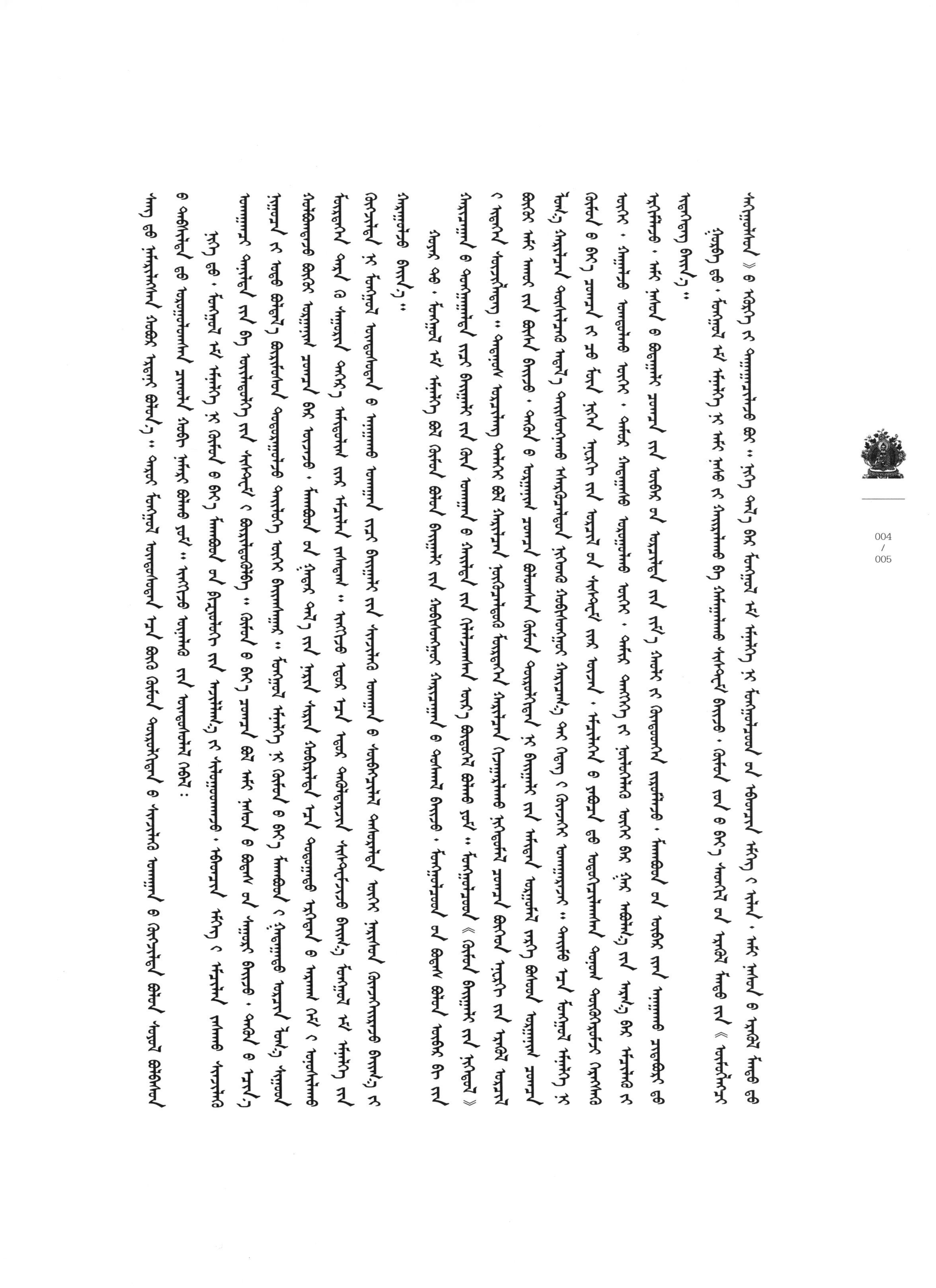

[illegible] 》 [illegible] ᠪᠠᠢᠨ᠎ᠠ ::

[illegible] 《 [illegible] ᠪᠠᠢᠨ᠎ᠠ ::

[illegible] ᠪᠠᠢᠨ᠎ᠠ ::

[illegible]

[illegible] :

[illegible]

[illegible]

[illegible]

[illegible]

[illegible]

[illegible]

[illegible]

[illegible]

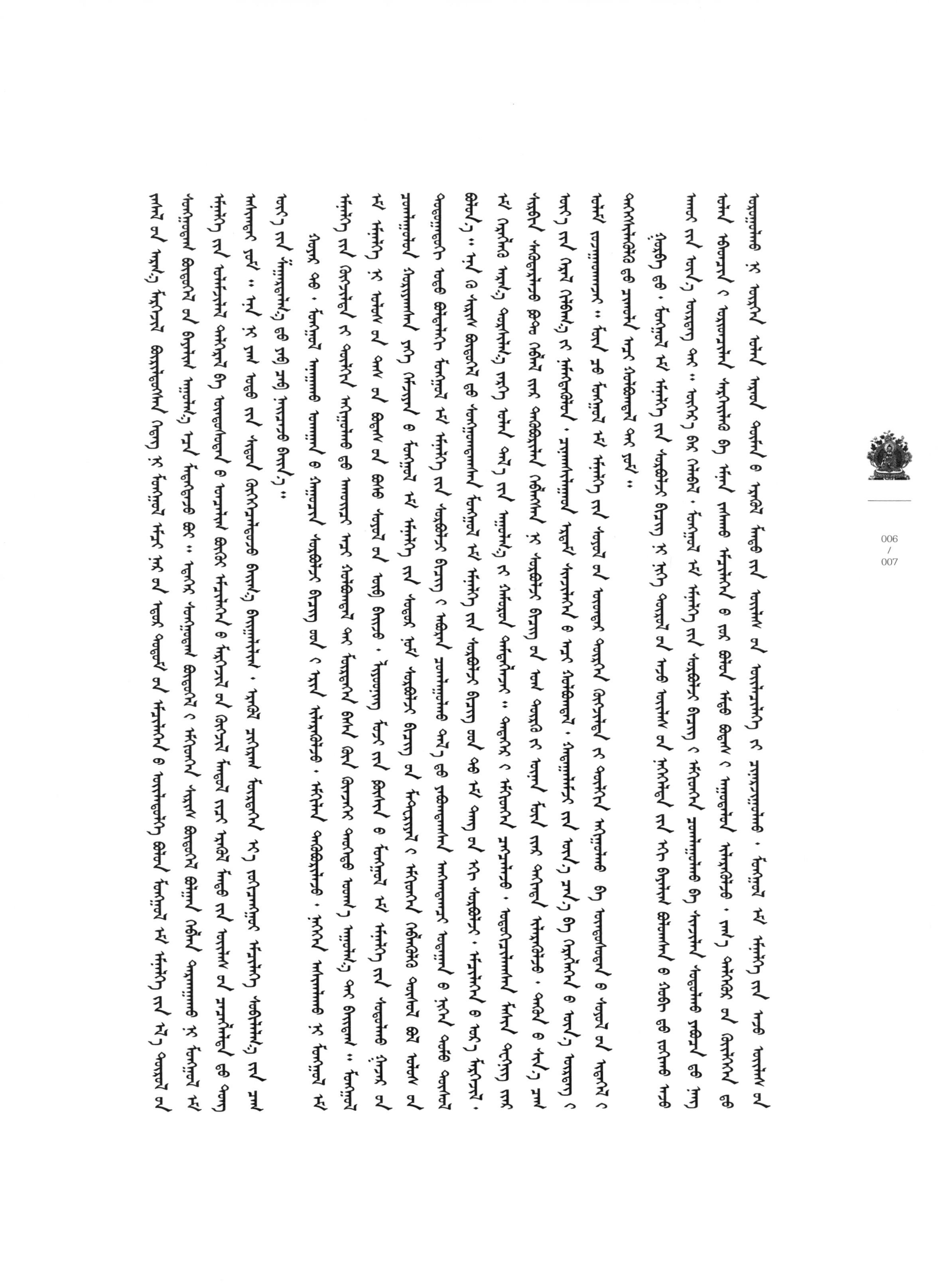

ᠳᠡᠪᠰᠢᠯᠲᠡ ᠶᠢ ᠳᠡᠯᠭᠡᠷᠡᠭᠦᠯᠬᠦ ᠳᠦ ᠲᠤᠰᠠᠯᠠᠬᠤ᠂ ᠪᠦᠬᠦ ᠮᠣᠩᠭᠣᠯ ᠬᠡᠯᠡ ᠪᠢᠴᠢᠭ ᠤᠨ ᠰᠤᠷᠭᠠᠯᠲᠠ ᠶᠢᠨ ᠴᠢᠨᠠᠷ ᠢ ᠳᠡᠭᠡᠭᠰᠢᠯᠡᠭᠦᠯᠬᠦ ᠳᠦ ᠲᠤᠰᠠᠯᠠᠨ᠎ᠠ᠂ ᠮᠡᠳᠡᠯᠭᠡ ᠶᠢᠨ ᠪᠦᠲᠦᠴᠡ ᠶᠢ ᠪᠠᠶᠠᠵᠢᠭᠤᠯᠬᠤ ᠳᠤ ᠴᠢᠬᠤᠯᠠ ᠠᠴᠢ ᠬᠣᠯᠪᠣᠭᠳᠠᠯ ᠲᠠᠢ ᠪᠣᠯᠤᠨ᠎ᠠ ::

ᠰᠠᠶᠢᠬᠠᠨ ᠪᠡᠷ᠂ ᠬᠡᠪᠯᠡᠯ ᠦᠨ ᠬᠣᠷᠢᠶ᠎ᠠ ᠶᠢᠨ ᠳᠠᠷᠤᠭ᠎ᠠ ᠪᠠ ᠮᠡᠷᠭᠡᠵᠢᠯ ᠦᠨ ᠬᠦᠮᠦᠰ ᠦᠨ ᠬᠠᠮᠲᠤ ᠬᠦᠴᠦᠯᠡᠯ ᠢ ᠰᠢᠩᠭᠡᠭᠡᠭᠰᠡᠨ ᠦᠷ᠎ᠡ ᠪᠣᠯᠤᠨ᠎ᠠ :: ᠮᠣᠩᠭᠣᠯ ᠬᠡᠯᠡ ᠪᠢᠴᠢᠭ ᠤᠨ ᠰᠤᠷᠭᠠᠯᠲᠠ ᠶᠢᠨ ᠰᠤᠷᠭᠠᠭᠤᠯᠢ ᠶᠢᠨ ᠪᠠᠭᠰᠢ ᠨᠠᠷ ᠤᠨ ᠬᠠᠮᠲᠤ ᠵᠢᠯ ᠦᠨ ᠠᠵᠢᠯ ᠲᠤᠷᠰᠢᠯᠭ᠎ᠠ ᠪᠣᠯᠤᠭᠰᠠᠨ ᠰᠠᠶᠢᠨᠰᠢᠶᠡᠯᠳᠡ ᠪᠡᠷ ᠰᠠᠶᠢᠨ ᠤ ᠬᠡᠷᠡᠭ ᠢ ᠳᠠᠭᠤᠰᠬᠠᠬᠤ ᠪᠡᠷ ᠬᠠᠮᠲᠤ ᠰᠠᠭᠤᠷᠢᠯᠠᠭᠰᠠᠨ ᠪᠠᠶᠢᠨ᠎ᠠ :: ᠲᠡᠷᠡ ᠪᠣᠯ ᠰᠤᠷᠭᠠᠭᠤᠯᠢ ᠶᠢᠨ ᠮᠣᠩᠭᠣᠯ ᠬᠡᠯᠡ ᠪᠢᠴᠢᠭ ᠤᠨ ᠬᠢᠴᠢᠶᠡᠯ ᠦᠨ 《ᠰᠤᠷᠭᠠᠭᠤᠯᠢ ᠶᠢᠨ ᠮᠣᠩᠭᠣᠯ ᠬᠡᠯᠡ ᠪᠢᠴᠢᠭ ᠤᠨ ᠰᠤᠷᠭᠠᠯᠲᠠ ᠶᠢᠨ ᠨᠣᠮ ᠤᠨ ᠪᠠᠶᠢᠭᠤᠯᠭ᠎ᠠ ᠶᠢᠨ ᠰᠤᠷᠭᠠᠯᠲᠠ ᠶᠢᠨ ᠲᠥᠯᠦᠪᠯᠡᠭᠡ 》 ᠶᠢᠨ ᠰᠠᠭᠤᠷᠢ ᠳᠡᠭᠡᠷ᠎ᠡ᠂ ᠰᠤᠷᠭᠠᠯᠲᠠ ᠶᠢᠨ ᠬᠢᠴᠢᠶᠡᠯ ᠦᠨ ᠬᠡᠷᠡᠭᠯᠡᠭᠡᠨ ᠦ ᠠᠭᠤᠯᠭ᠎ᠠ ᠪᠣᠯᠤᠨ ᠪᠠᠭᠰᠢ ᠨᠠᠷ ᠤᠨ ᠬᠡᠷᠡᠭᠴᠡᠭᠡ ᠶᠢ ᠪᠠᠳᠤᠯᠠᠭᠰᠠᠨ ᠳᠠ ᠬᠤᠪᠢ ᠶᠢ ᠰᠤᠷᠭᠠᠭᠤᠯᠢ ᠶᠢᠨ ᠪᠠᠭᠰᠢ ᠨᠠᠷ ᠤᠨ ᠬᠡᠷᠡᠭᠯᠡᠬᠦ ᠳᠦ ᠵᠣᠷᠢᠭᠤᠯᠤᠨ ᠪᠠᠶᠢᠨ᠎ᠠ ::

2018 ᠣᠨ ᠤ 6 ᠰᠠᠷ᠎ᠠ

《ᠰᠤᠷᠭᠠᠭᠤᠯᠢ ᠶᠢᠨ ᠮᠣᠩᠭᠣᠯ ᠬᠡᠯᠡ ᠪᠢᠴᠢᠭ ᠤᠨ ᠰᠤᠷᠭᠠᠯᠲᠠ ᠶᠢᠨ ᠨᠣᠮ ᠤᠨ ᠪᠠᠭᠰᠢ ᠶᠢᠨ ᠬᠡᠷᠡᠭᠯᠡᠬᠦ ᠨᠣᠮ》 ᠤᠨ ᠨᠠᠶᠢᠷᠠᠭᠤᠯᠬᠤ ᠳᠤᠭᠤᠶᠢᠯᠠᠩ

总序

蒙古族是一个历史悠久而又富于传奇色彩的民族。蒙古民族在漫长的历史进程中，形成了博大精深、绚丽多彩的民族文化样态，在居住、饮食、服饰、语言、文字、歌舞、艺术、医药、卫生等多个方面，积累下了丰富的成果，形成了自己的传统。这些传统文化的每一部分，都是凝结天地精气、承传祖先遗训的美丽造物，更是不断吐故纳新、汇聚历史风云的精华结晶。

蒙医药是蒙古民族文化百花园中的绚丽的一枝，它与蒙古族文化的其他部分一起构成了蒙古族文化博大精深的内涵体系，共同把蒙古族文化的百花园装扮得分外美丽。蒙医药源于上古，成于元代，兴于明清，盛于当代，是中华民族传统医学中的瑰宝，在中国杏林中独树一帜。

蒙古族自古以游牧为生，生活在寒冷又干旱、半干旱的草原，主要以牛羊肉和乳制品为食，平日里的骑马放牧、转场迁徙和战时纵马驰骋，极易造成摔伤、骨折、战伤等外伤。这样的气候条件、地理条件、饮食条件和生活情形，促使蒙古族的先民不断体察与大自然中动物、植物的关系，对动植物的营养、毒性等性能和防病治疗等作用，形成了初步的认识和掌握；把在长期狩猎、游牧、农耕生产和迁徙、征战中积累起来的与疾病伤害做斗争的感受和经验，加以分析和总结，从而发明了极具地域特点和民族特色的诊治技术，如灸疗术、整骨术、震脑术以及策格（酸马奶）疗法等。这是蒙医药学的萌芽和雏形阶段。

到了元代，蒙医药学获得了长足发展。这一方面是由于中原内地医学与蒙医药的相互滋养和促进，另一方面，元代蒙医药学获得体制性政策保障，在承袭唐宋时期医疗制度的基础上，国都设立太医院，各地设立惠民局，大力扶持和推广蒙医蒙药，从而为蒙医药的全方位发展提供了良好条件。在原有基础上，骨伤科等蒙古族传统医疗技术获得了新的发展和提高。与此同时，通过博采众长，集思广纳，深入研究，蒙古族先民早已归纳出来的“疾病的本质为寒、热两种”的认识，即“寒热学说”，以及人体解剖知识、药物知识、急救知识和传染病预防知识等传统蒙医药的理论认识得到了进一步丰富和充实。元太医忽思慧撰写的《饮膳正要》是记录蒙医学饮食疗法内容的第一部典籍。这些都为16世纪后蒙医蒙药走向成熟奠定了坚实基础。

明清时期，随着藏医学的《四部医典》和古代印度医学的部分理论陆续传入蒙古地区，蒙医药学得以合理吸收藏医学和印度医学的精华，基础理论研究和临床治疗实践都上升到了新的高度。蒙古族的先民以藏医学及古代印度医学的“五元学说”为借鉴和出发点，以“三根和七素”作为理论基础，兼而吸收中医药知识，并结合蒙古地区的特点和民间疗法，创建了以传统的“寒热学说”为核心主导的独立的蒙医学理论体系。伊喜巴拉珠尔在他的《甘露四部》中，把传统的蒙古骨伤整治术和创伤医疗术，从“创伤医疗术”“脱臼复位术”“骨伤疗法”“震脑疗法”等几个具体的角度，进行了详细的理论阐述和操作说明，内容甚为丰满，提出了“六基症”“寒症”“十大要症”等独特理论。与此同时，在临床治疗经验日渐丰富的基础上，形成了具有民族特点的独特的医疗诊治体系。蒙古族的骨伤整治技术更是独到而神奇，著名蒙医绰尔济莫尔根以其精湛的外科诊治技术享誉漠南，被载入《清史稿》。而他仅仅是众多蒙古族“神医”中的典型代表而已。随着黄教在蒙古的兴盛，规模较大的寺庙都设有曼巴扎仓，这不仅是当地的医疗中心，也是学习和研究藏医、蒙医理论的基地，培养了大批蒙医蒙药人才。地处东部的蒙古勒津（今辽宁阜新），素有“蒙医药发祥地”之称，早在1669年瑞应寺兴建之初，寺内就设有曼巴扎仓。蒙医药理论研究方兴未艾，对蒙药的性味功能也有了更深刻的认识，《认药白晶鉴》《识药学》《蒙药正典》三大蒙药学代表性著作应运而生。《秘诀方海》收载有内、外、妇、儿、五官及热病、传染病等临床各科的3000余种药方，尤其是《甘露四部》在蒙医药学的基础理论探究和传统疗法的整理方面做出了创造性的贡献，奠定了近代蒙医药学理法方药的基础。总之，理论和实践相互印证、相互促进的良好局面的形成，是这一时期蒙医药学发展的一大特征。

新中国成立，迎来了蒙医蒙药发展的新纪元。在党和国家民族政策的光辉照耀下，蒙医蒙药获得了大踏步的发展。据不完全统计，新中国成立以来，不仅建立了许多新的蒙医医疗机构和研究机构，而且也成立了许多蒙医学校，设置蒙医药专业，有计划、有步骤地培养蒙医药人才。如新中国成立后第一所蒙医学校就是著名蒙医古拿巴达拉在辽宁蒙古勒津（阜新）瑞应寺主持建立的。1958年内蒙古医学院在全国西医药院校中第一个设立了蒙医专业本科。1980年在通辽成立了内蒙古民族医学院，1987年更名为内蒙古蒙医学院，2000年与通辽地区其他两所高校合并组建了内蒙古民族大学。2016年通辽市被命名为“中国蒙医药之都”，蒙医药的发展，形成了新的格局，新的境界。在继承传统的基础上，古老的蒙医药体系不断吸收新的时代精华，活力频注，生机勃发，在与国际水平和现代科技接轨方面，在协同化、规模化、科学化、信息化、产业化发展等方面，不断探索和迈进。

纵观蒙医蒙药发展历程，深深感到她是蒙古民族文化宝库，乃至人类文化宝库里的珍宝，散发着璀璨夺目的光芒。蒙医蒙药是蒙古族人民对人类科学进步、文明发展进程做出的极大贡献。

第一，蒙医蒙药是对人体生理机制及疾病治疗的科学认识体系和实践体系。人体是生命的物质基础，一个蕴藏着无数奥秘的神奇所在。蒙医把人体看作是与外界直接联系的有机整体，通过身体表面的细微变化诊察体内的疾病，并在此基础上辨证施治。自成体系、日渐成熟的蒙医蒙药反映着蒙古民族在医学领域的探究深度。

第二，蒙医蒙药是人与大自然辩证关系的折射，是蒙古人在物我关系、自然哲学探究高度的表征。蒙古人信仰“天人一脉”，相信宇宙是个相互联系、彼此制约的系统，是一个能量循环共生的生态圈，人是这个生态圈里的有机部分，与动物、植物等其他部分都有着相生相抵又相依相宜的关系。蒙医把人体本身也看作是一个自我能量循环系统，蒙医的很多治疗手段（比如骨伤术），不使用仪器，不开刀破肤，不打钢钉，不伤元气，全靠手法技术医治的前提，是对个体生命自我循环规律的尊重、顺应和对自愈能力的信任。

第三，蒙医蒙药是生命的珍爱与呵护系统，承担着民众身心健康的“保护神”的使命。一方面，蒙医蒙药反映着蒙古人战胜疾病侵袭、维护生命健康的爱心和仁怀，另一方面，蒙医蒙药反映着蒙古人既诚于顺应自然，又勇于利用自然，并在与自然的关系中，发展出为我所用的实际效能、实际价值的能力。蒙医蒙药是蒙古人源远流长的创新意识和创新能力的实证和“活化石”。

蒙医药学在其发展的各个历史时期形成的文献典籍，不仅是蒙古民族的优秀文化遗产，也是蒙医药学丰富内容的主要载体。为展示蒙医药学博大精深的内容，更好地保护、传承和利用民族优秀文化遗产，辽宁民族出版社组织辽宁省阜新蒙医药研究所和内蒙古民族大学蒙医药专家学者，将辽宁省阜新蒙医药研究所馆藏部分古籍文献进行整理，并影印出版《中国蒙医药古籍影印珍本》。

《中国蒙医药古籍影印珍本》（丛书），共7卷本，包括《兰塔布》《甘露精要八支秘诀续. Ⅰ》《甘露精要八支秘诀续. Ⅱ》《痘症精言》（蒙古文版）、《格体全录》《蒙古文手抄普济杂方》《蒙古文手抄本一药方》，内容涵盖了蒙医药基础理论、临床经验、药物药理、药物方剂、自然疗法等多个层面。

《中国蒙医药古籍影印珍本》的出版，意义重大。

第一，有利于弘扬民族医术，造福人类健康。蒙医药在治病救人、保健益生方面，具有一套科学和谐的理念和独到神奇的技术方法，而这些既体现在蒙医医生的日常医疗活动中，也积淀于各种蒙医药典籍中。将这些典籍集中整理出版，有利于蒙医药学的传播，有利于民族医术的弘扬，更有益于人类健康。这与当下人们追求自然、健康、和谐的医疗保健效果的时代需求，是相契合的。

第二，有利于蒙医药古籍文献的发掘整理利用，以促进蒙医药的振兴和发展，具有强劲的现实意义和深远的历史意义。蒙医药是国家级非物质文化遗产，将辽宁省阜新蒙医药研究所馆藏的大量蒙医药古籍文献资料整理出版，是目前为止国内首个关于蒙医药古籍抢救类大型出版项目。本丛书收录的蒙医药古籍文献中记录了大量医药资源、诊疗技术、用药经验，对其进行整理、梳理，利用现代科学仪器来扫描影印出版，能真实展现古籍原貌，从而让古老典籍焕发时代光彩，极具学术价值、收藏价值和应用价值，有利于促进蒙医药文化的长足发展，提升文化自信。

第三，蒙医药古籍文献作为一种产业开发的资源，具有一定的经济价值。从蒙医药古籍文献整理和研究中挖掘更多的有效预防和治疗疾病的方剂和药物，并将其投入市场，不仅可以为人民群众的健康提供服务，还能带动蒙医药的产业化发展，创造出可观的经济效益，并进而带动民族地区其他行业的发展，加速和谐社会建设进程。

第四，蒙医药古籍文献是中华民族宝贵的文化遗产，是中华文化的重要组成部分，抢救和保护民族古籍，对于传承和弘扬中华优秀传统文化，扩大中华优秀传统文化影响，具有重要意义。党的十九大报告指出："深入挖掘中华优秀传统文化蕴含的思想观念、人文精神、道德规范，结合时代要求继承创新，让中华文化展现出永久魅力和时代风采。"

《中国蒙医药古籍影印珍本》编辑委员会

2018年6月

General Preface

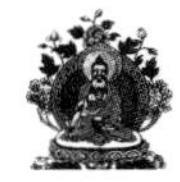

The Mongolian nationality is a legendary ethnic group with a long history. In the long history process, Mongolians have developed broad, profound and gorgeous cultural patterns in many aspects, such as living, diet, clothing, language, writing, dance, art, medicine and health, which has accumulated tremendous achievements and formed its unique tradition. Each part of this traditional culture is the beautiful creation that condenses the world essence and the ancestral teachings; it is also the cream and crystallization that encourage constant innovations and gather the experience of big historical events.

Mongolian Medicine, is the gorgeous one in the Mongolian cultural garden. With other flowers in this cultural garden, it develops a broad and full Mongolian connotation system, making the garden extraordinarily beautiful. Mongolian Medicine, which originated in ancient times, formed in the Yuan Dynasty, developed in the Ming and Qing dynasties, and flourished in the contemporary era, is the treasure of traditional Chinese Medicine and the unique one in the Chinese medical field.

Mongolians have lived a nomadic life since ancient times. They lived in the cold, arid or semi-arid grassland, and fed on beef, mutton, and dairy products. Riding, grazing, migrating and fast gallop during the war made them easy to suffer from various injuries like bruises, fractures, and war wound. Under such climatic, geographical, dietary and living conditions, Mongolian ancestors insistently observed the relationship between animals and plants in nature, and initially mastered the nutrition, toxicity of animals and plants and their functions to prevent and cure of diseases. Through analyzing and summarizing the experience that has been accumulated to fight against diseases during the long period of hunting, nomadism, agricultural production, migration, and fighting, the Mongolian people invented a series of treatments inclusive of regional and ethnic characteristics. For example, fire therapy to resist cold and dampness, osteopathy featured by bone setting and skull setting, as well as dietotherapy like kumiss therapy based on the nutrition of the dairy product. This period is the bud and embryonic stage of Mongolian medical science.

In the Yuan Dynasty, Mongolian Medicine had made great progress for two reasons. First, the mainland Medicine and Mongolian Medicine nourished and promoted each other mutually. Second, Mongolian Medicine received institutional political security in the Yuan Dynasty. Followed the medical system in the Tang and Song dynasties, the government of the Yuan Dynasty set up The Imperial Hospital and The Medical Institute of Benevolence to support and promote Mongolian Medicine, thus providing a suitable condition for the all-round development of Mongolian Medicine. On the original basis, the traditional Mongolian medical technologies such as orthopedics and traumatology had gained new progress. At the same time, by absorbing, drawing upon all useful opinions and in-depth research, the Mongolian ancestors had already summed up the understanding that "the origins of disease are no more than cold and fever", thus inventing and enriching "Theory of Cold and Fever" and other traditional Mongolian medical theory, such as human anatomy knowledge, medicine knowledge, first-aid knowledge and infectious disease prevention knowledge. Yuan Imperial doctor Husihui's *Yinshan Zhengyao* is the first book of Mongolian medical dietotherapy, which laid the foundation for the maturity of Mongolian Medicine after the 16th century.

In the Ming and Qing dynasties, with the introduction of Tibetan *Rgyud bzhi* and some ancient Indian medical theories, Mongolian Medicine reasonably absorbed the essence of Tibetan Medicine and Indian Medicine. Therefore, its basic theoretical research and clinical treatment practice had reached a new level. Taking Tibetan Medicine and ancient Indian Medicine's "Wuyuan Xueshuo" as references and starting points, on the theoretical basis of "Three Roots and Seven Elements", absorbing the knowledge of traditional Chinese Medicine, and combining the characteristics of Mongolian region and folk therapy, the Mongolian people created an independent Mongolian medical theory system, in which "Theory of Cold and Fever" plays the core leading role. In Ixibalazhuer's book *Ganlu Tetralogy*, he theoretically and practically elaborated the traditional Mongolian Bone Injury Treatment from many specific perspectives, such as "Trauma Surgery", "Dislocation Reduction", "Bone Injury Therapy", "Shaking Brain Therapy",etc. The contents were very substantial, in which the special theories of "Six Basic Diseases", "Cold Diseases", "Top Ten Major Symptoms" were proposed. At the same time, on the basis of the increasingly rich experience of clinical treatment, a unique medical treatment system with ethnic characteristics came into being. Mongolian Bone Injury Treatment is extremely unique and magical. Mongolian medical expert Chuerjimorgen was famous for the exquisite precision of his treatment in surgery. Thus, he was written into *Draft History of the Qing Dynasty.* He is but a typical representative of the large number of Mongolian "Miracle Doctors". With the prosperity of Yellow Sect in the Mongolian region, temples in large-scale all equipped with Mamba Raseng. Mamba Raseng is not only the medical center, but also the base for studying and researching the theories of Mongolian and Tibetan Medicine. It has cultivated a great number of talents in this field. Mongoliajin located in the Eastern part (now Liaoning Fuxin), is known as "The Birthplace of Mongolian Medicine". As early as 1669, Ruiying Temple was built and equipped with Mamba Raseng. Research on Mongolian Medicine theories was just unfolding. Mongolian doctors also achieved more profound understanding of the nature and flavor of Mongolian drugs. Under such situation, three typical masterpieces of Mongolian Medicine appeared. They are *Baijing Drug Recognition and Discrimination*, *Recognition of Drugs*, *Mongolian Medicine Canon.* Another famous book *Magic Code and Recipe* selected more than 3000 prescriptions for internal, external, women, children, facial features, fever and infectious diseases. Especially *Ganlu Tetralogy* which made a creative contribution to exploring the basic theories and sorting the traditional therapies laid a solid foundation for the modern Mongolian Medicine. In a word, the situation that theory and practice mutually confirm and promote each other was a major characteristic of the Mongolian Medicine development in this period.

The founding of New China ushered in a new era of Mongolian Medicine progress. Under the brilliant care of our Party and State, Mongolian Medicine dramatically developed. Preliminary statistics show that, many new Mongolian medical institutions, research centers as well as Mongolian Medicine schools were established to cultivate Mongolian talents purposefully and designedly. For example, the first Mongolian Medicine school was built in Mongoliajin (Fuxin) Ruiying Temple in Liaoning Province by a famous Mongolian doctor Badara. In 1958, Inner Mongolia Medical College, which is famous as a West Medicine college, firstly set up Mongolian Medicine department. In 1980, Inner Mongolian National Medical College was established in Tongliao and renamed Mongolian Medical College of Inner Mongolia in 1987, and expanded as Inner Mongolia University for Nationalities after merging other two colleges in 2000. In 2016, Tongliao was entitled "Mongolian Medicine Capital of China". A new pattern and a new state for the development of Mongolian Medicine came into being. On the basis of inheriting its tradition, ancient Mongolian Medicine absorbs the essence of the contemporary era, brimming over with vigor and vitality. It insistently explores and progresses in many aspects such as the connection with global society and modern science and technology, as well as its collaboratization, scientization, scale expansion, informatization and industrialization.

From an overview of the development history of Mongolian Medicine, it can be drawn that she is a priceless treasure of Mongolian culture, and even the treasure of human culture, exuding dazzling light. It is Mongolians' great contribution to the development of human science and the development of civilization.

First, Mongolian Medicine is a scientific understanding system and practical system of human physiological mechanism and disease treatment. Human body is the material basis of life, a place containing countless mysteries. Mongolian Medicine takes the human body as an organic whole that is directly related to the outside world. Disease can be correctly diagnosed and dialectically treated through the subtle changes in the body. The Mongolian Medicine, coming from ancient times, establishing her own system, becoming mature and perfect, reflects the depth of the exploration Mongolian people have done in the field of medical science.

Second, Mongolian Medicine is the reflection of the dialectical relationship between man and nature, and it is the symbol of Mongolians' exploration level in the relationship between man and nature, and natural philosophy. The Mongolians believe in the theory that man is a part of nature. They believe that the universe is an interrelated and restricted system, and it is a symbiotic ecological circle of balanced energy. Human being is an organic part of this ecological circle, keeping a contrarious and dependent relationship with animals and plants. Mongolian Medicine takes the human body as a self-energy circulatory system. There are numerous treatments in Mongolian Medicine (such as Bone Injury Therapy), free from instruments, operations, steel nails and avoiding devitalizing patients. All these treatments are based on manipulative therapy, reflecting Mongolian Medicine's respect for human beings' self-circulation law and confidence for their self-cure ability.

Third, Mongolian Medicine is the precious and caring system of life, bearing the mission of protecting people's physical and mental health. On one hand, Mongolian Medicine reflects the Mongolians' love of conquering the disease and safeguarding the health of life. On the other hand, Mongolian Medicine reflects that Mongolians sincerely obey the rules of nature and bravely make use of nature. In the relationship between man and nature, they develop their abilities of taking every advantage of nature to maximize the actual effects and practical value. Mongolian Medicine is the robust evidence and the "living fossil" of the Mongolian people's long history of innovation and creation.

Ancient and classical works appeared in different period in the process of the Mongolian Medicine development are not only the precious heritage of Mongolian culture, but also the great carrier of the rich content of Mongolian Medicine. In order to show the broad and profound Mongolian Medicine, to better protect, inherit and make use of this precious heritage, Liaoning Nationality Publishing House photocopied and published *Rare Photocopy of Chinese Mongolian Medicine Ancient Book* by organizing the scholars of Liaoning Fuxin Mongolian Medicine Research Institute and Inner Mongolia University for Nationalities to sort the ancient and classical works kept in Liaoning Fuxin Mongolian Medicine Research Institute.

Rare Photocopy of Chinese Mongolian Medicine Ancient Book (series) consists of seven volumes, including *Man Ngag Lhan Thabs*, *The Secret Tantra of Nectar Essence Eight Branches (i.e. Rgyud bzhi) I*, *The Secret Tantra of Nectar Essence Eight Branches (i.e. Rgyud bzhi) II*, *The Fine Words of Smallpox*, *Completely Record of Body*, *Mongolian Manuscripts of Cure-all Prescriptions* and *Mongolian Manuscripts of Prescriptions*. It covers the basic theories of medicine, clinical experience, pharmacology, prescriptions, natural therapies and many other aspects.

It is of profound significance to publish the *Rare Photocopy of Chinese Mongolian Medicine Ancient Book*.

First, it helps to carry forward National Medicine to benefit human health. Mongolian Medicine saves lives and cures of diseases with a set of scientific and harmonious ideas and unique and magical technical methods. These are not only embodied in the daily therapeutic activities of Mongolian Medicine doctors, but also accumulated in various Mongolian Medicine classics. Centralization and publication of these classics are conducive to the spread of Mongolian Medicine, to the promotion of National Medicine and human health. This is in harmony with the demand of the contemporary time that people pursue the pure, healthy and harmonious health care.

Second, it is beneficial to the exploitation and utilization of ancient literature of Mongolian Medicine in order to promote Mongolian Medicine's rejuvenation and development, which has strong practical significance and far-reaching historical significance. Mongolian Medicine is a state-level intangible cultural heritage. Editing and publishing a large number of Mongolian Medicine ancient literature from Liaoning

Fuxin Mongolian Medicine Research Institute is the first large-scale project on the rescue of Mongolian Medicine ancient classics in our country. This book contains a mass of medical resources, diagnosis and treatment technologies and medication experience. Sorting and photocopying this great work with modern scientific instruments can truly display these ancient classics and let them glow splendid brilliance, which is of great academic value, collection value and application value. It is also contributes to the rapid development and increasing self-confidence of Mongolian Medicine culture.

Third, as a kind of cultural resource, the ancient literature of Mongolian Medicine has certain economic value. During the process of sorting and researching these ancient classics, some prescriptions and medicine that can effectively cure of and prevent diseases were discovered. Putting them into the market, not only can provide service for people's health keeping, but also can drive the development of Mongolian Medicine industrialization, creating considerable economic benefits, promoting the development of other industries in ethnic areas and accelerating the process of building a harmonious society.

Fourth, the ancient literature of Mongolian Medicine is the precious cultural heritage of China, and is an important part of Chinese culture. Rescuing and protecting national ancient books is of great significance for inheriting and carrying forward Chinese excellent traditional culture and expanding the influence of Chinese excellent traditional culture. The 19th National Congress of the Communist Party of China pointed out: "Dig into the ideas, spirit and moral norms of Chinese elite traditional culture. Inherit and innovate Chinese elite traditional culture to meet the requirements of the contemporary era. Let Chinese culture show its permanent charm and time features."

Rare Photocopy of Chinese Mongolian Medicine Ancient Book

Editorial Committee

June, 2018

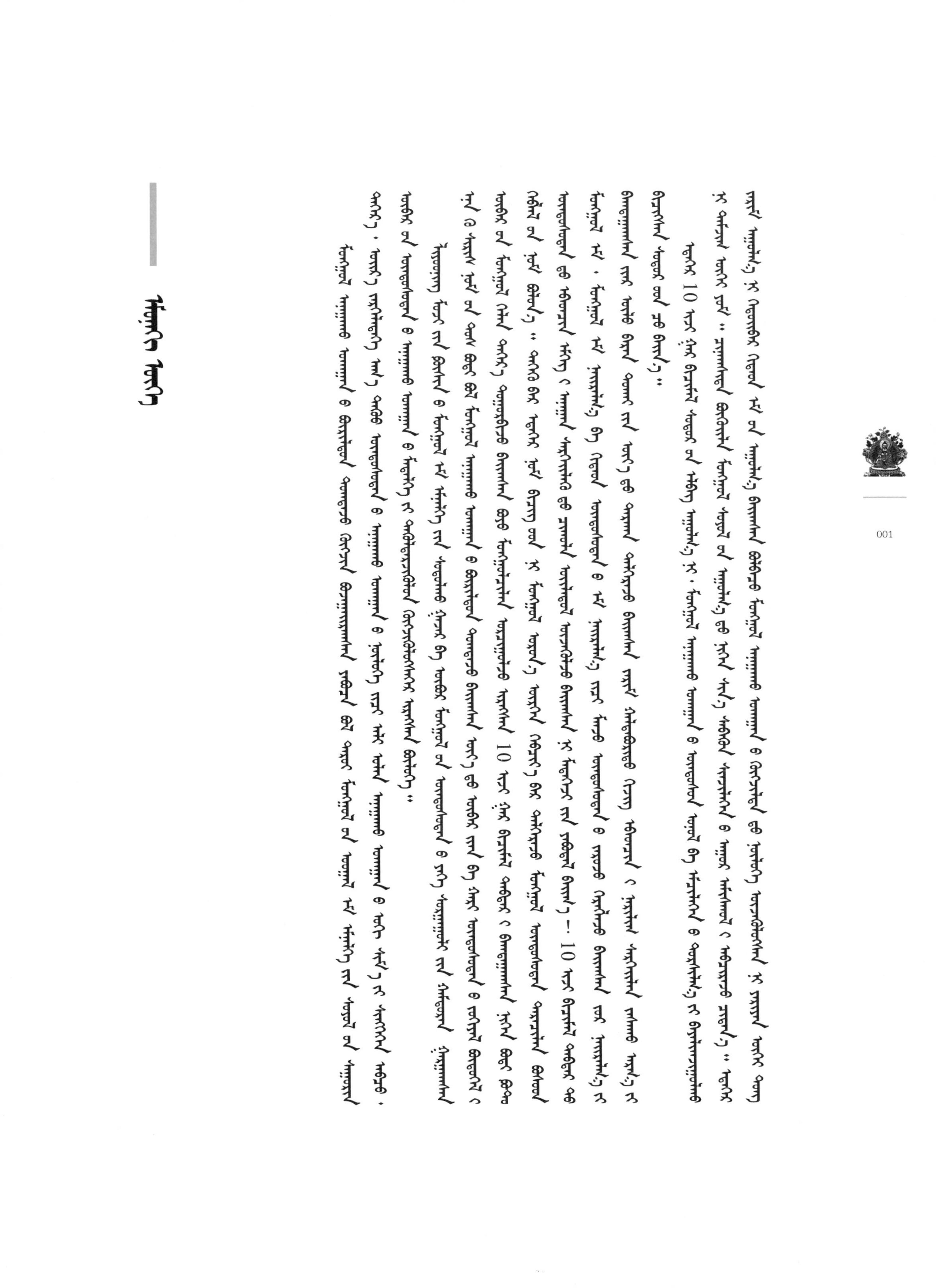

ᠡᠮᠦᠨᠡᠬᠢ ᠦᠭᠡ

[illegible]

[illegible]

[illegible]

[illegible]

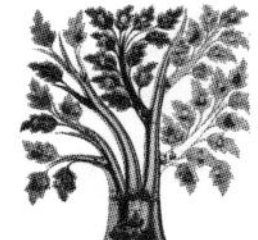

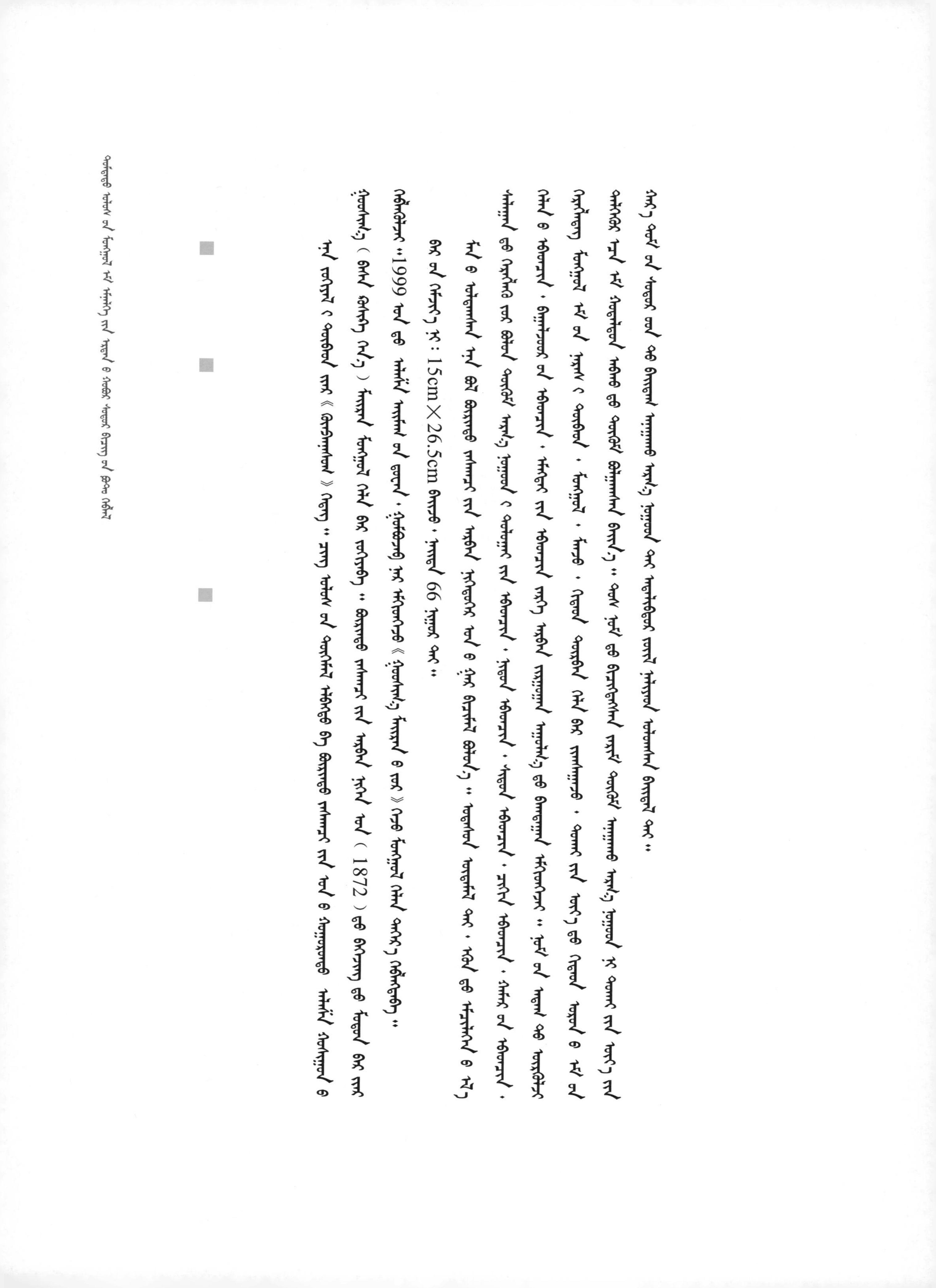

[illegible]

[illegible] ([illegible]) [illegible] (1872) [illegible]

[illegible] ::1999 [illegible] 《[illegible]》 [illegible] ::

[illegible]: 15cm×26.5cm [illegible] 66 [illegible] ::

[illegible]

Mongolian Manuscripts of Cure-all Prescriptions

蒙古文手写本普济杂方

1

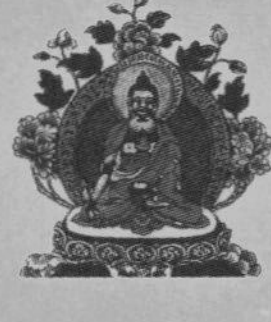

[illegible] ::

[illegible] ::

[illegible] ::

[illegible] ::

[illegible] ::

[illegible] ::

[illegible] ::

[illegible] ::

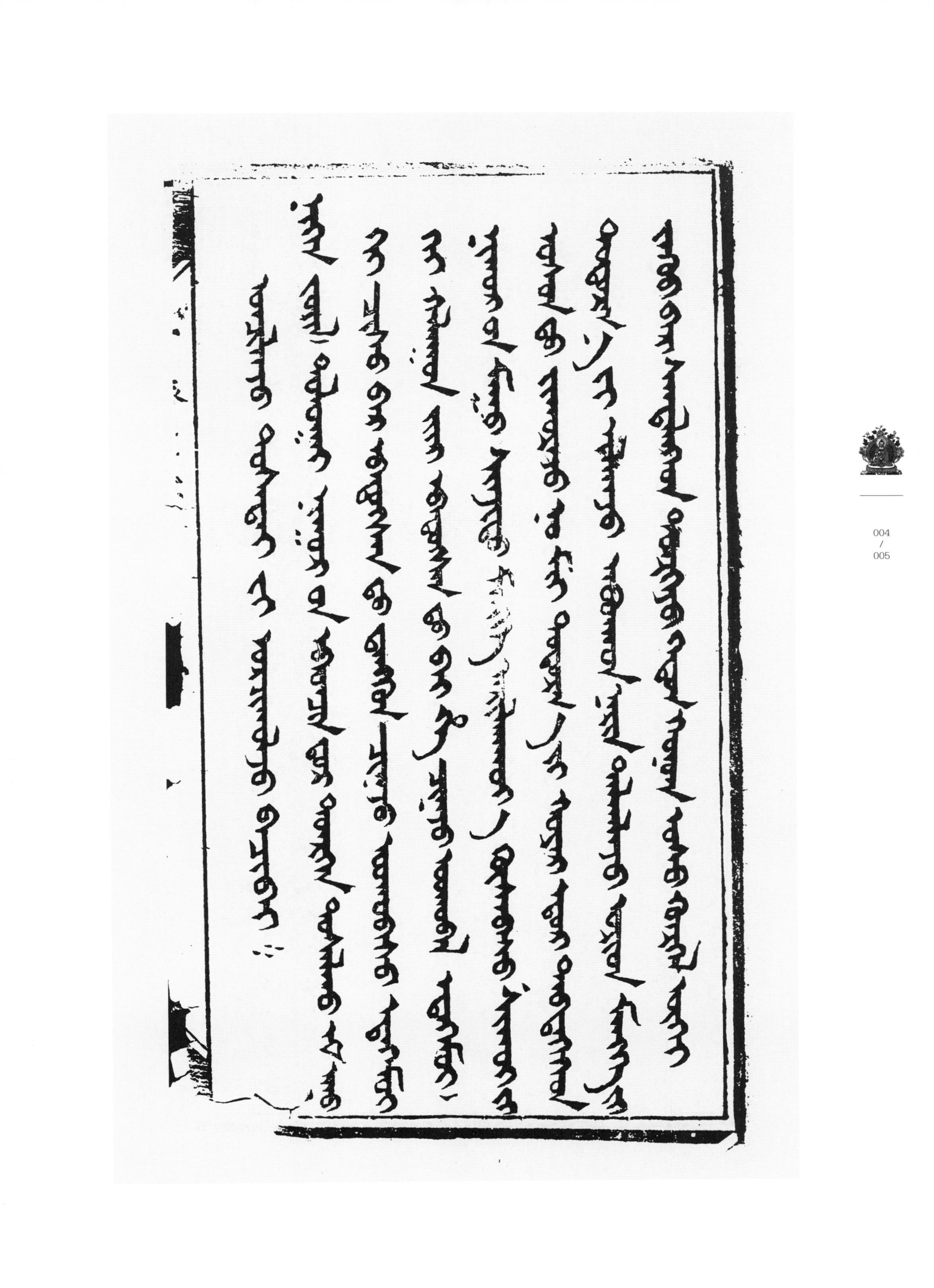

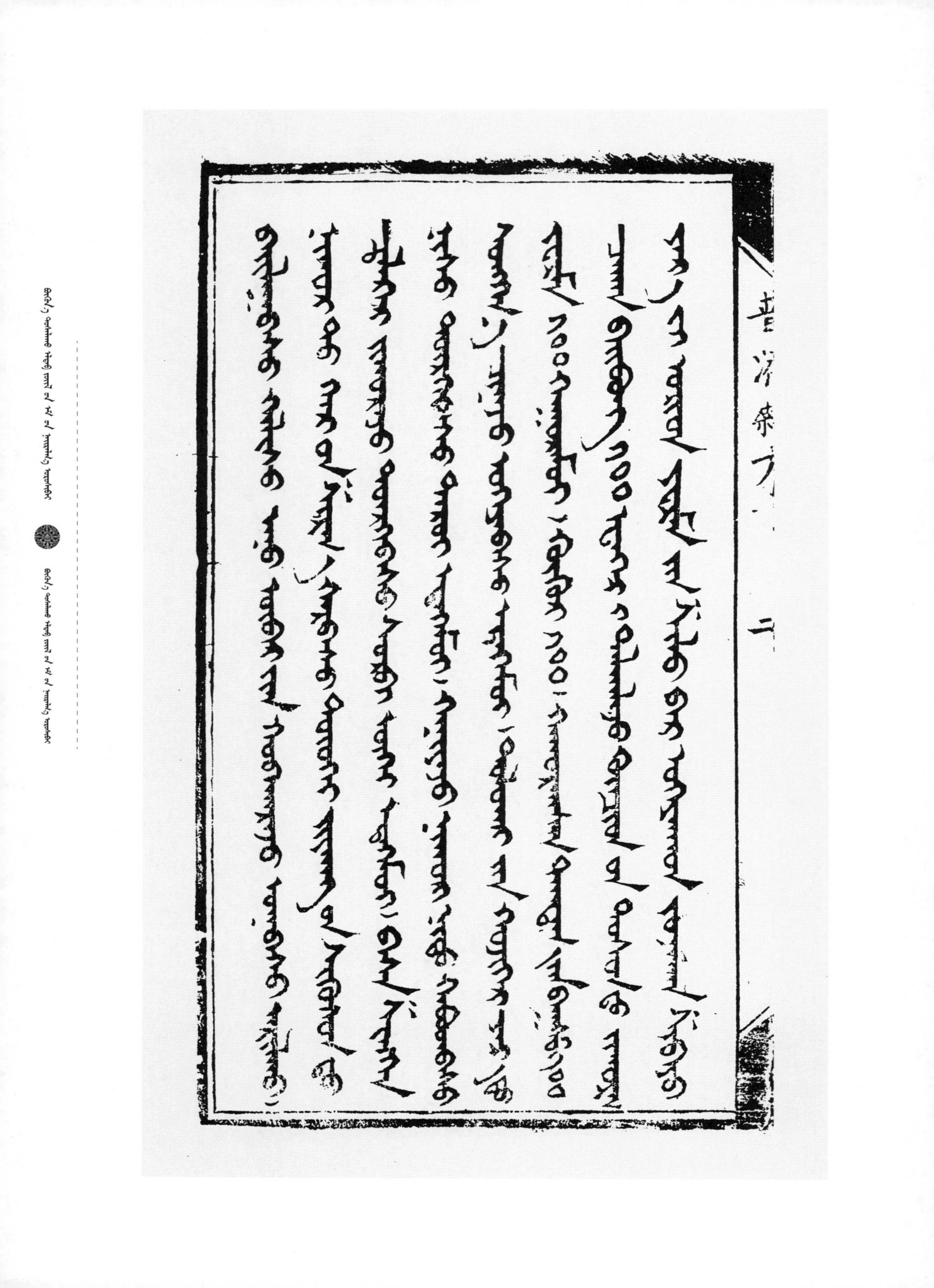

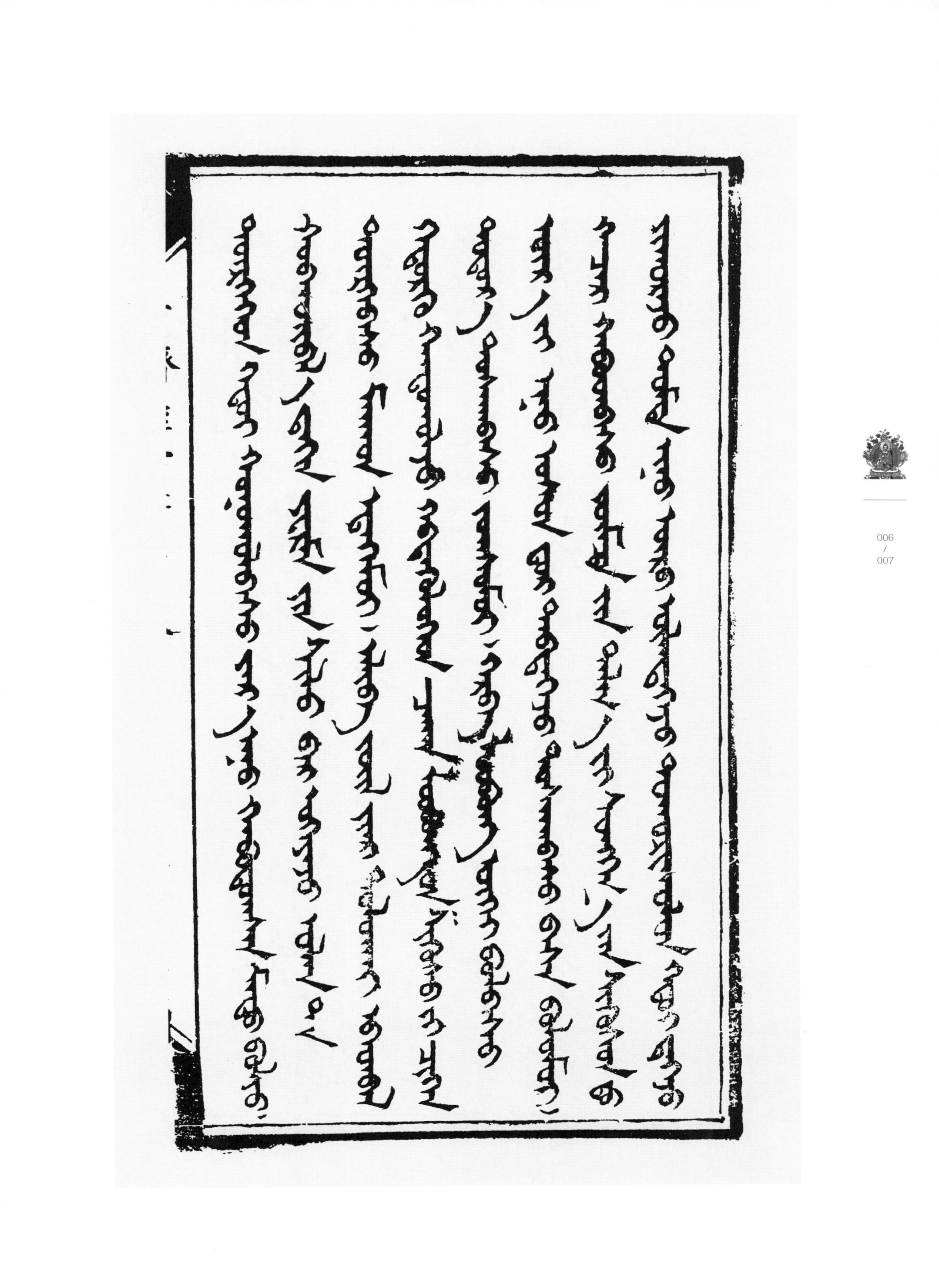

普濟雜方

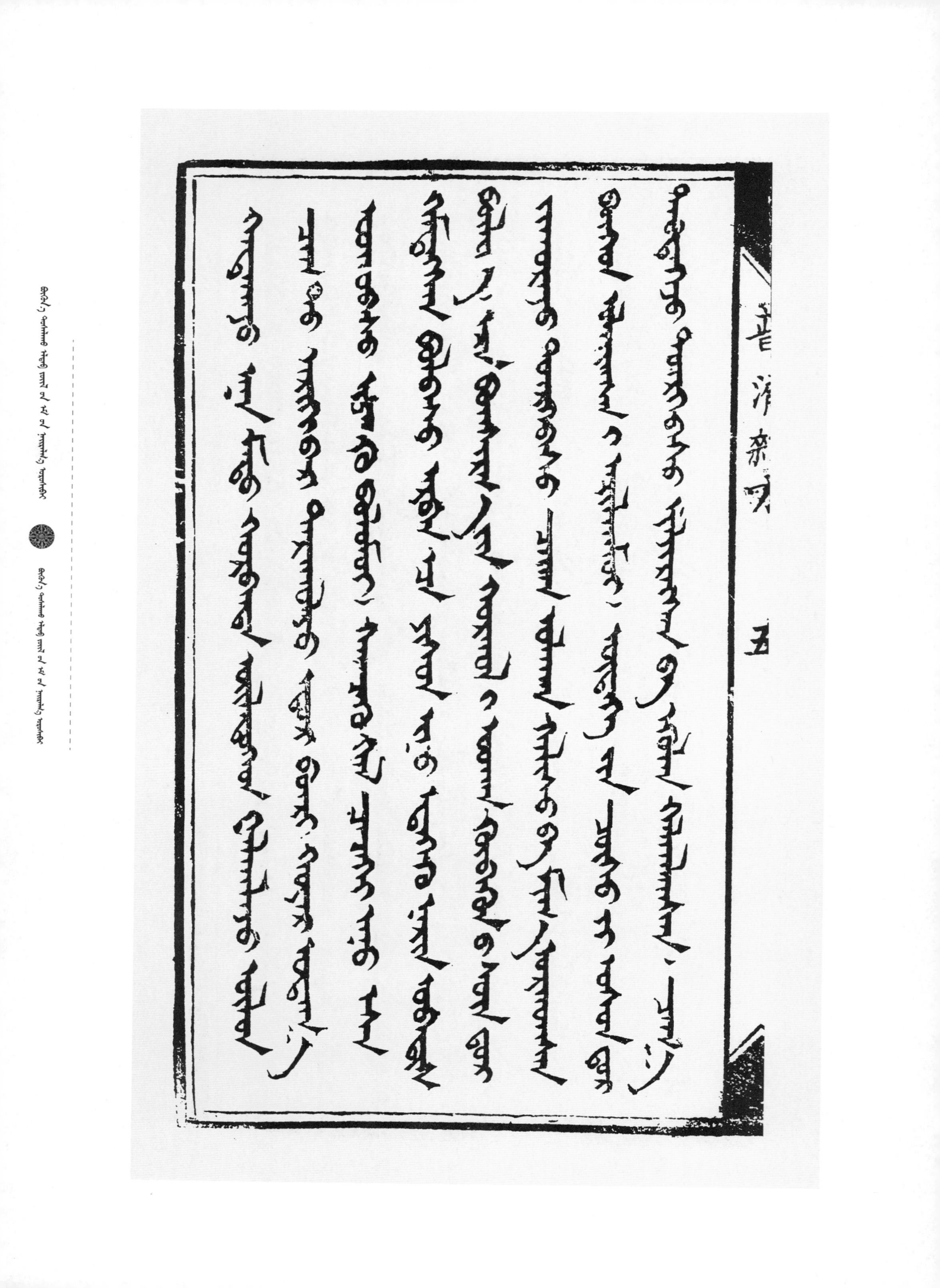

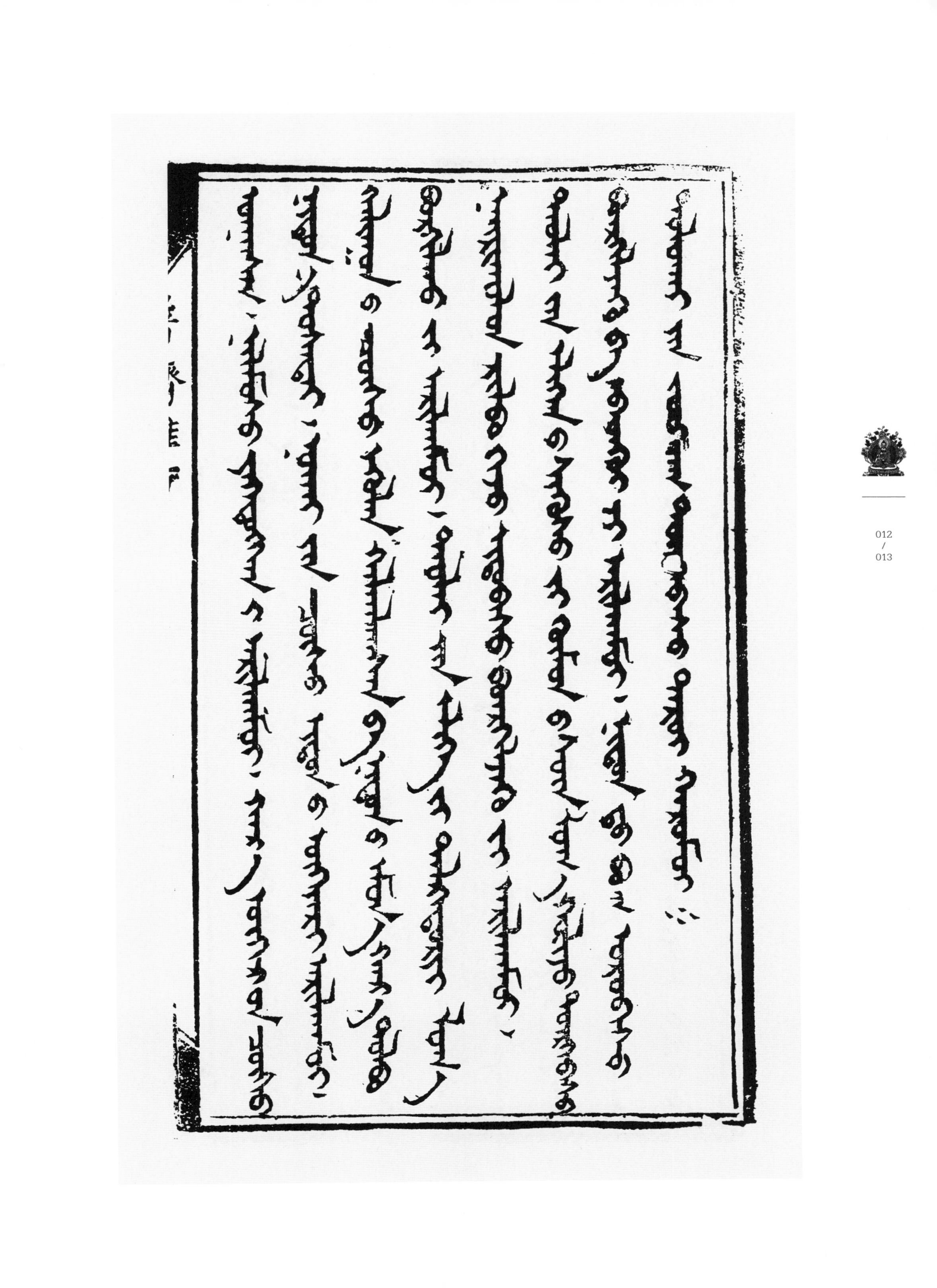

[illegible]

[illegible]

[illegible]

[illegible]

[illegible]

[illegible]

[illegible]

[illegible] ᠄᠄

[illegible]

[illegible]

[illegible]

[illegible]

[illegible]

[illegible]

[illegible]

[illegible]

[illegible]

[illegible]

[illegible]

[illegible]

[illegible]

[illegible]

[illegible]

[illegible]

[illegible]

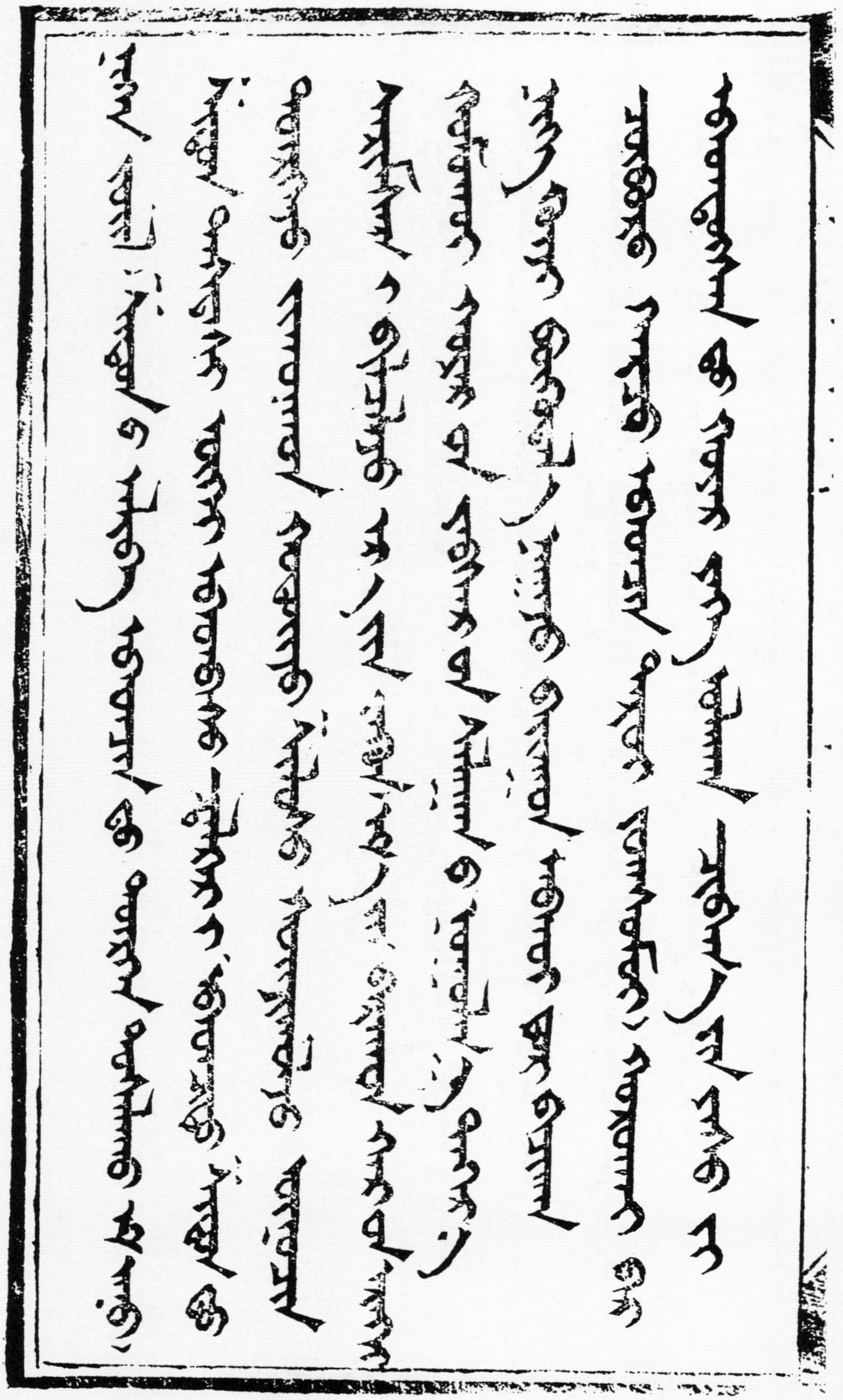

普濟雜方　二

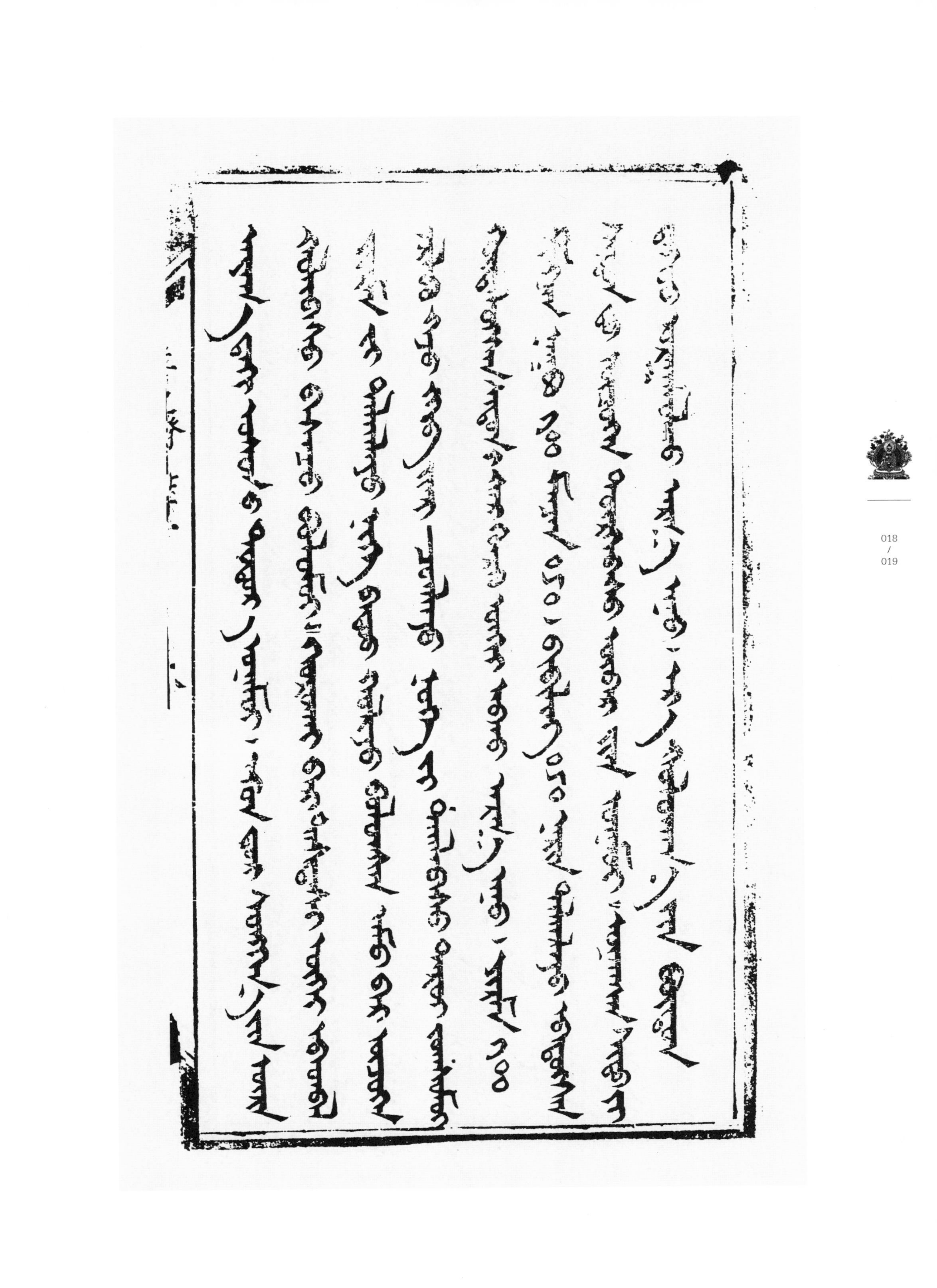

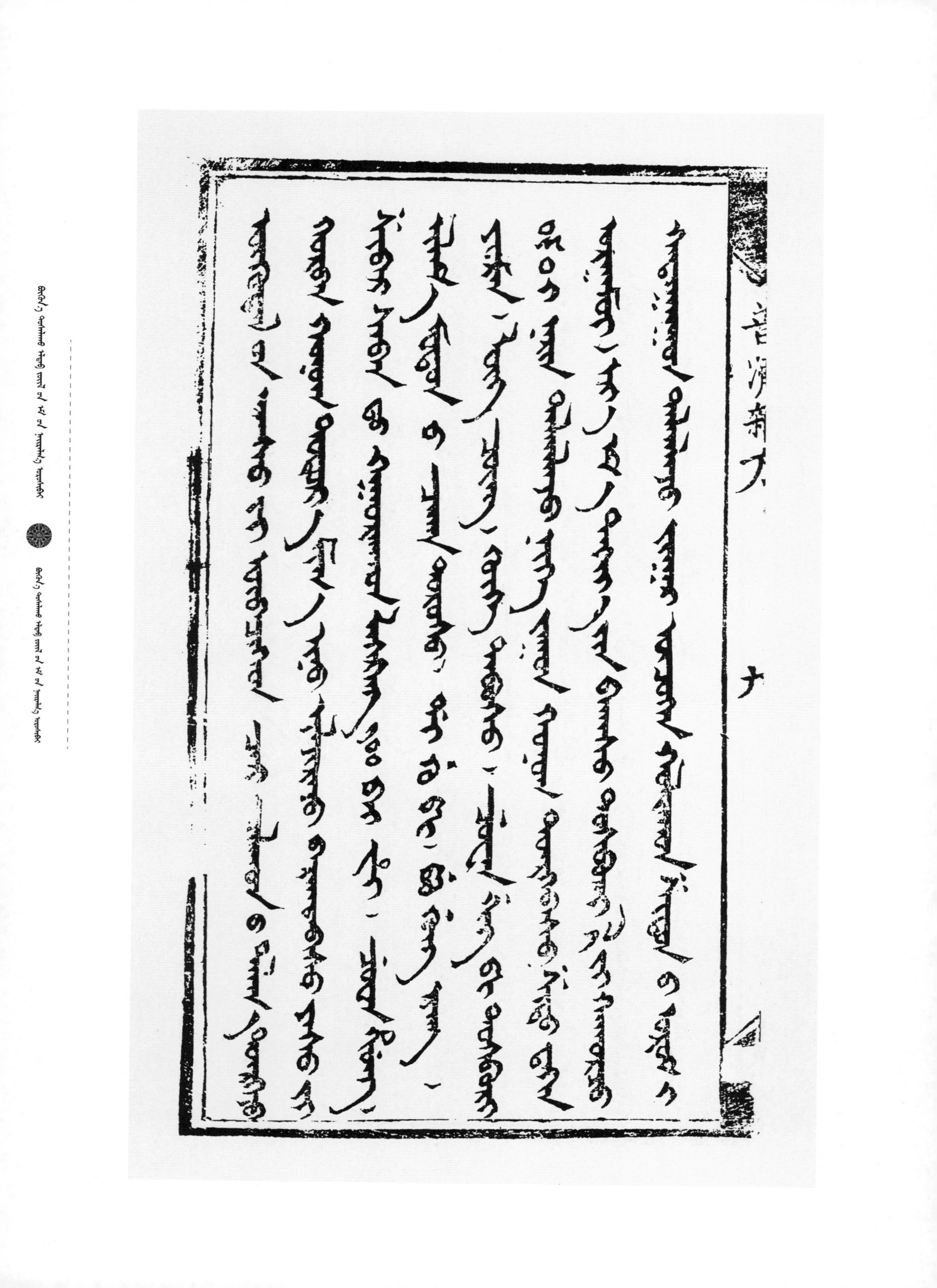

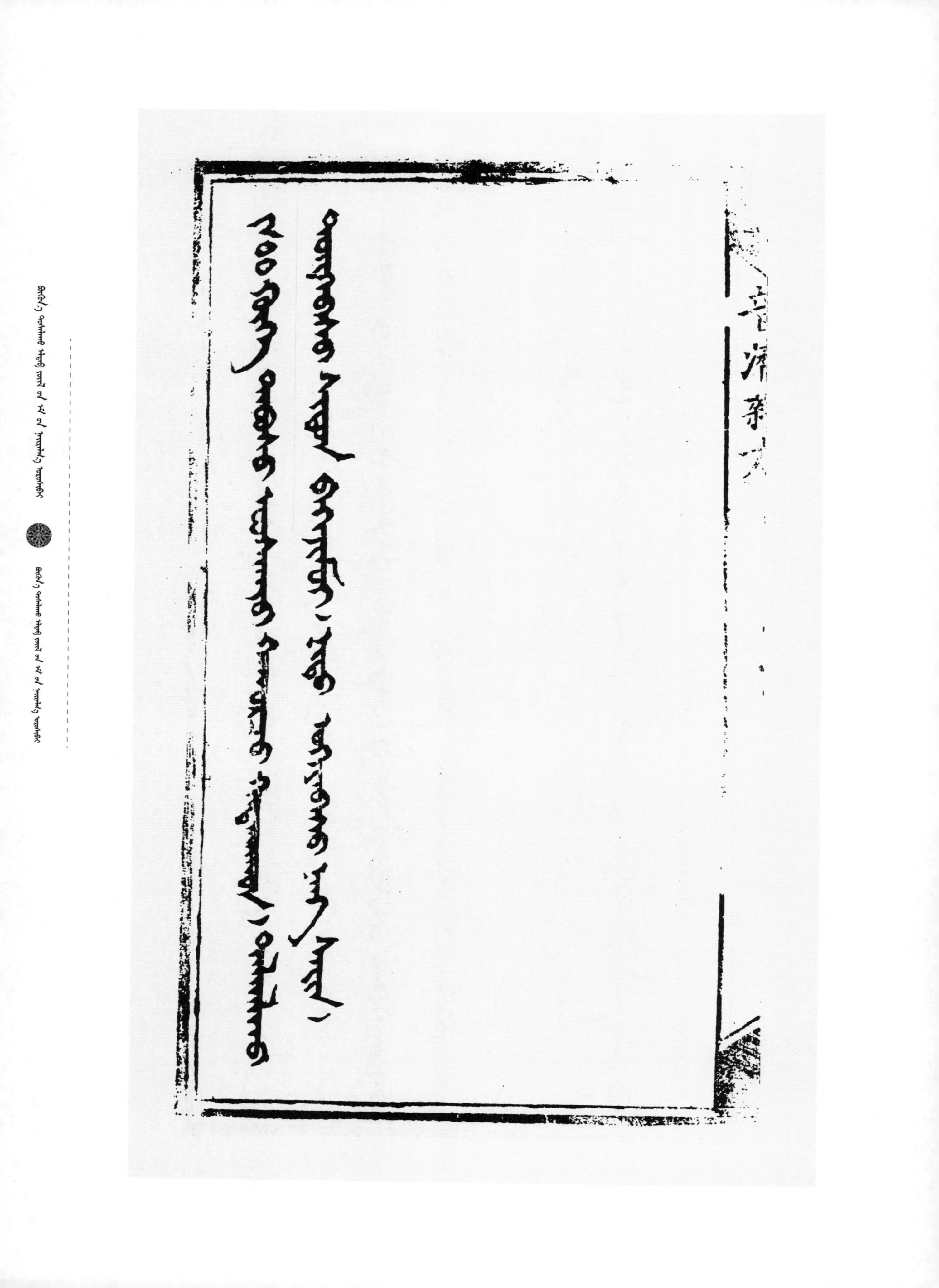

[illegible]

[illegible]

音清新文

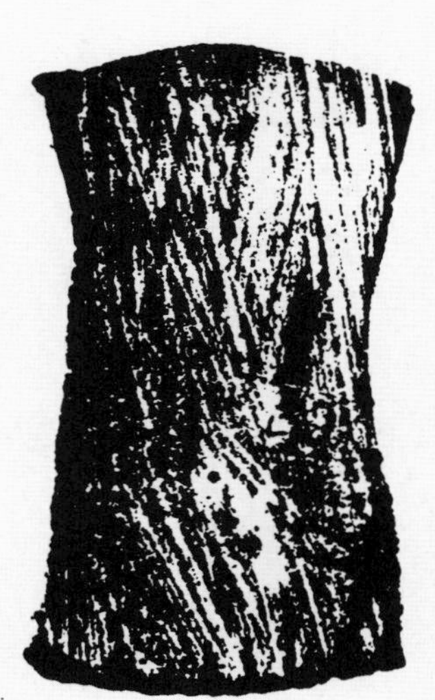

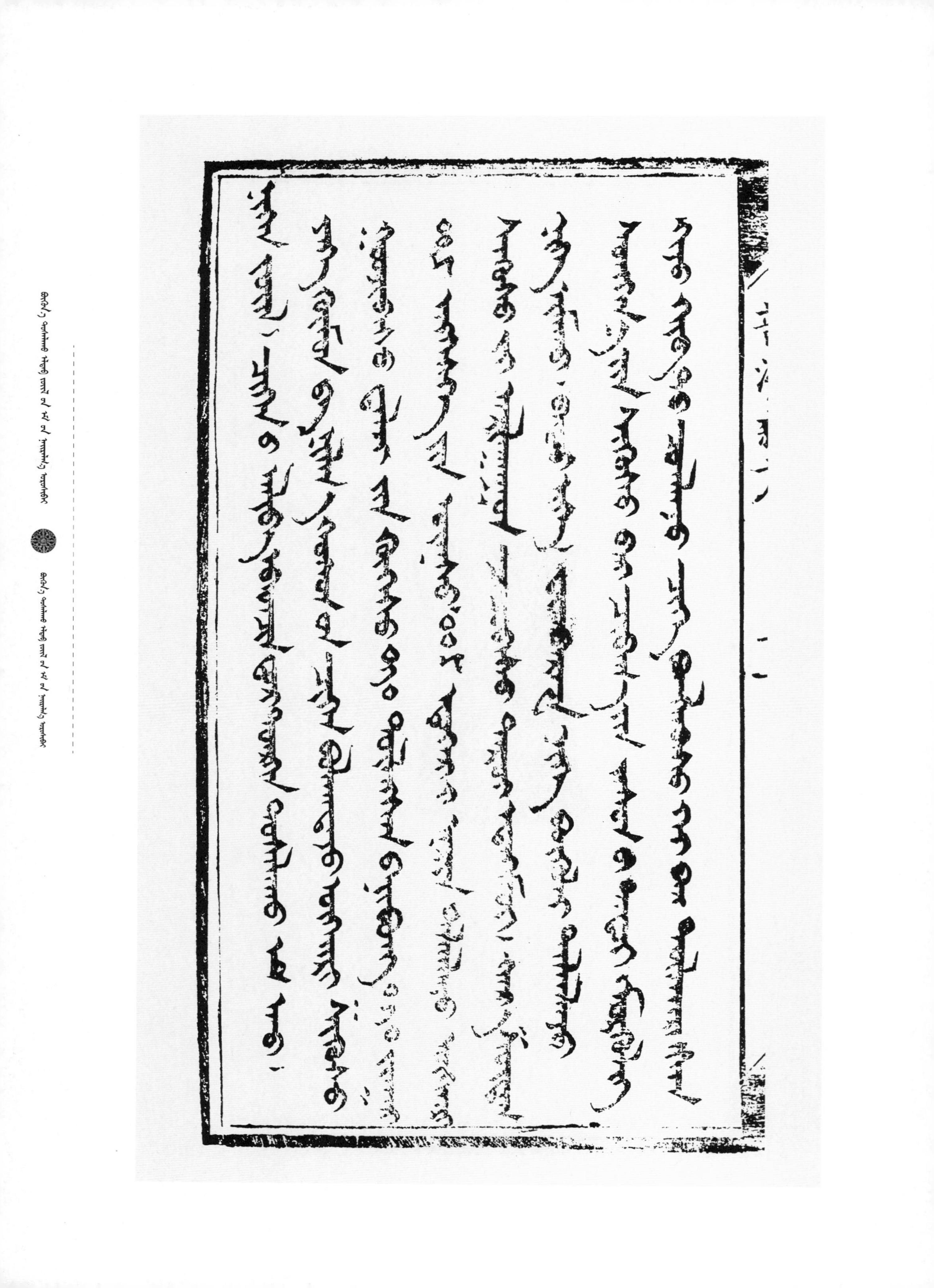

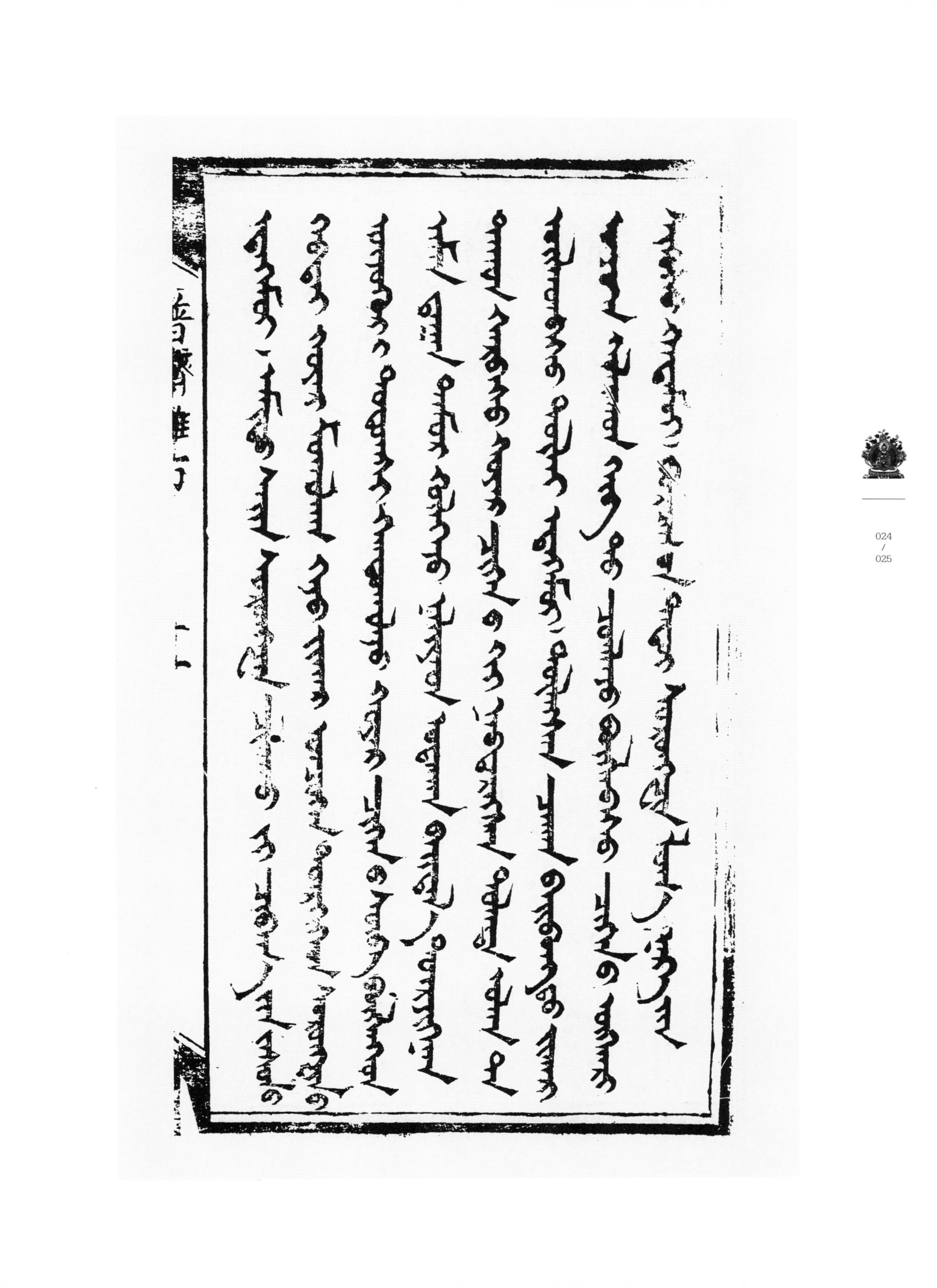

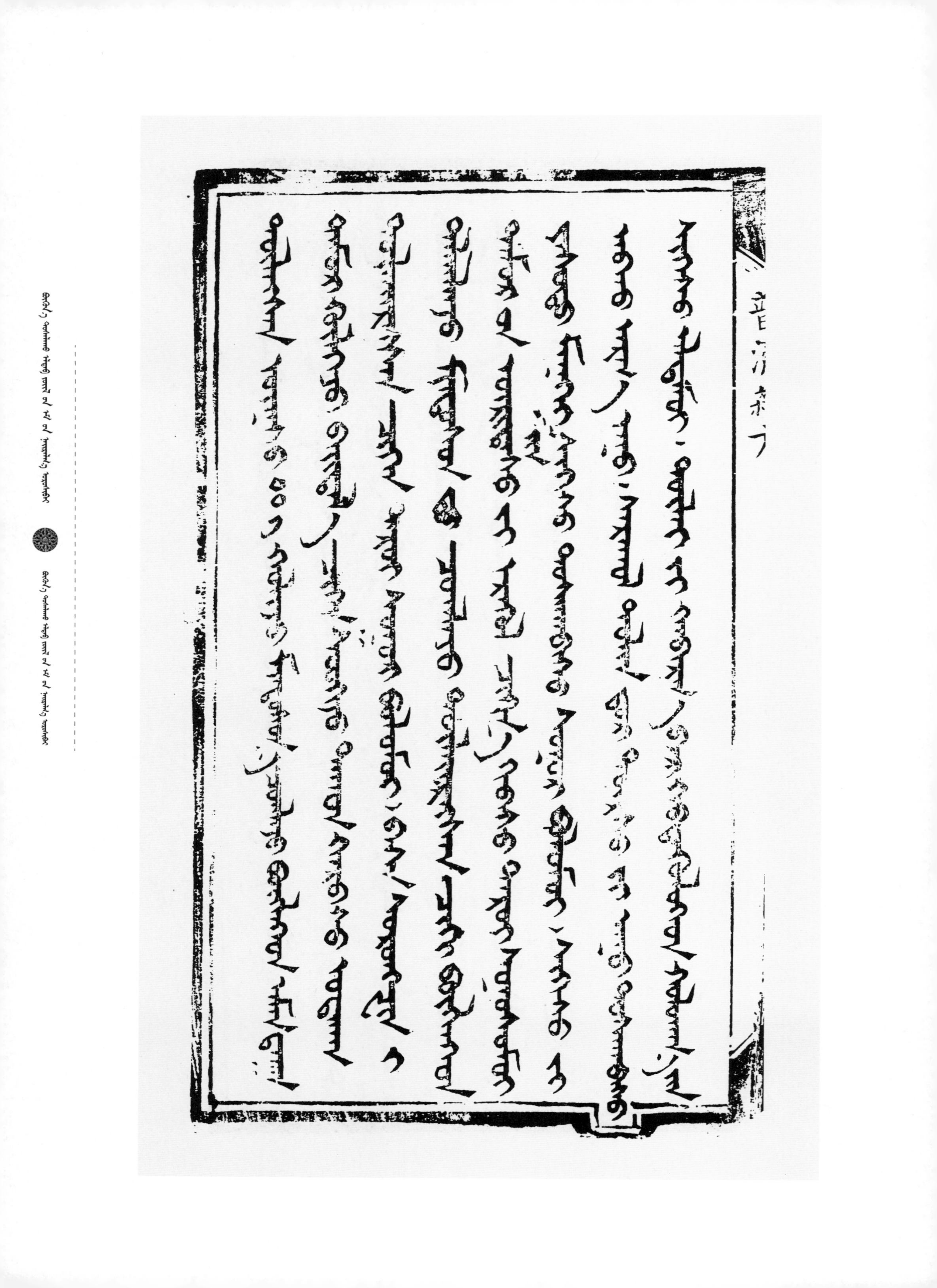

音[illegible]

[illegible]

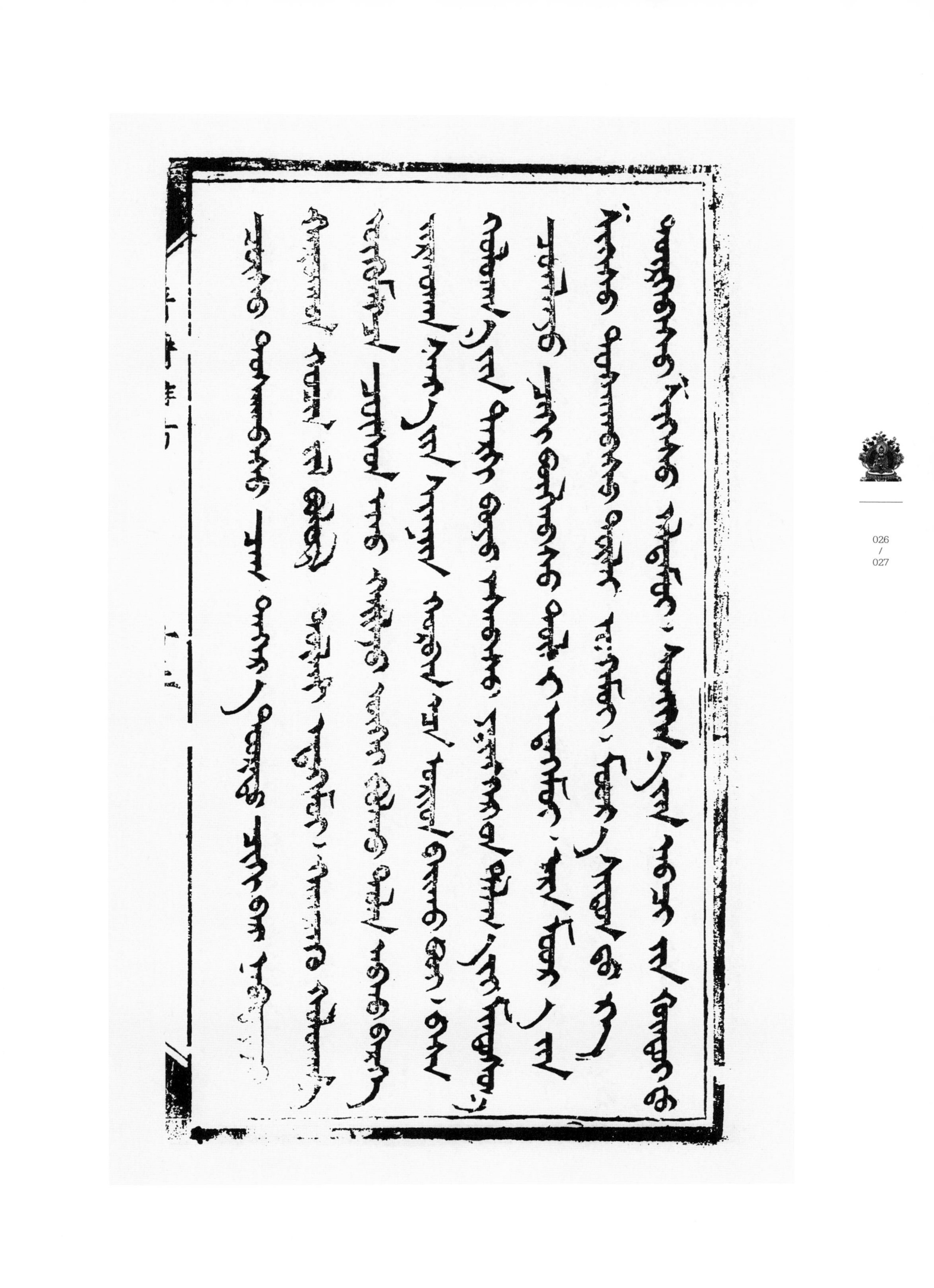

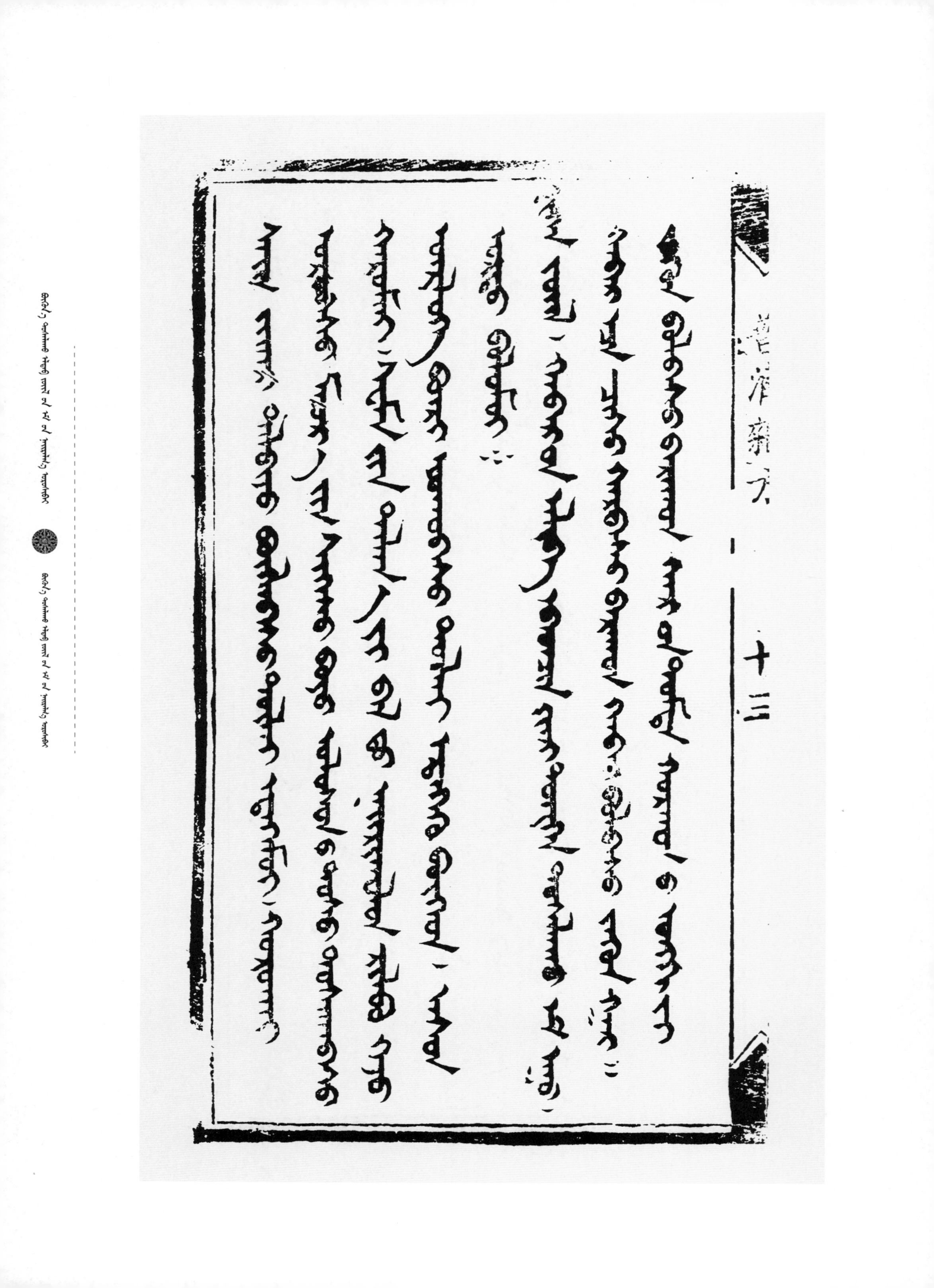

[illegible]

[illegible]

[illegible]

[illegible]

[illegible]

[illegible]

[illegible]

[illegible]

[illegible]

[illegible]

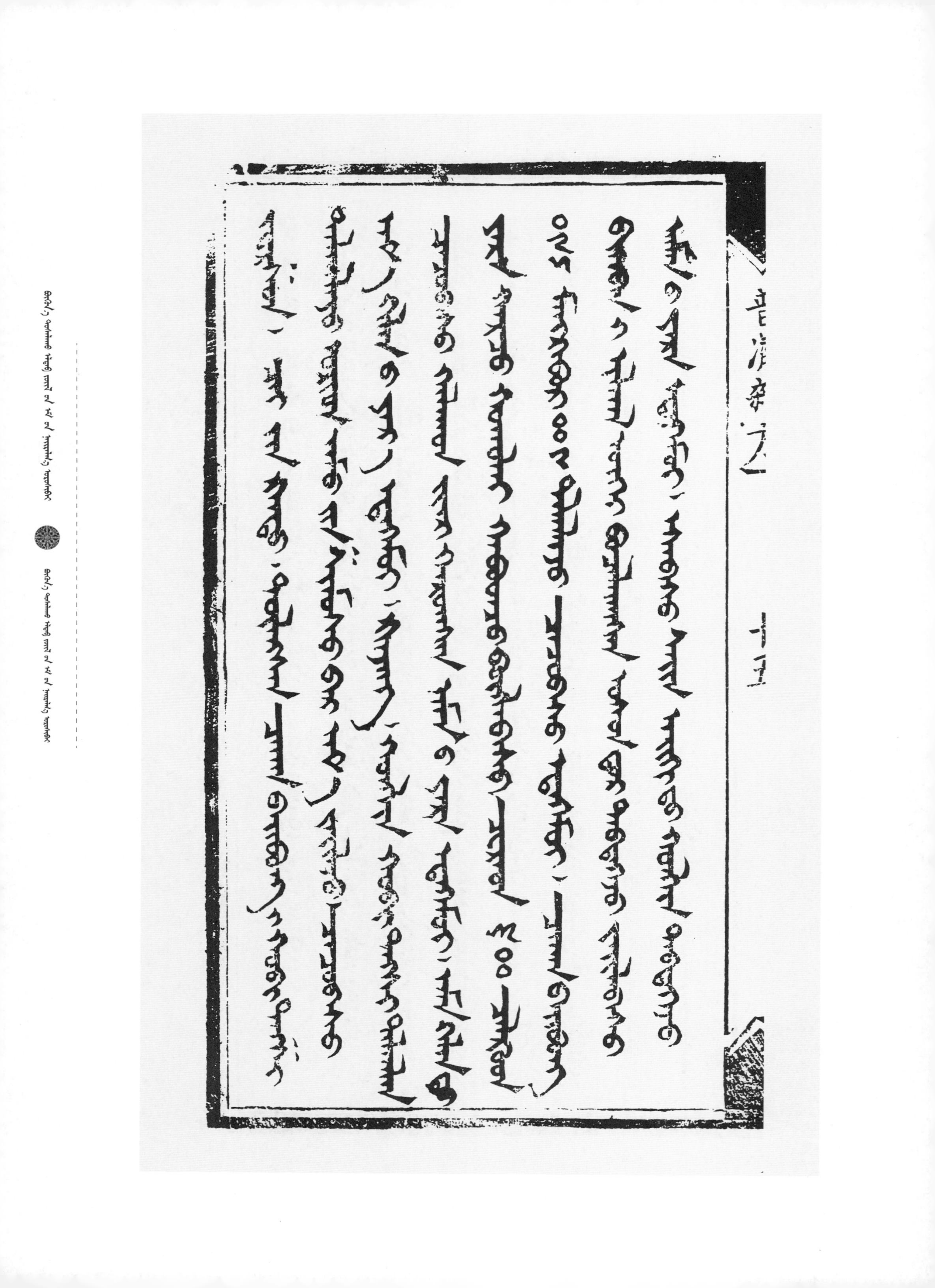

[illegible]

[illegible]

[illegible]

[illegible]

[illegible]

[illegible]

[illegible]

[illegible]

[illegible]

[illegible]

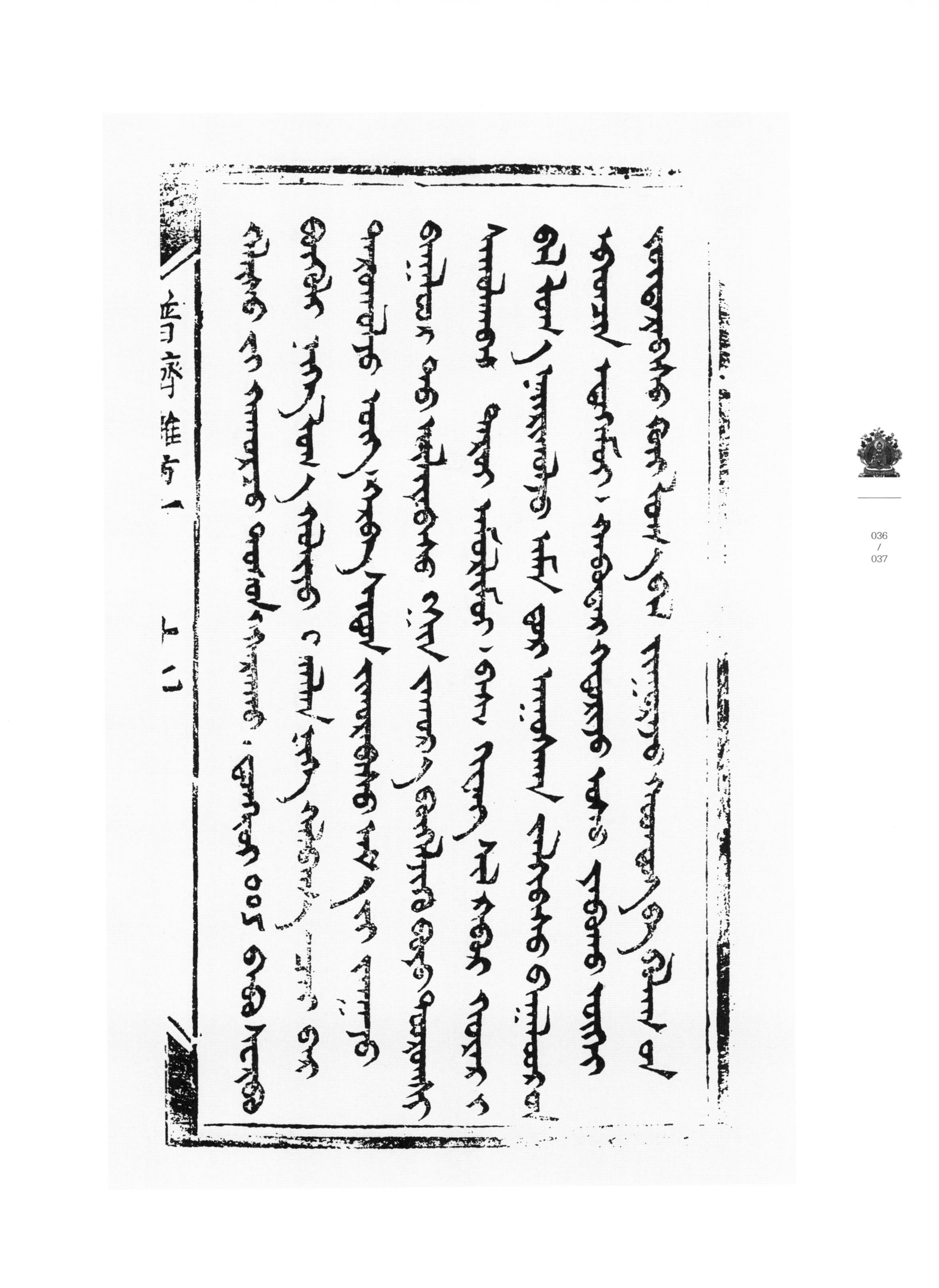

[illegible]

[illegible]
[illegible]
[illegible]
[illegible]
[illegible]
[illegible]
[illegible]
[illegible]

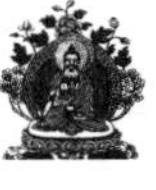

[illegible]

[illegible]

[illegible]

[illegible]

[illegible]

[illegible]

[illegible]

[illegible]

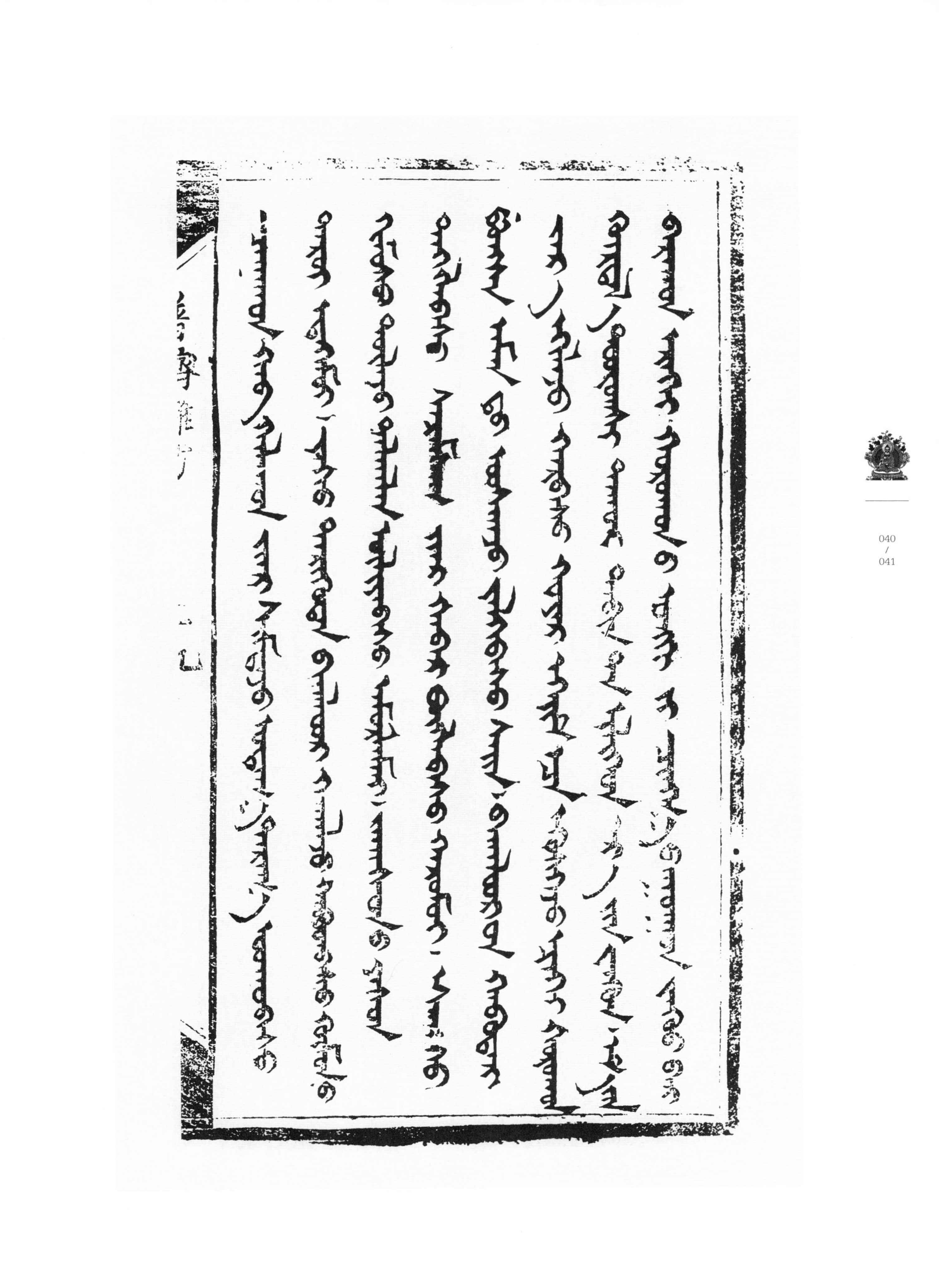

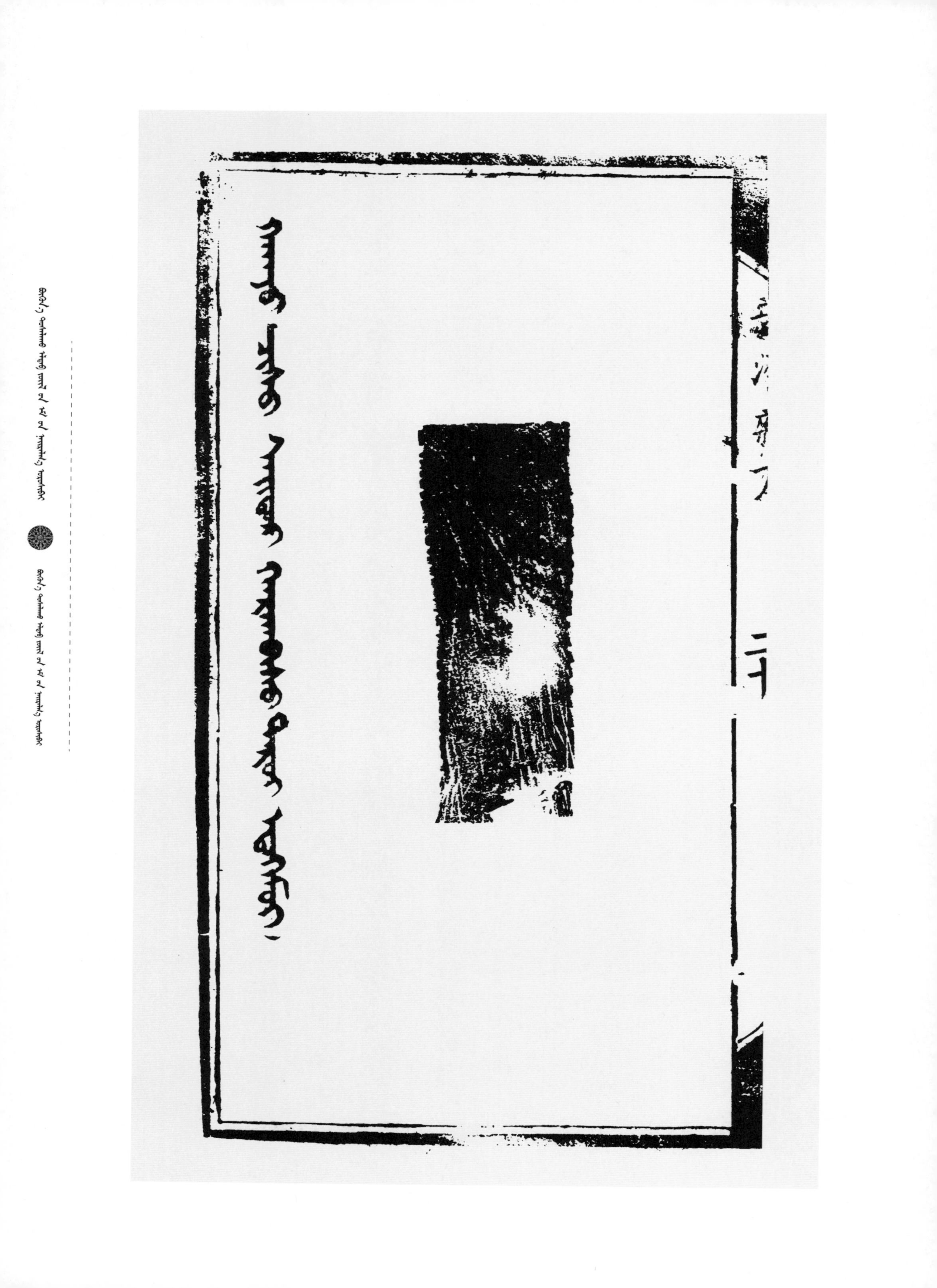

[illegible]

蒙漢齊文 二十

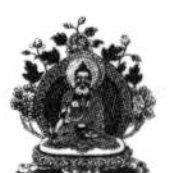

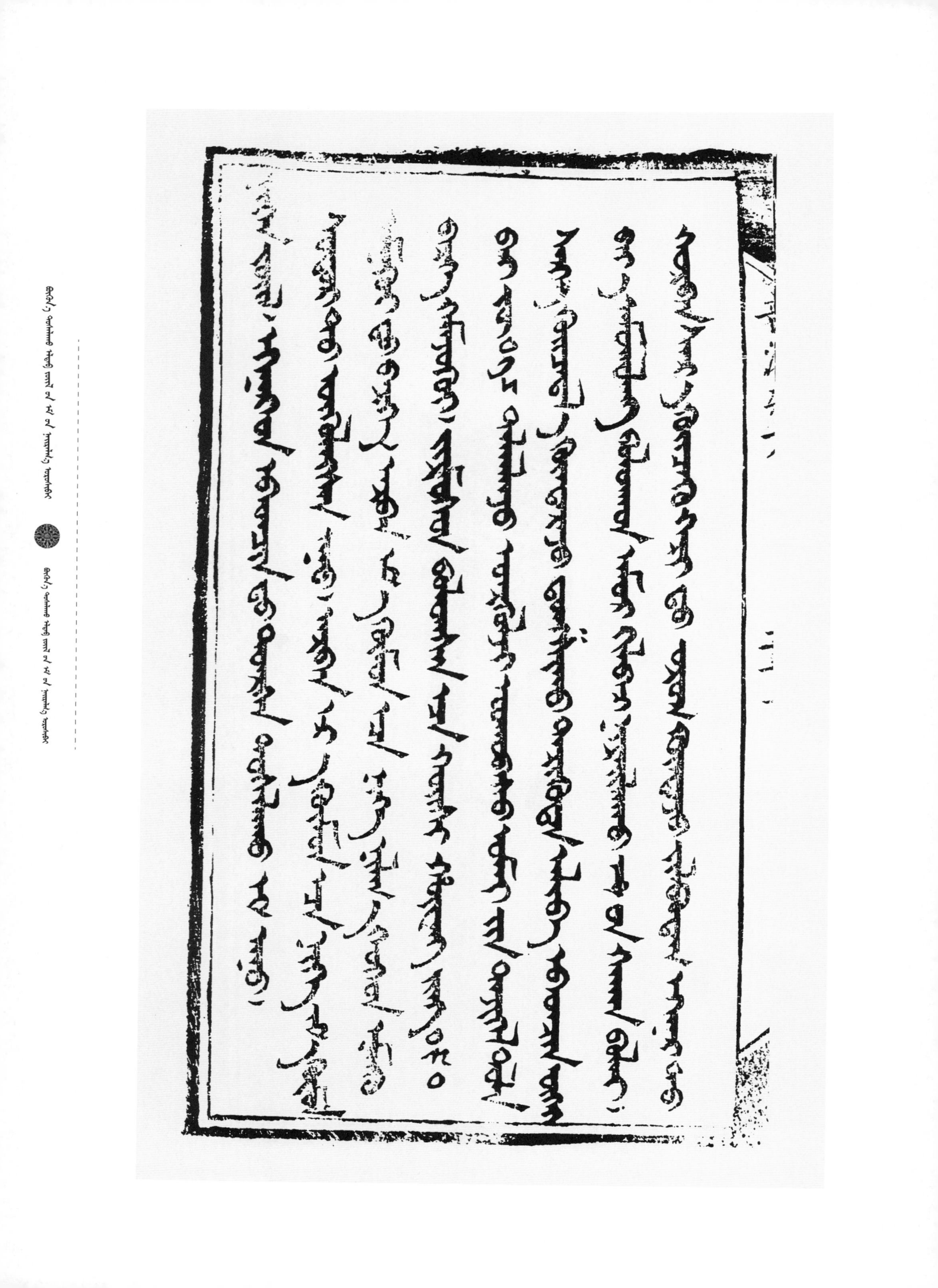

[illegible]

[illegible]

[illegible]

[illegible]

[illegible]

[illegible]

[illegible]

[illegible]

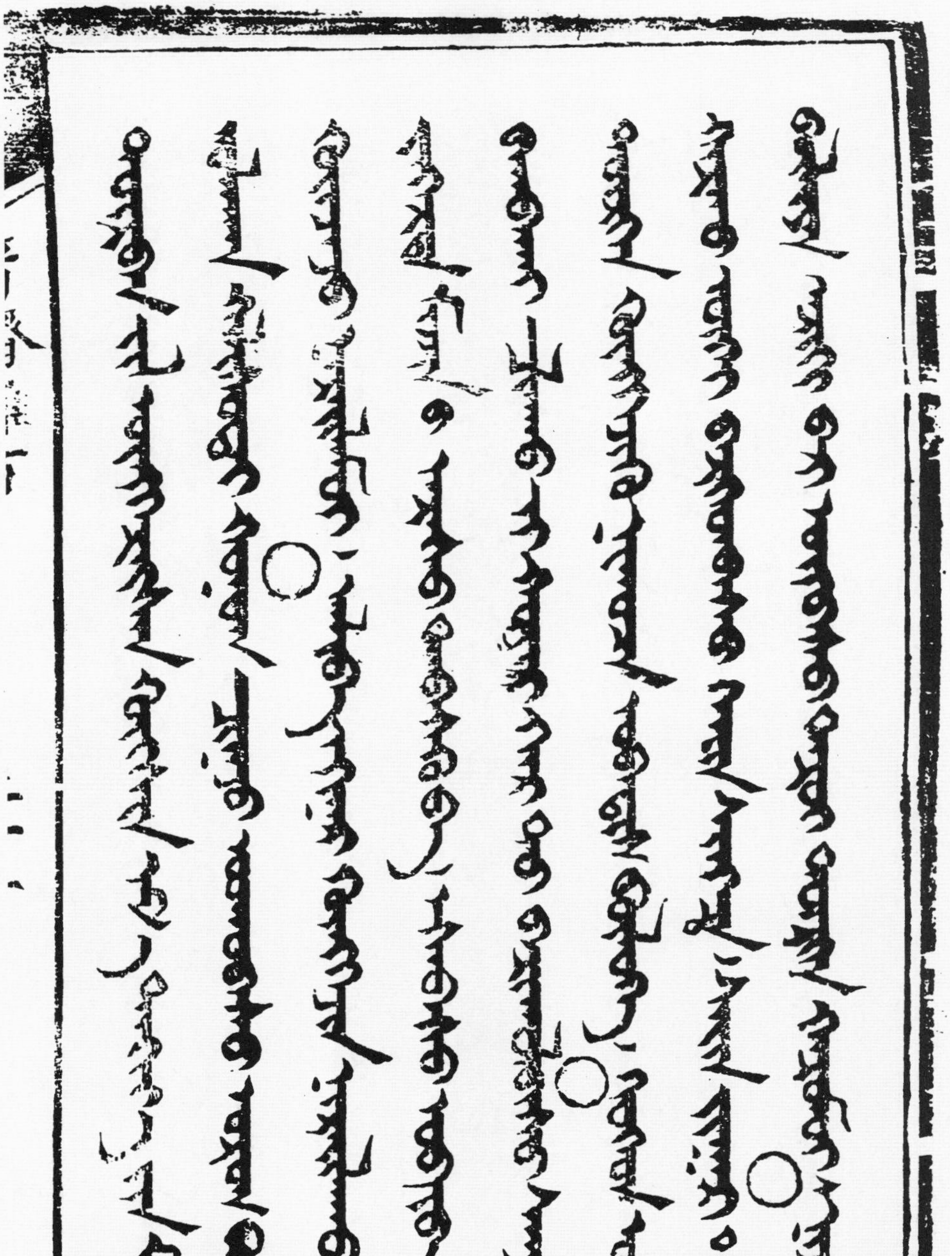

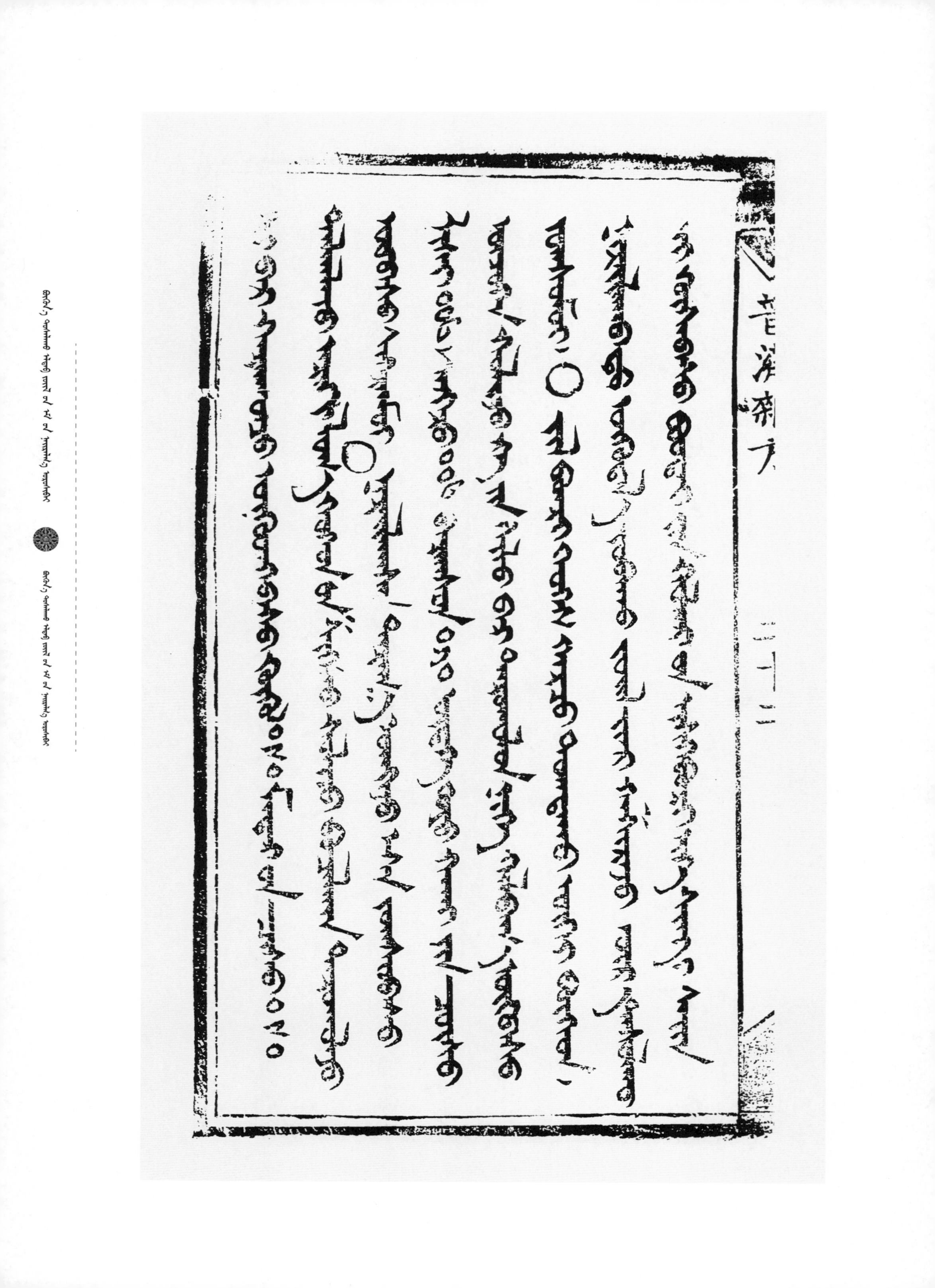

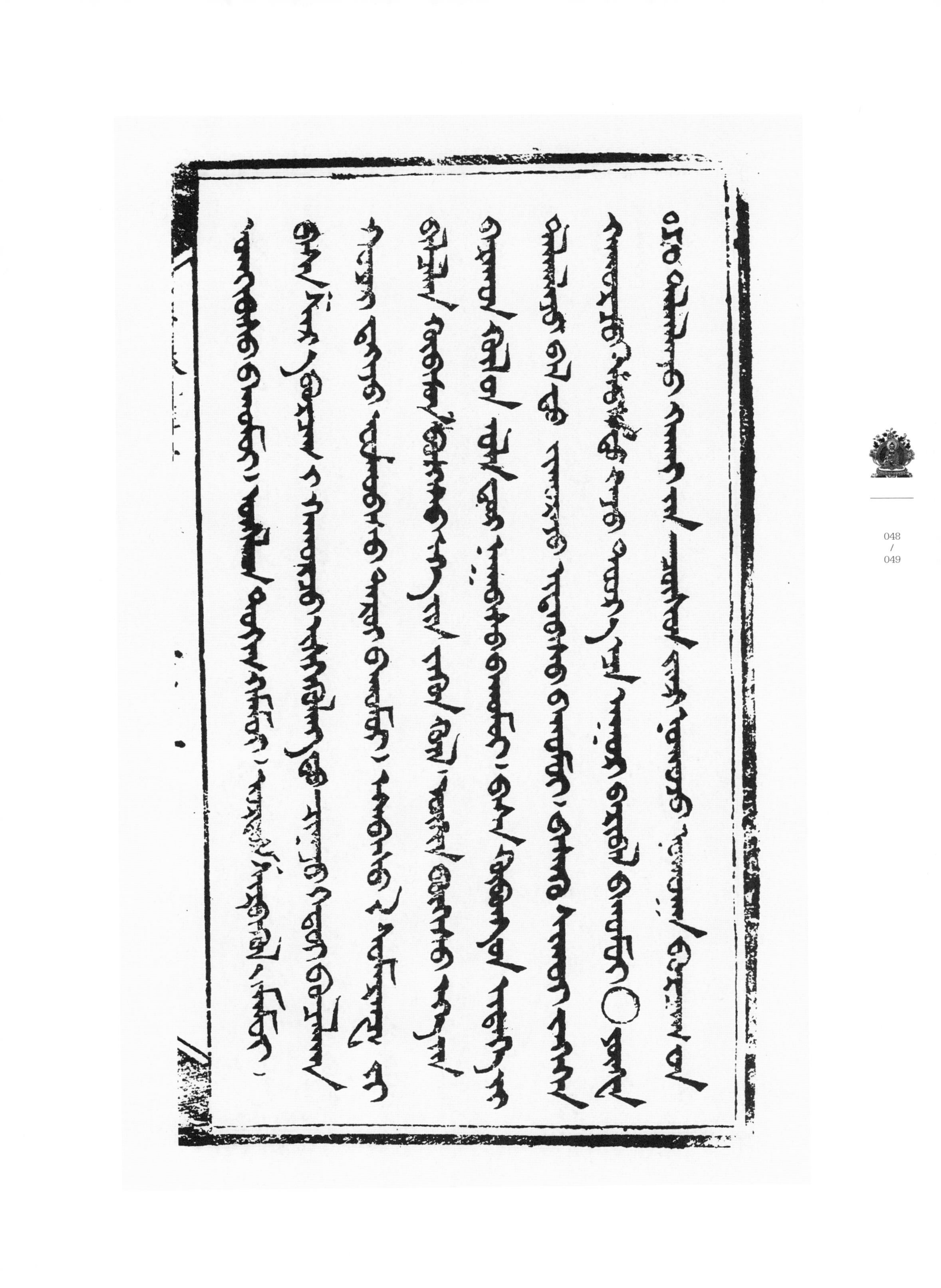

[illegible] [illegible]

[illegible]
[illegible]
[illegible]
[illegible]
[illegible]
[illegible]
[illegible]
[illegible]
[illegible]

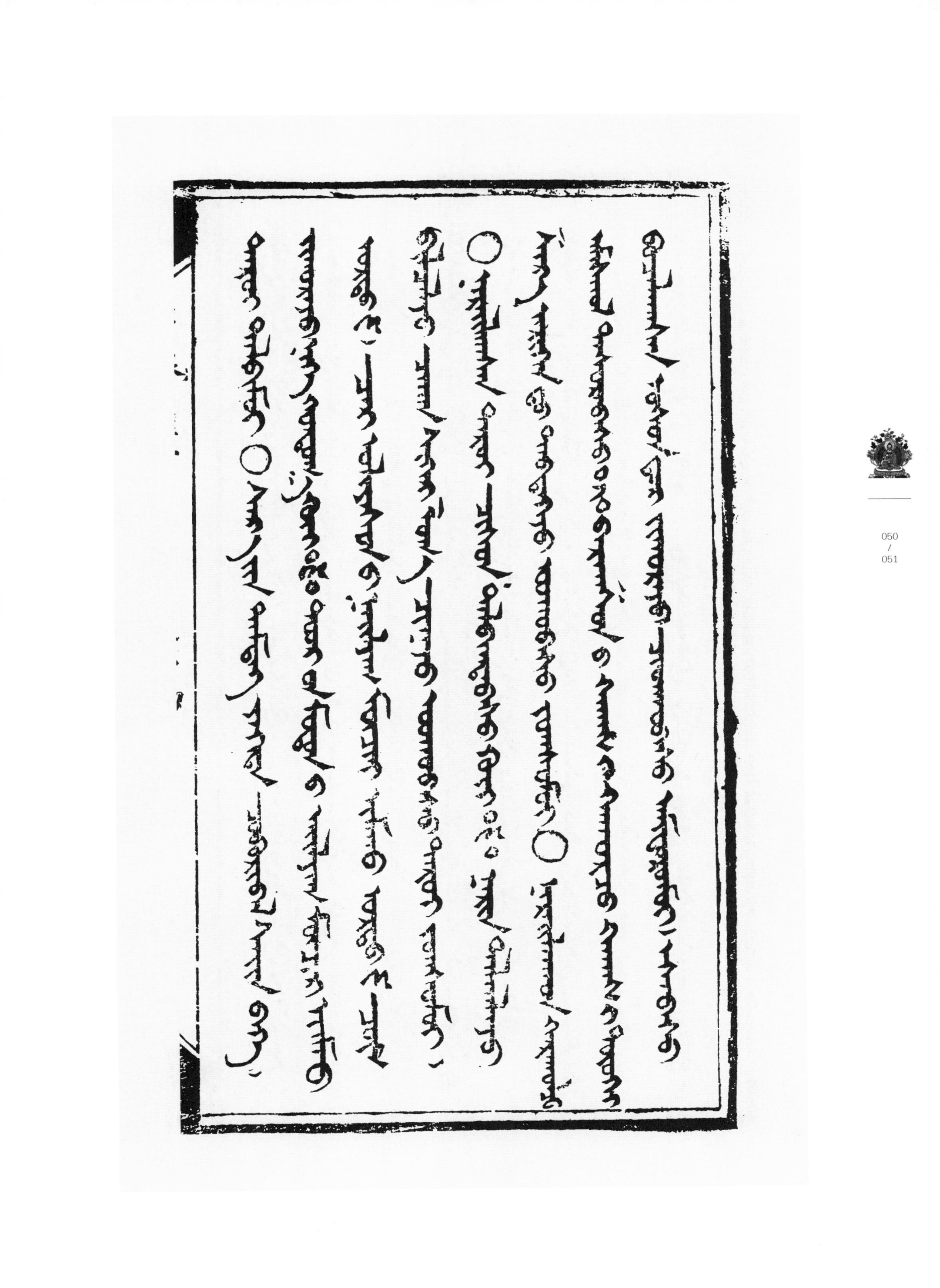

[illegible]

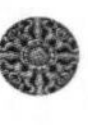

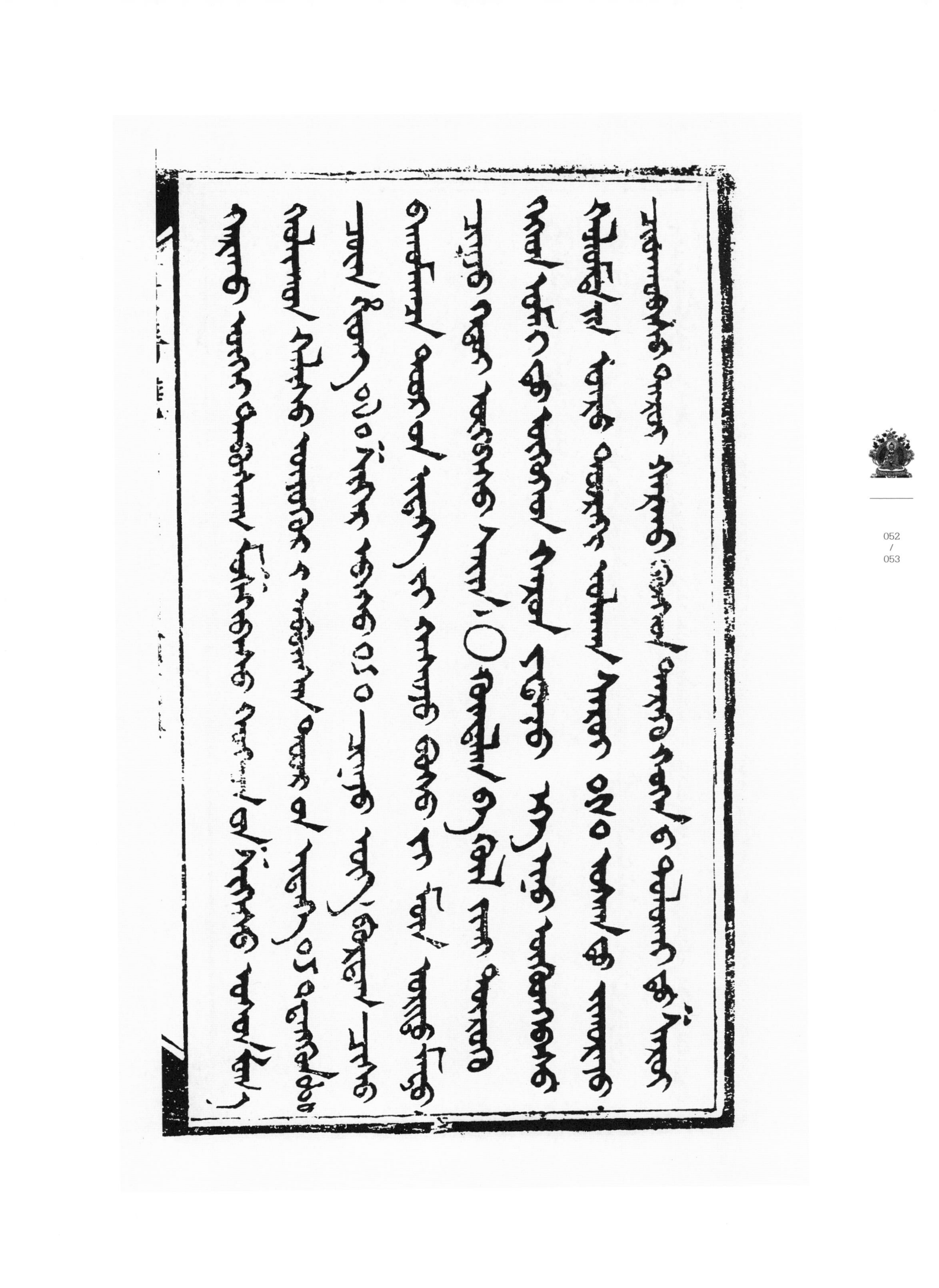

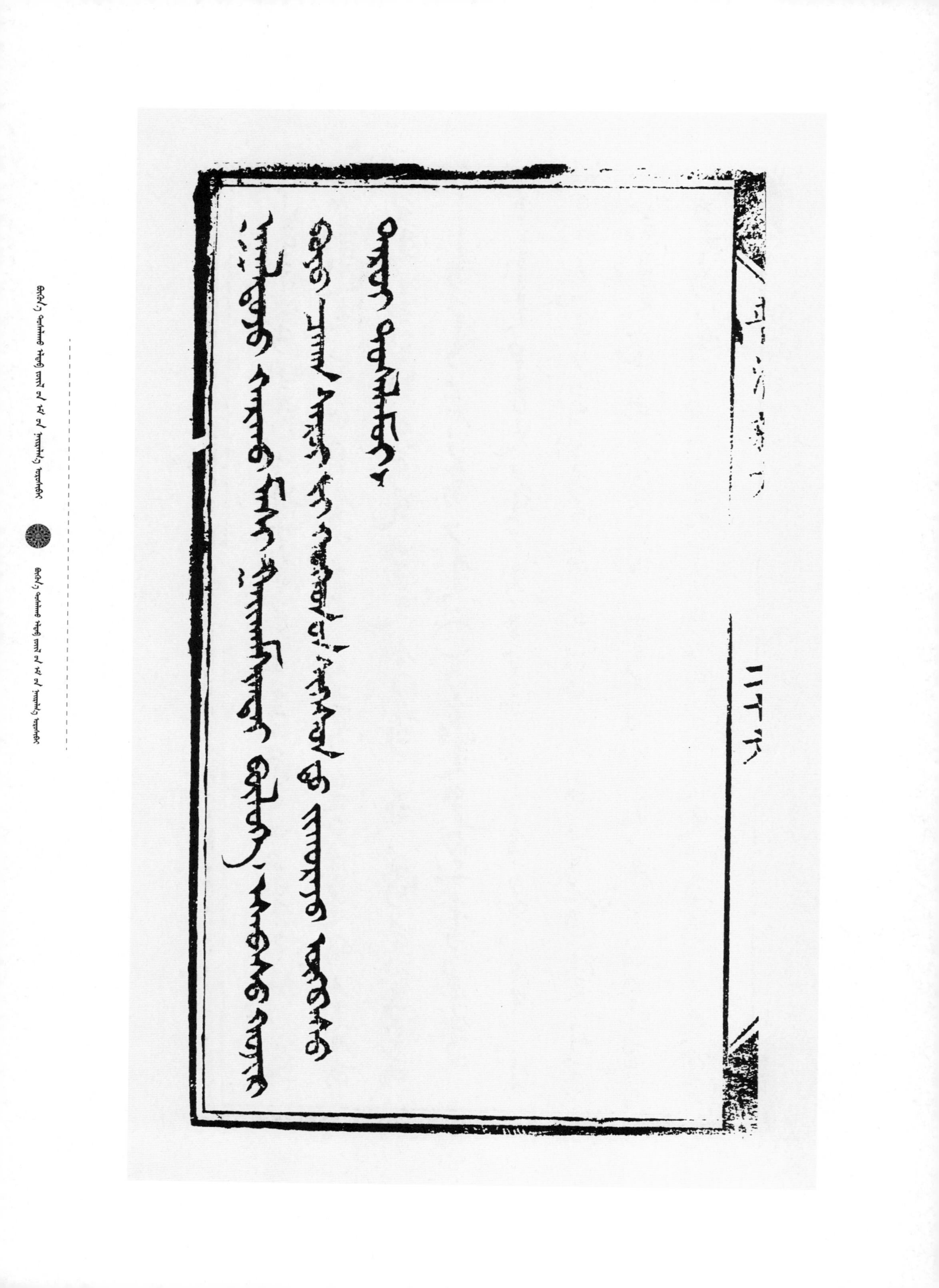

[illegible]

[illegible]

[illegible]

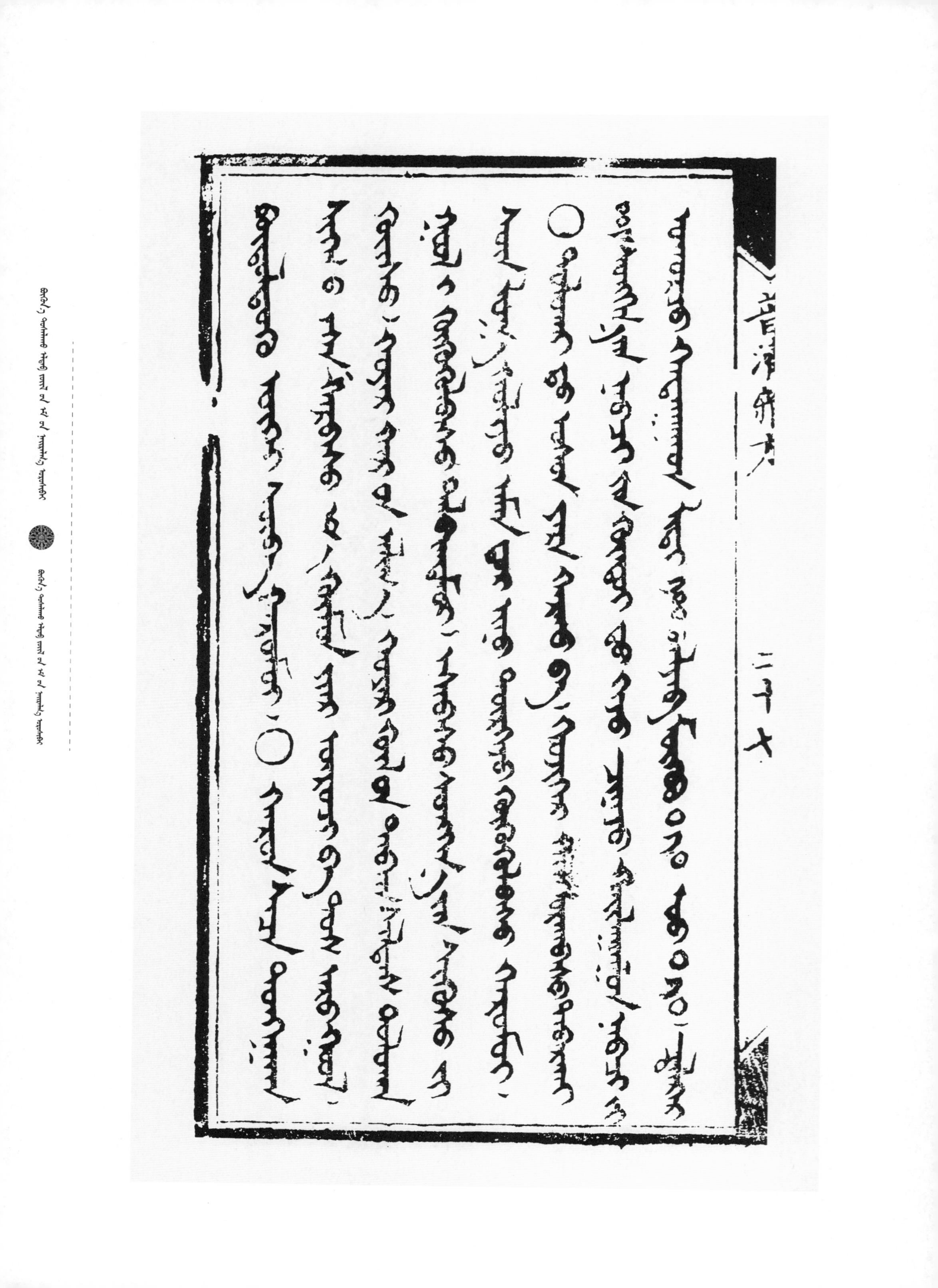

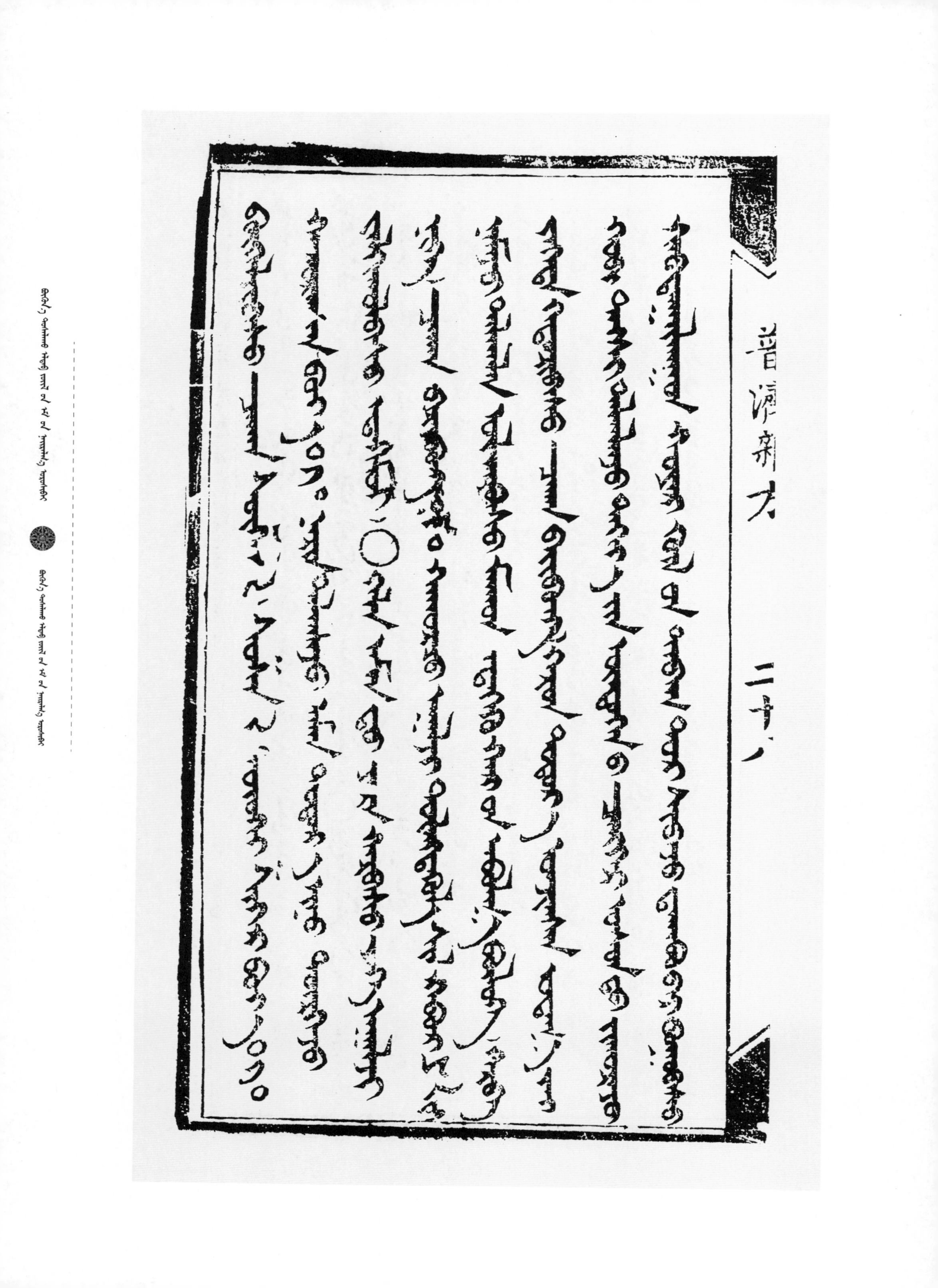

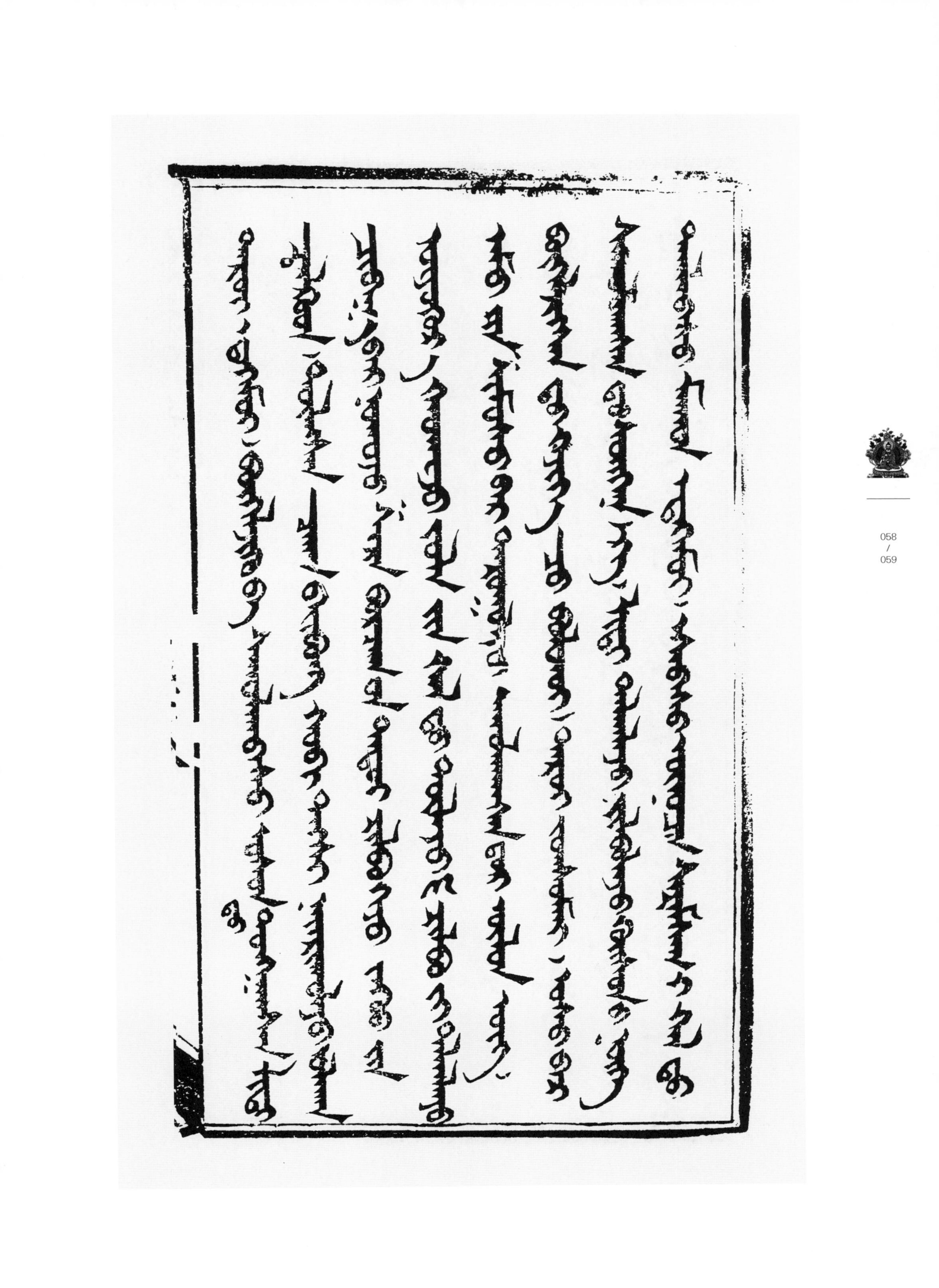

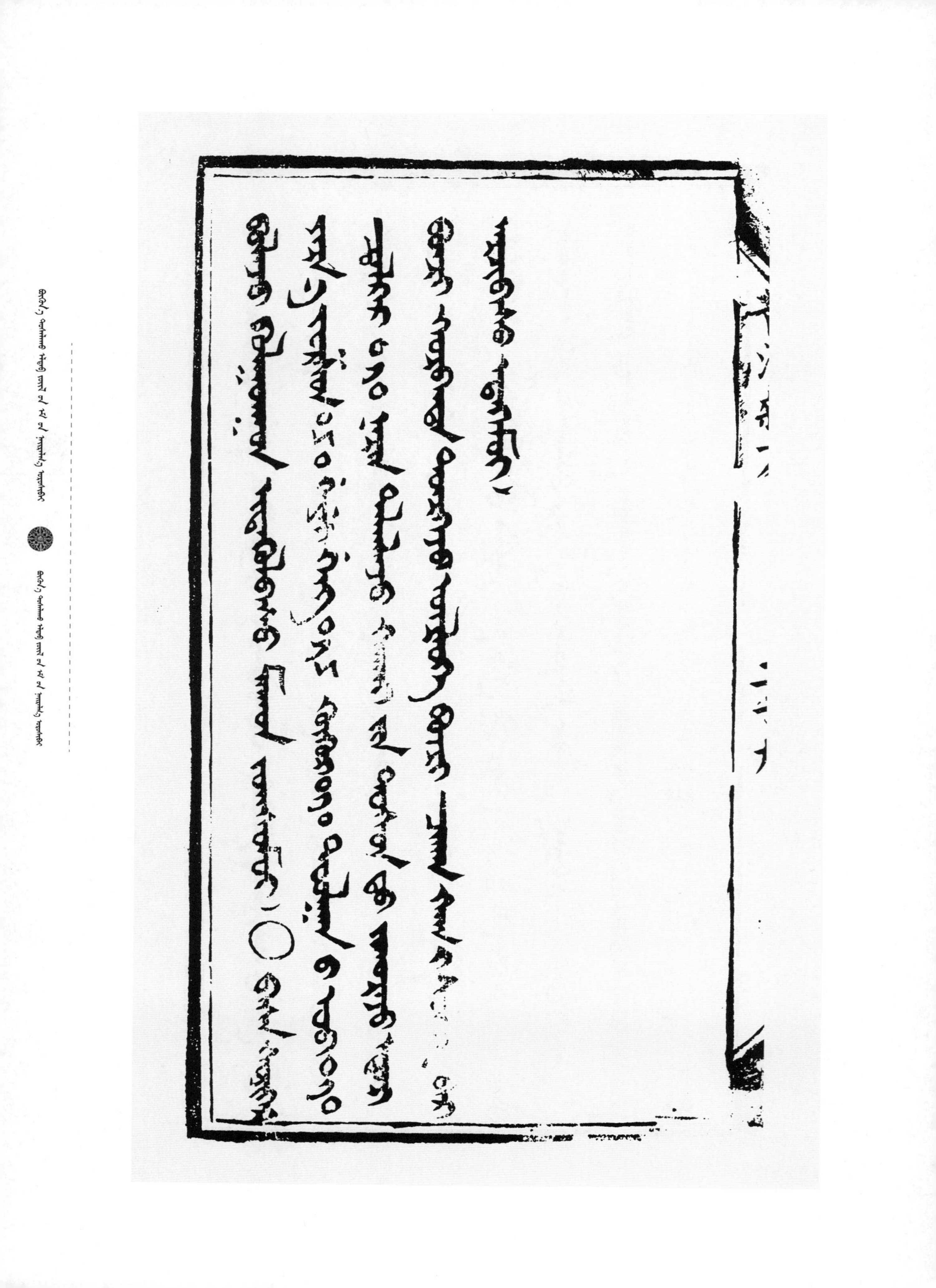

[illegible]

[illegible]

[illegible]

[illegible]

[illegible]

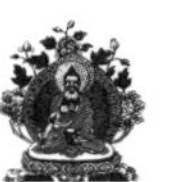

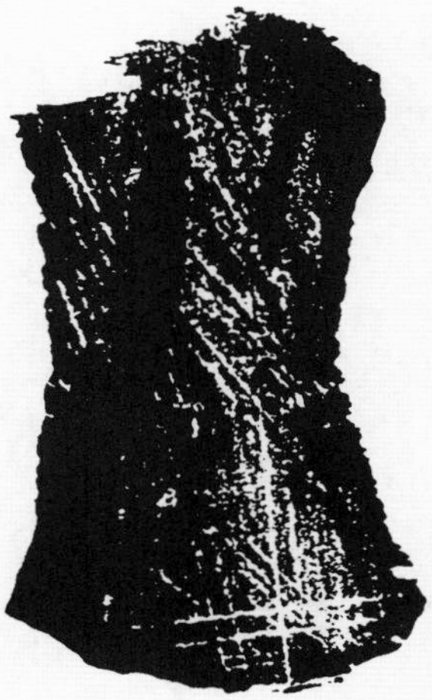

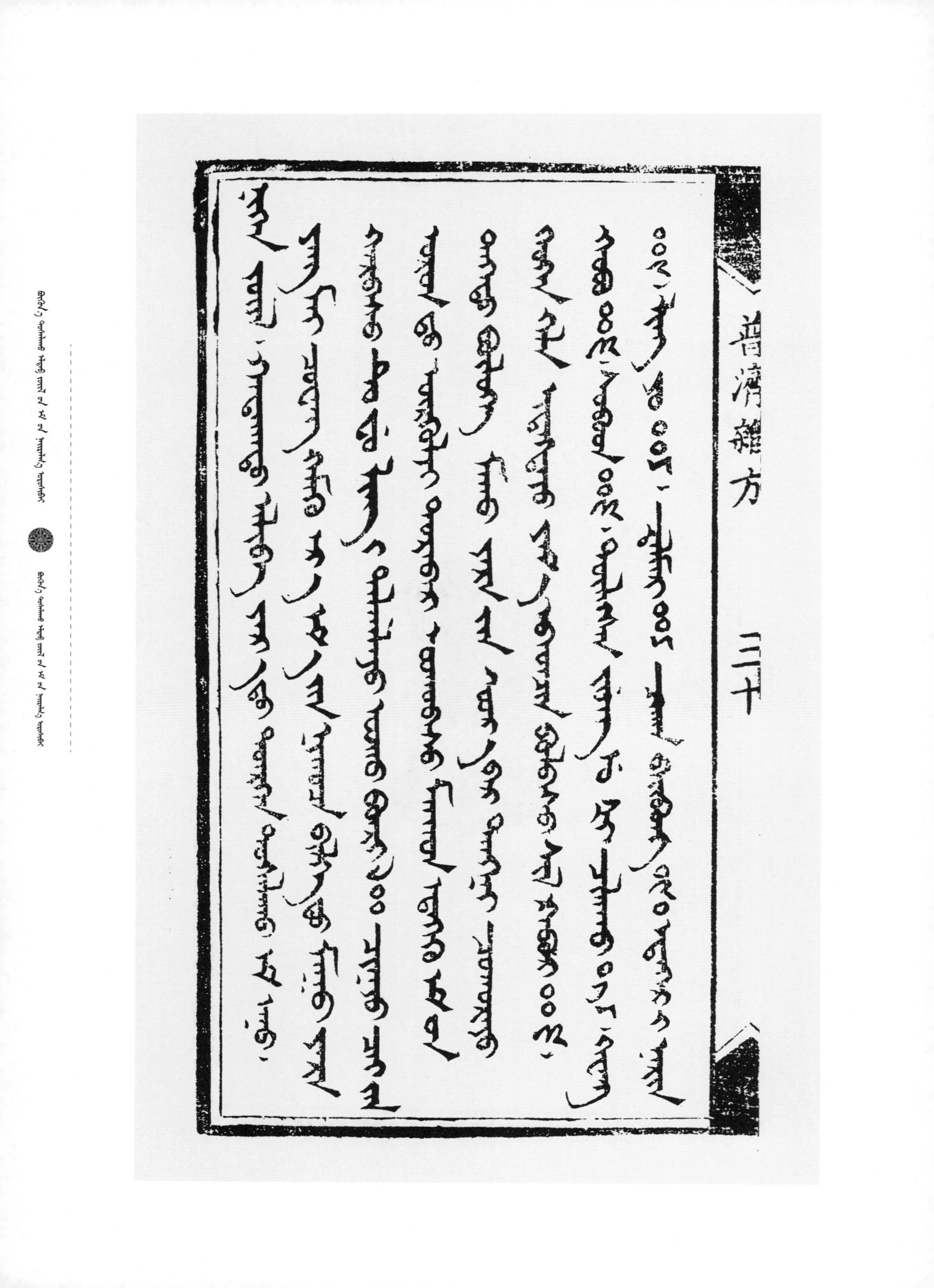

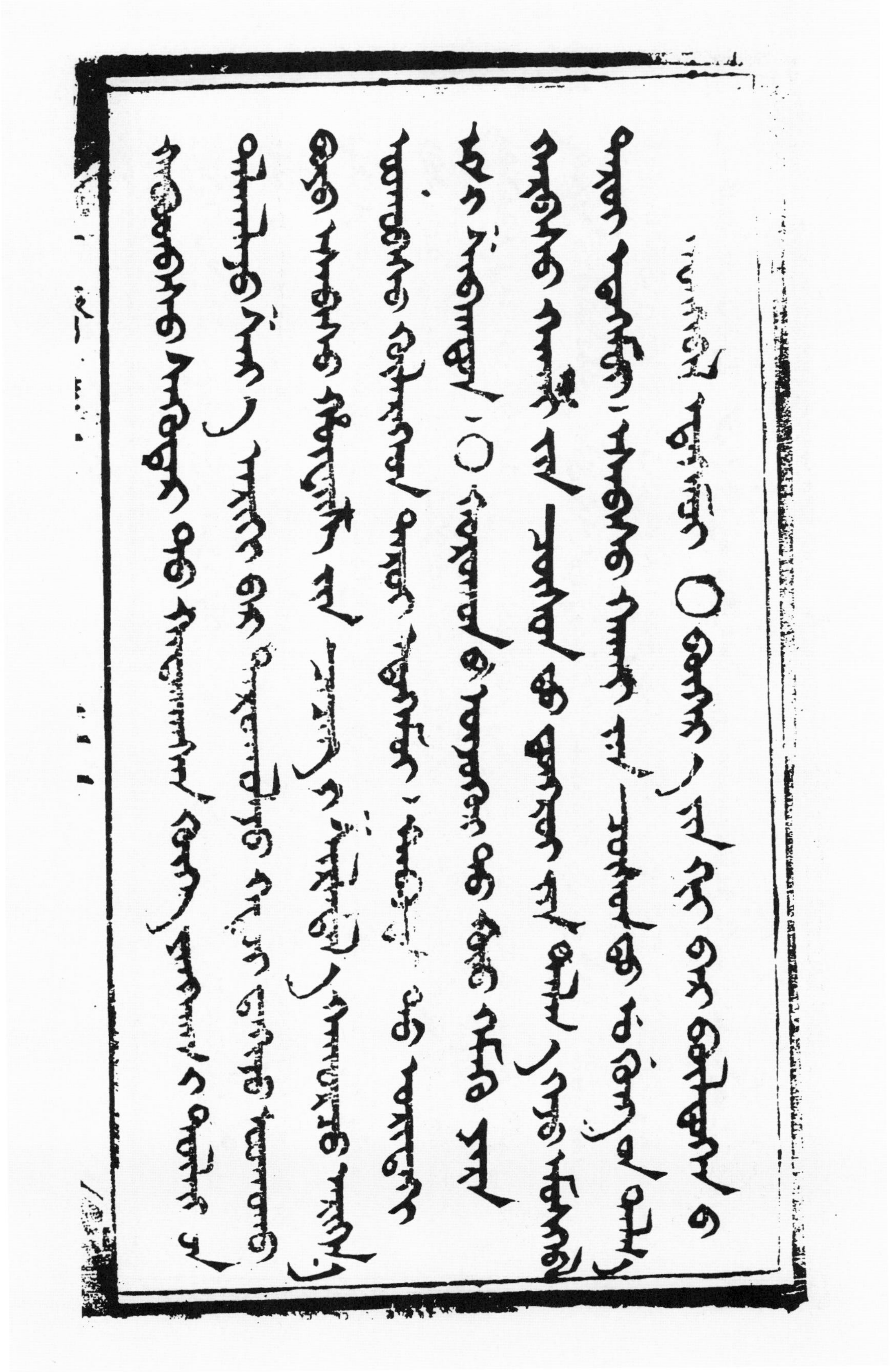

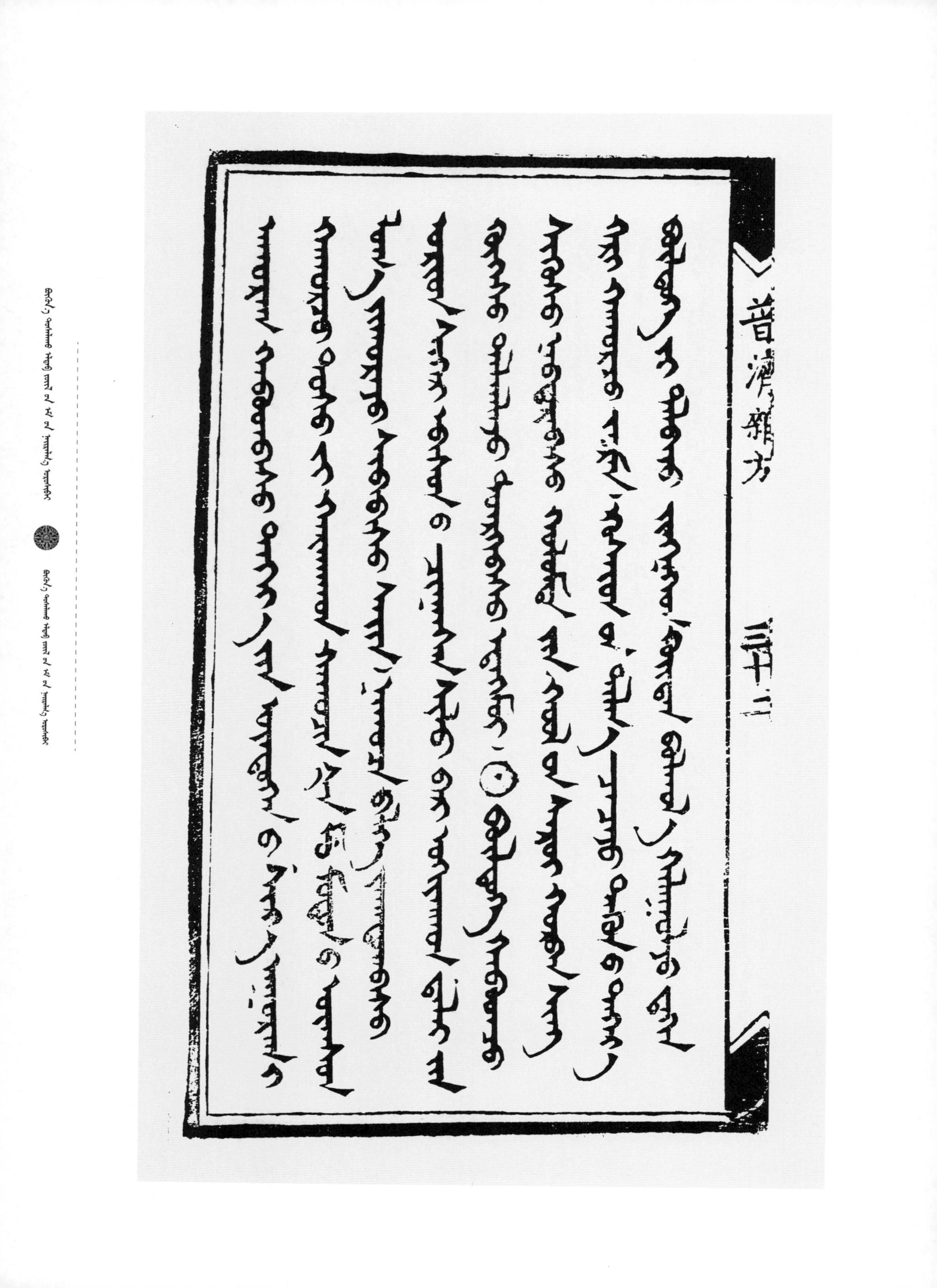

[illegible]

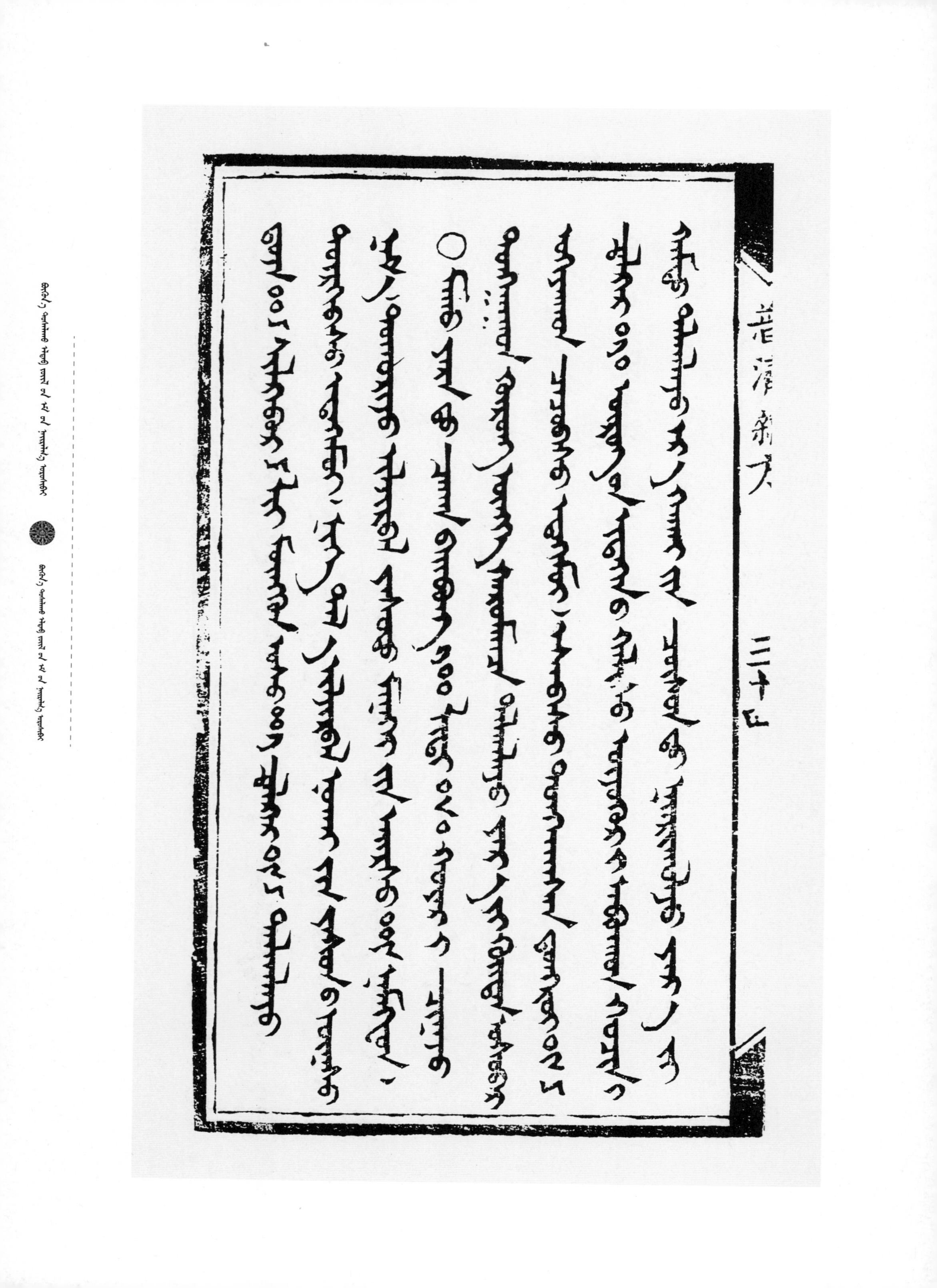

[illegible]

[illegible]

[illegible]

[illegible]

[illegible]

[illegible]

[illegible]

[illegible]

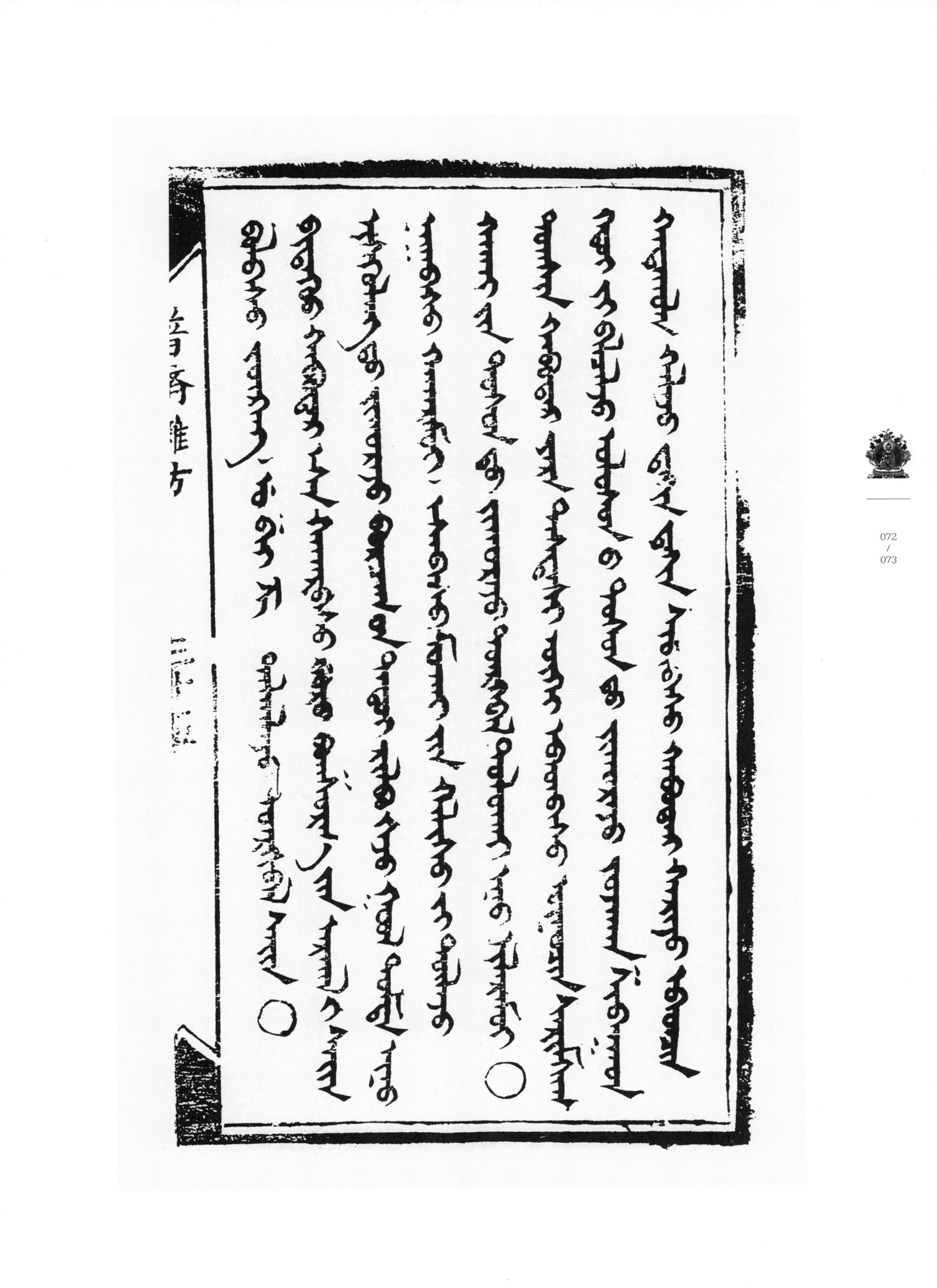

普濟雜方

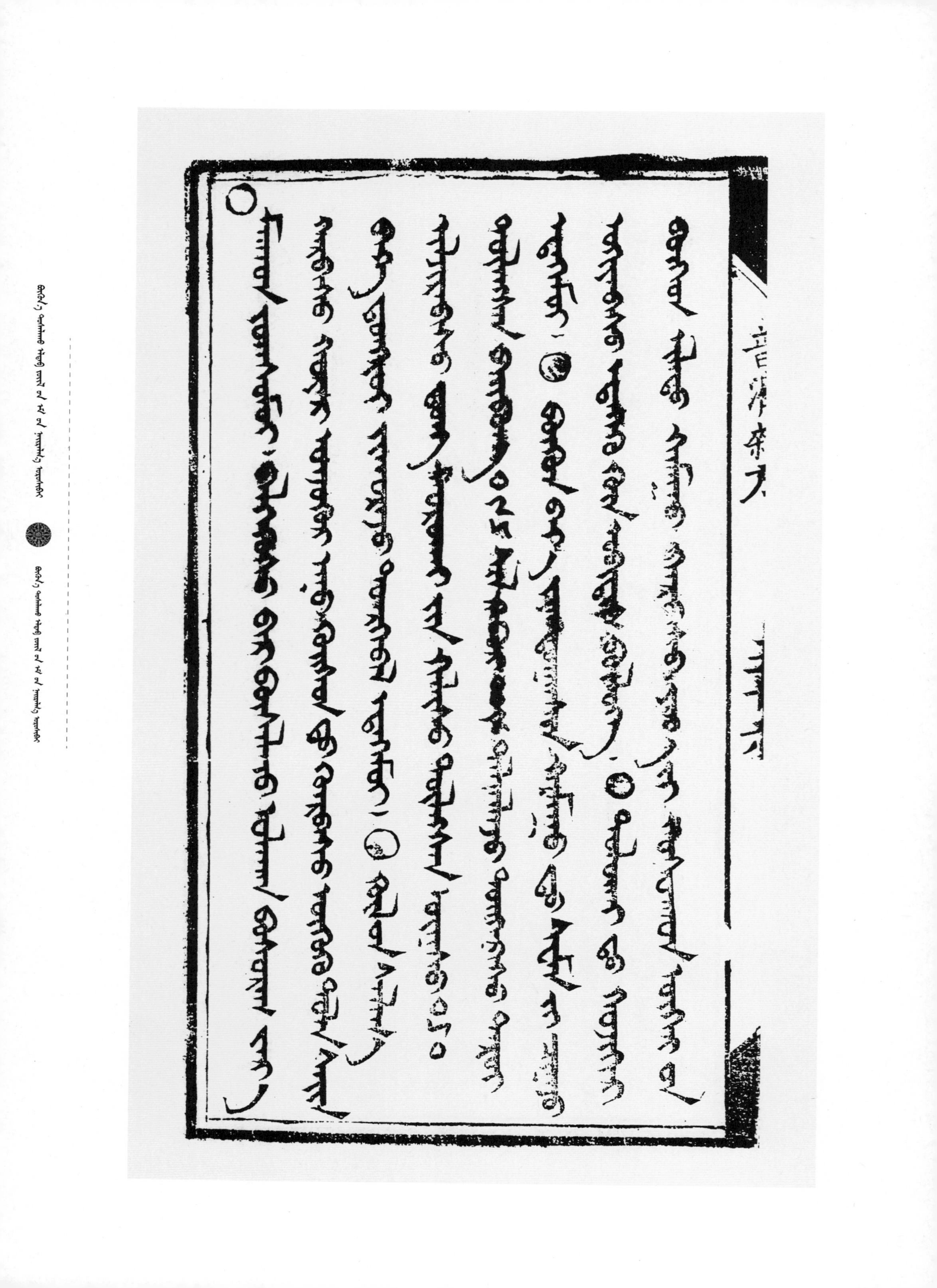

[illegible]

[illegible]

[illegible]

[illegible]

[illegible]

[illegible]

[illegible]

[illegible]

[illegible]

[illegible]

[illegible]

[illegible]

[illegible]

[illegible]

[illegible]

[illegible]

[illegible]

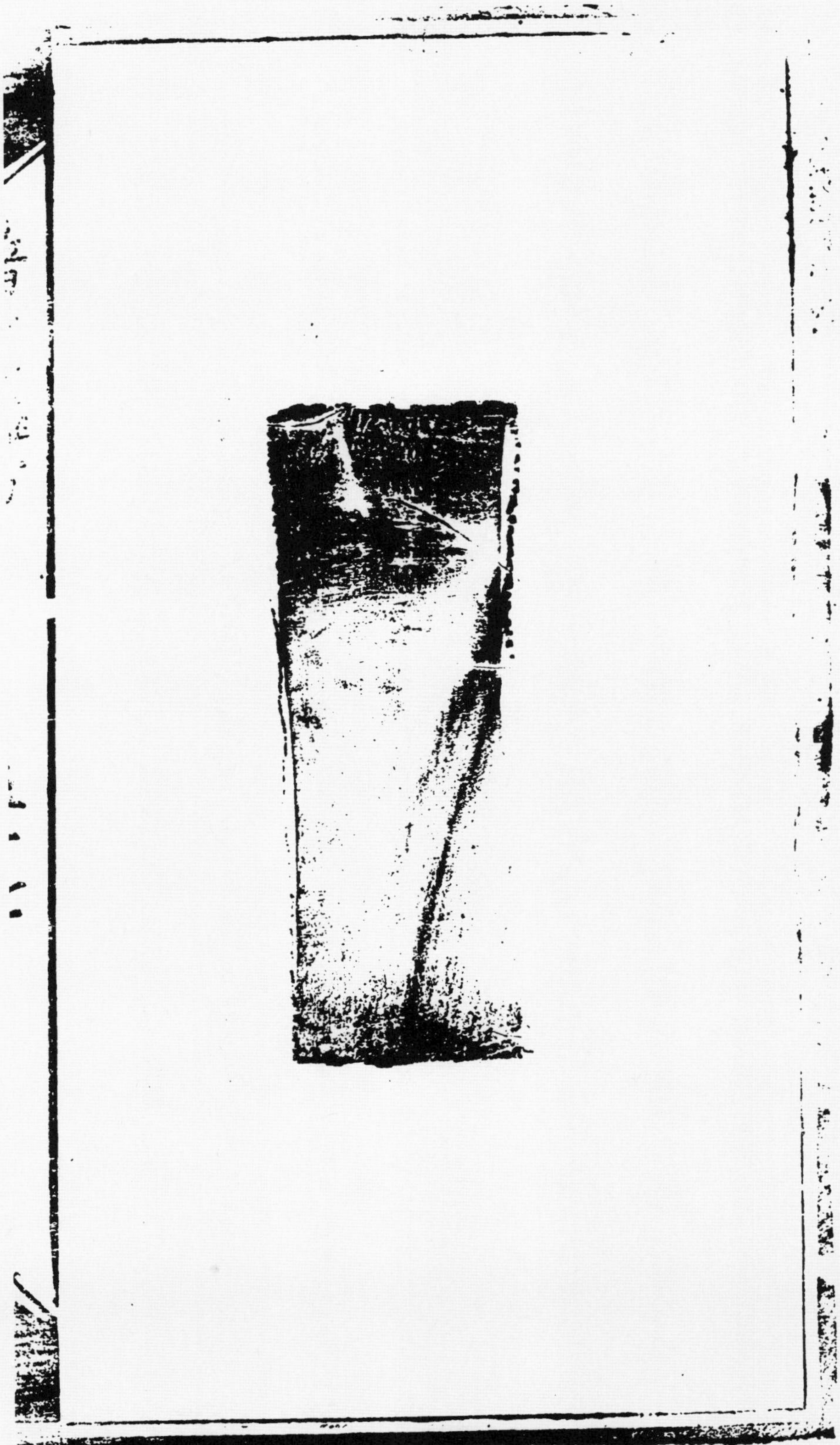

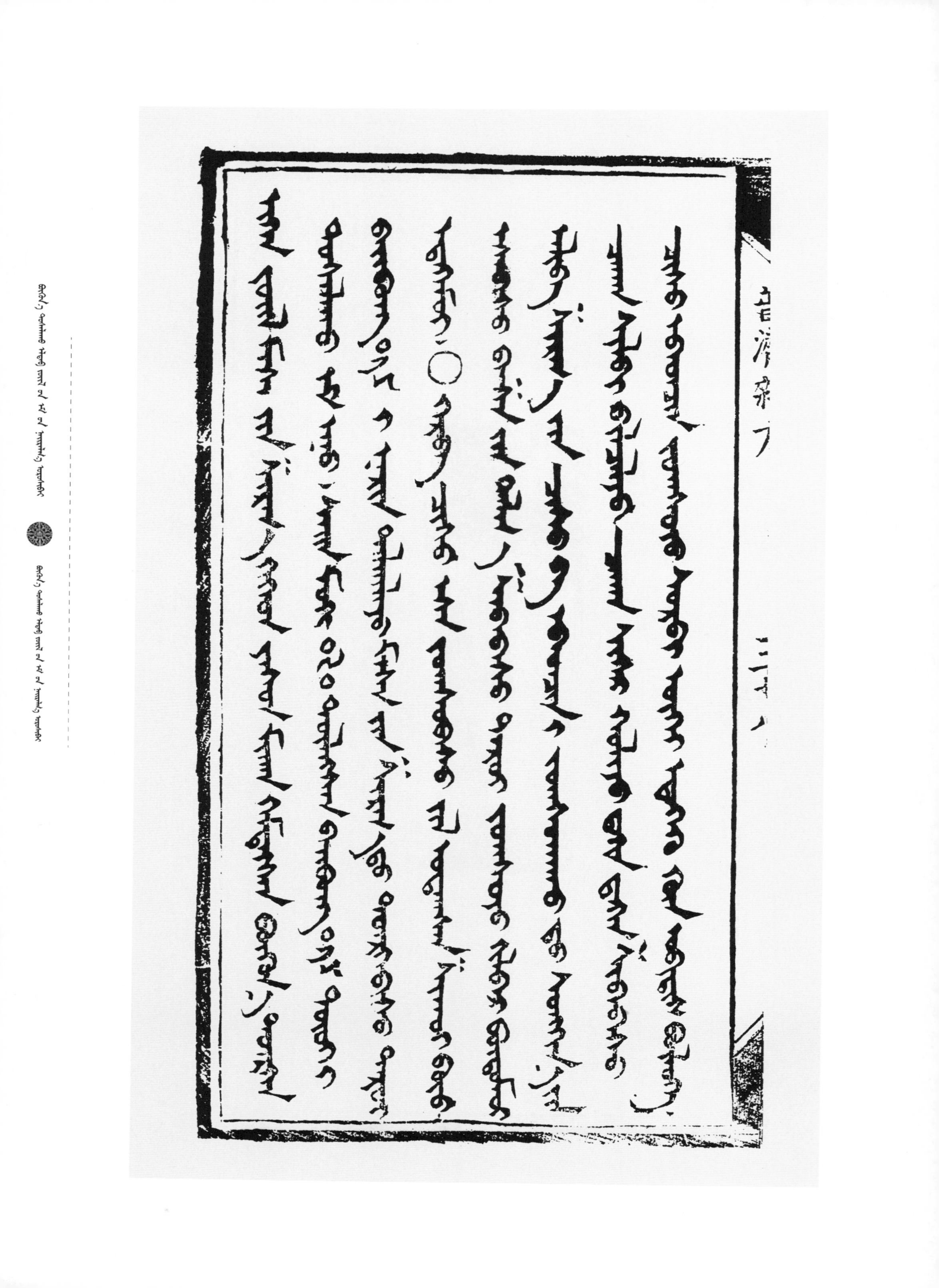

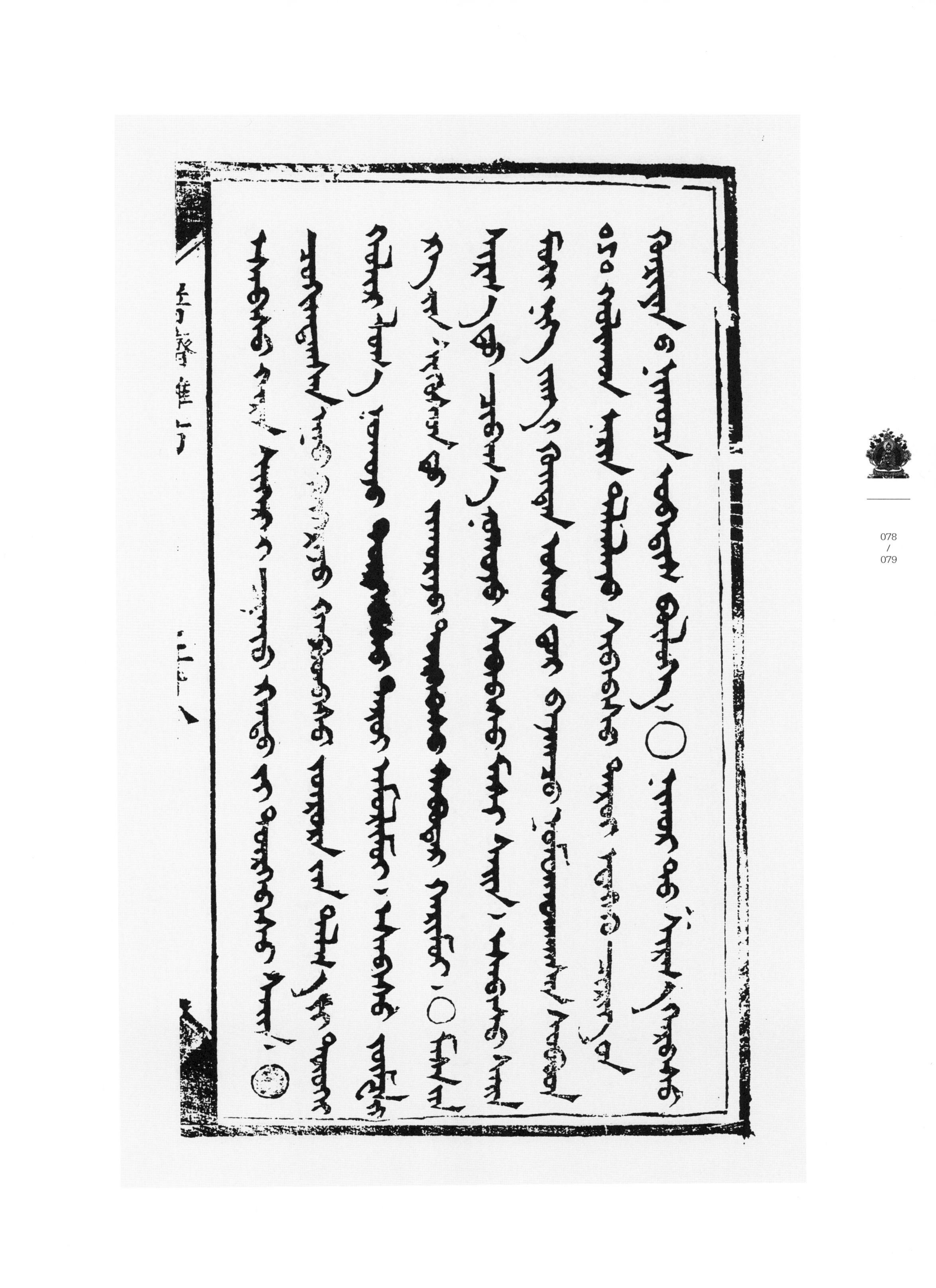

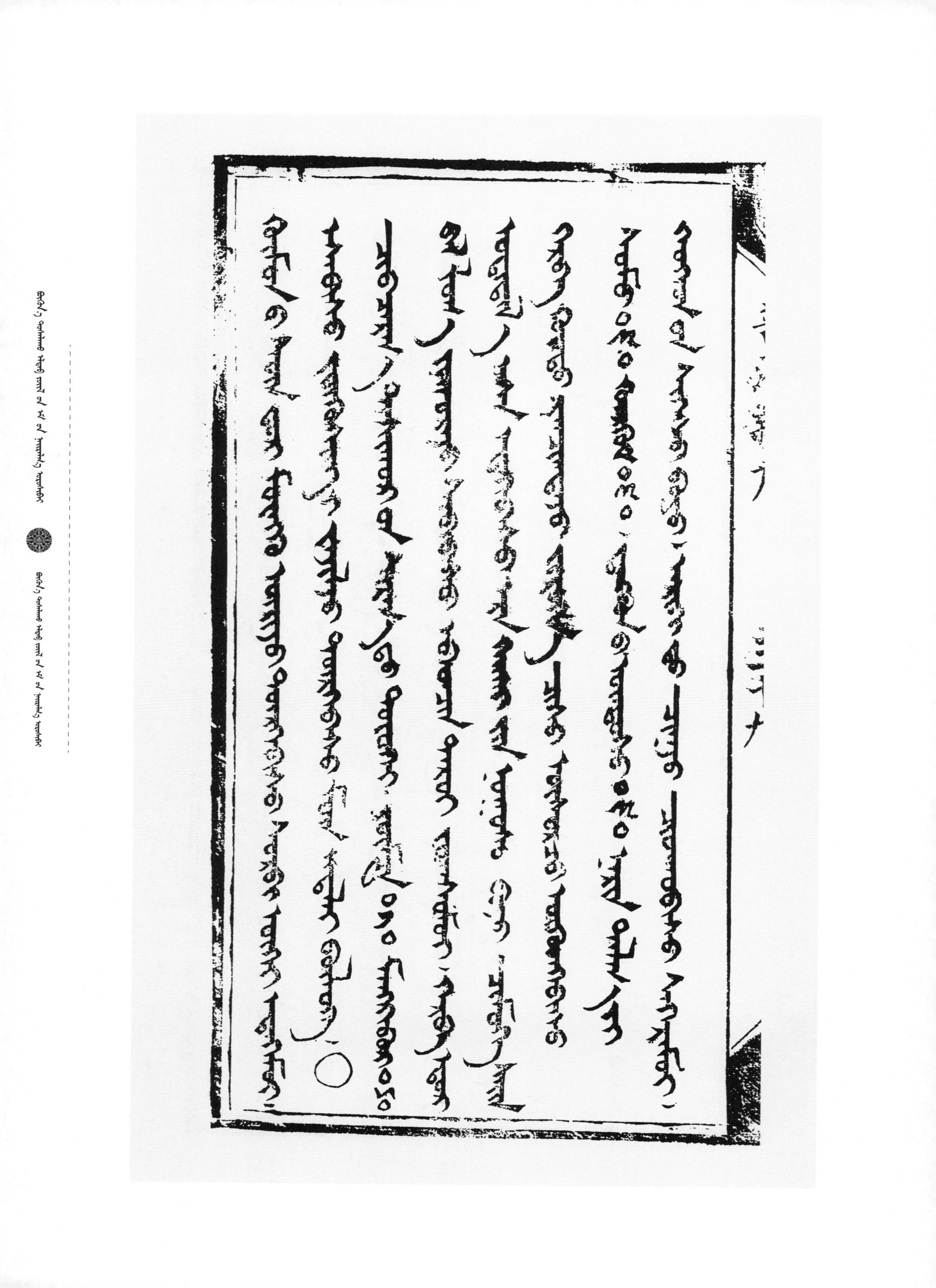

[illegible]

[illegible]

[illegible]

[illegible]

[illegible]

[illegible]

[illegible]

[illegible]

[illegible]

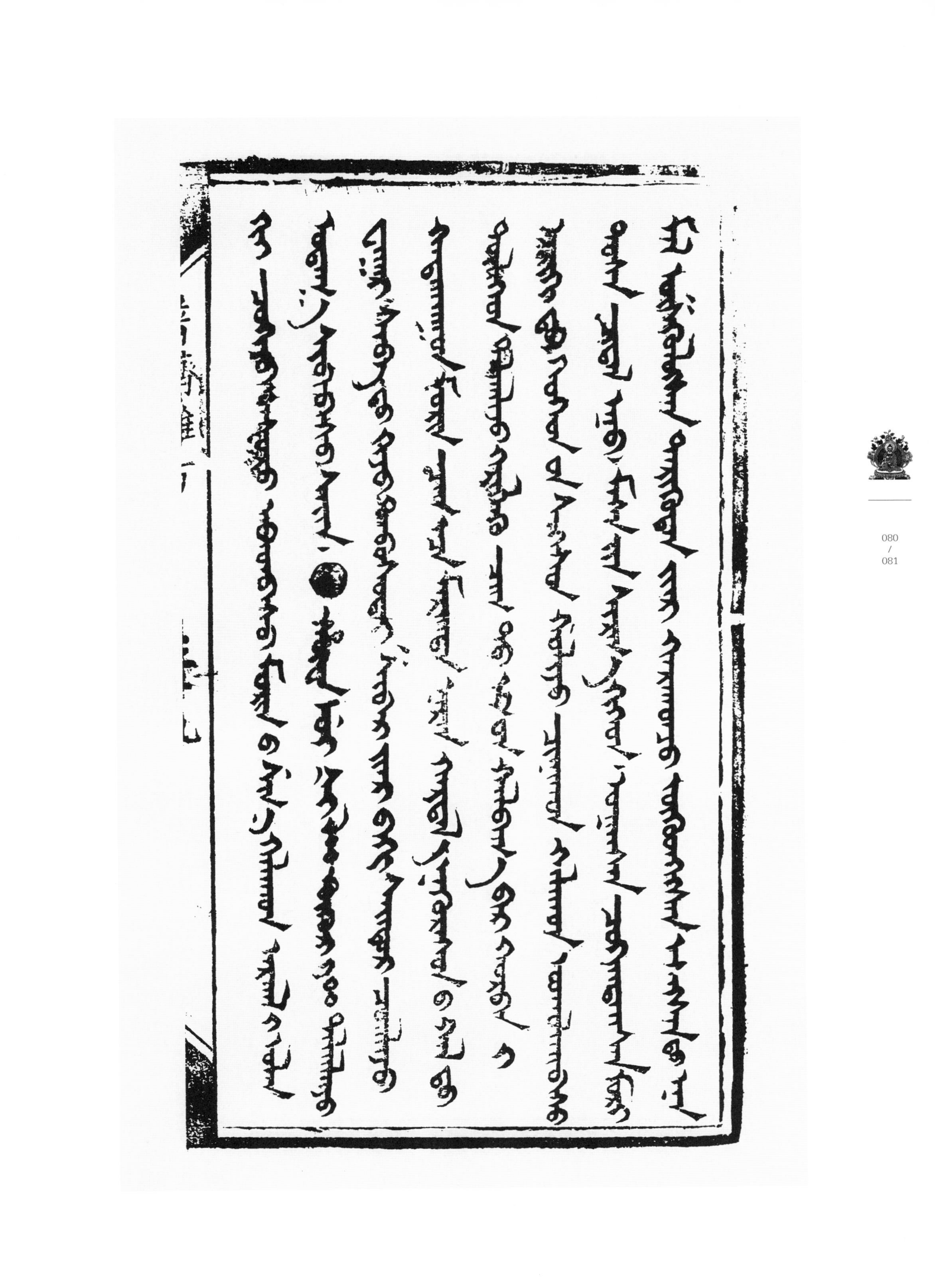

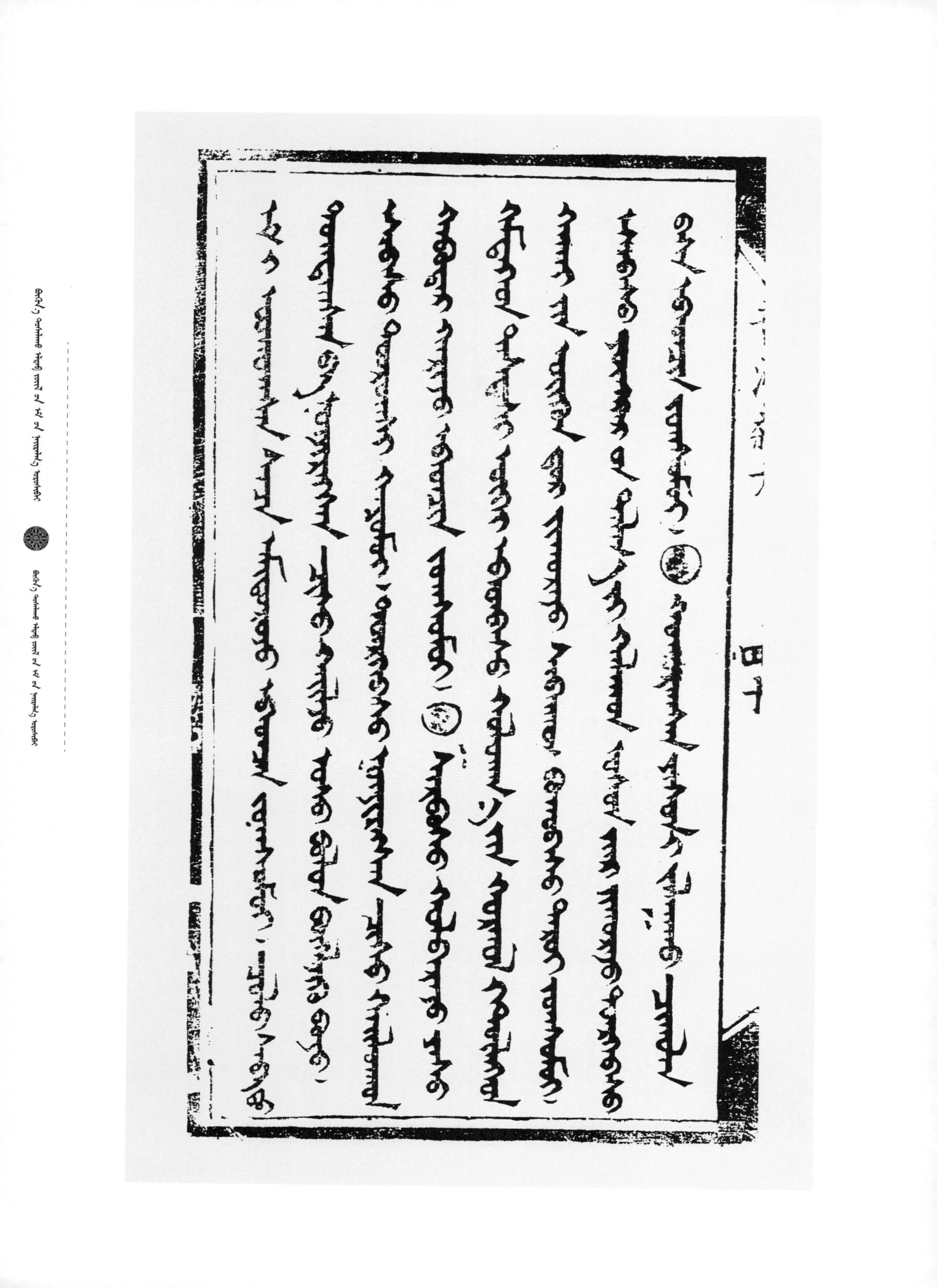

四十

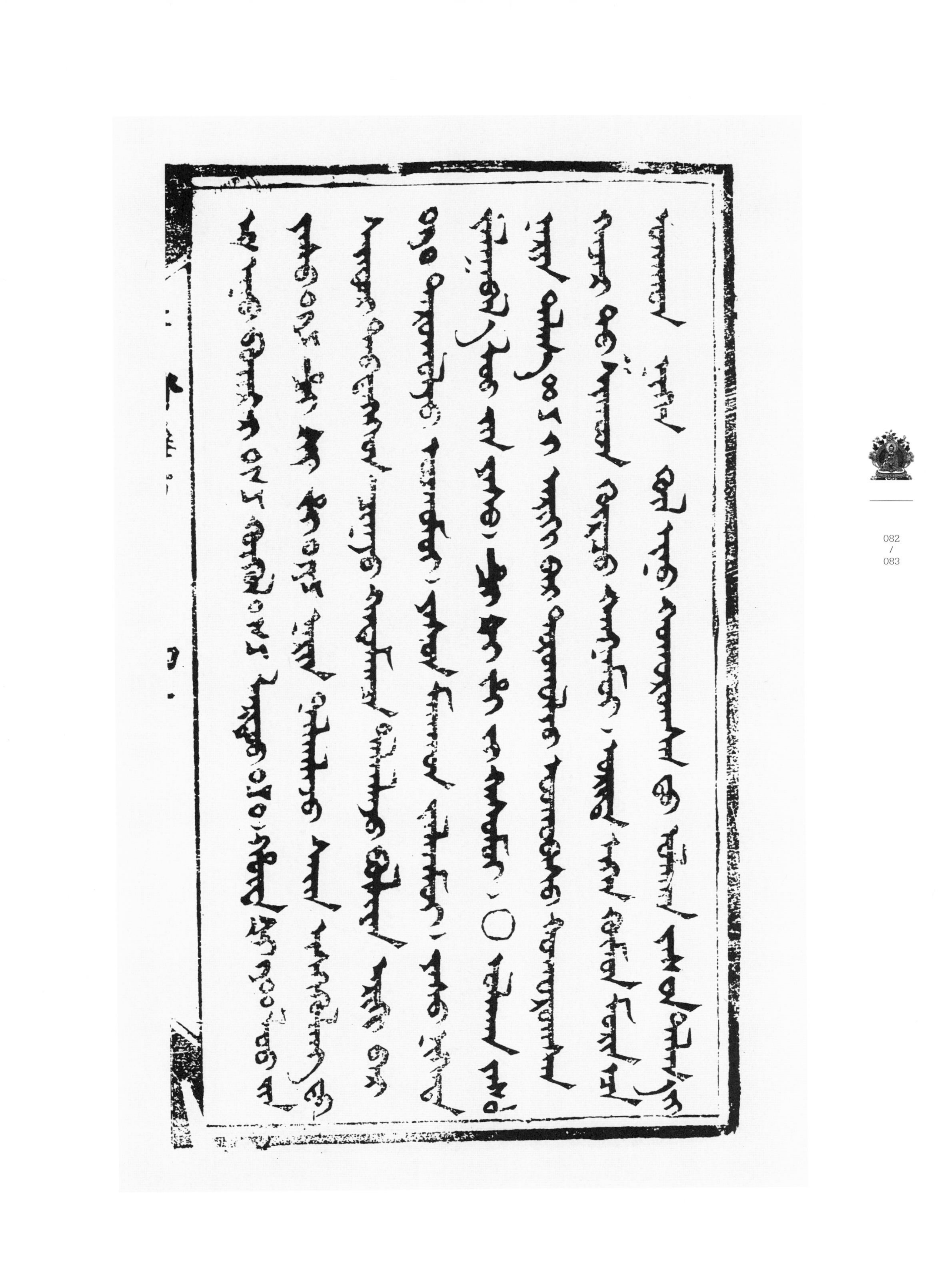

[illegible]

[illegible]

[illegible]

[illegible]

[illegible]

[illegible]

[illegible]

[illegible]

[illegible]

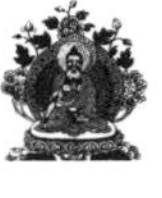

[illegible]

[illegible]

[illegible]

[illegible]

[illegible]

[illegible]

[illegible]

[illegible]

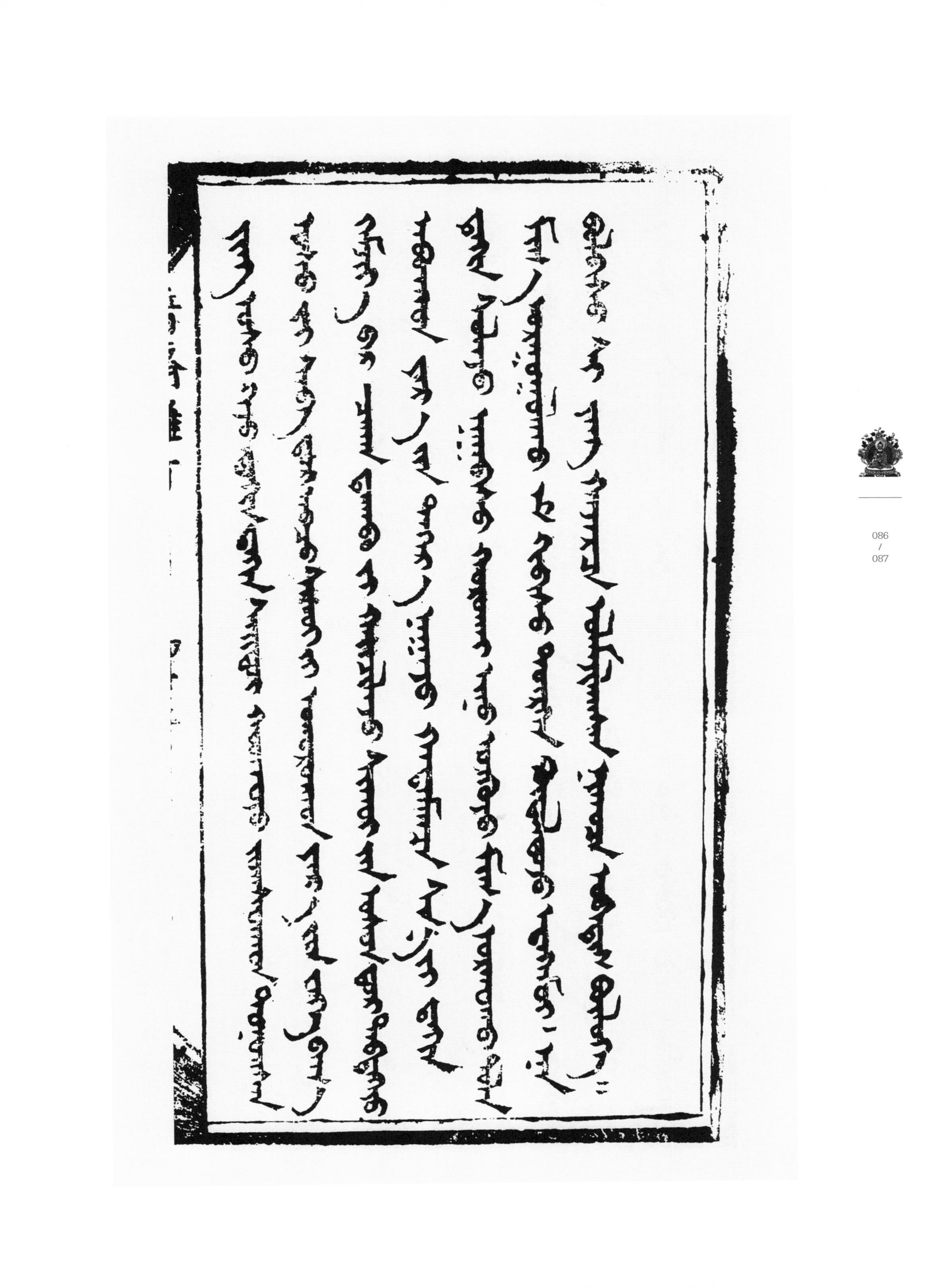

[illegible]

◎ [illegible]

[illegible]

[illegible]

[illegible] ◎ [illegible]

[illegible]

[illegible]

[illegible]

[illegible]

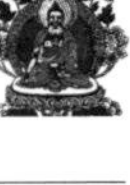

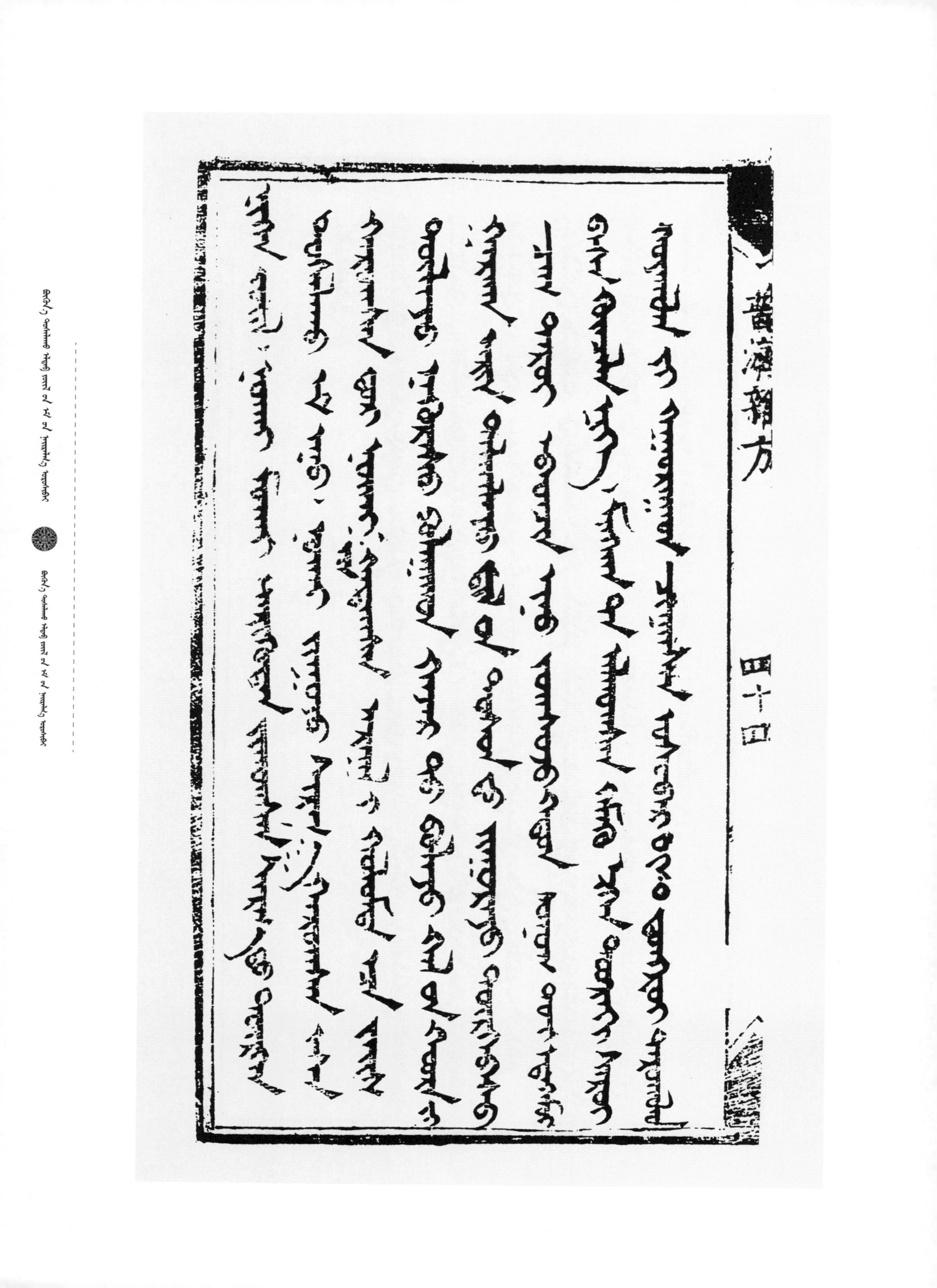

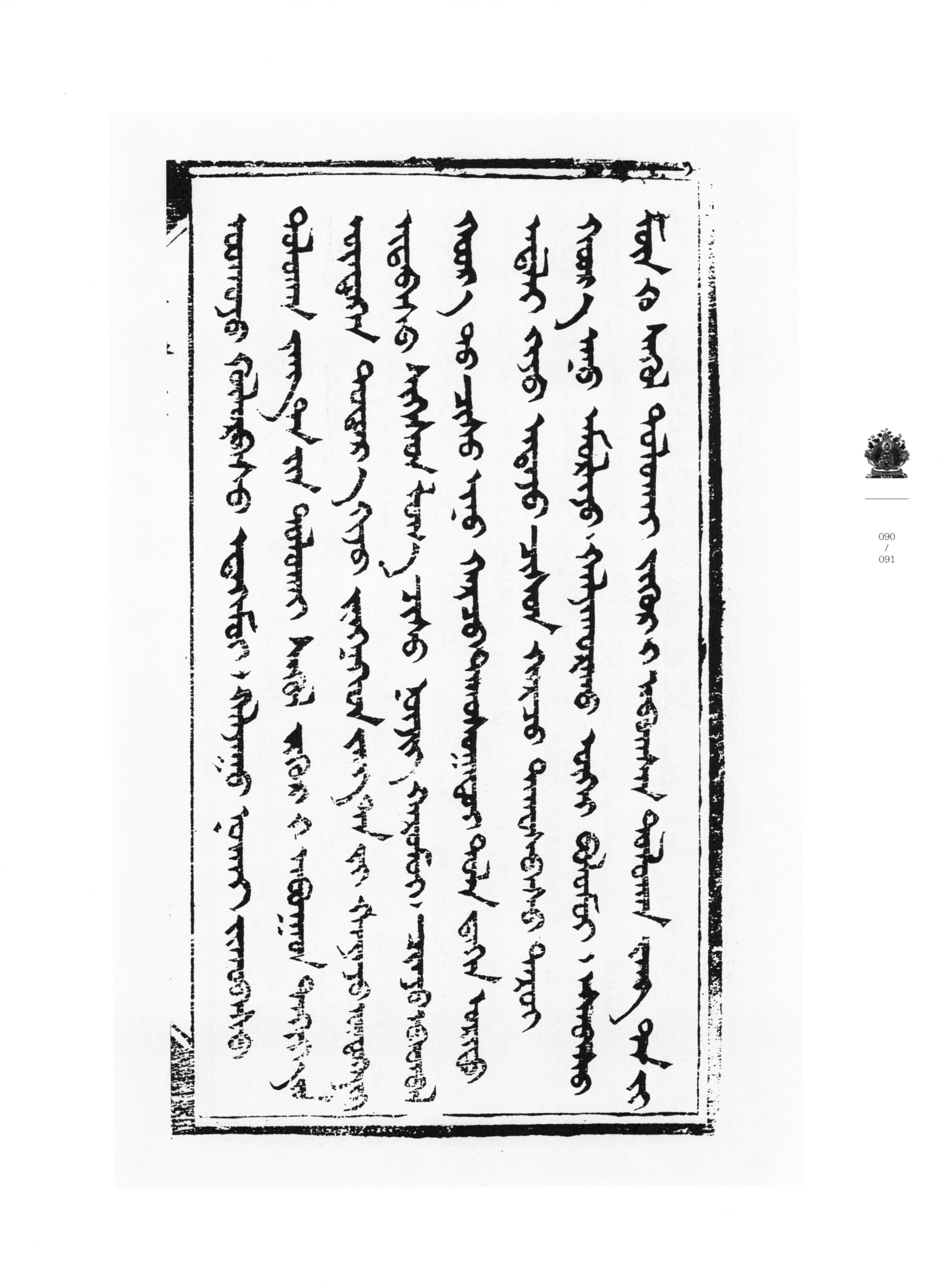

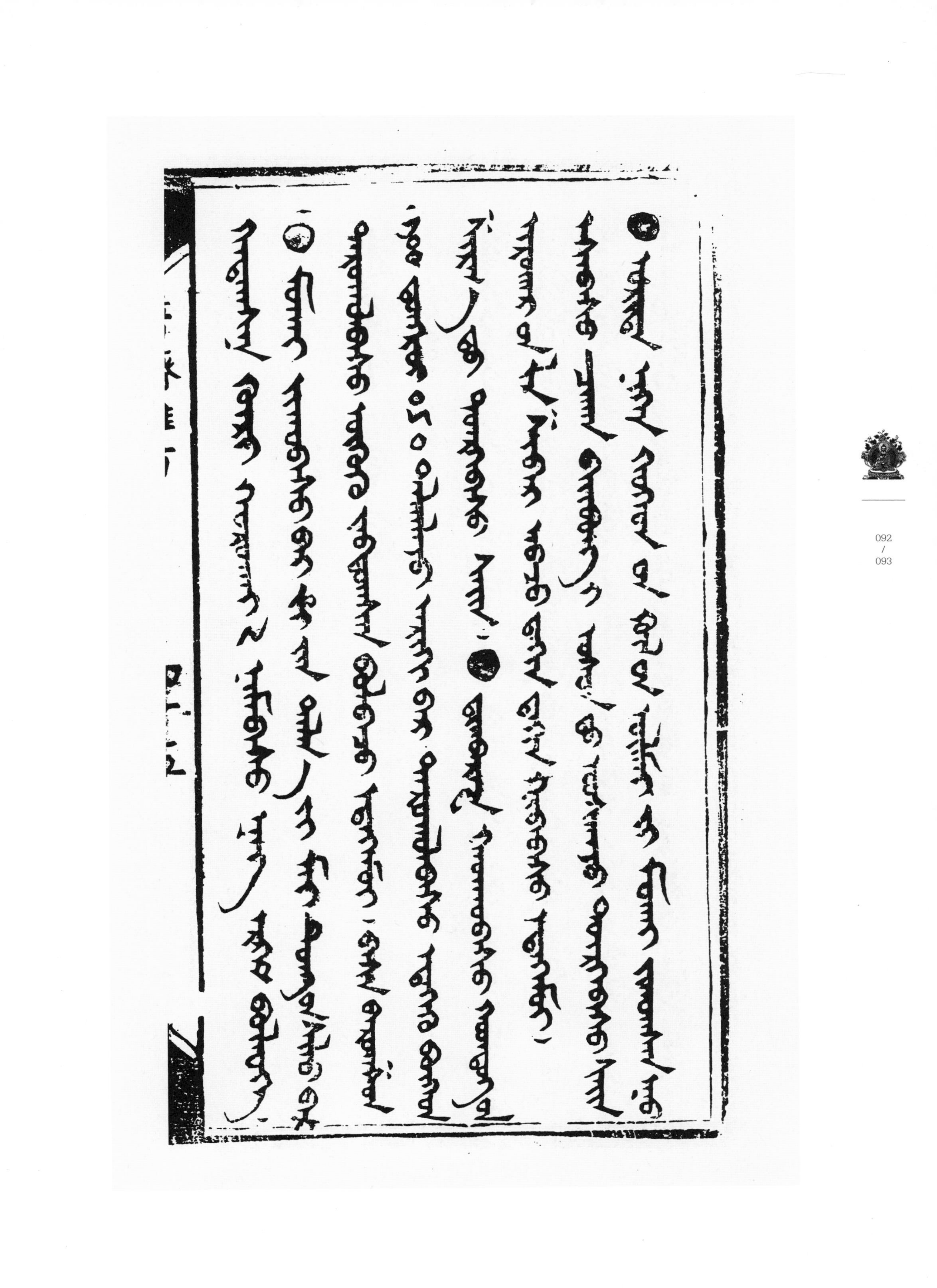

[illegible] ::

[illegible]

[illegible]

[illegible]

[illegible]

[illegible]

[illegible]

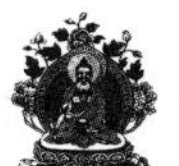

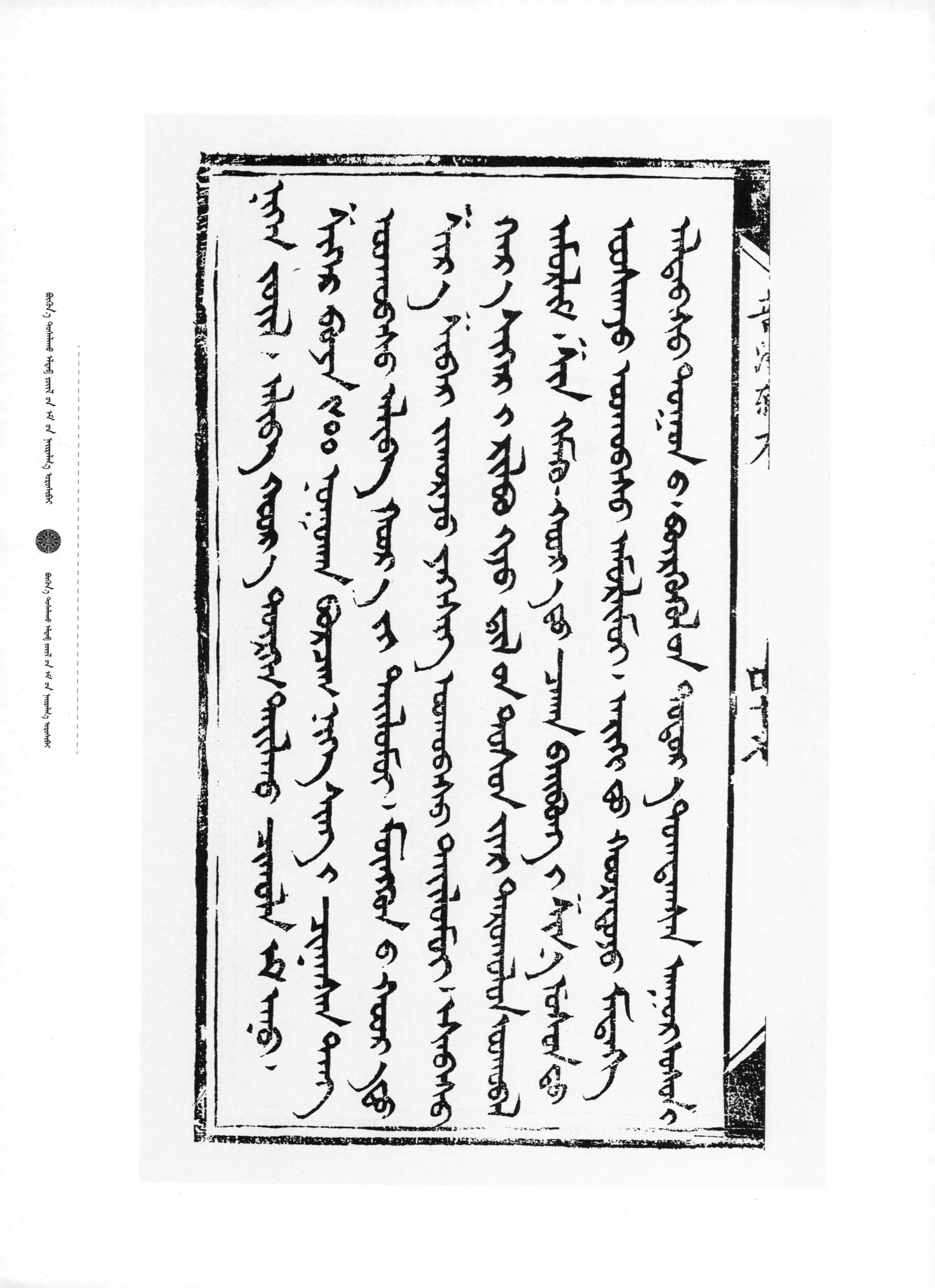

[illegible]

[illegible]

[illegible]

[illegible]

[illegible]

[illegible]

[illegible]

[illegible]

[illegible]

[illegible]

[illegible]

[illegible]

[illegible]

[illegible]

[illegible]

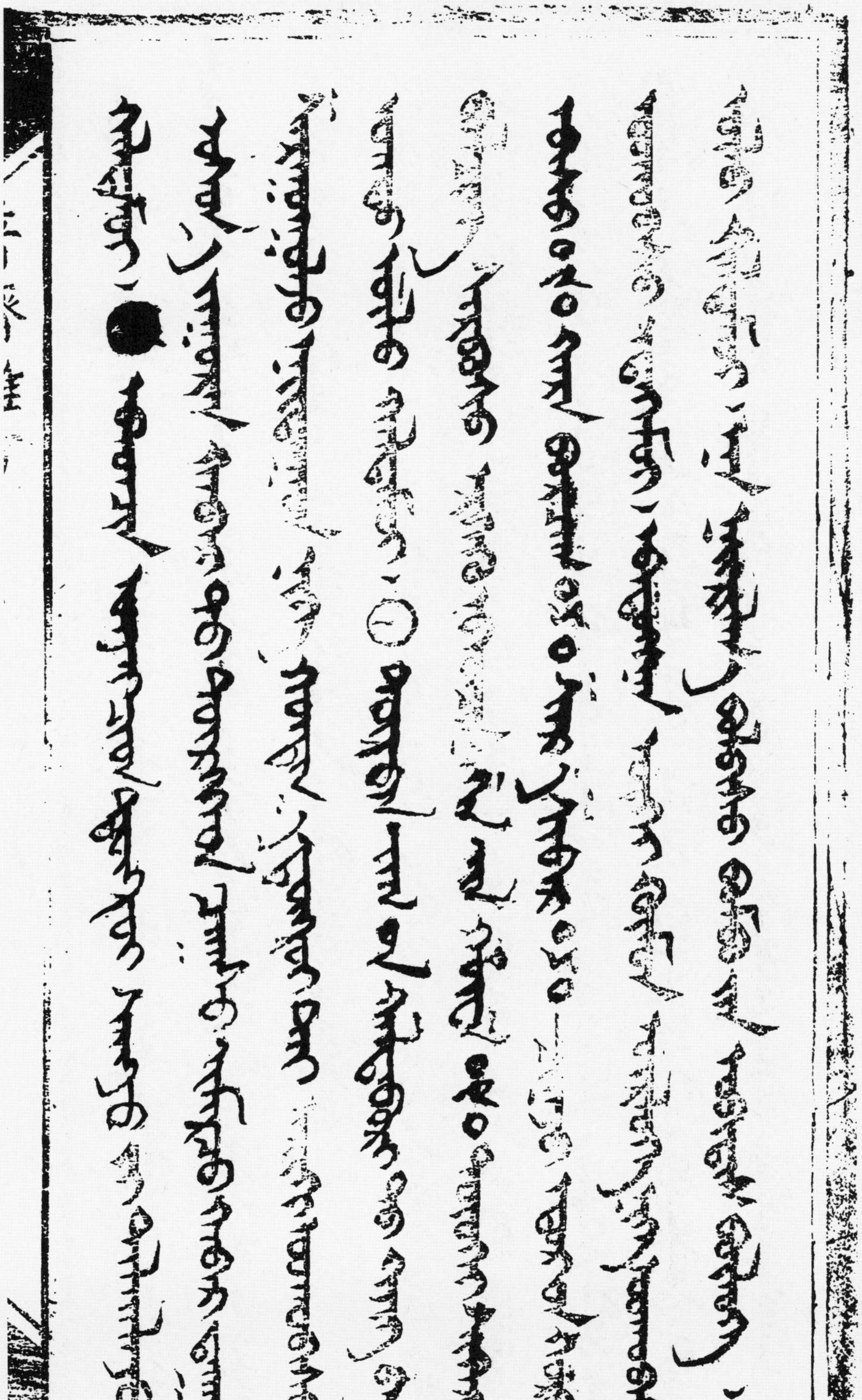

[illegible]

[illegible]

[illegible]

[illegible]

[illegible]

[illegible]

[illegible]

[illegible]

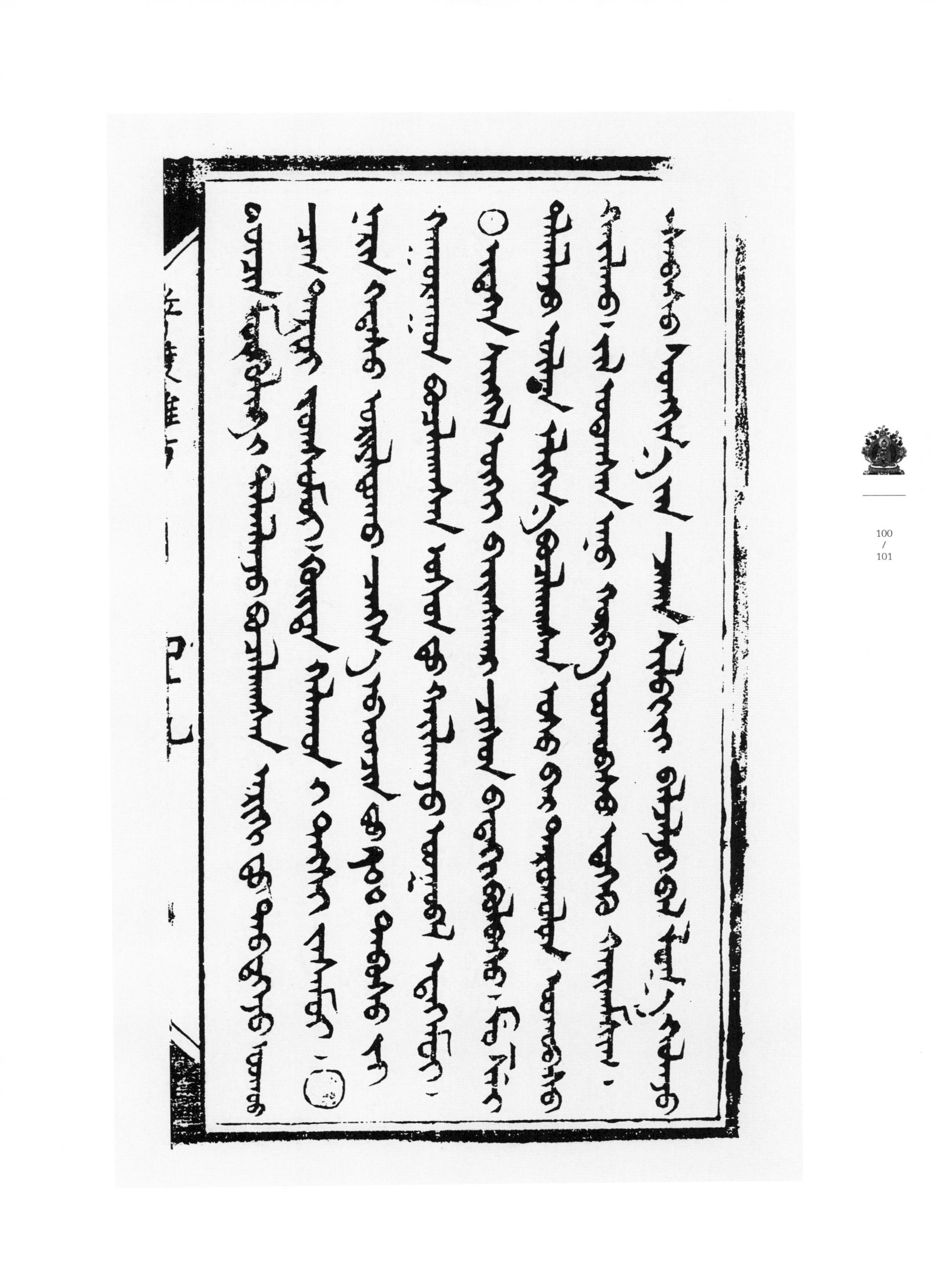

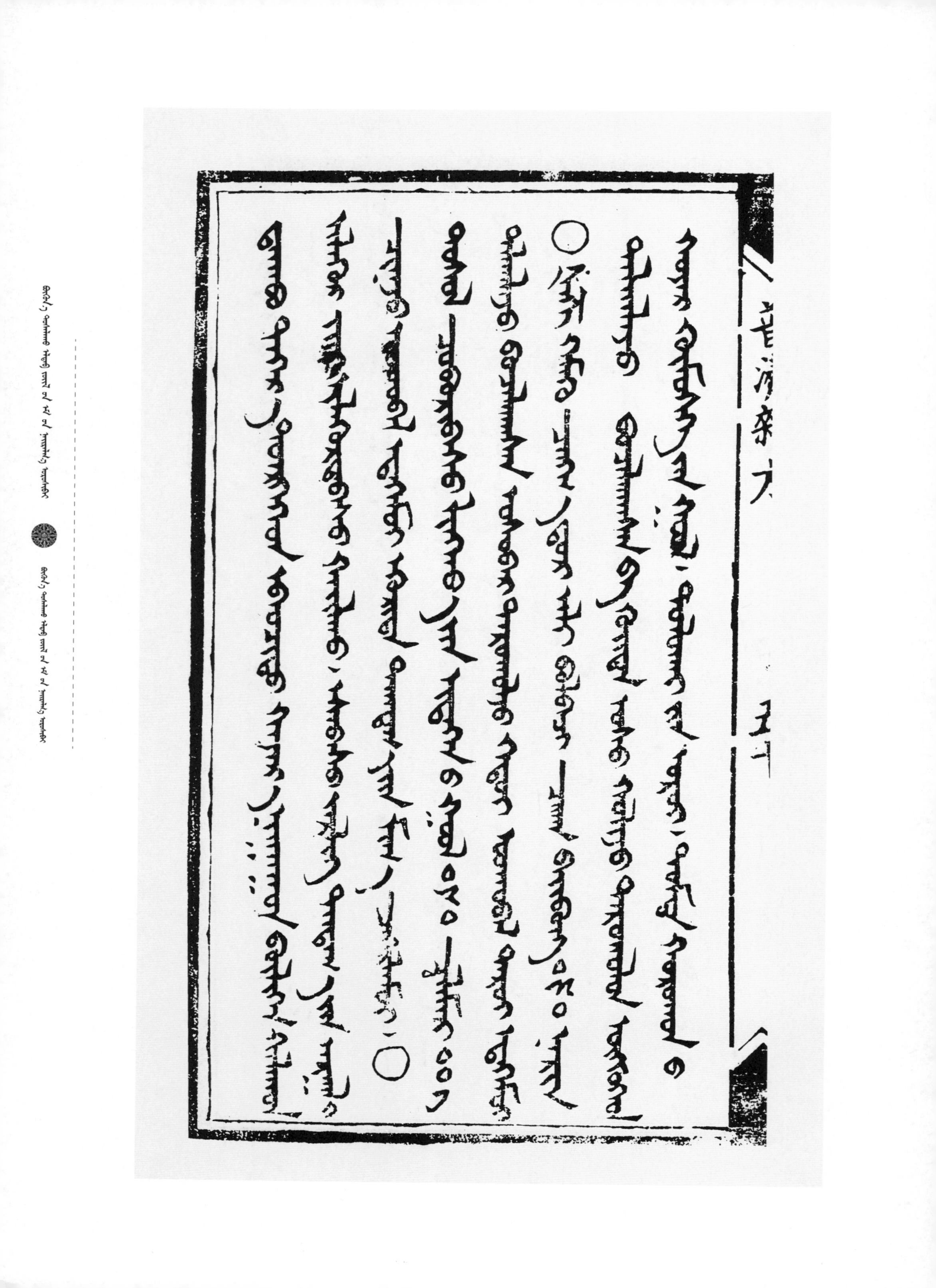

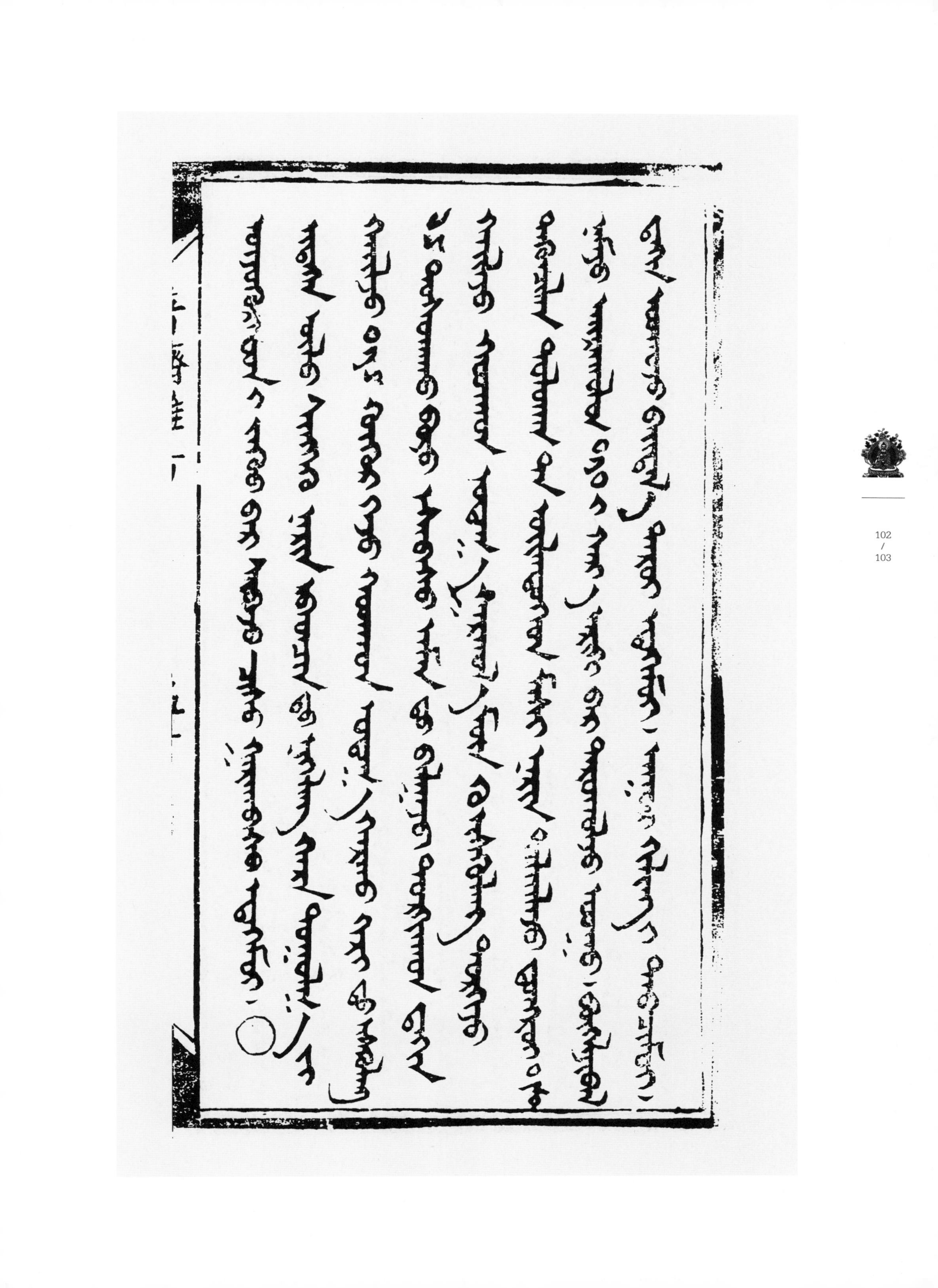

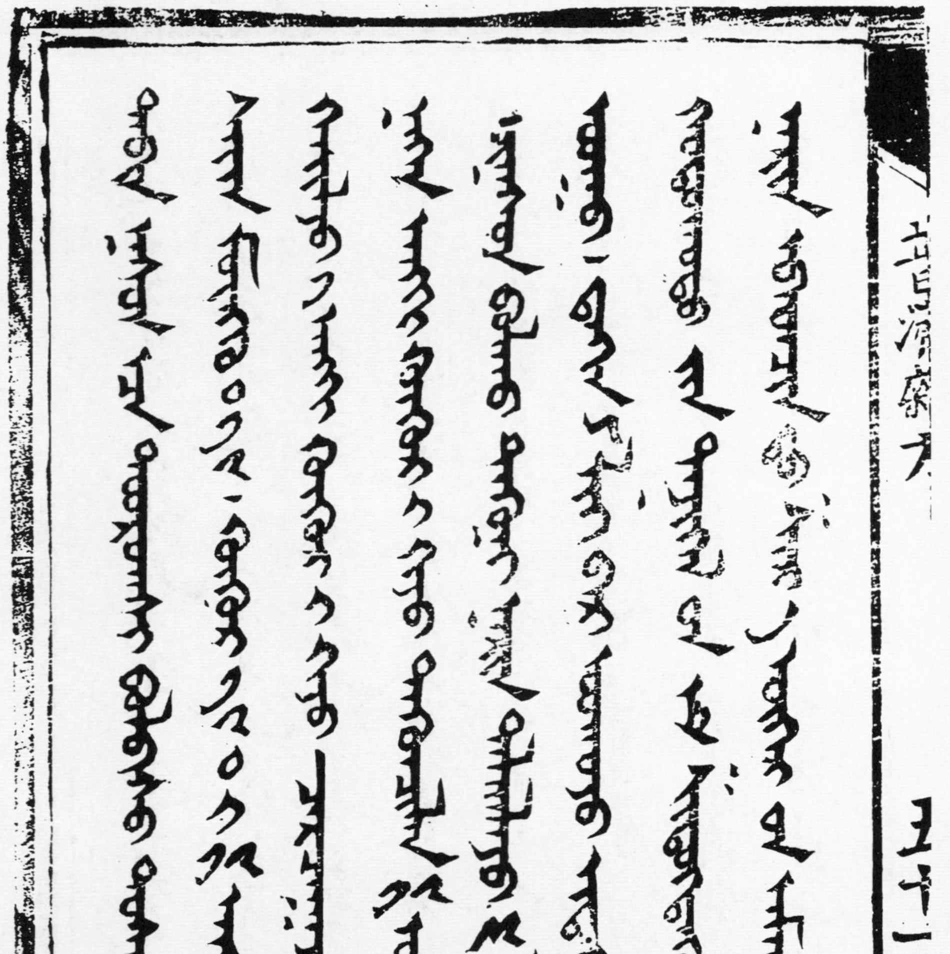

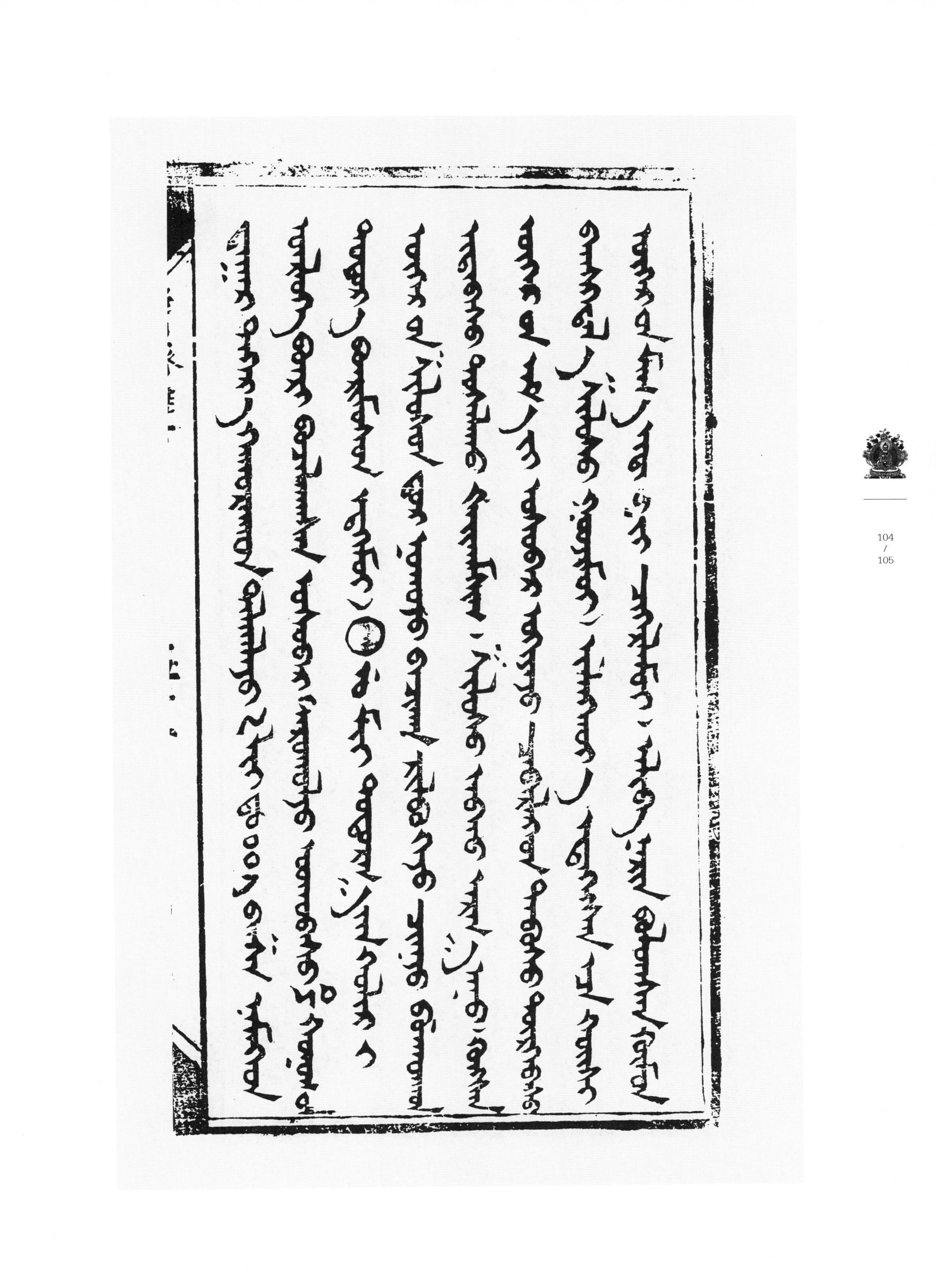

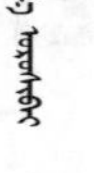

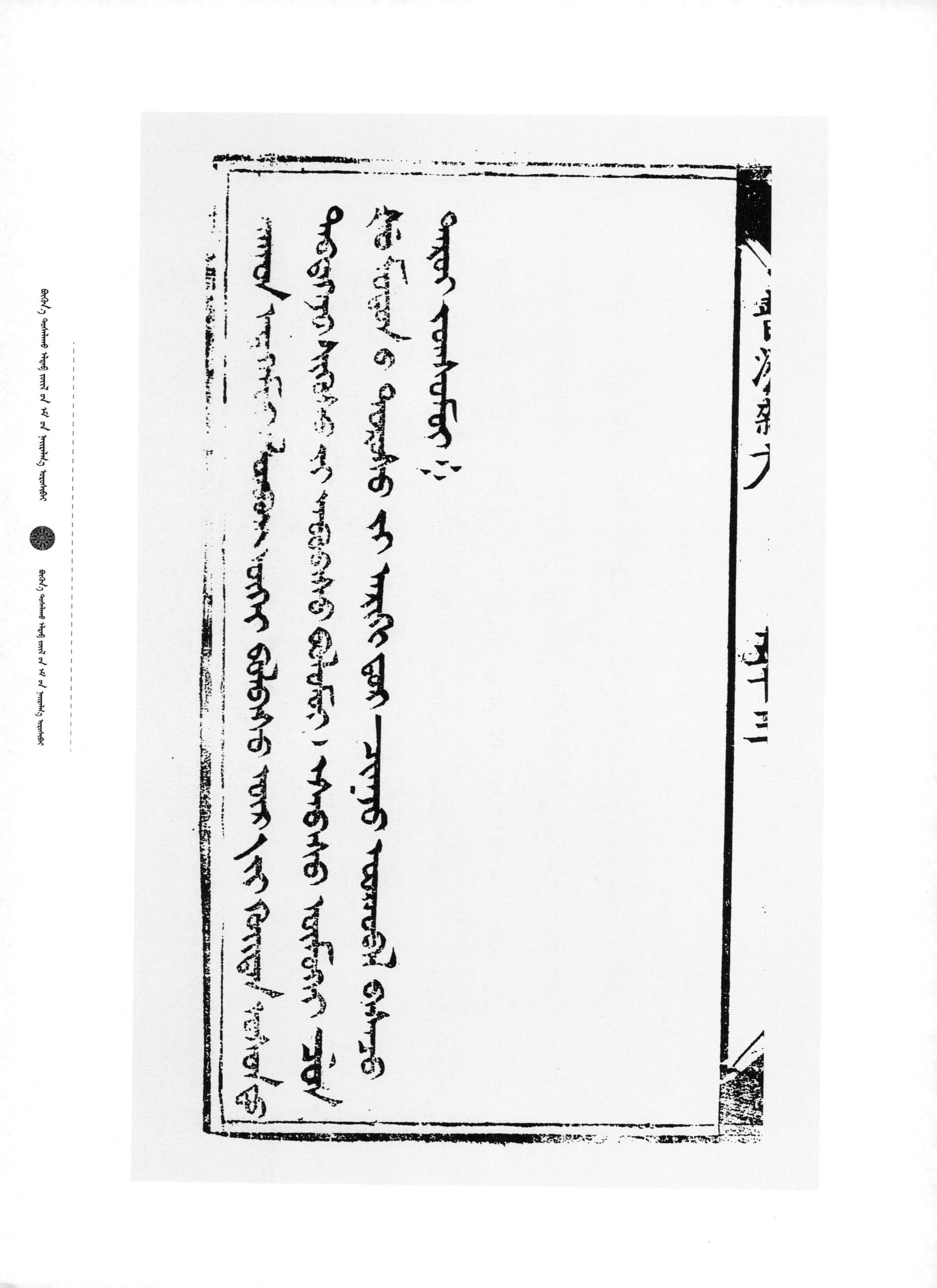

[illegible]

[illegible]

[illegible]

[illegible]

[illegible]

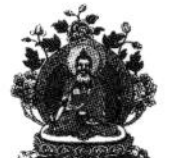

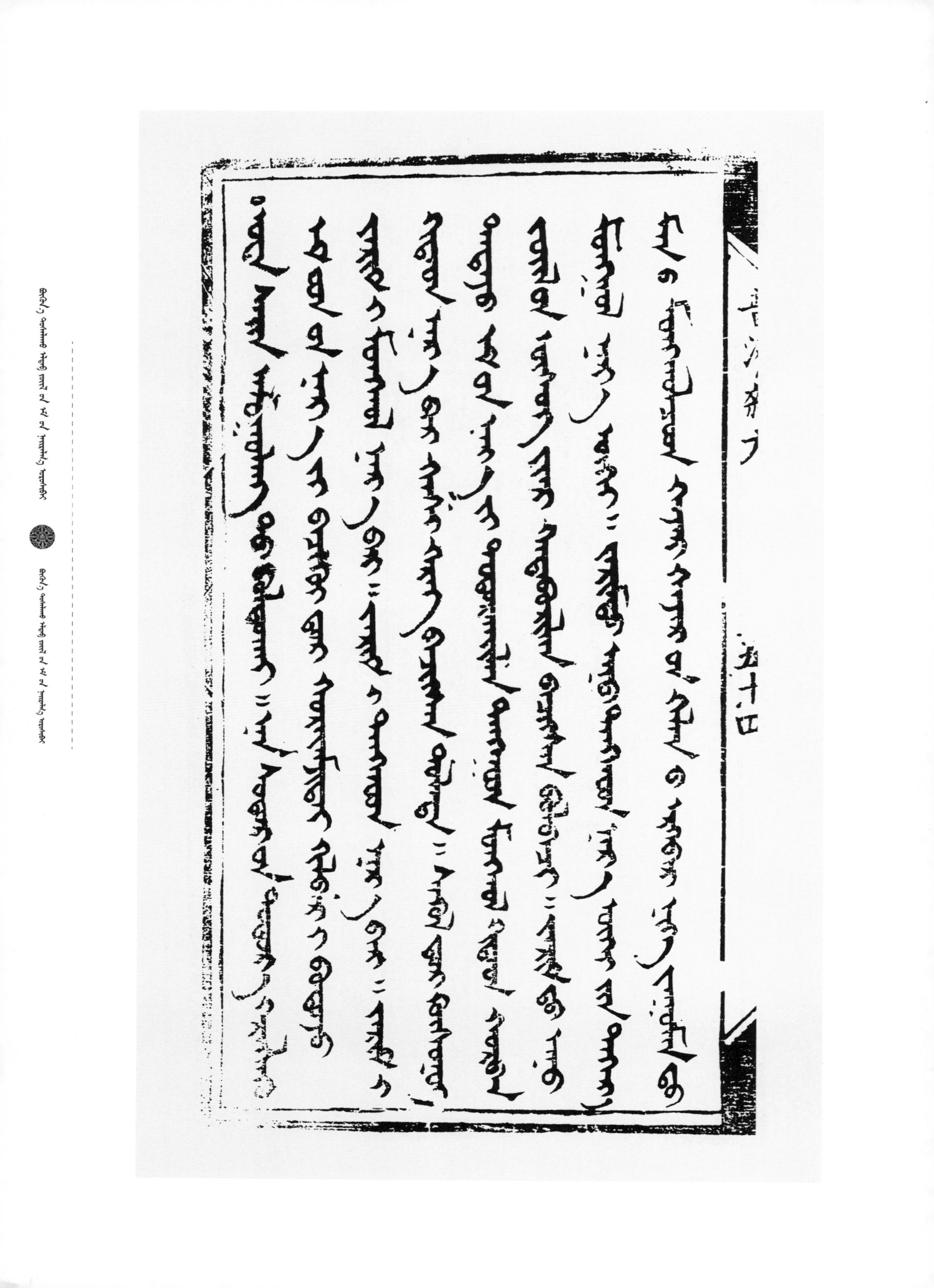

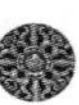

皂礬	輕粉	珍珠
紅礬	硼砂	硃砂
石灰	白礬	辛紅銀硃

滑石	硇砂	冰片
滋石	火硝	朝腦
膽礬	雄黃	青塩

鉛粉	紅銅	龍骨
黃丹	鉛	石燕子
中乳石	蚌	銀

没藥	水銀	牙硝
乳香	官粉	硫黄
蜂房		寒水石

百草霜

ཐང་ཤིང་
松香

麥門冬

ཨུཏྤལ
菊花

ཇ་དར།
兒茶

རྒྱ་མཚོའི་ལྦུ་བ།
海票硝

ལུག་མིག
菊花

血竭

虎

蓮子	燈草	大黃
薄荷	苦參	黃連
當歸	菖蒲	甘草

པའི་ཏི། 白芷	མཛོ་སྨྲེས། 蘼木	ཉུངས་མ། 蔓菁
ཁྲུ་ཡན་ཤྲུང་། 川芎	སེར་ཙན་ནག་པོ 細辛	ལ་ཕྱར་ 相附
ཏི་ཀུ་པི། 地骨皮	ཚོལ་ལེར་ཤིང་ 槐樹	སྐྱེར་ཤུན། 黄栢皮

白术	土茯苓	麻黄
蒼术	黄精	鬱金
兎絲草	支子 山查	番木鱉

藏文	汉文
ཐང་ཤིང་།	松樹
[illegible]	桑樹
[illegible]	杉木
ཨ་ག་རུ།	沉香
[illegible]	商陸
[illegible]	桔梗
ཤིང་ཚ།	肉桂
[illegible]	槐樹
ལྕང་མ།	柳樹

五倍子	人參	蕉葉
木賊。錯草	半夏	栢楊
山藥	金銀花	當參丹參

穚麦	桃子	核桃
小米 谷米	梨	杏子
黄米	西瓜	棗子 △

烏梅	黑糖 老糖	白果
胡蔴	柿子	白糖 洋糖
芝蔴	白果	氷糖

紅豆	黑豆	益母草
生姜	黃豆	蒺藜
姜片子	綠豆	沙苑蒺藜

丁香	大回香	乾姜
肉桂	胡椒	良姜
草果	花椒	小回香

海槿皮	ཛཱ་ཏི 肉荳蔻	པི་པི་ལིང 蓽撥
མ་ནུ 青木香	གོ་ཡུ 梹榔	ཡུང་བ 姜黄
海桐皮	牙皂	སུག་སྨེལ 白荳蔻

ཙོང་། 葱	སེ་འབྲུ། 石榴	བའི་ཡོ་ཇུ་ག། 百藥煎
ལ་ཕུག 白蘿卜	ཕུ་གུང་ཡིང 蒲公陰	སྨན་ཆས། 草烏
ཨ་ཙི་ཀོ 茄子	པ་ཏོག 巴豆	ཡུ་ཀྱི་ཤིར 三七 山漆

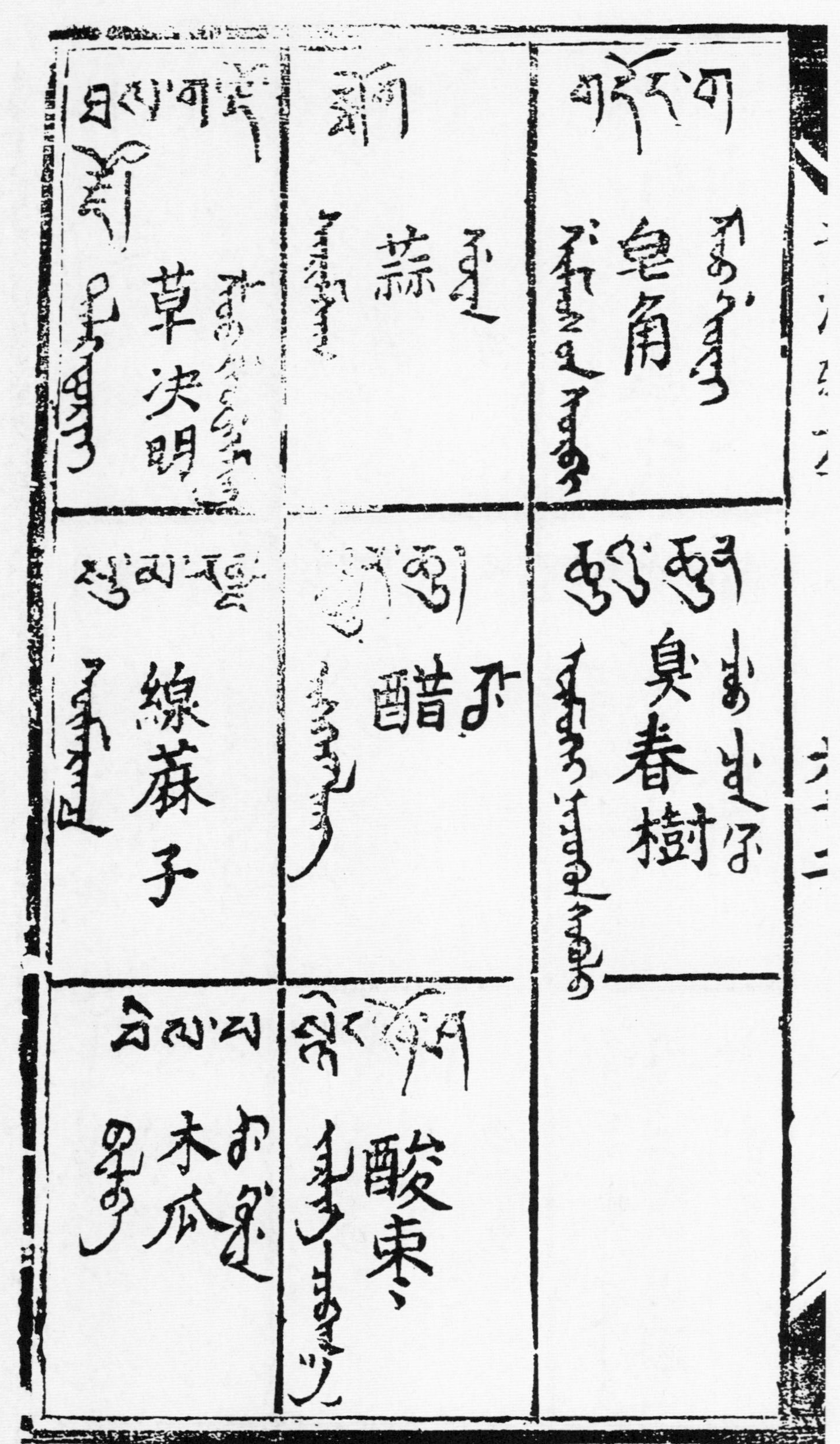
皂角
蒜
草决明
臭春樹
醋
線蔴子
酸棗
木瓜

兔	鴿糞	鷄
犀	牛	家雀
麝香	猪	胎髮

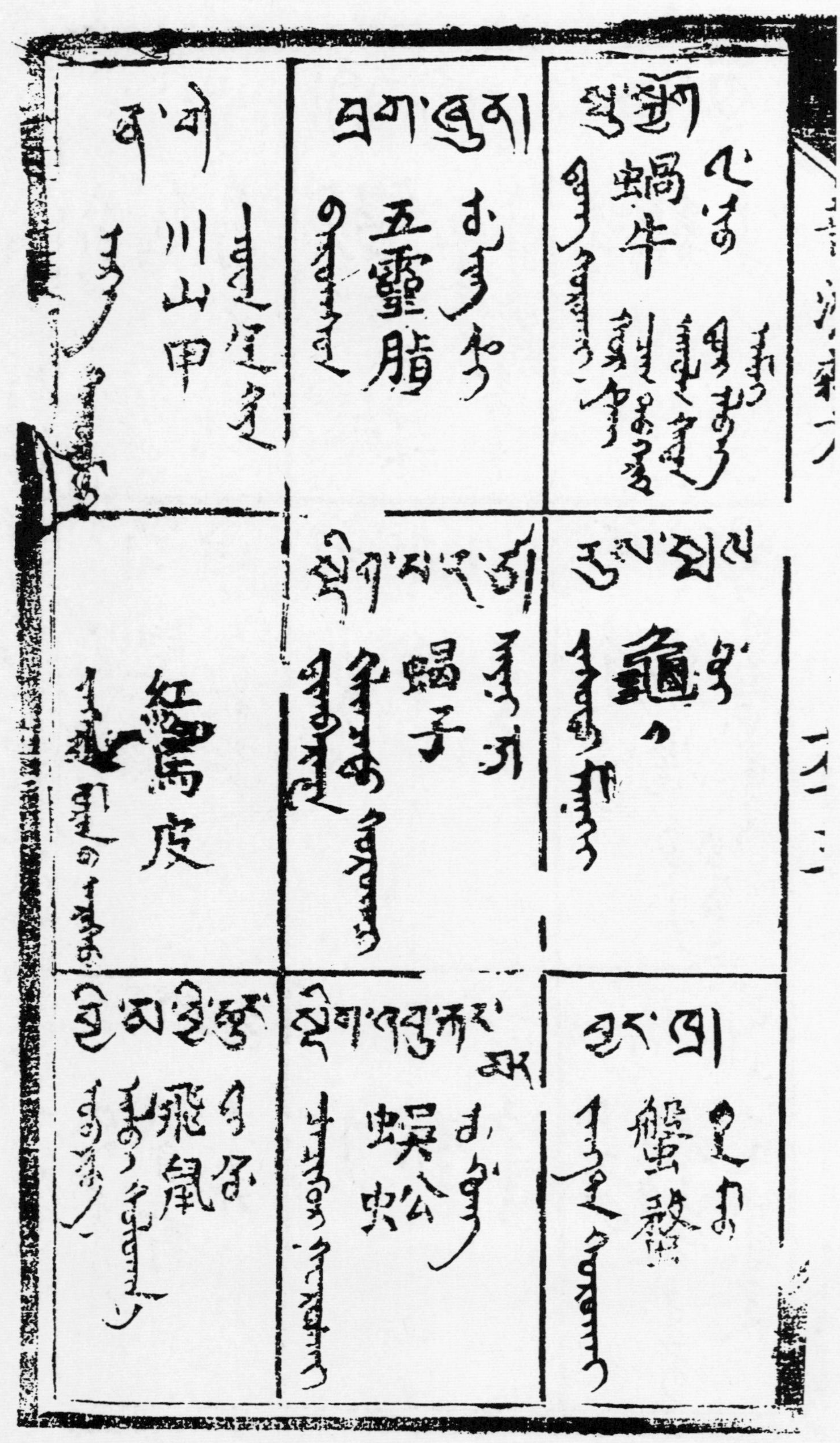

蝸牛

龜

蟹螯

五靈脂

蝎子

蜈蚣

川山甲

紅鶴皮

飛鼠

སྦྲུལ་ཤ། 蛇肉	སྡོམ། 蜘蛛	ངང་པ། 鵝
གླང་ཆེན། 象	ཏི་ཏི་ཡི་ཕྲུག 胡燕	བལ་སྦུར། 蜣螂
སྦྲང་བུ། 蜂	སྲམ། 獺	ཤང་ཤང་ཏེ། [illegible]

[illegible] 學集 二三

錢	兩	蜜
斤	分	
升	釐	

生	蒸	煮
熟	熬	揚
煎	滾	燒炙

[illegible]

[illegible] ᠄᠄

[illegible] ᠄᠄

[illegible] ᠄᠄

[illegible] ᠄᠄

[illegible] ᠄᠄

[illegible] ᠄᠄

[illegible] ᠄᠄

[illegible]

[illegible]

[illegible]

[illegible]

[illegible]

[illegible]

[illegible]

[illegible]

[illegible]

京都

大清同治十二年吉月日

御前行走阿拉善和碩親王襍下梅林章京高世格情因畧識漢字自各便方內擇取有驗

述治雜病藥方指要藩譯蒙古字語刊刻成本將板交給東西廟擺賣新

舊滿蒙漢書之蕭姓收存印本發賣為此謹告咸知矣

ᠨᠡᠶᠢᠲᠡᠯᠡᠭᠰᠡᠨ [illegible] ::

[illegible] ::

[illegible] ::

[illegible] ᠦᠨᠡᠲᠦ ᠪᠠᠷᠢᠮᠲᠠ [illegible]

ᠲᠤᠰ ᠳᠡᠪᠲᠡᠷ [illegible] :: [illegible] 《 [illegible] 》 [illegible]

[illegible] : 24cm×26.5cm [illegible], [illegible] 55 [illegible] ::

ᠲᠤᠰ ᠳᠡᠪᠲᠡᠷ [illegible] ᠦᠨᠡᠲᠦ ᠪᠠᠷᠢᠮᠲᠠ ᠪᠣᠯᠤᠨ᠎ᠠ ::

Mongolian Manuscripts of Cure-all Prescriptions

蒙古文手抄本普济杂方

2

○ [illegible]

[illegible]

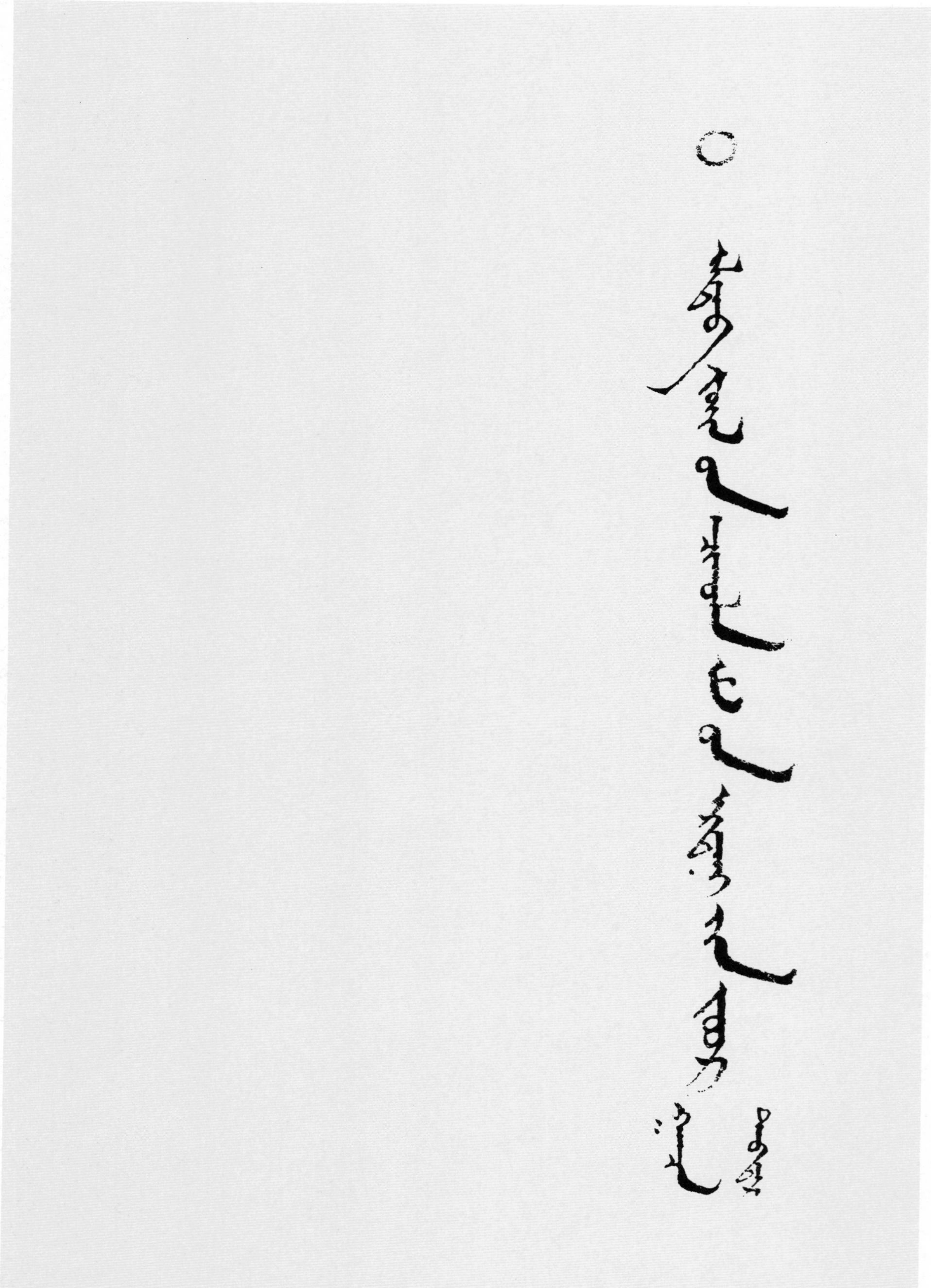

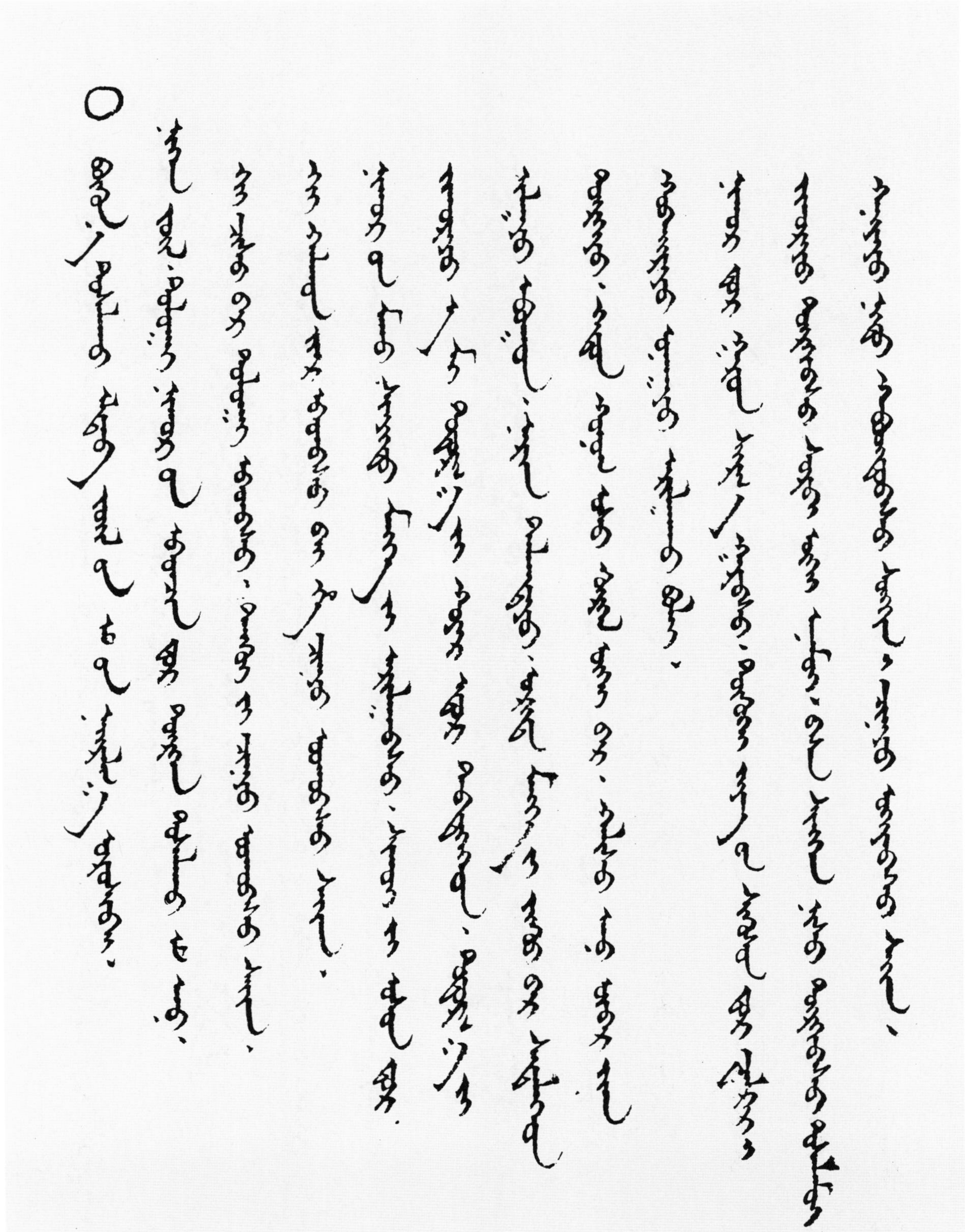

[illegible]
[illegible]
[illegible]
[illegible]
[illegible]
[illegible]
[illegible]
[illegible]
[illegible]
[illegible]
[illegible]
[illegible]

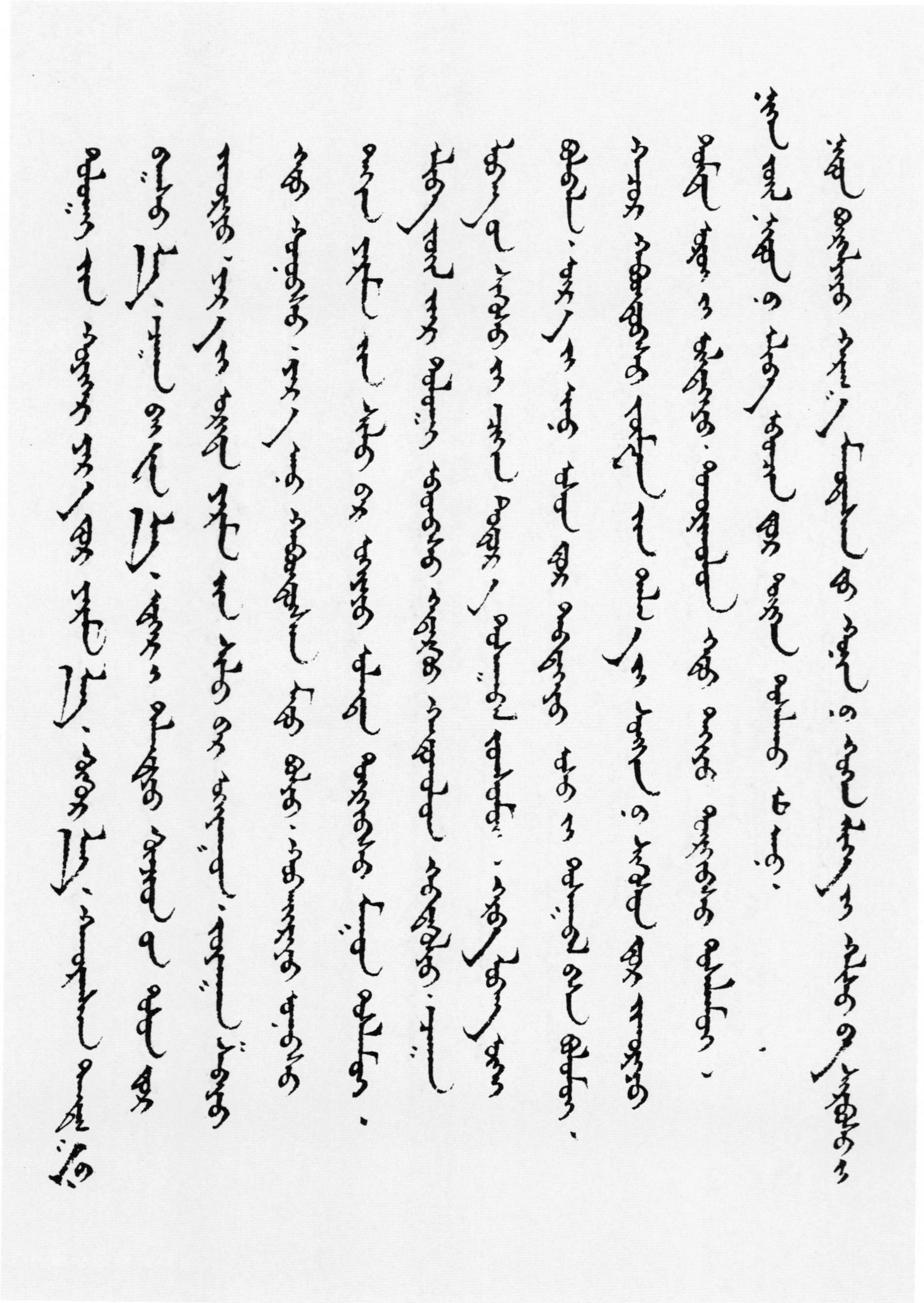

[illegible]
[illegible]
[illegible]
[illegible]

[illegible]
[illegible]
[illegible]
[illegible]

[illegible]
[illegible]
[illegible]

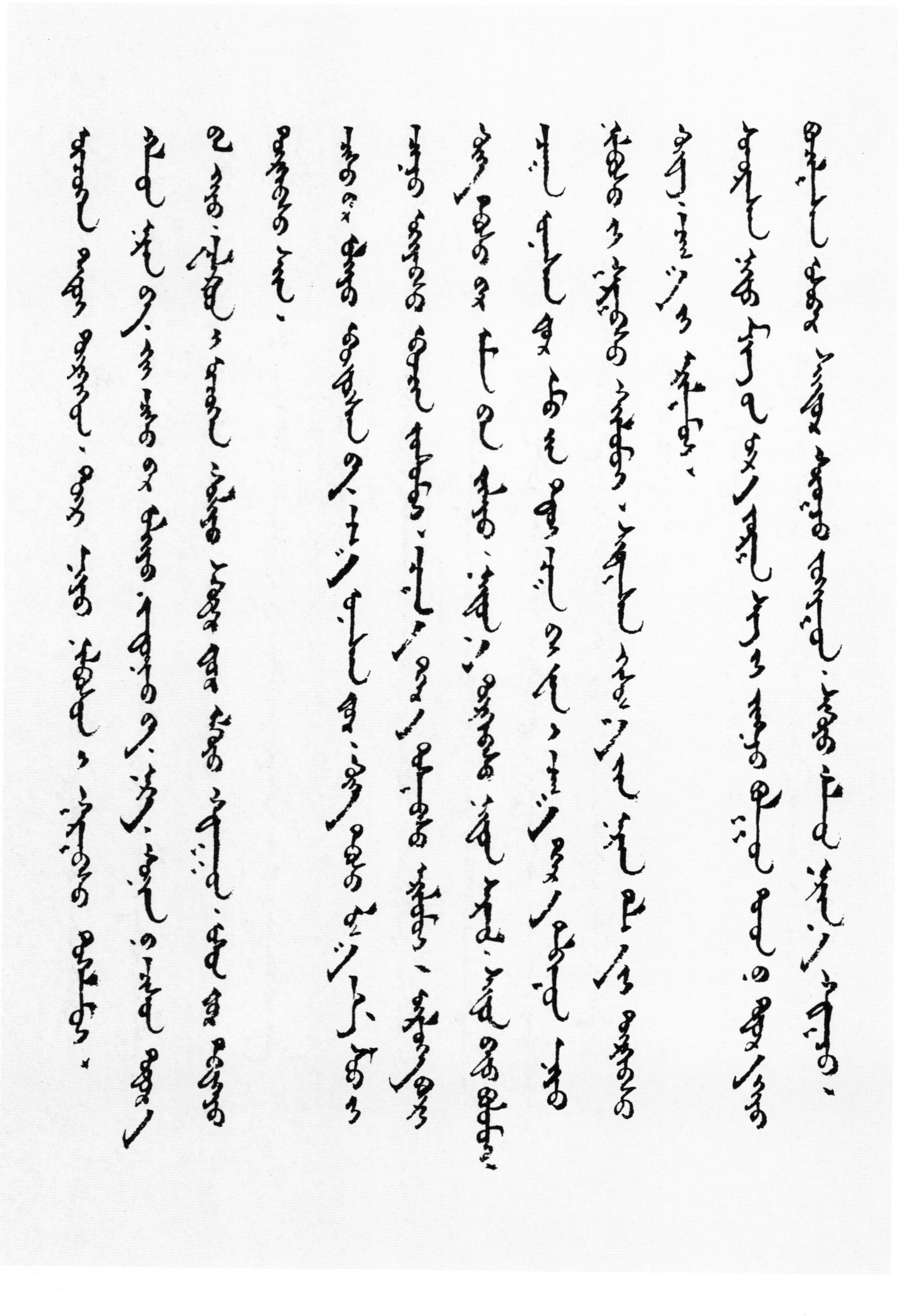

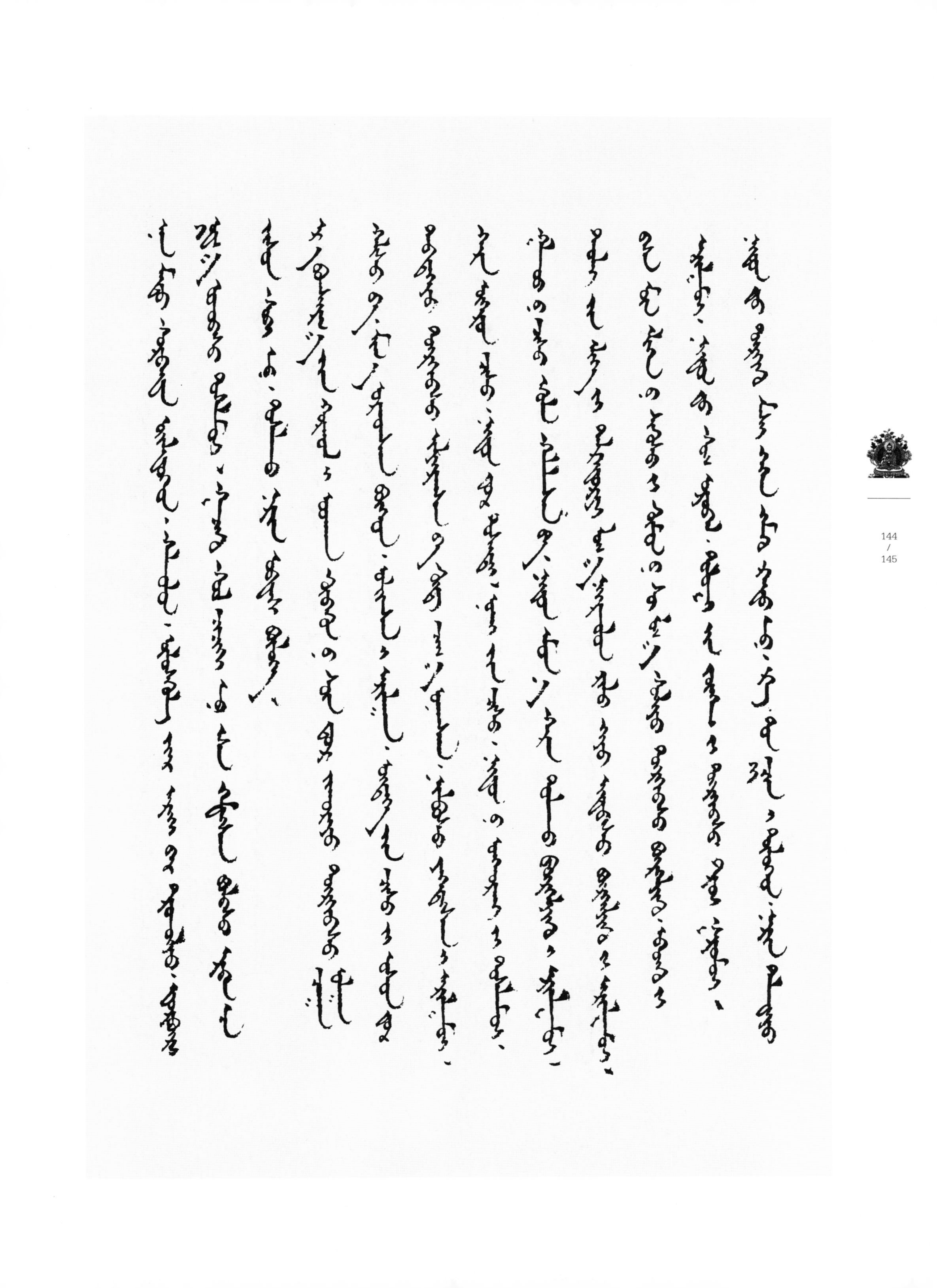

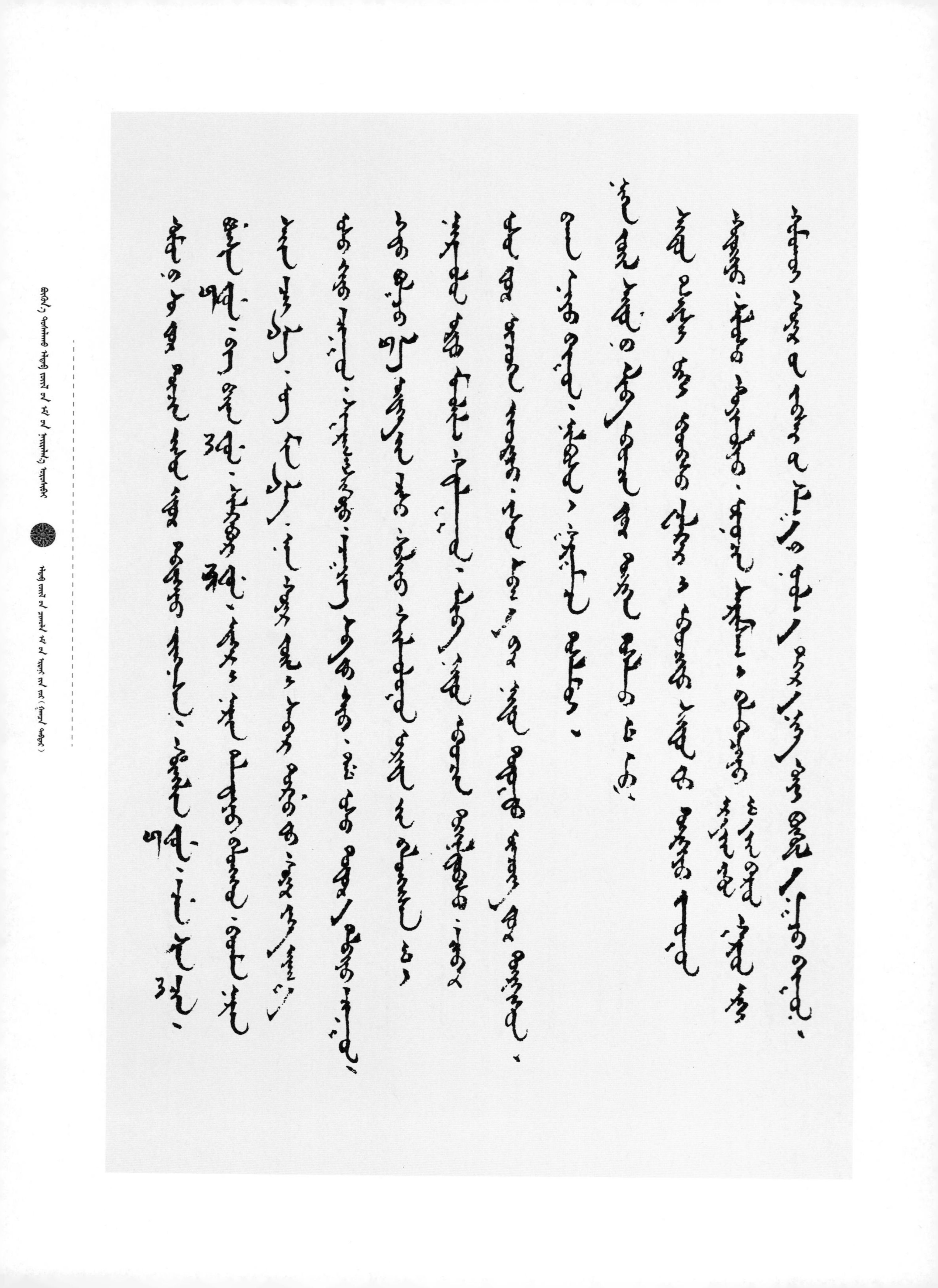

[illegible]

[illegible]

[illegible]

[illegible]

[illegible]

[illegible]

[illegible]

[illegible]

[illegible]

[illegible]

[illegible]

[illegible]

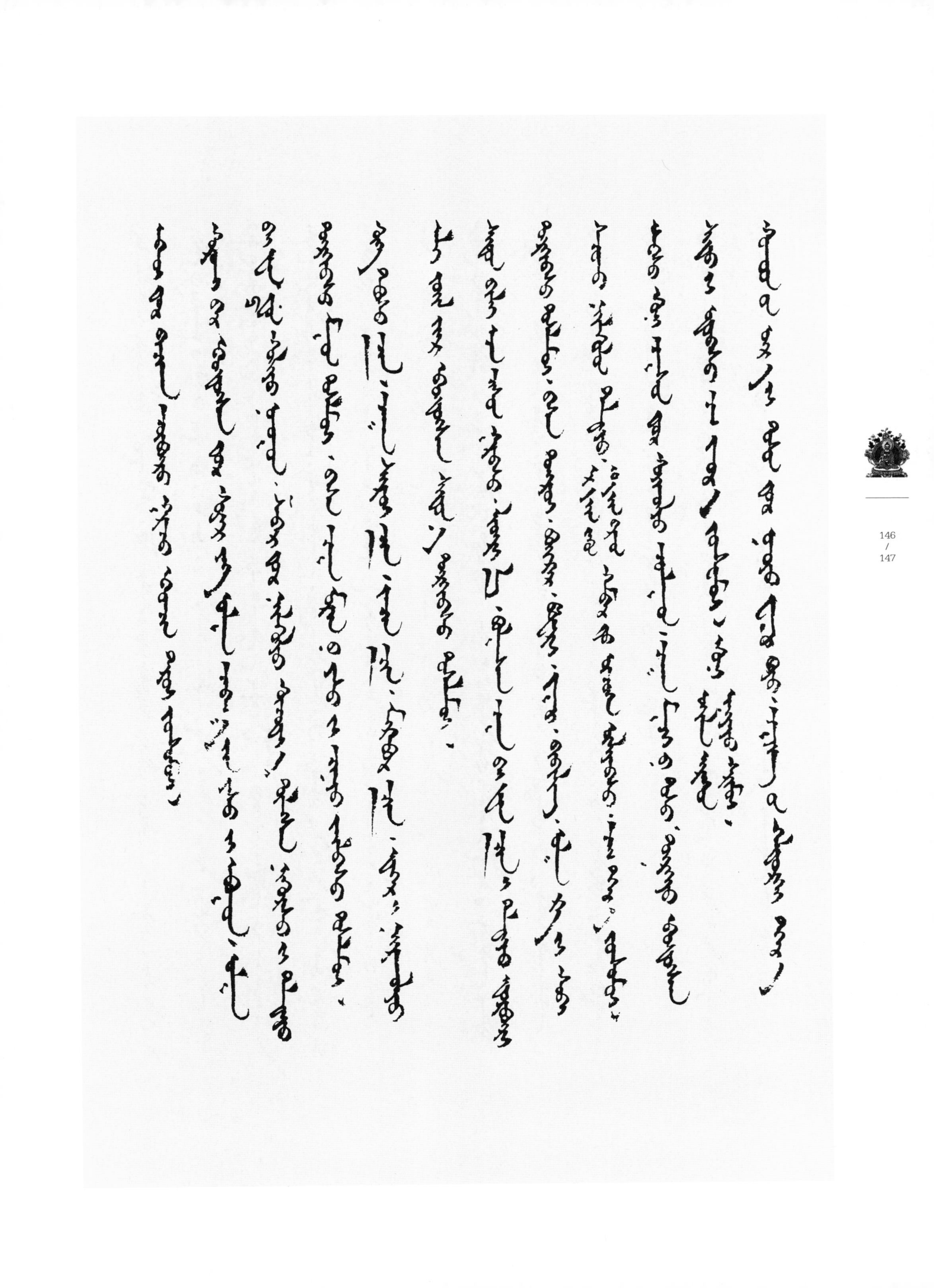

[illegible]

[illegible]

[illegible]

[illegible]

[illegible]

[illegible]

[illegible]

[illegible]

[illegible]

[illegible]

[illegible]

[illegible]

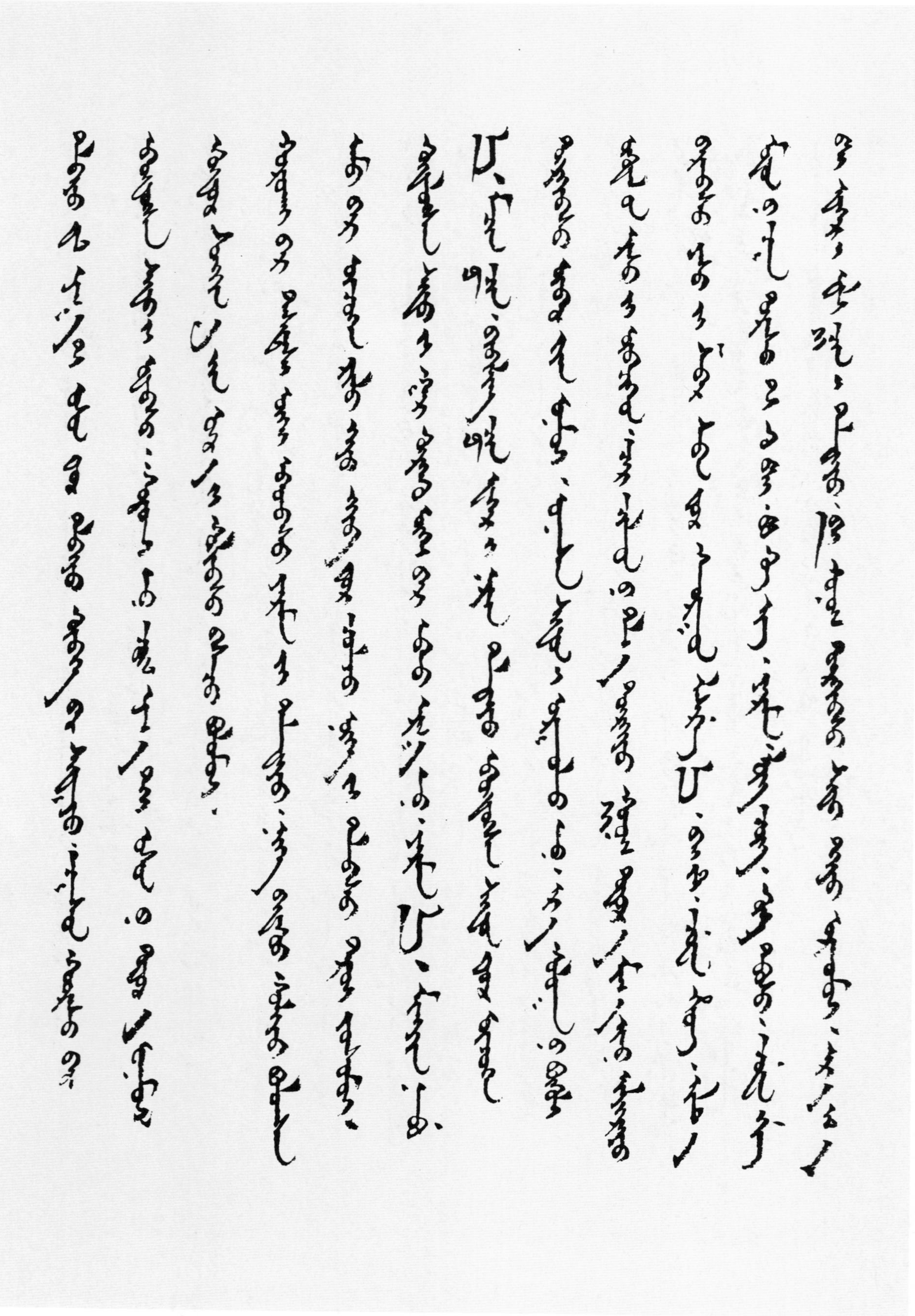

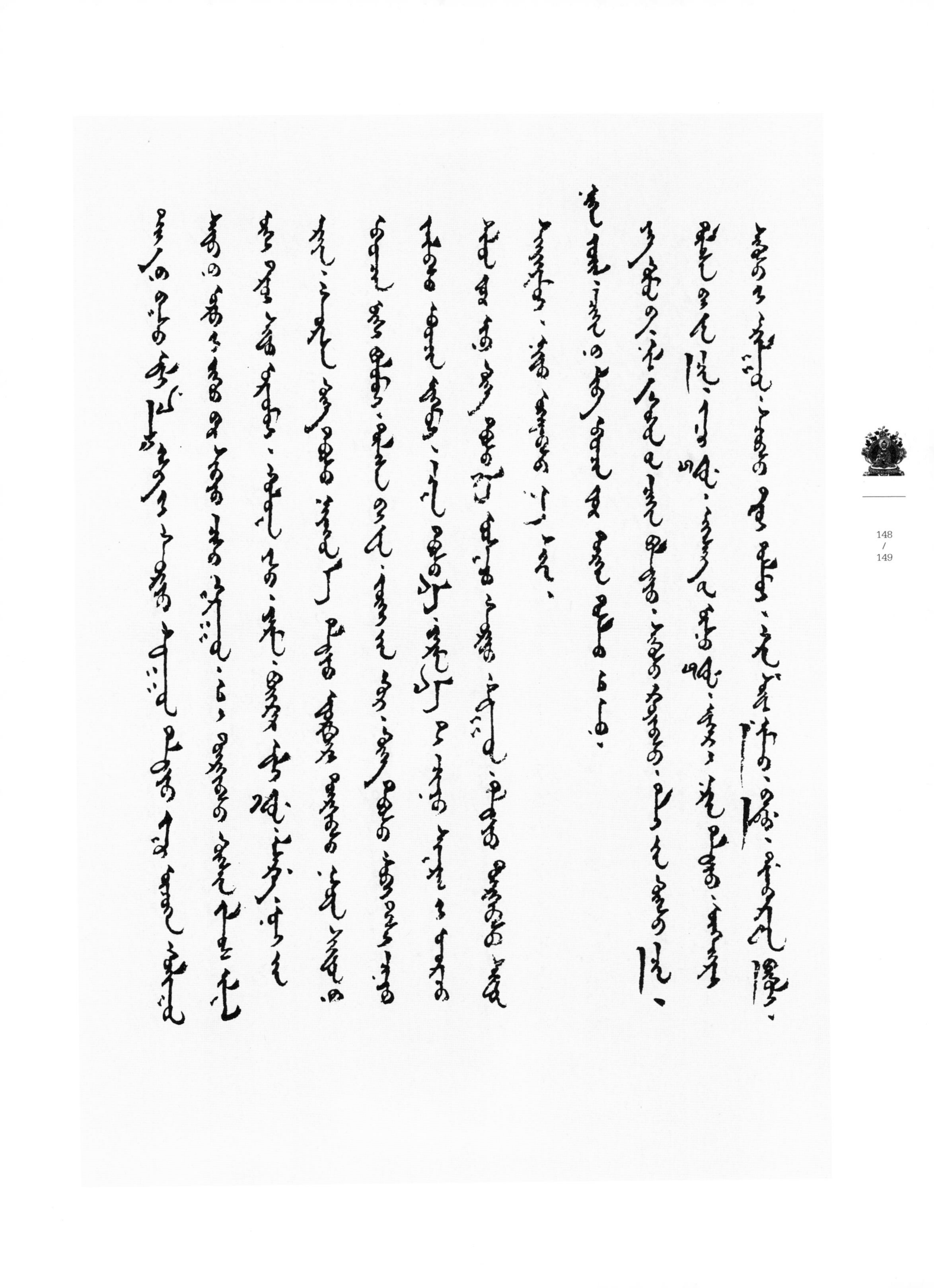

[illegible]
[illegible]
[illegible]
[illegible]
[illegible]
[illegible]
[illegible]
[illegible]
[illegible]
[illegible]
[illegible]
[illegible]
[illegible]

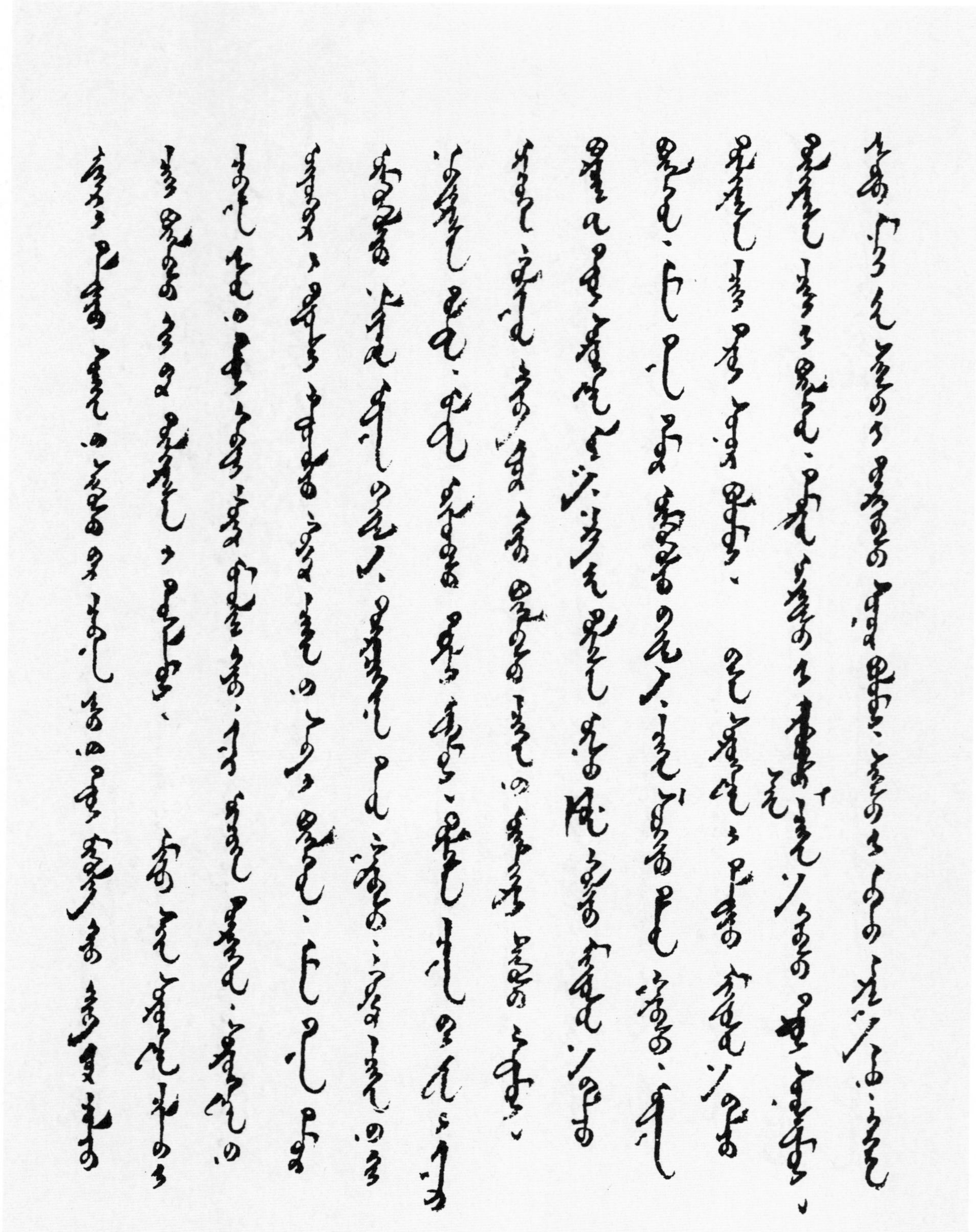

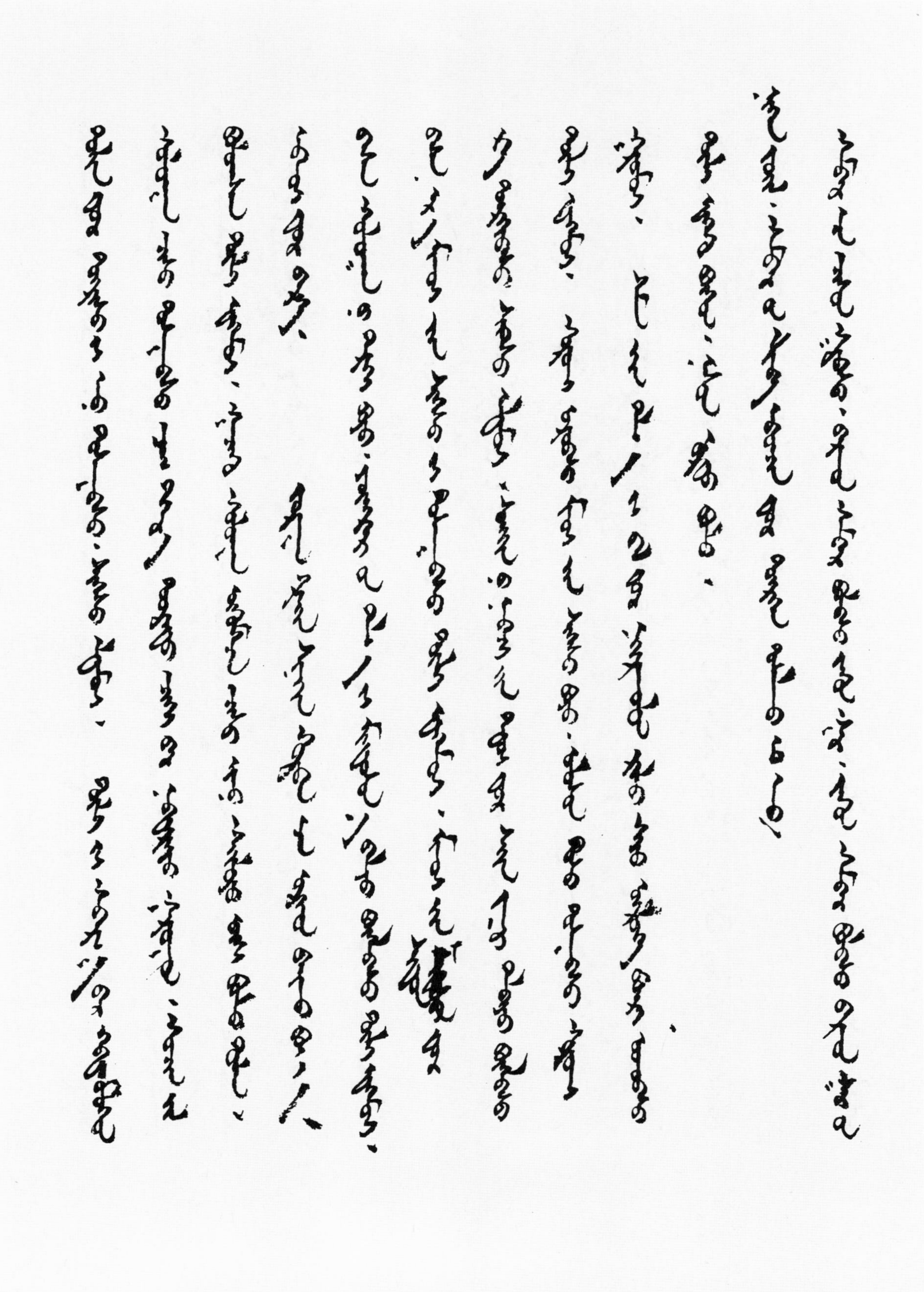

[illegible]

[illegible]

[illegible]

[illegible]

[illegible]

[illegible]

[illegible]

[illegible]

[illegible]

[illegible]

[illegible]

[illegible]

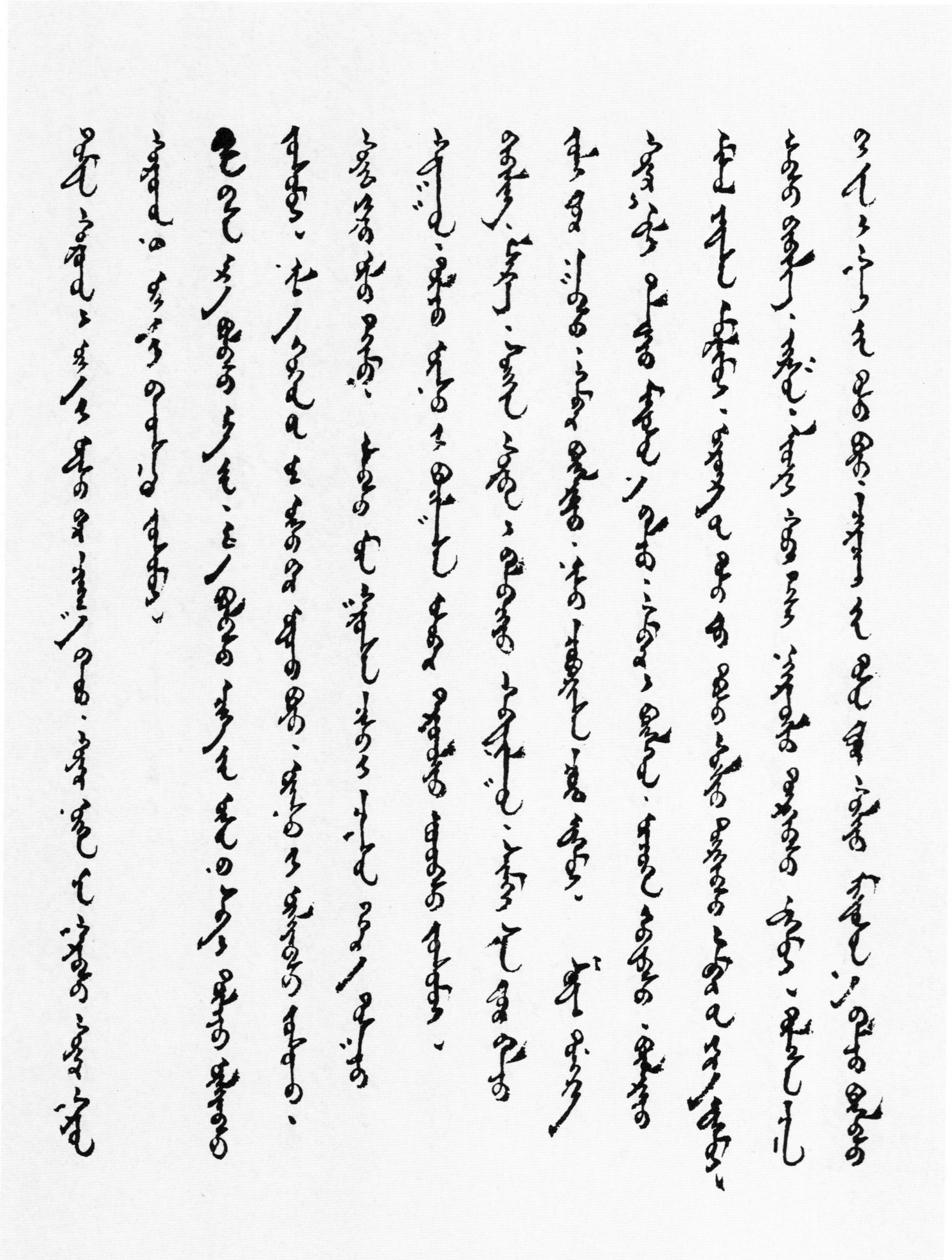

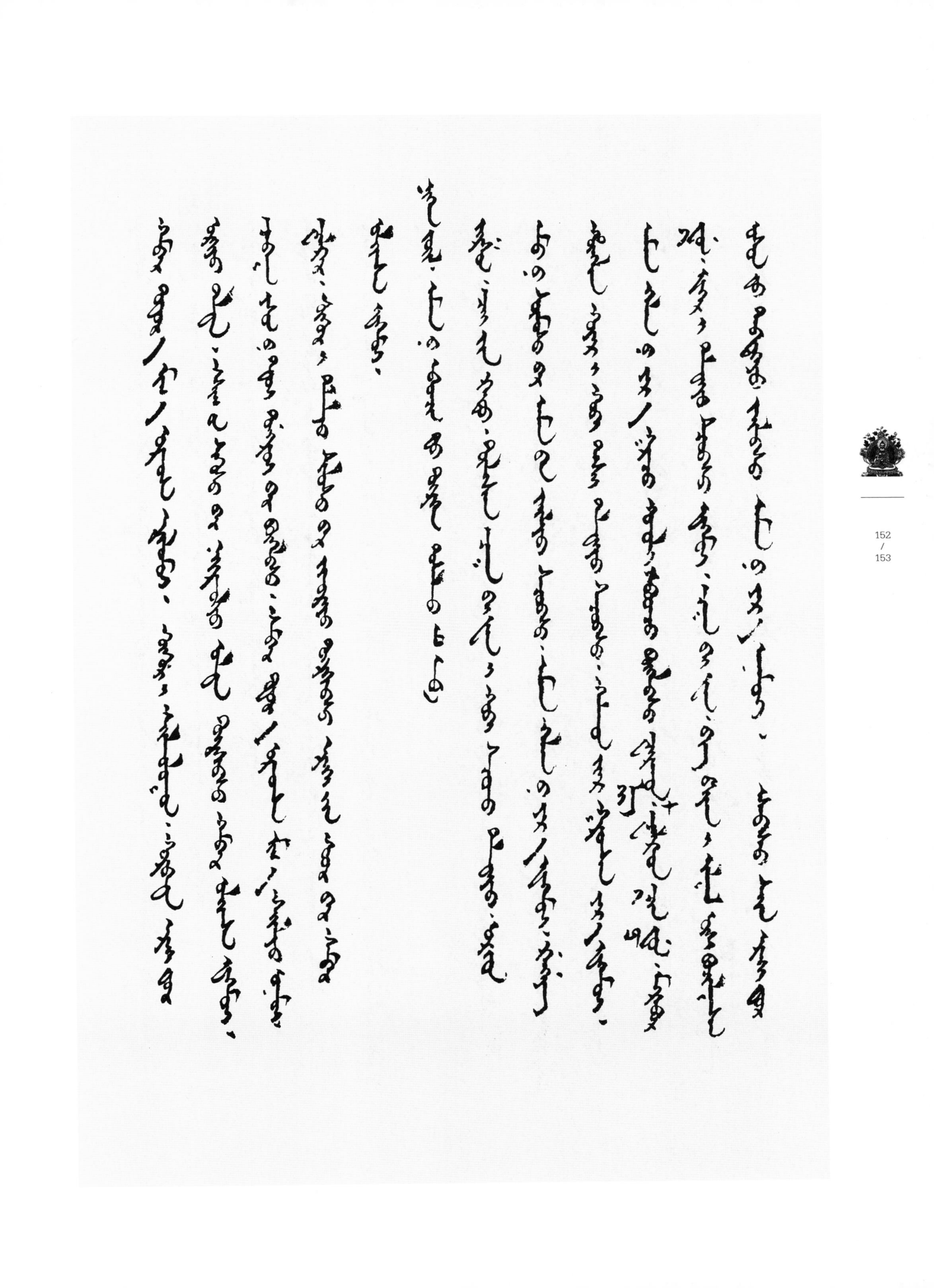

[illegible]

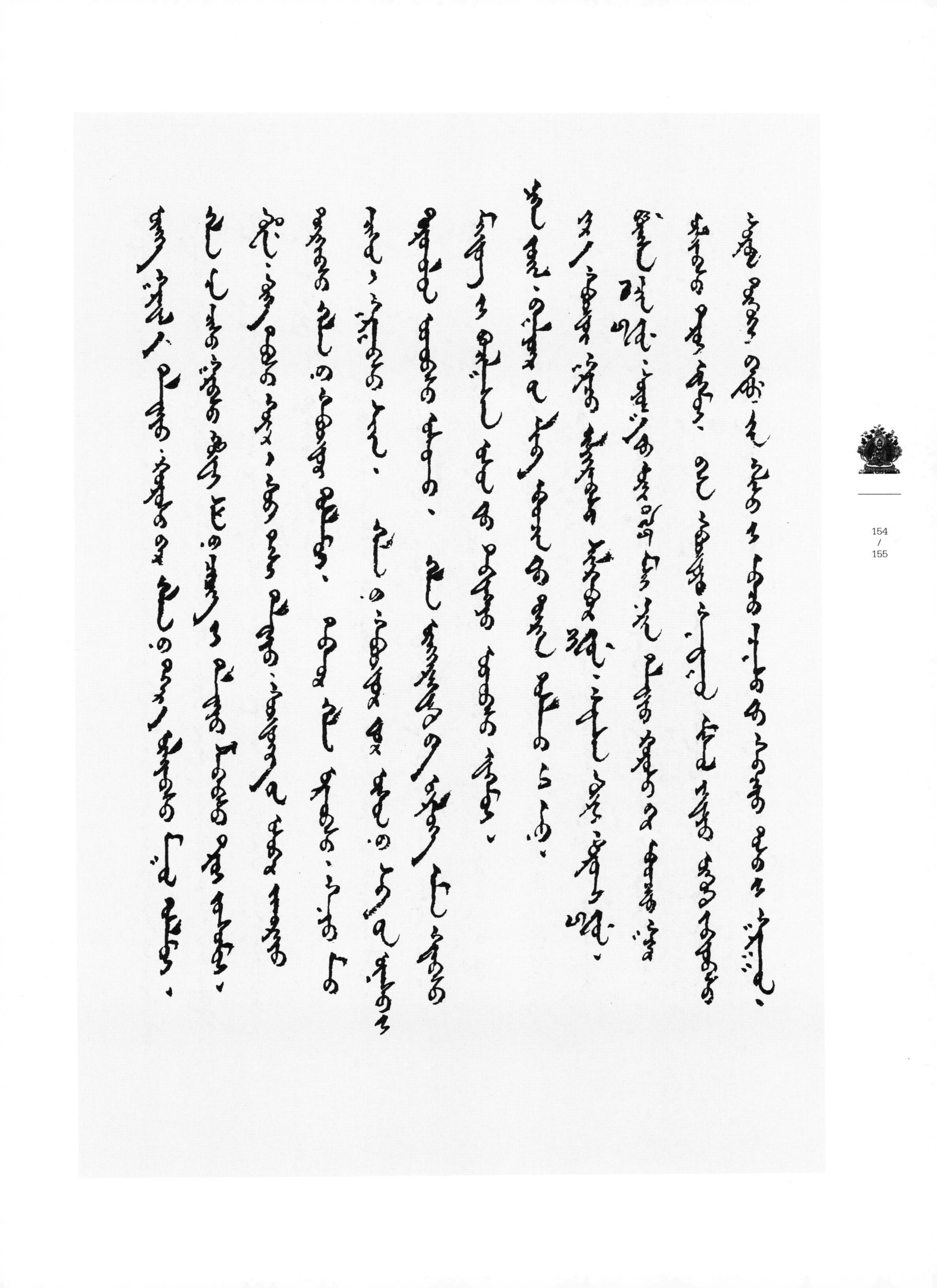

[illegible]

[illegible]

[illegible]

[illegible]

[illegible]

[illegible]

[illegible]

[illegible]

[illegible]

[illegible]

[illegible]

[illegible]

[illegible]

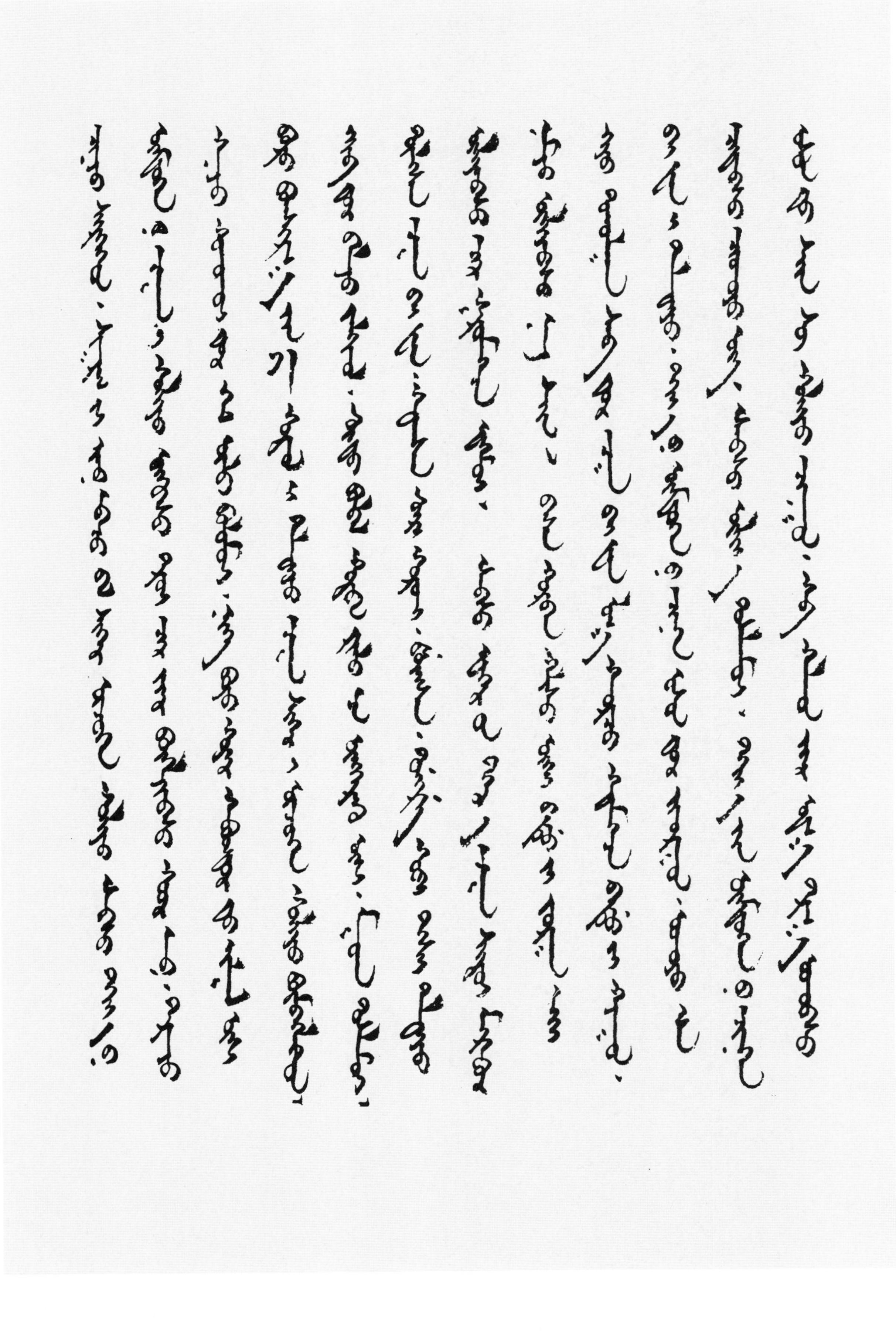

[illegible]

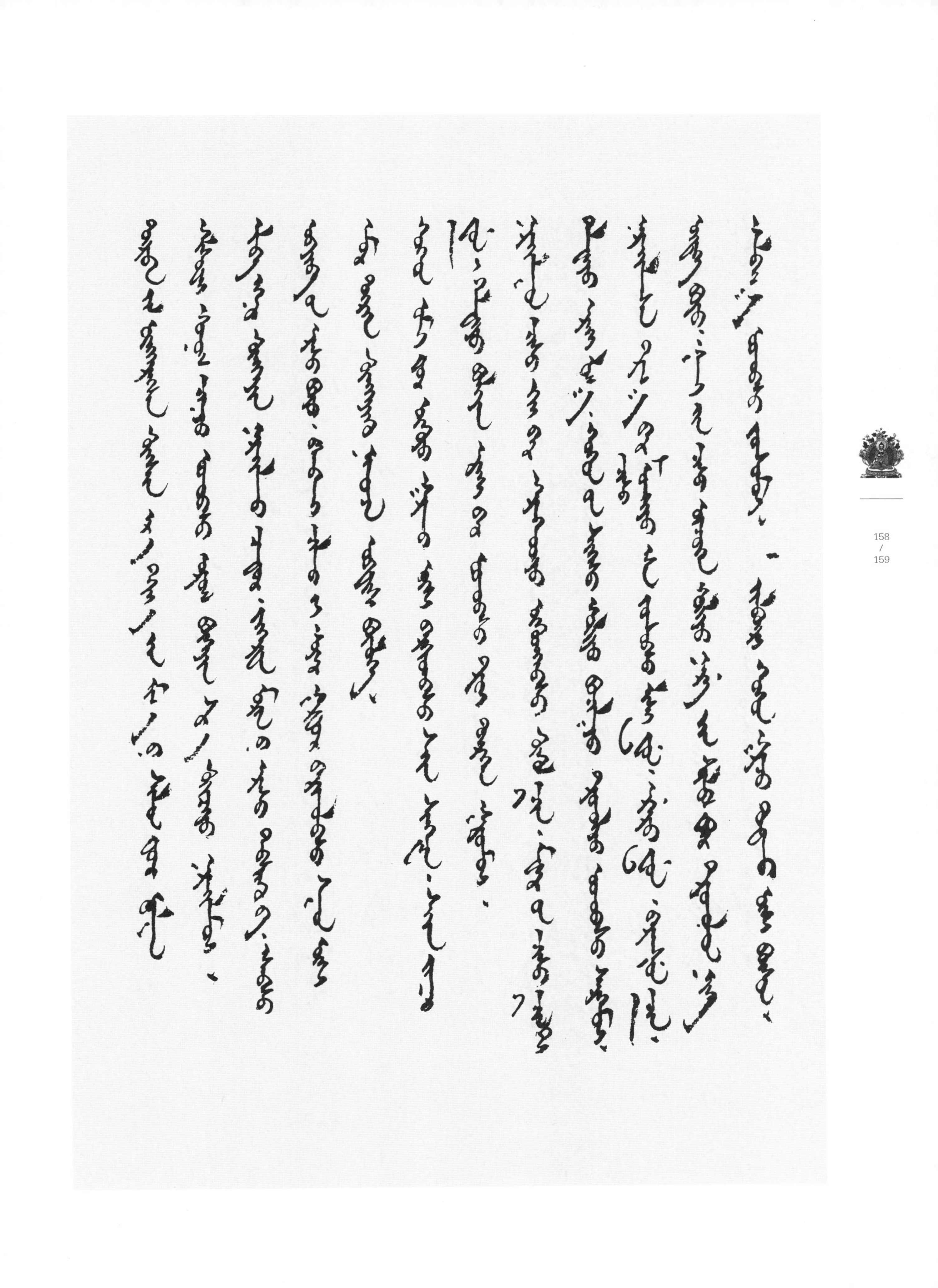

[illegible]
[illegible]
[illegible]
[illegible]
[illegible]
[illegible]
[illegible]
[illegible]
[illegible]
[illegible]
[illegible]
[illegible]

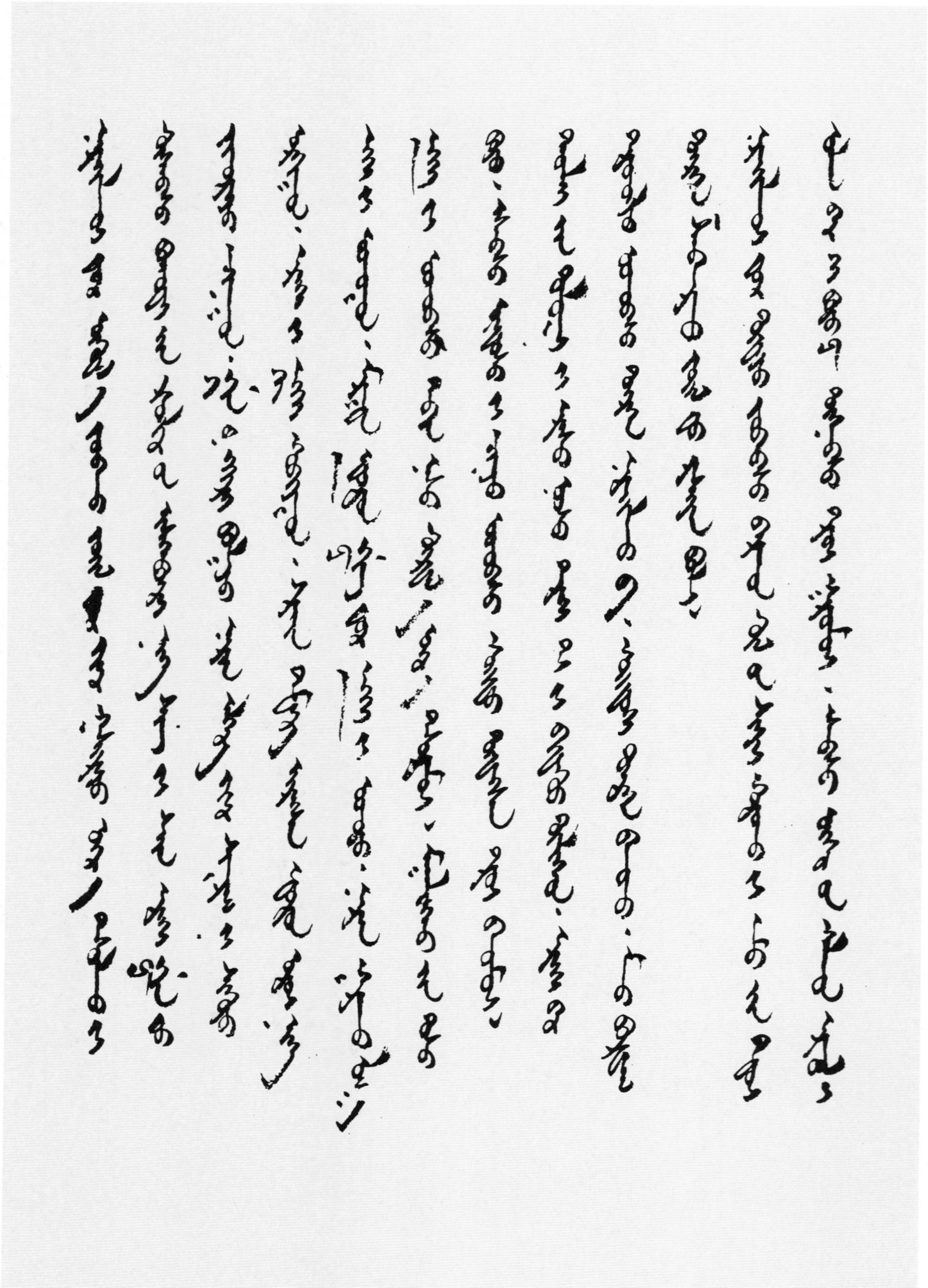

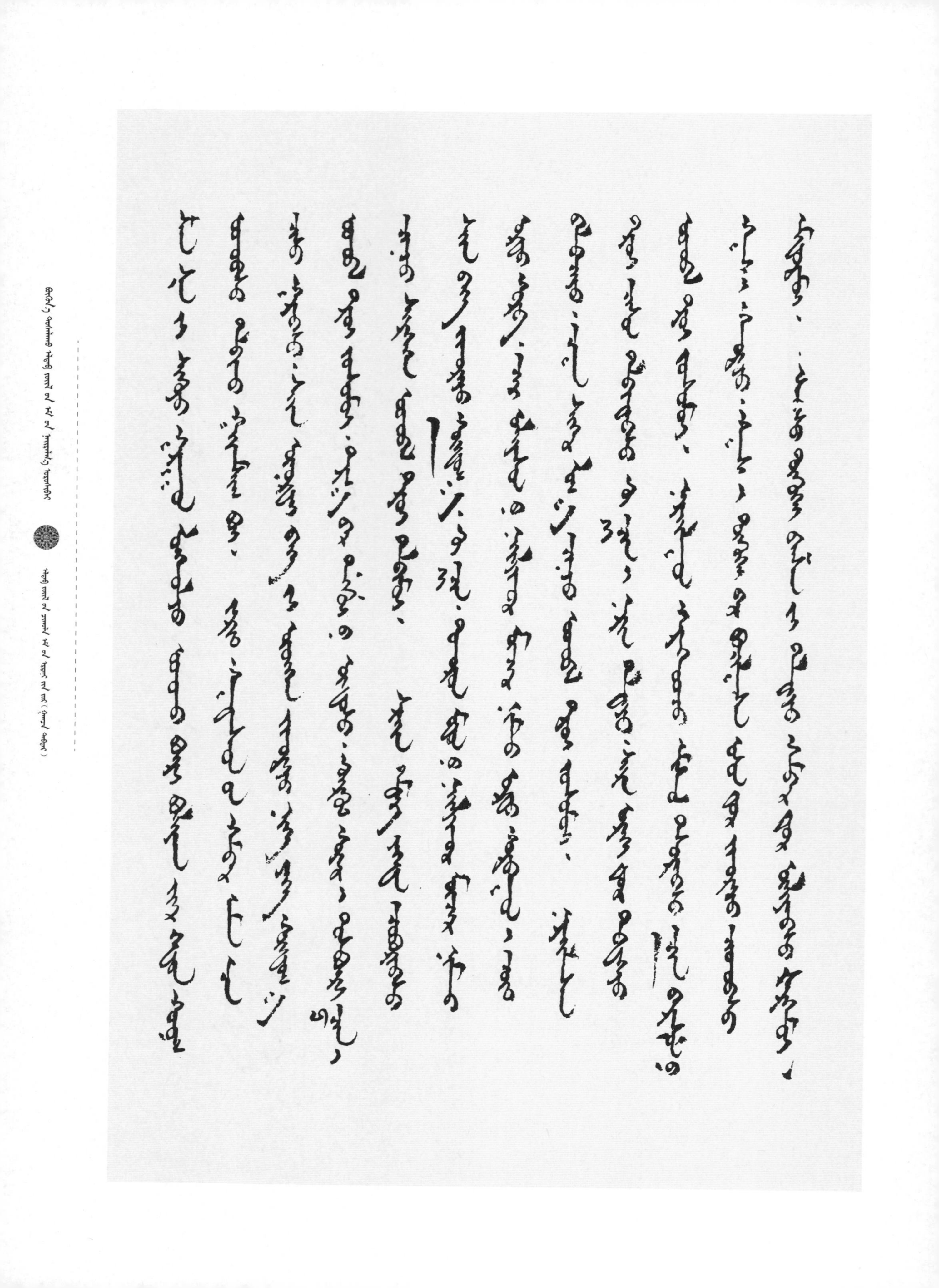

[illegible]

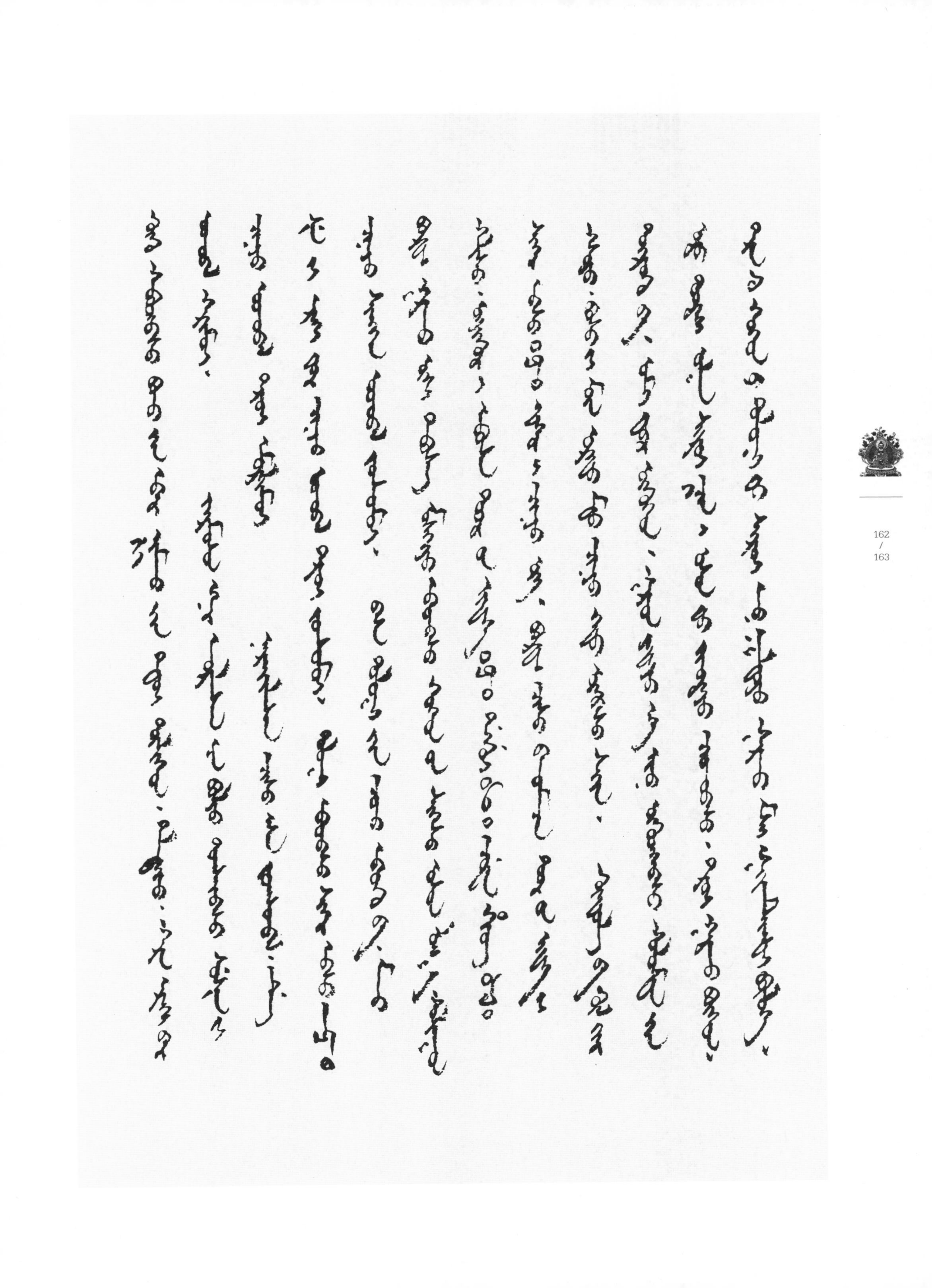

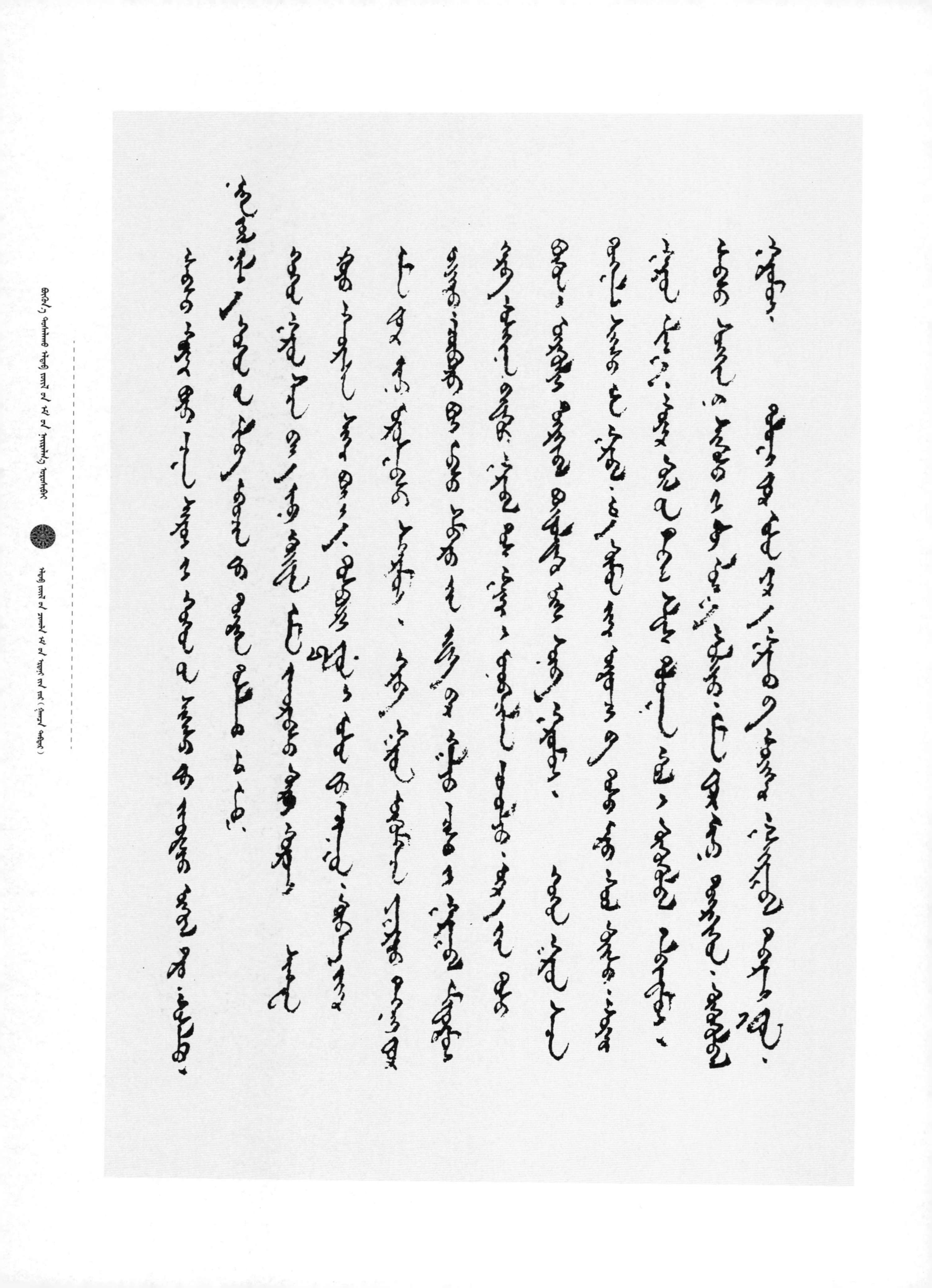

[illegible]

[illegible]

[illegible]

[illegible]

[illegible]

[illegible]

[illegible]

[illegible]

[illegible]

[illegible]

[illegible]

[illegible]

[illegible]

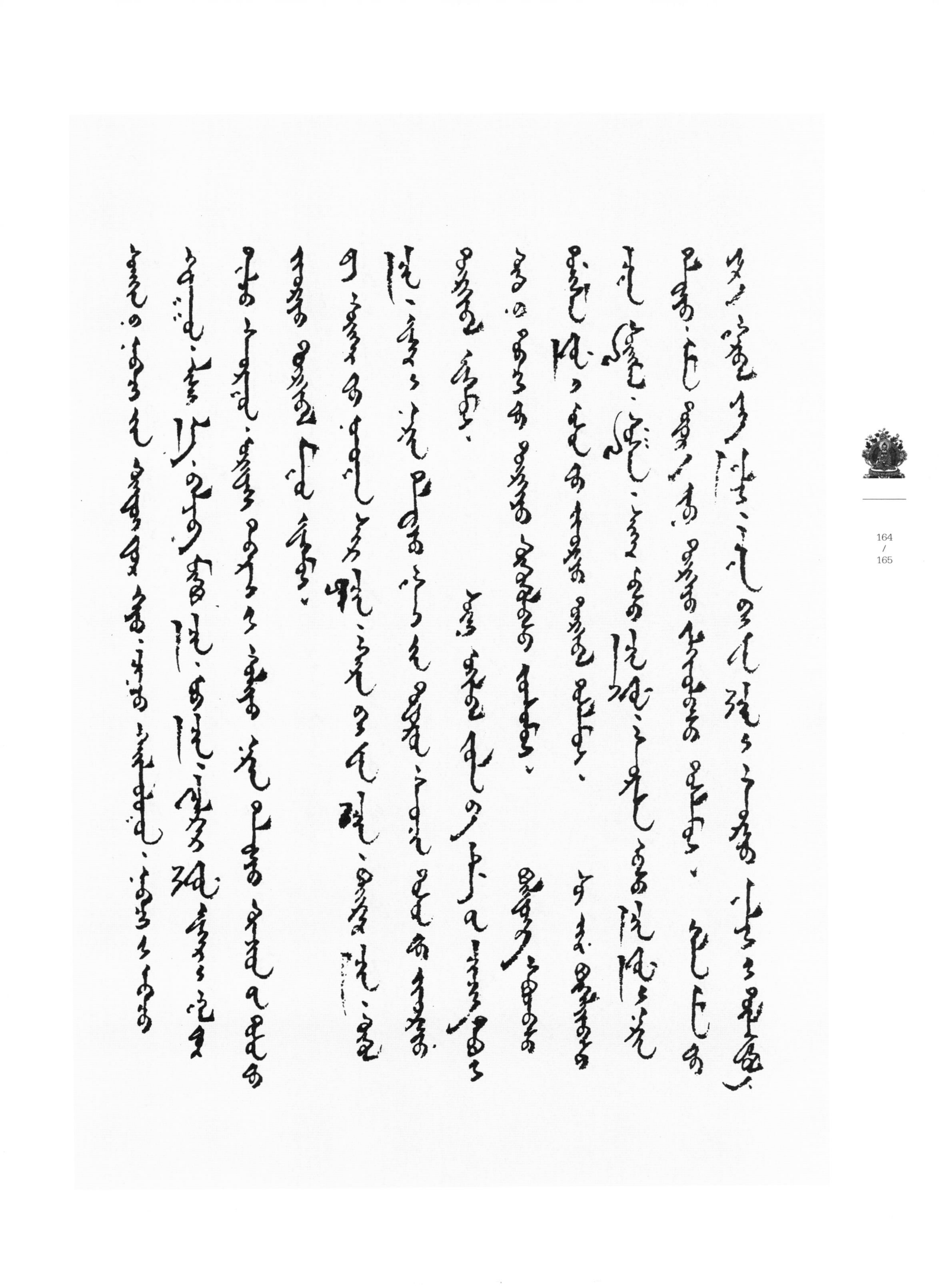

[illegible]

[illegible]

[illegible]

[illegible]

[illegible]

[illegible]

[illegible]

[illegible]

[illegible]

[illegible]

[illegible]

[illegible]

[illegible]

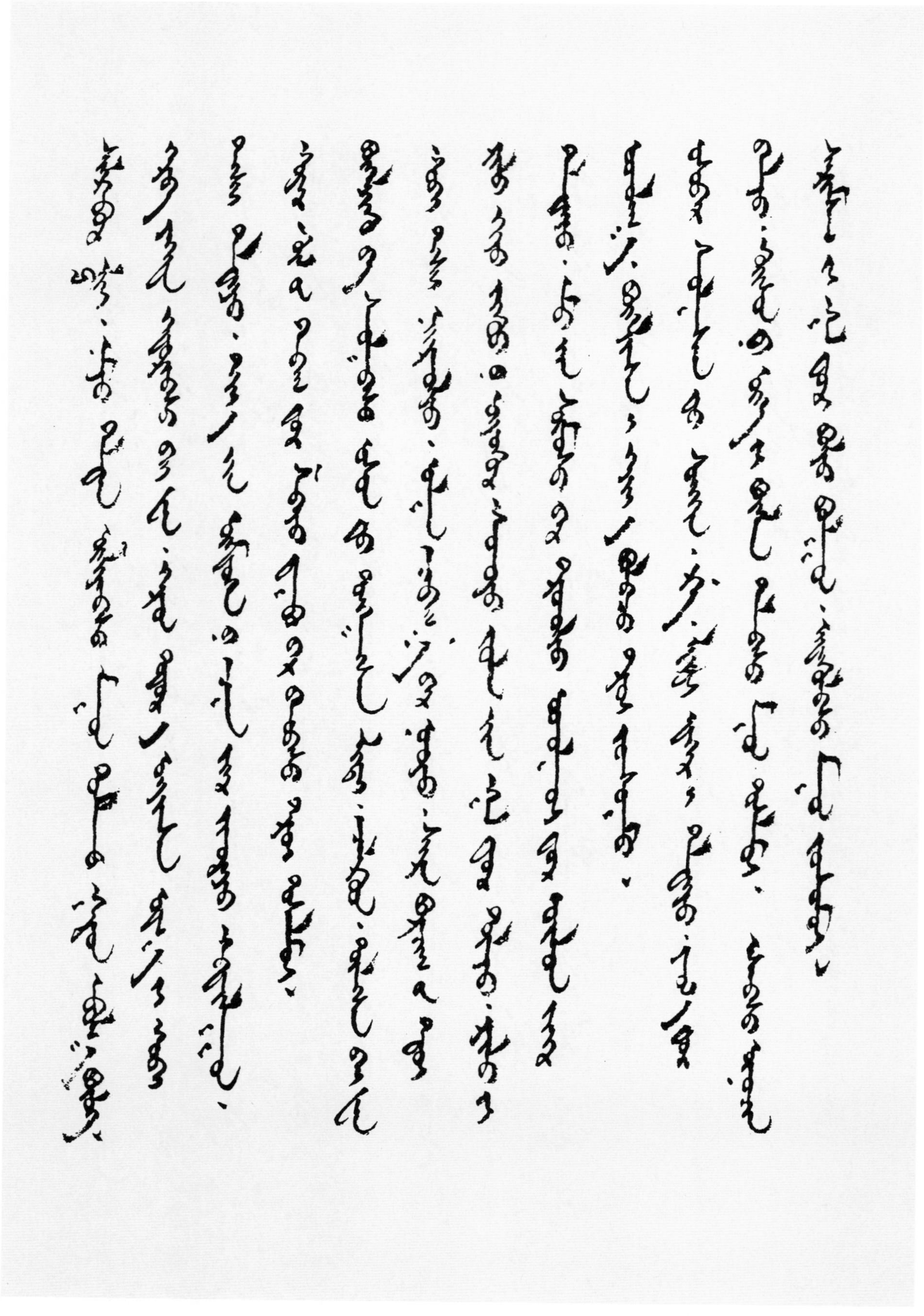

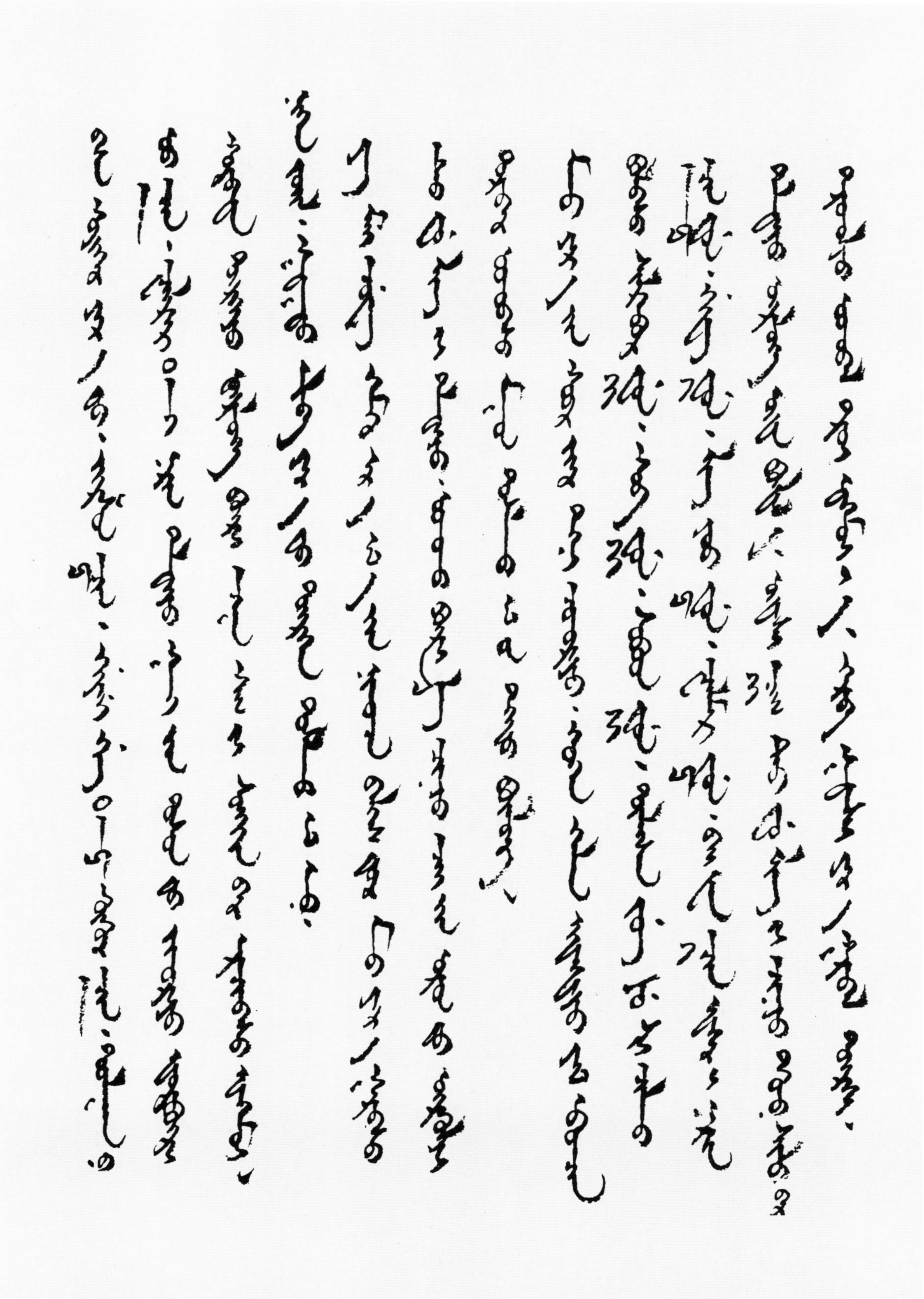

[illegible]
[illegible]
[illegible]
[illegible]
[illegible]
[illegible]
[illegible]
[illegible]
[illegible]
[illegible]
[illegible]
[illegible]
[illegible]

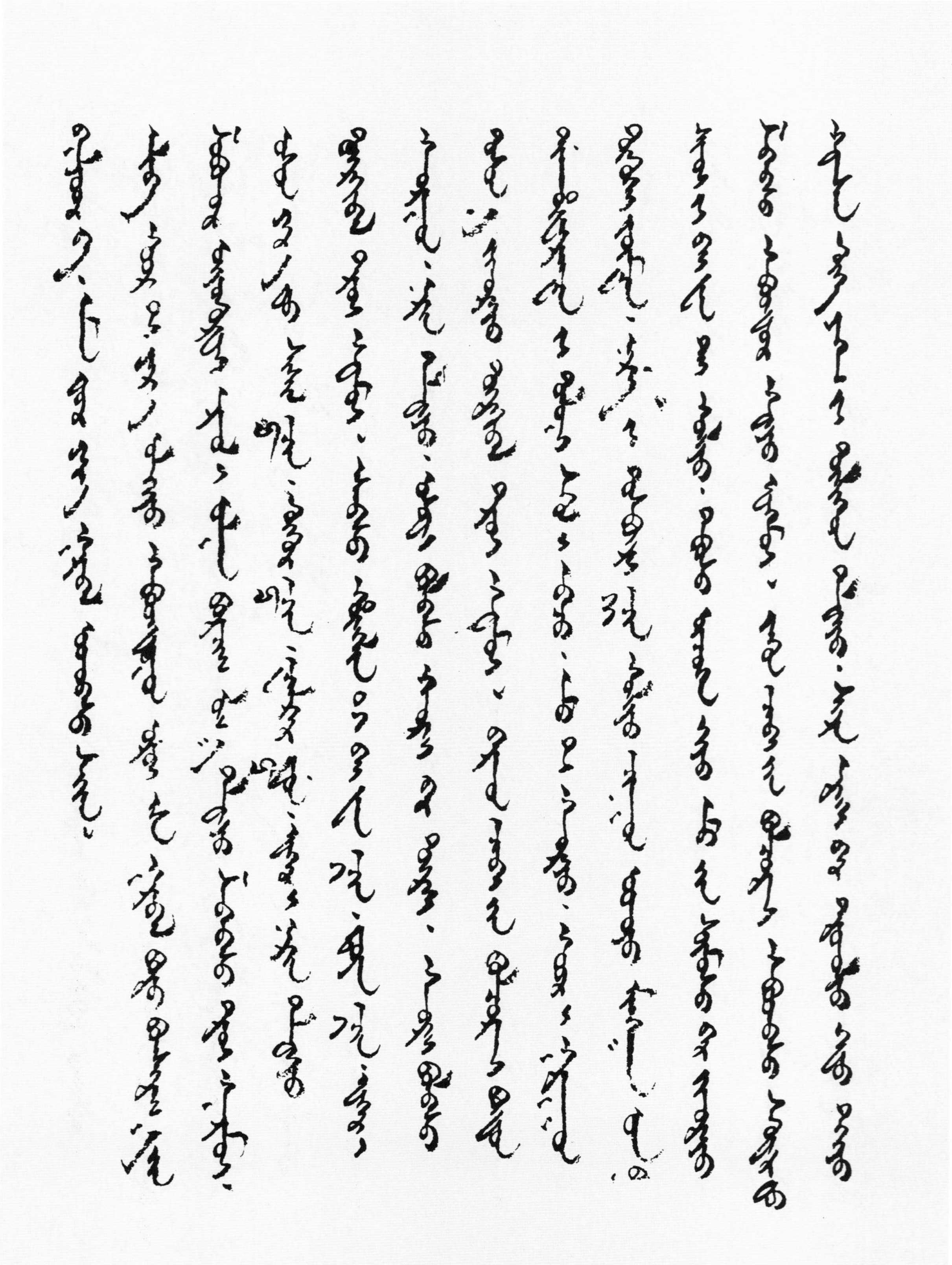

[illegible]

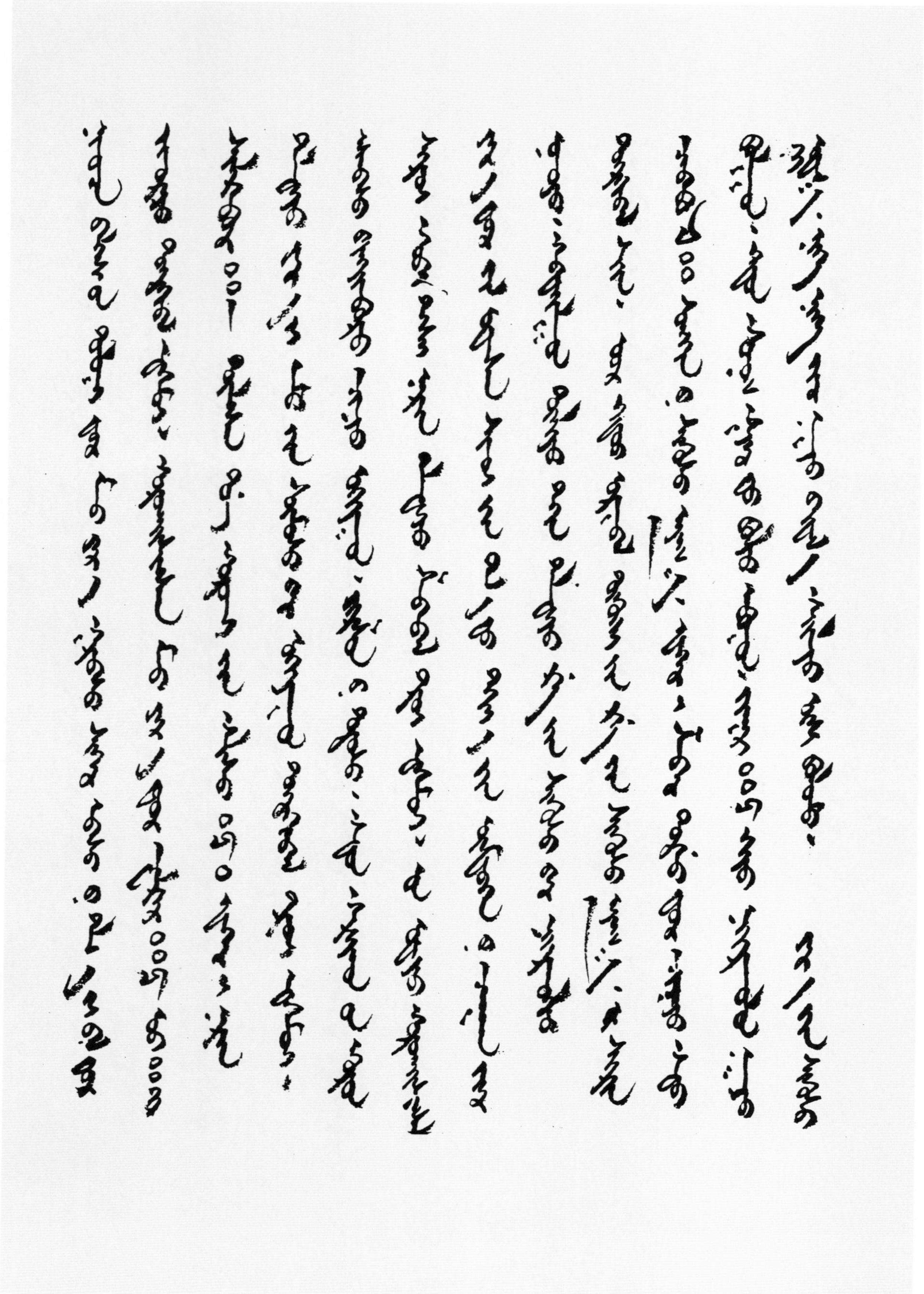

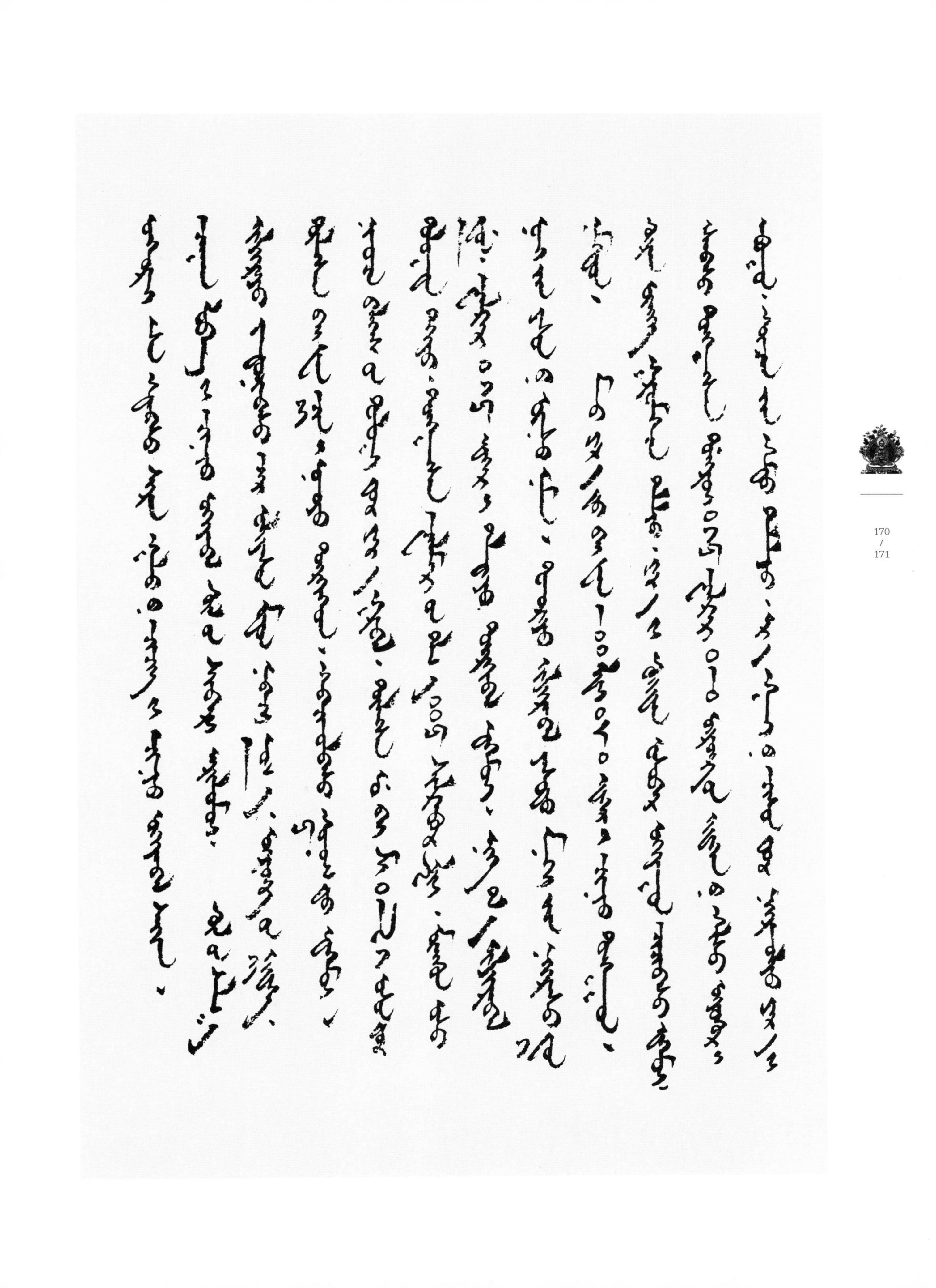

[illegible]

[illegible]

[illegible]

[illegible]

[illegible]

[illegible]

[illegible]

[illegible]

[illegible]

[illegible]

[illegible]

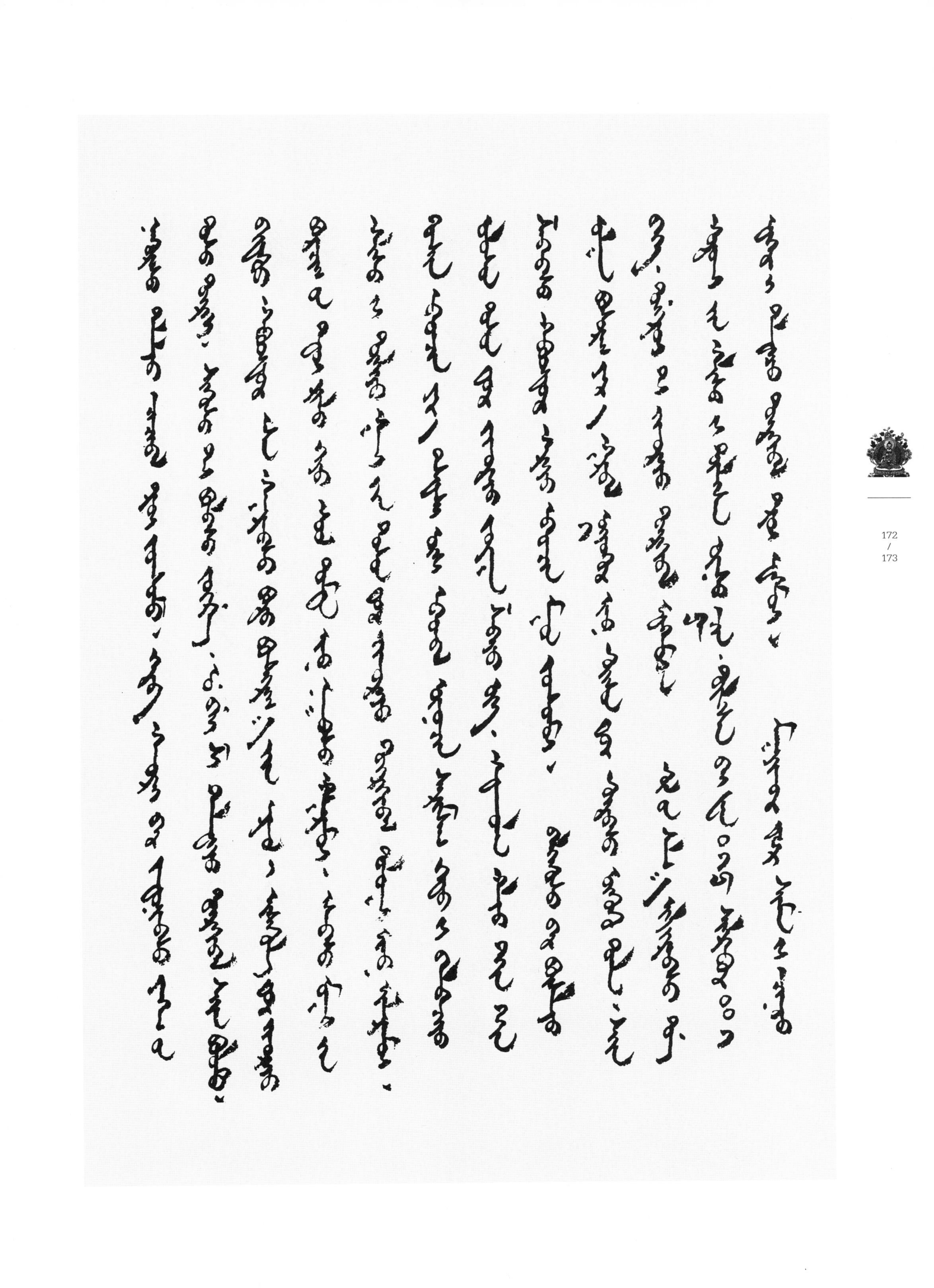

[illegible]

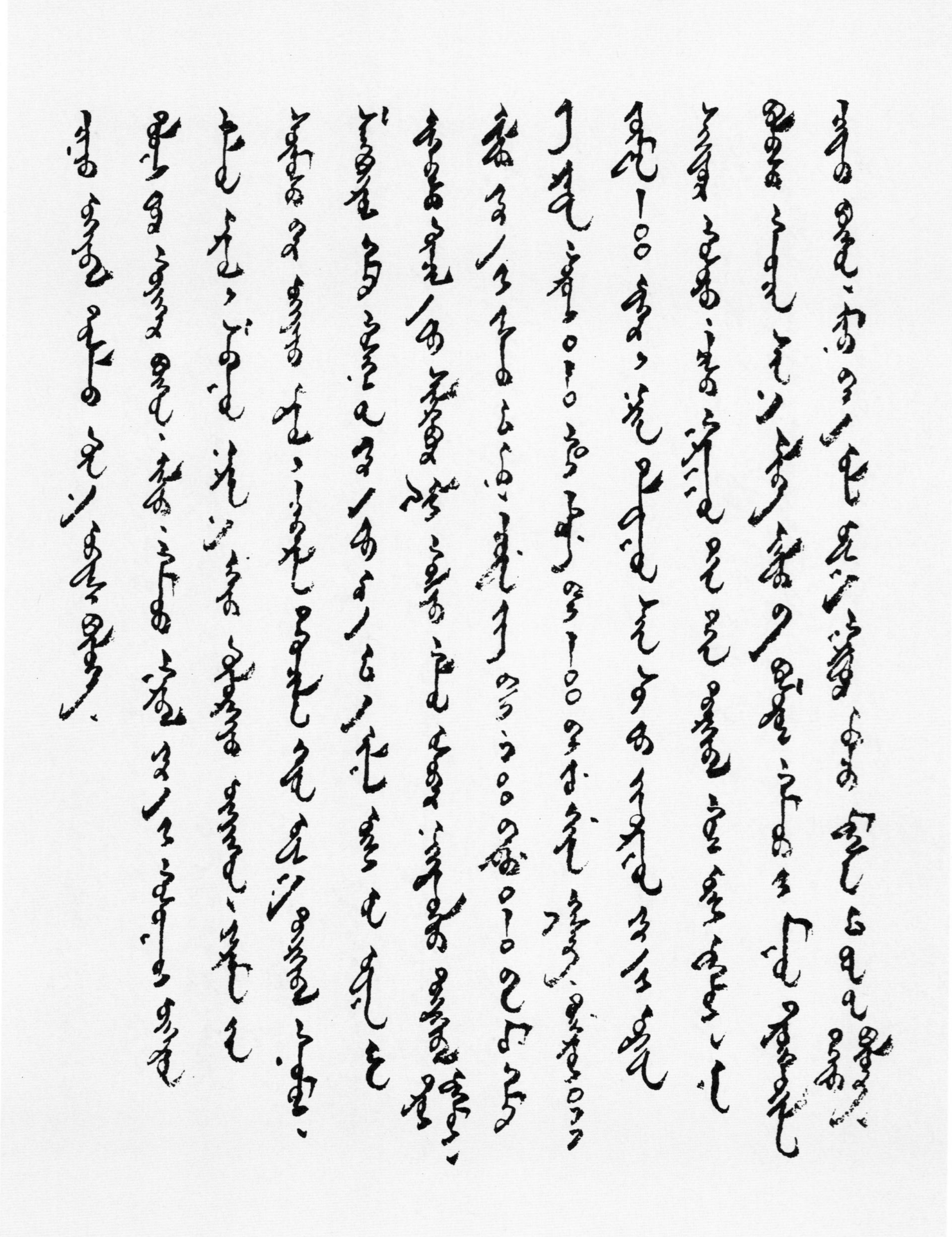

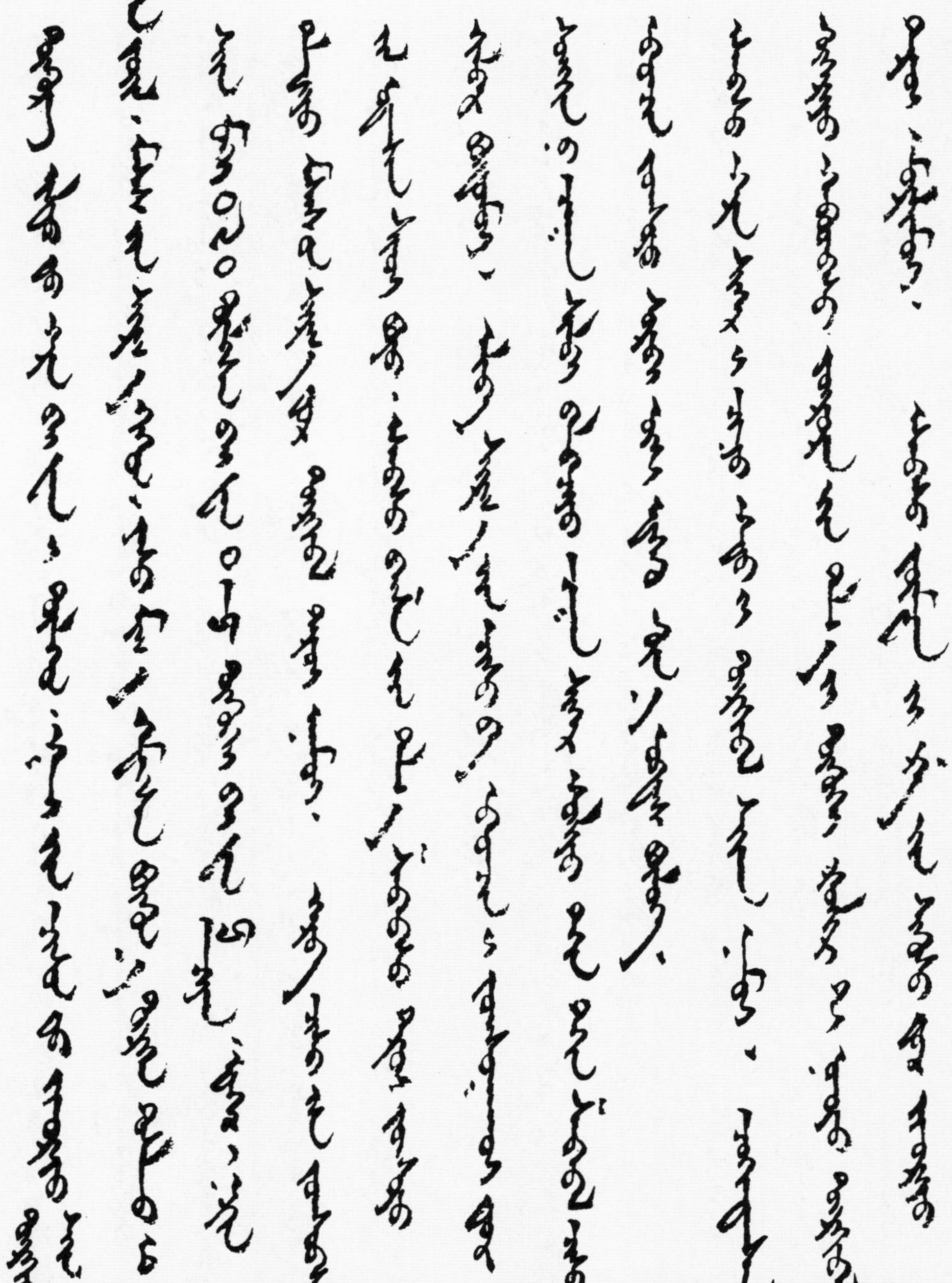

[illegible]

[illegible]

[illegible]

[illegible]

[illegible]

[illegible]

[illegible]

[illegible]

[illegible]

[illegible]

[illegible]

[illegible]

[illegible]

[illegible]

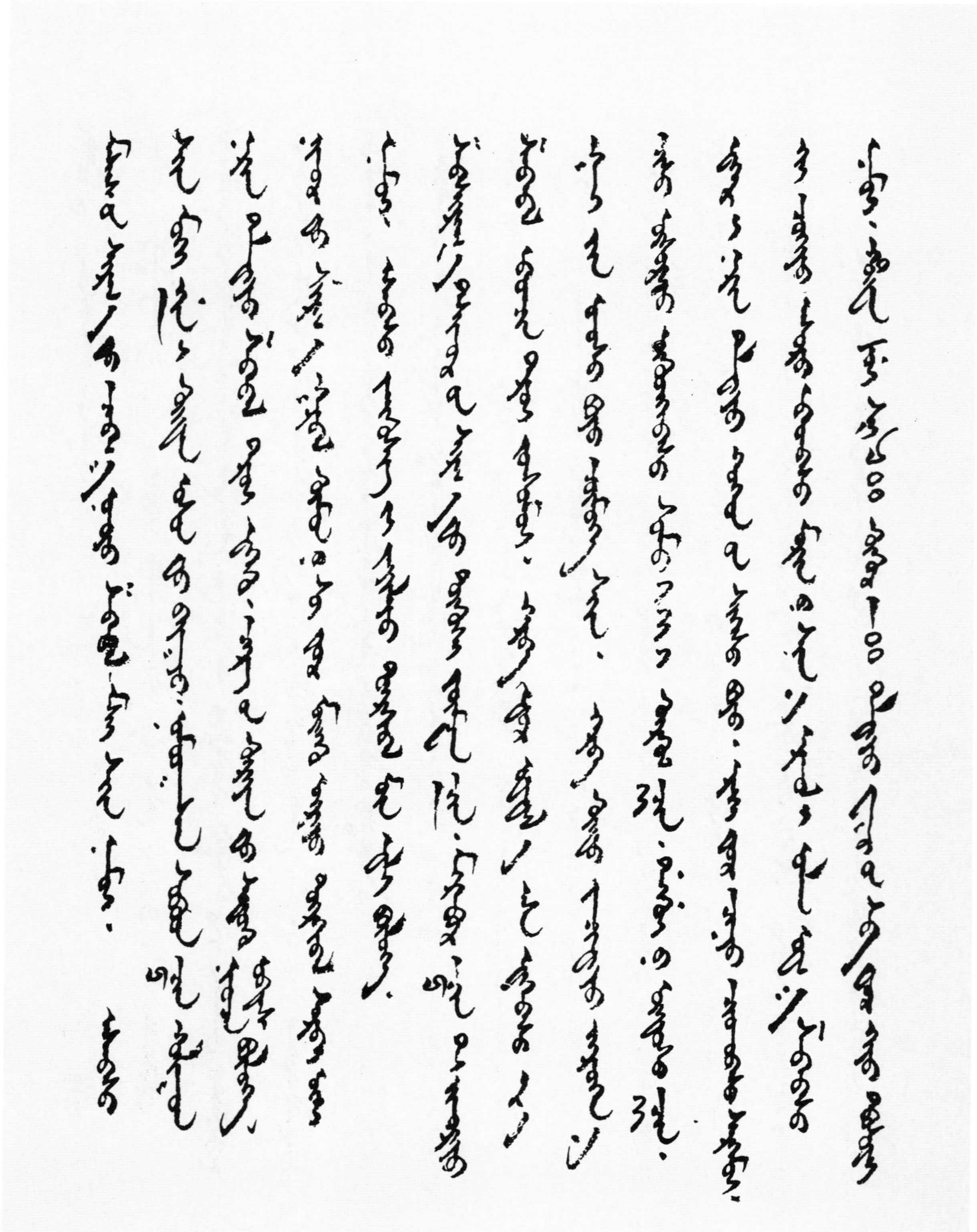

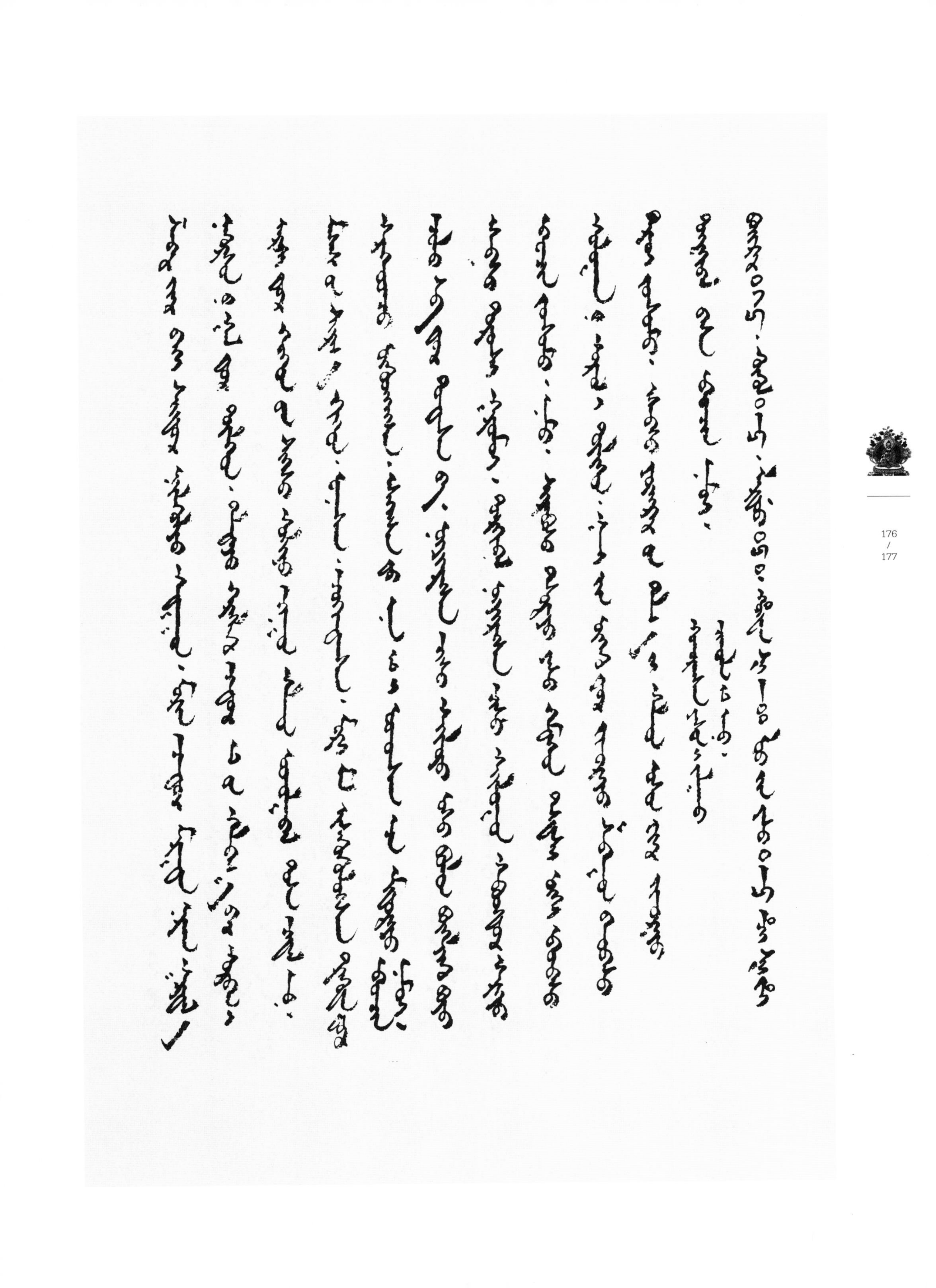

[illegible]

[illegible]

[illegible]

[illegible]

[illegible]

[illegible]

[illegible]

[illegible]

[illegible]

[illegible]

[illegible]

[illegible]

[illegible]

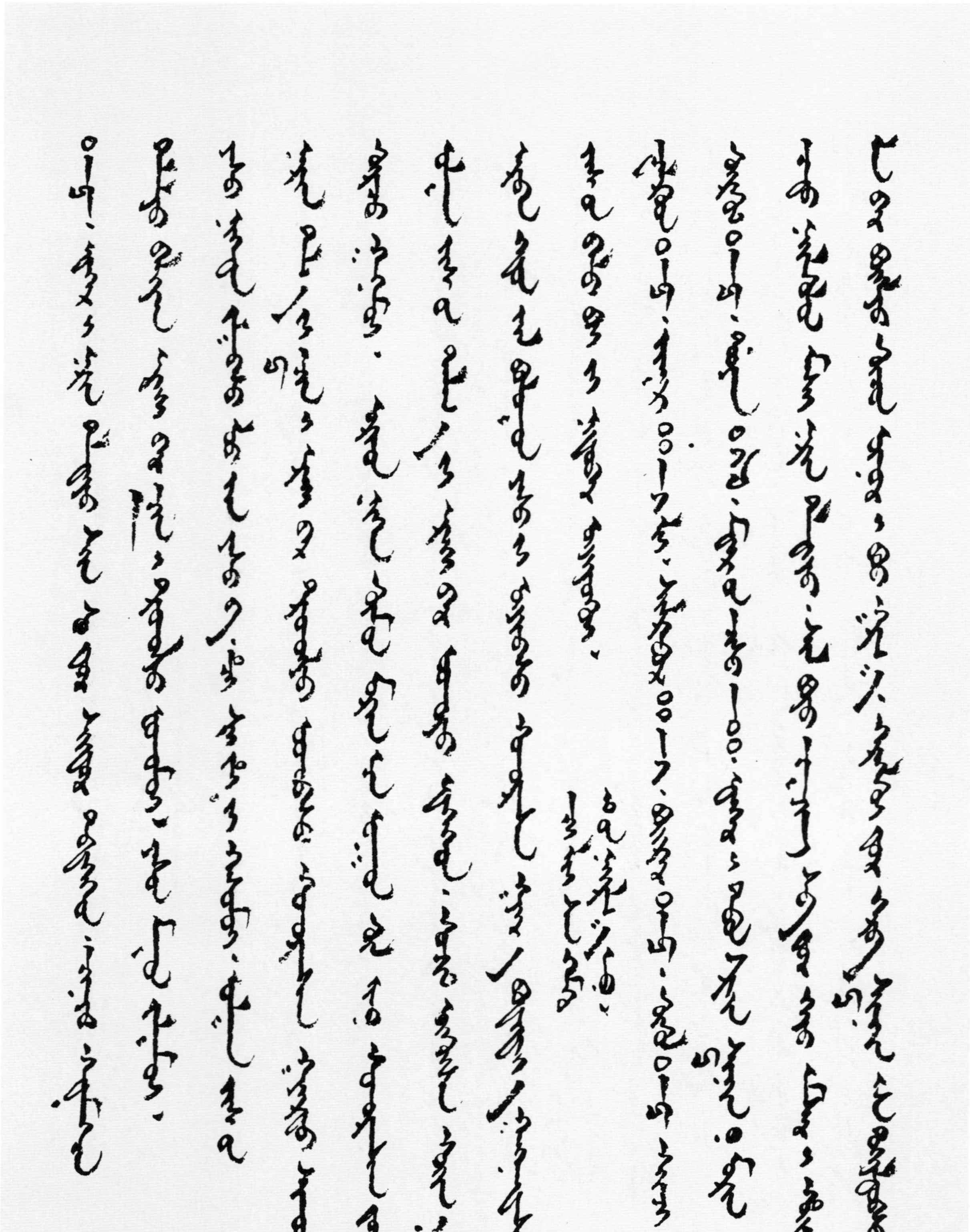

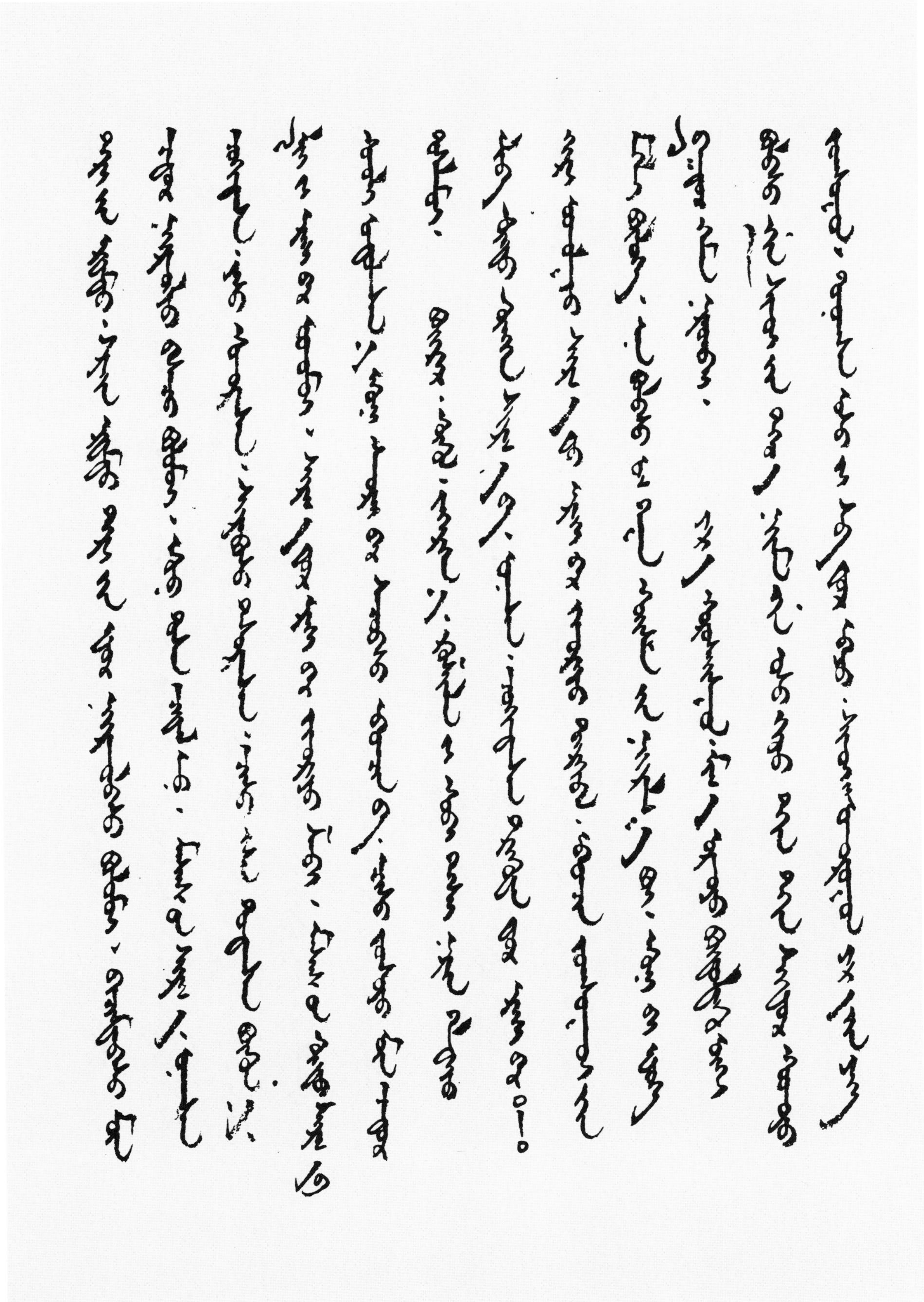

[illegible]

[illegible]

[illegible]

[illegible]

[illegible]

[illegible]

[illegible]

[illegible]

[illegible]

[illegible]

[illegible]

[illegible]

[illegible]

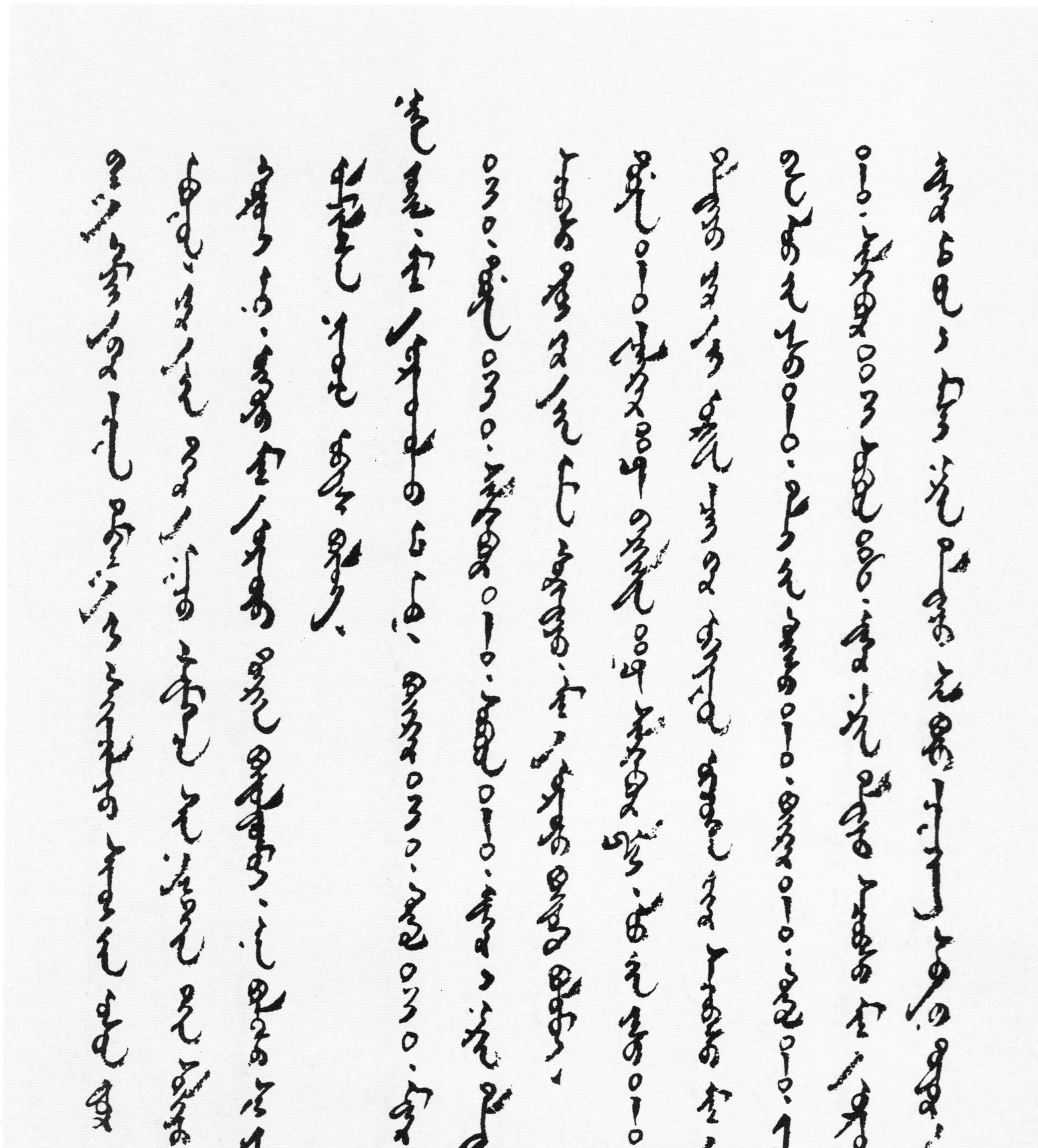

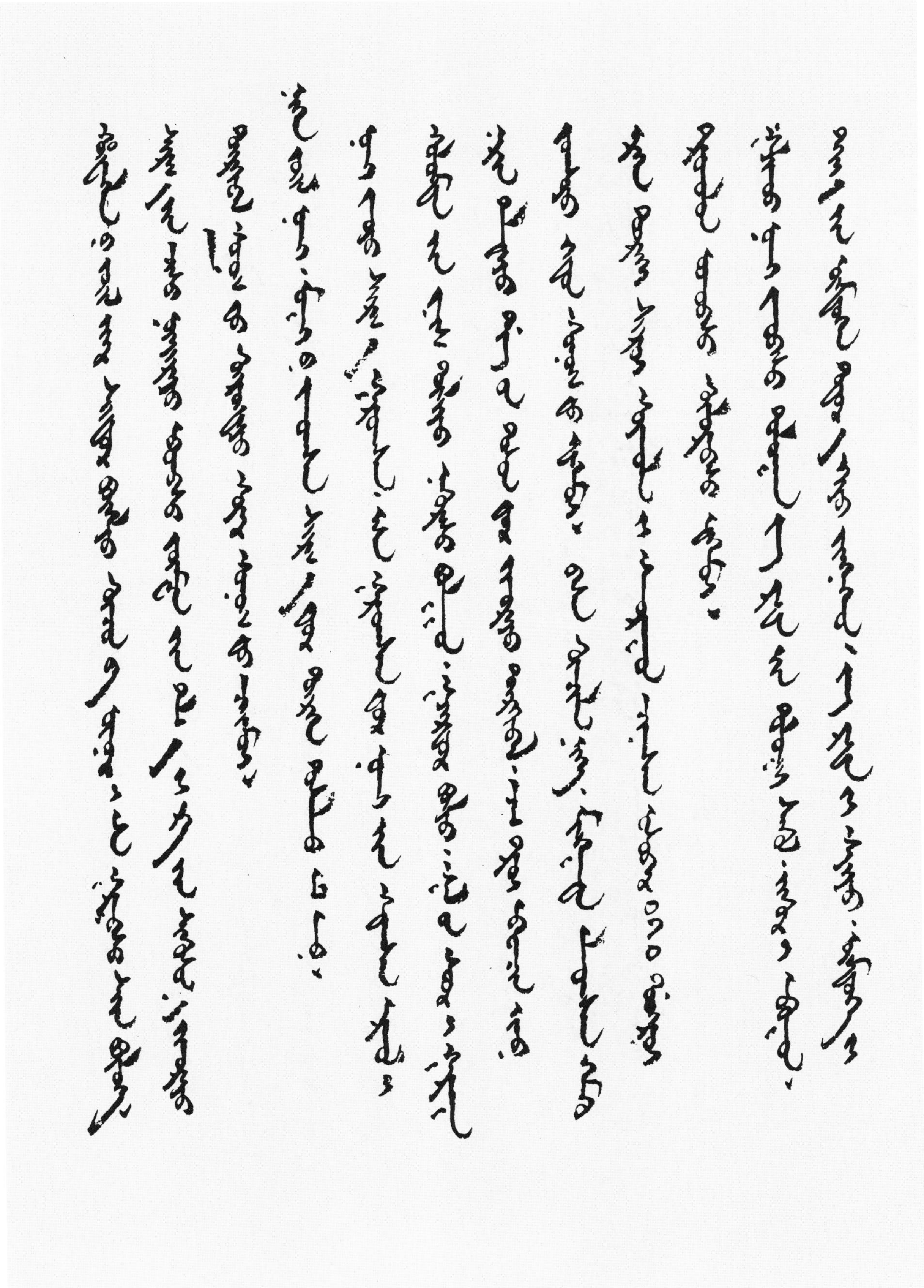

[illegible]

[illegible]

[illegible]

[illegible]

[illegible]

[illegible]

[illegible]

[illegible]

[illegible]

[illegible]

[illegible]

[illegible]

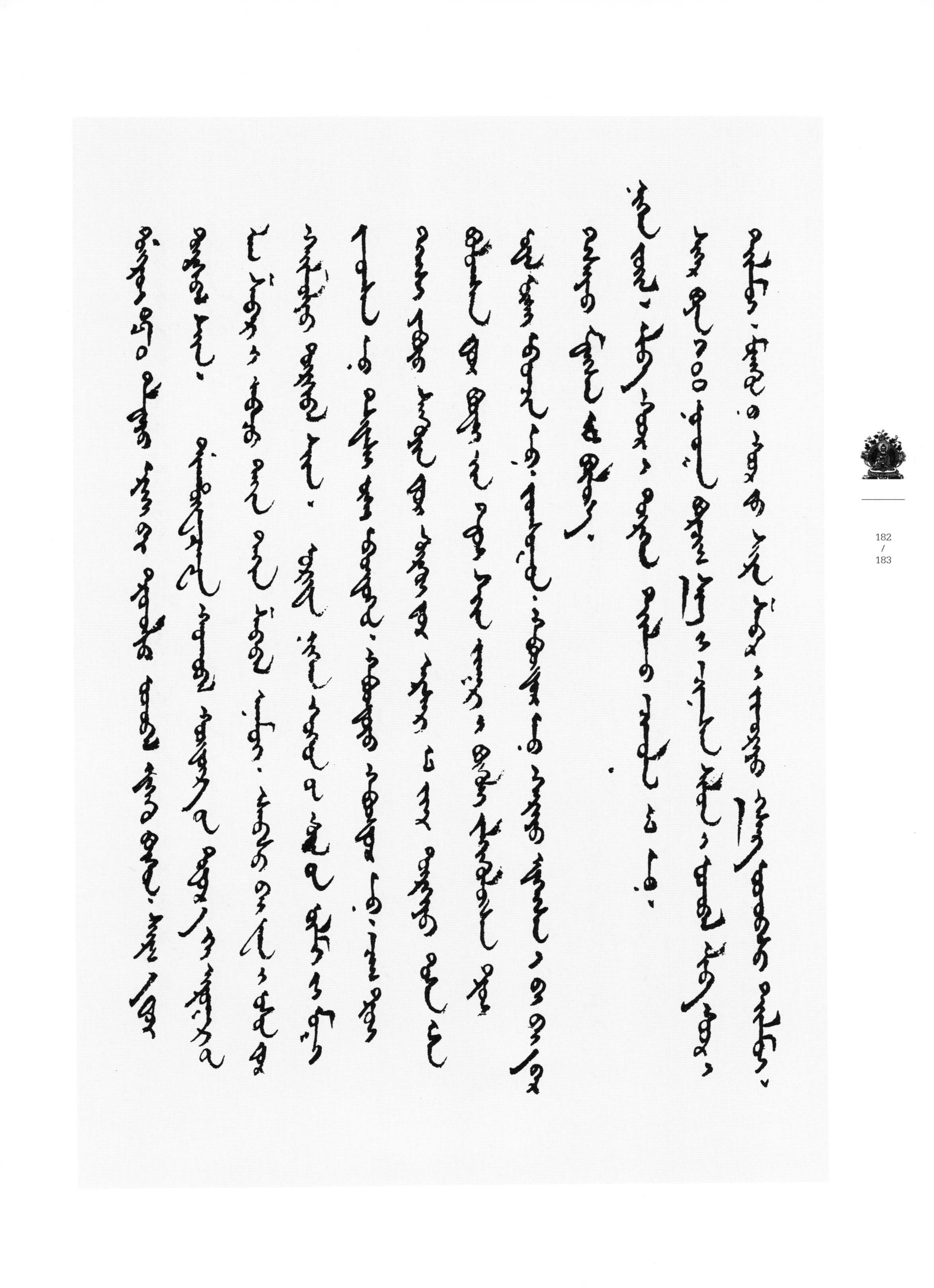

[illegible]

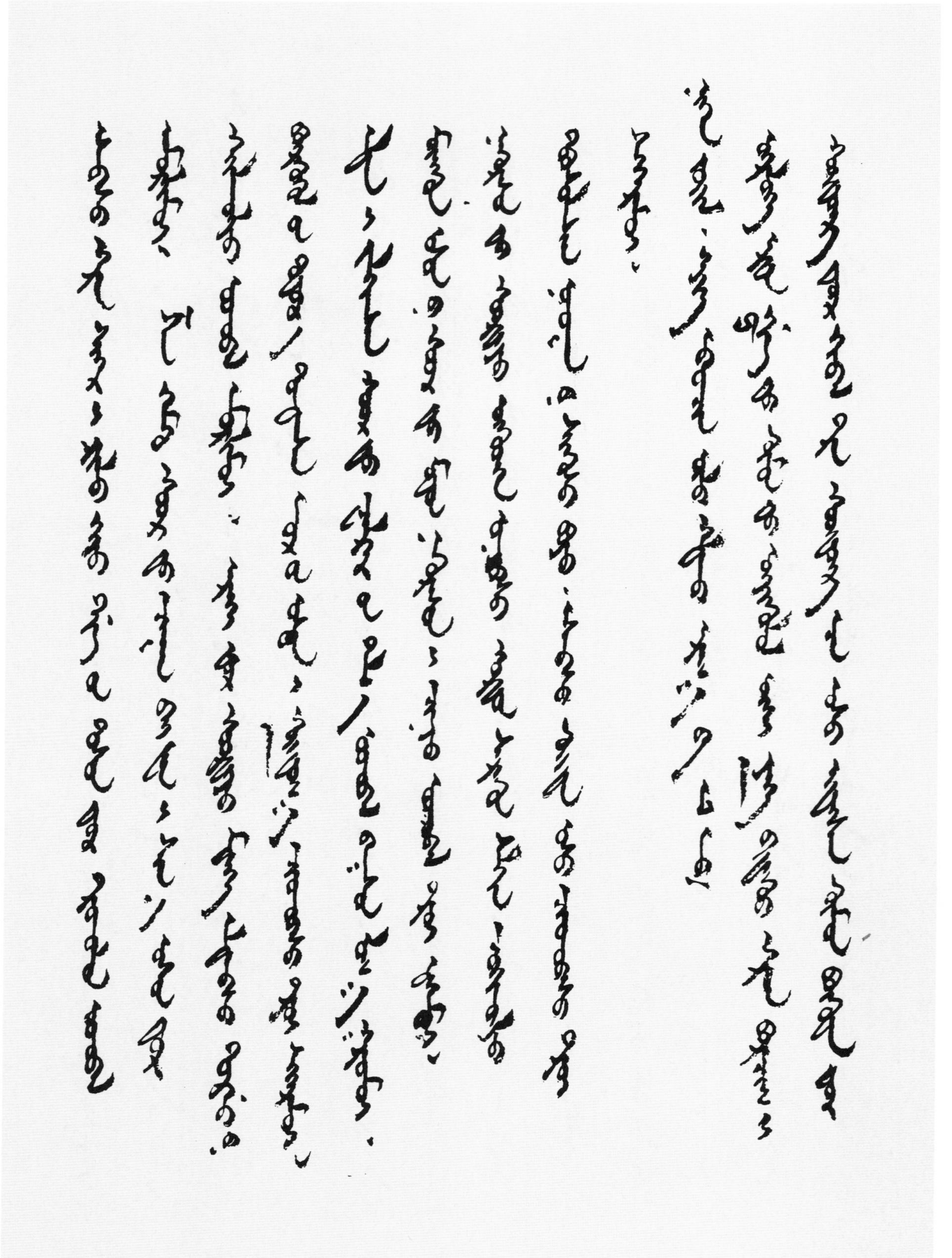

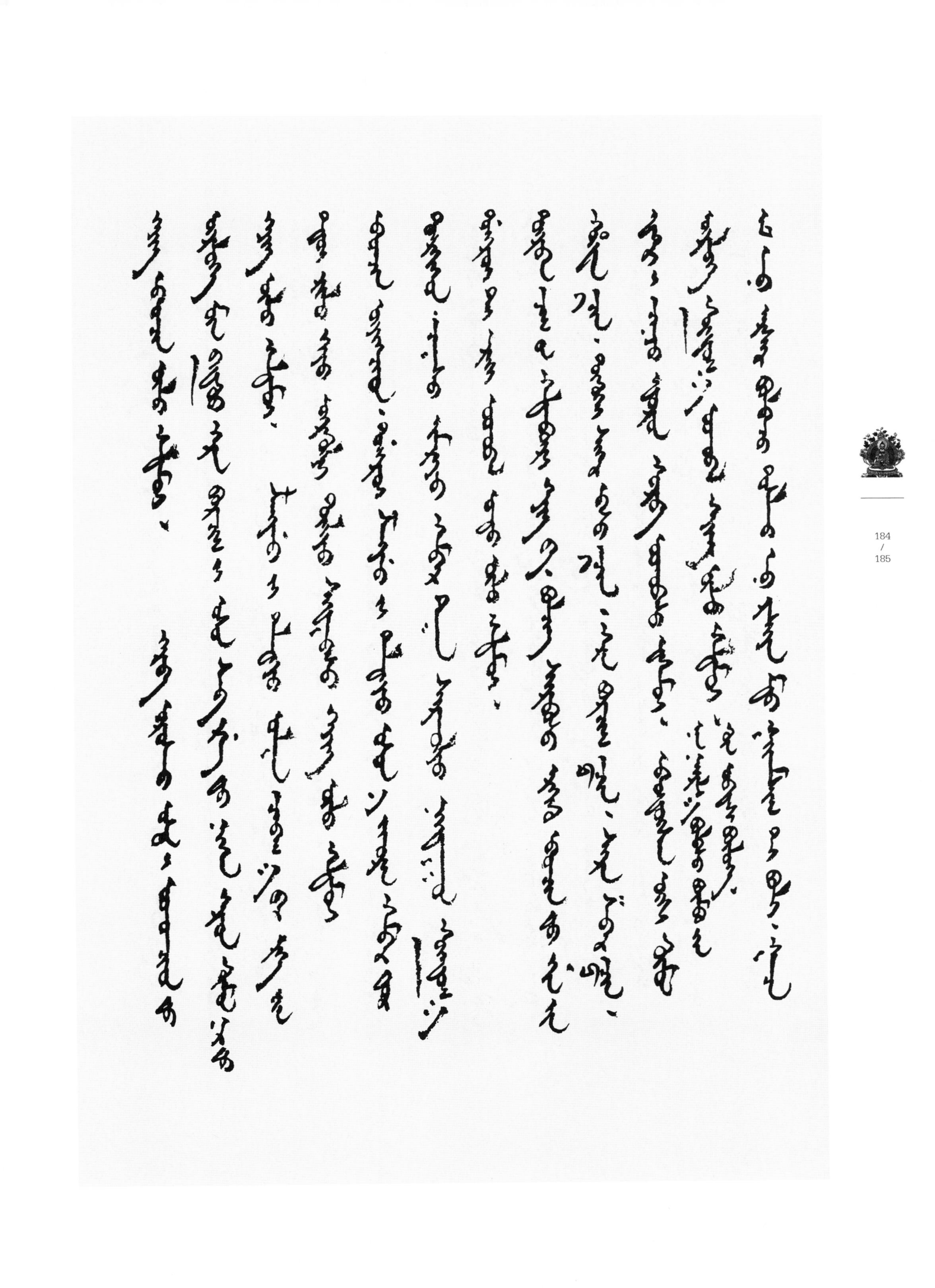

[illegible]
[illegible]
[illegible]
[illegible]
[illegible]
[illegible]
[illegible]
[illegible]
[illegible]
[illegible]
[illegible]
[illegible]

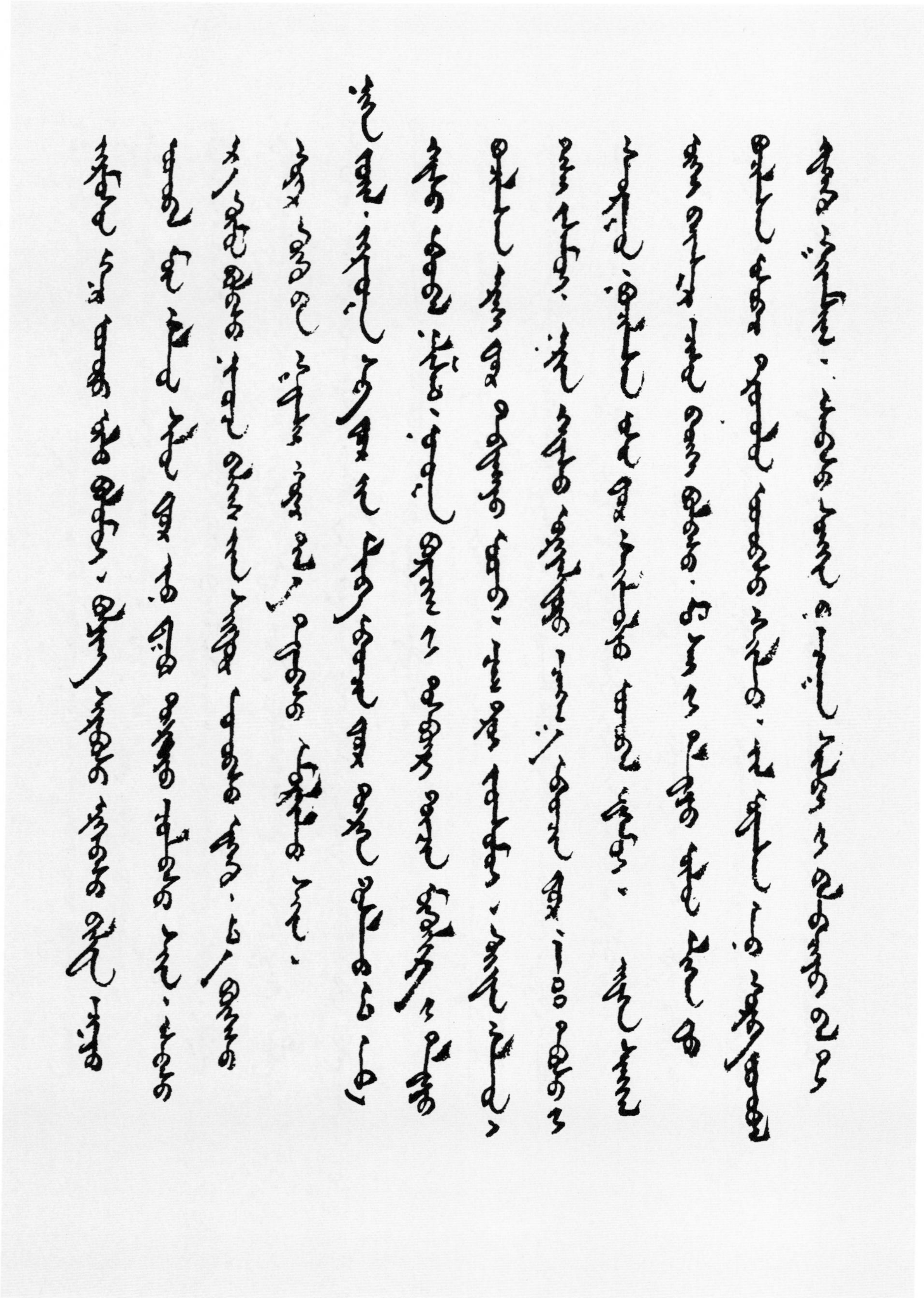

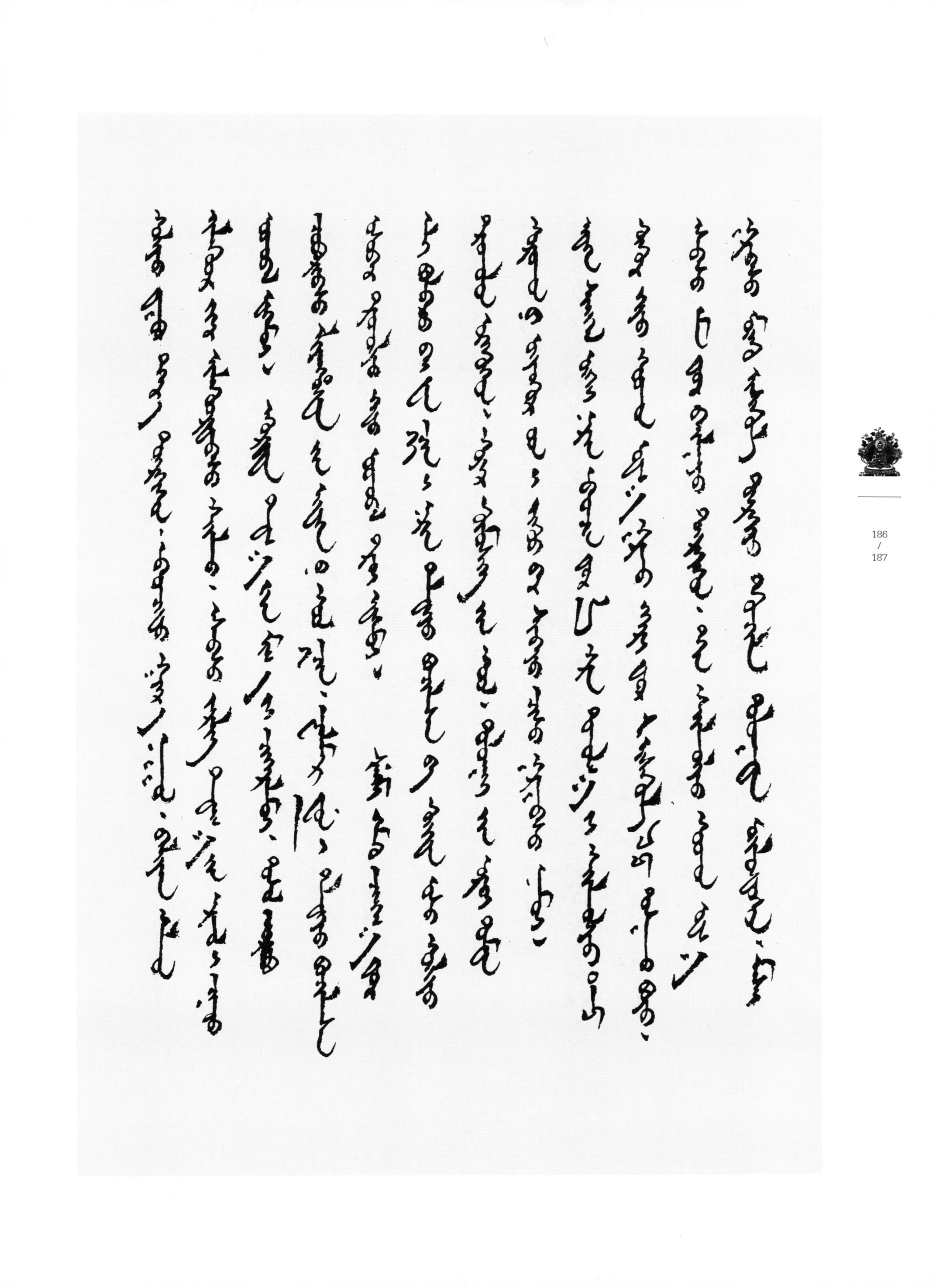

[illegible]
[illegible]
[illegible]
[illegible]
[illegible]
[illegible]
[illegible]
[illegible]
[illegible]
[illegible]
[illegible]
[illegible]

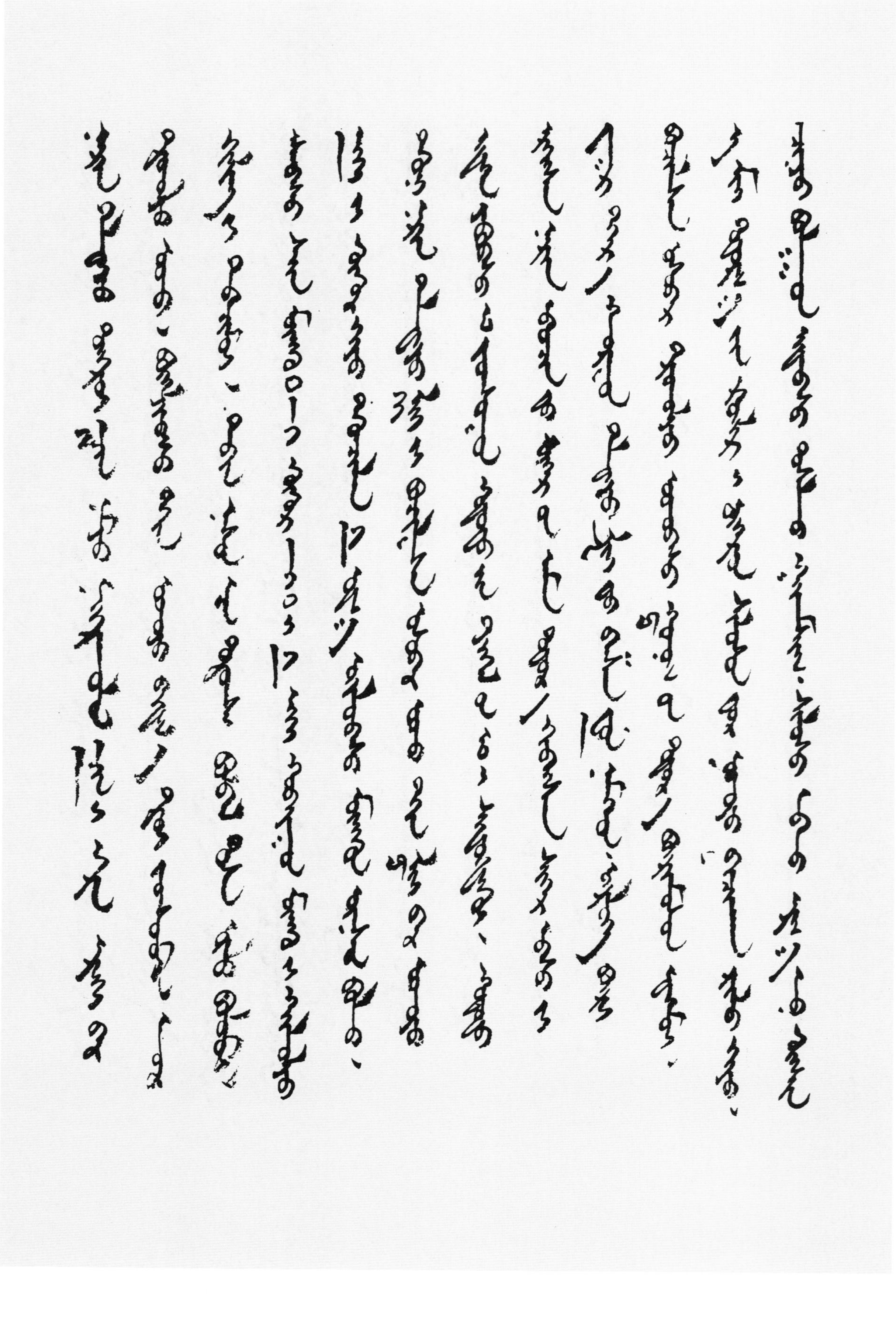

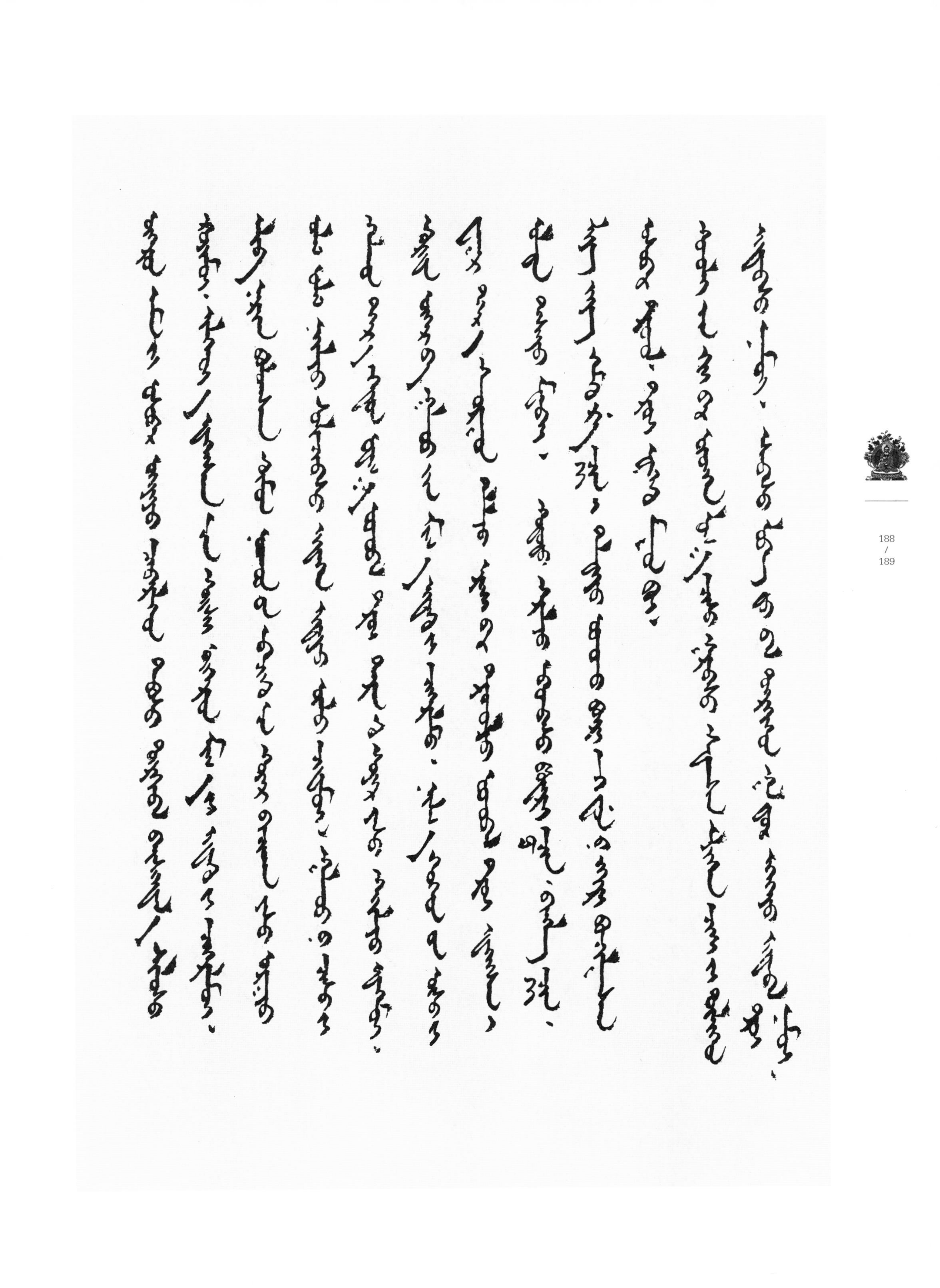

[illegible]

[illegible]

[illegible]

[illegible]

[illegible]

[illegible]

[illegible]

[illegible]

[illegible]

[illegible]

[illegible]

[illegible]

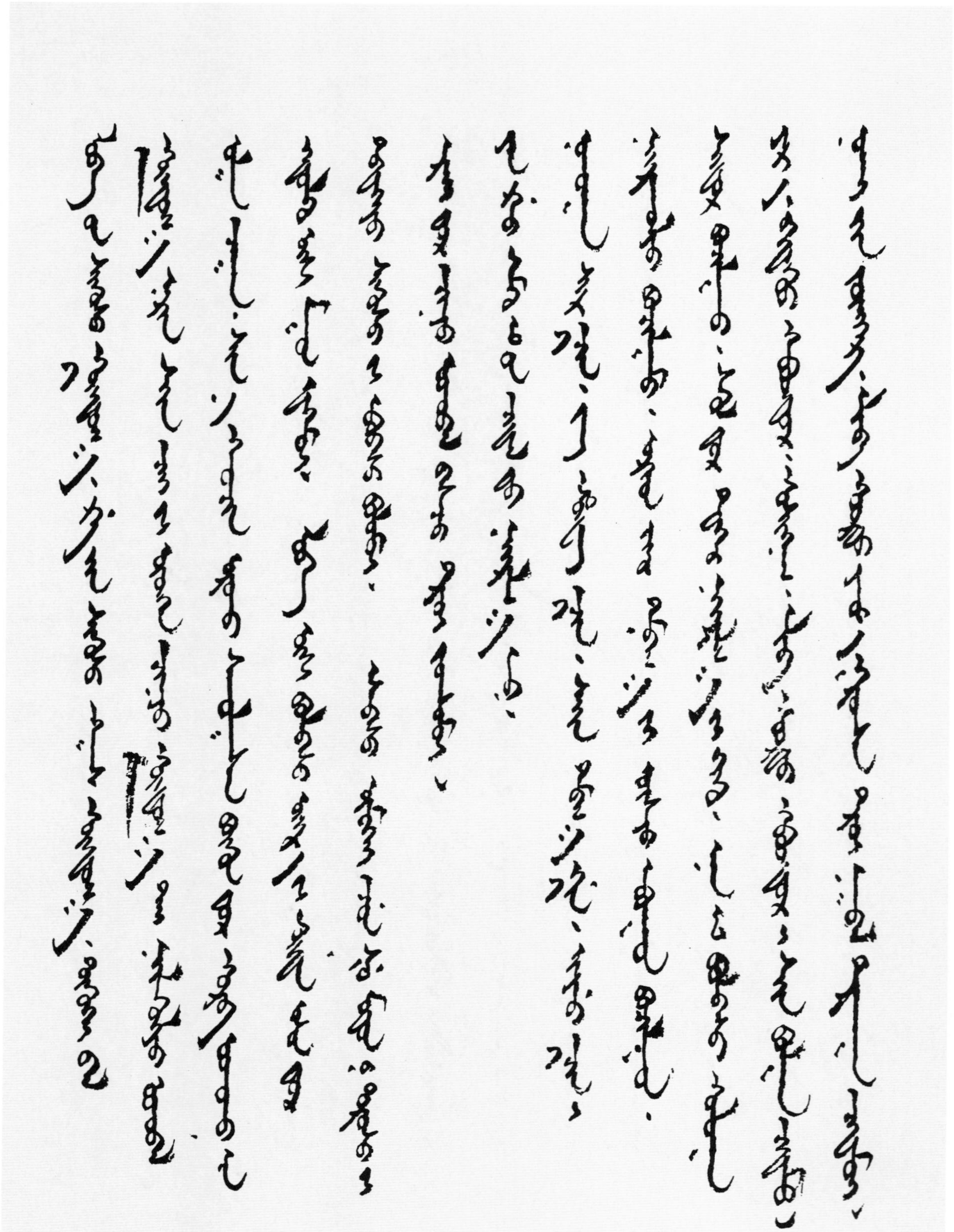

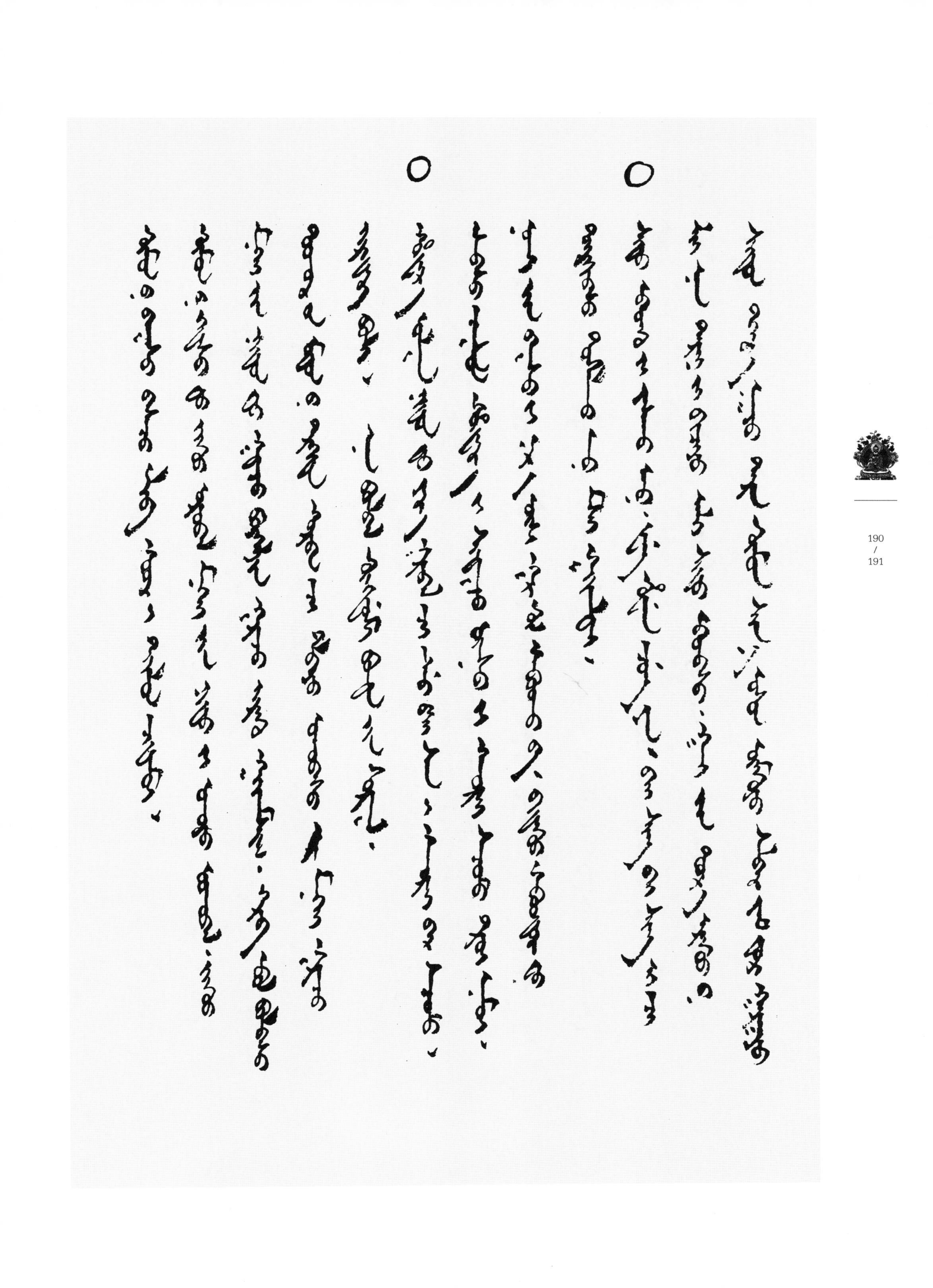

[illegible]

[illegible]

[illegible]

[illegible]

[illegible]

[illegible]

[illegible]

[illegible]

[illegible]

[illegible]

[illegible]

[illegible]

[illegible]

[illegible]

[illegible]

[illegible]

[illegible]

[illegible]

[illegible]

[illegible]

[illegible]

[illegible]

[illegible]

[illegible]

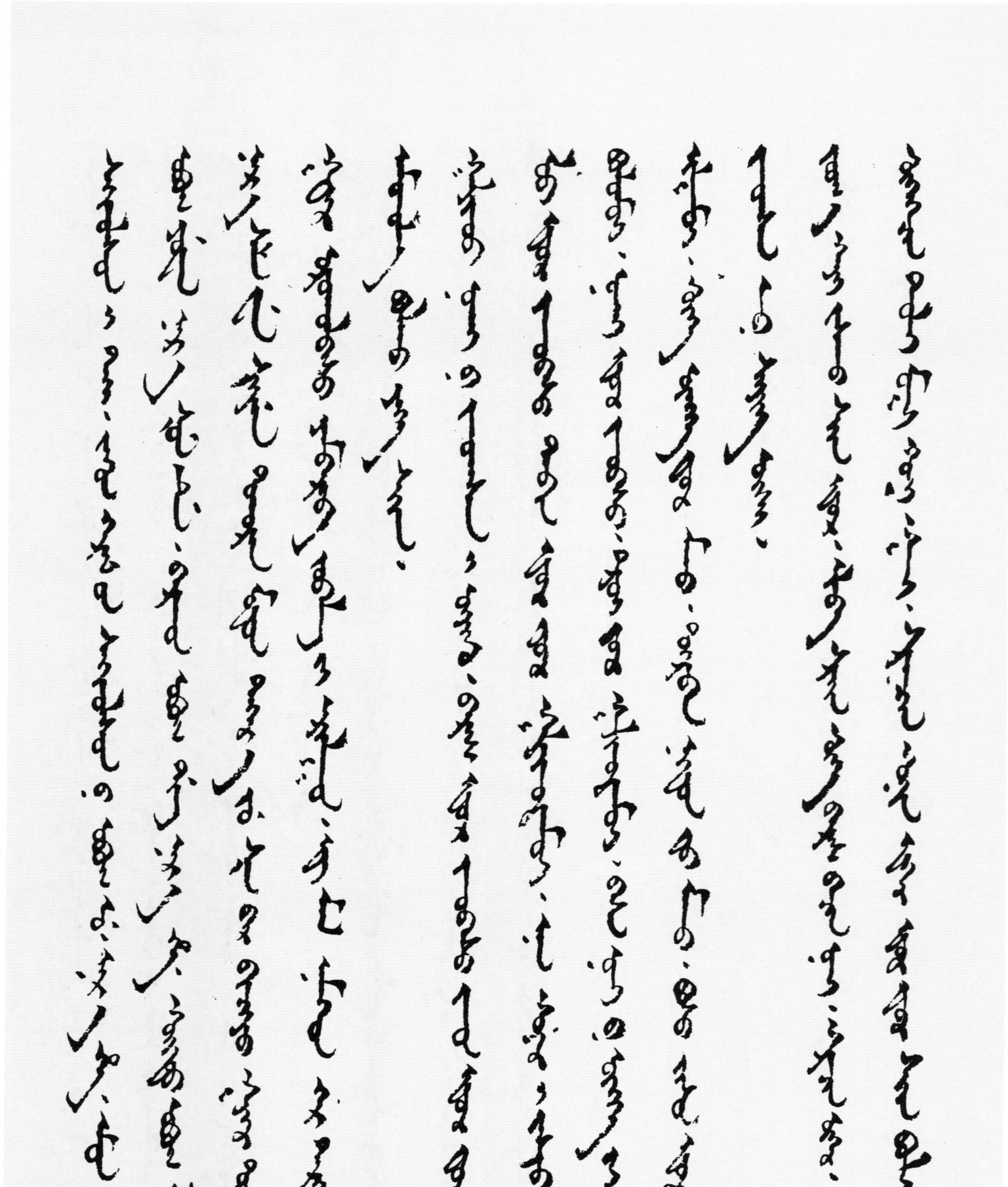

མཚལ་དཀར

[illegible]

མུ་ཏིག [illegible]	མཚུར་ནག [illegible]	རྡོ་ཐལ [illegible]	ཁྲི་མ་མོ [illegible]	རྡོ་ཁབ་ལེན [illegible]	ལྕ་ཁྲི [illegible]
མཚལ་རྡོར [illegible]	མཚུར་དམར [illegible]	ཧ་ཤིག [illegible]	ཐེ་ཚུ [illegible]	ཞིབ་པ་ཕ [illegible]	དངུལ་ཆུ [illegible]
མཚལ་དམར [illegible]	མཚུར་དཀར [illegible]	མར་ག་ཟུར [illegible]	ཕྱུང་རོས [illegible]	ཡ་ཁྲི [illegible]	[illegible]
ཡལ་ག་ཟུར [illegible]	ཚ་ལ [illegible]	ཆུ་སྨན [illegible]	ག་ཟུར [illegible]	མུ་ཟི་གསེར [illegible]	ཀུར་རུ་བི [illegible]
མཚལ་དཀར [illegible]	ཁྲོ་ཆུ [illegible]	འབྲུག་ཐུས [illegible]	ཞེས་དུག [illegible]	ལྷང་ཚེར [illegible]	རྒྱ་སྐྱ་ནག [illegible]

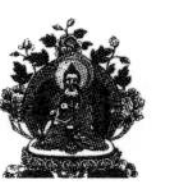

རྒྱ་སྤོས་དཀར	སྣུམ་ཚ	སྤྱ་རར་རྫིག་པ	རྡོར་ལེན	མིང་ཅན་མ་བོ	སྐྱེང་ཁུན
སྤུར་ཚང	སྨུ་ཞི ཐང་ཆུ	སྲེ་རྒྱལ	ཤིང་མངར	ཨ་བི་ཁ	ཚི་སྦྱུམ
སྟོད་ར་དཀར	རྗེ་ཛ	བརྒྱ་འབྲས	ལུང་མ	ཧར་ཀུན	དཔག་ཐོ་སེར་བོ
རྒྱ་མཚོ་སྦུ་བ	ཆུ་སྲིན་ཁྲག	ལ་ཕང	ཤུ་དག ཆུ་དག	ཡ་འཛི	ཀོ་ཁྲེ་ལ
སྤོས་ཤལ	ཏེར་ཚོ	སྐྱི་དྲི	མཛེ་སོ་ཤིང	སྦྲུལ་ཞན་ཤུར	ཚོས་སེར་ཤིང

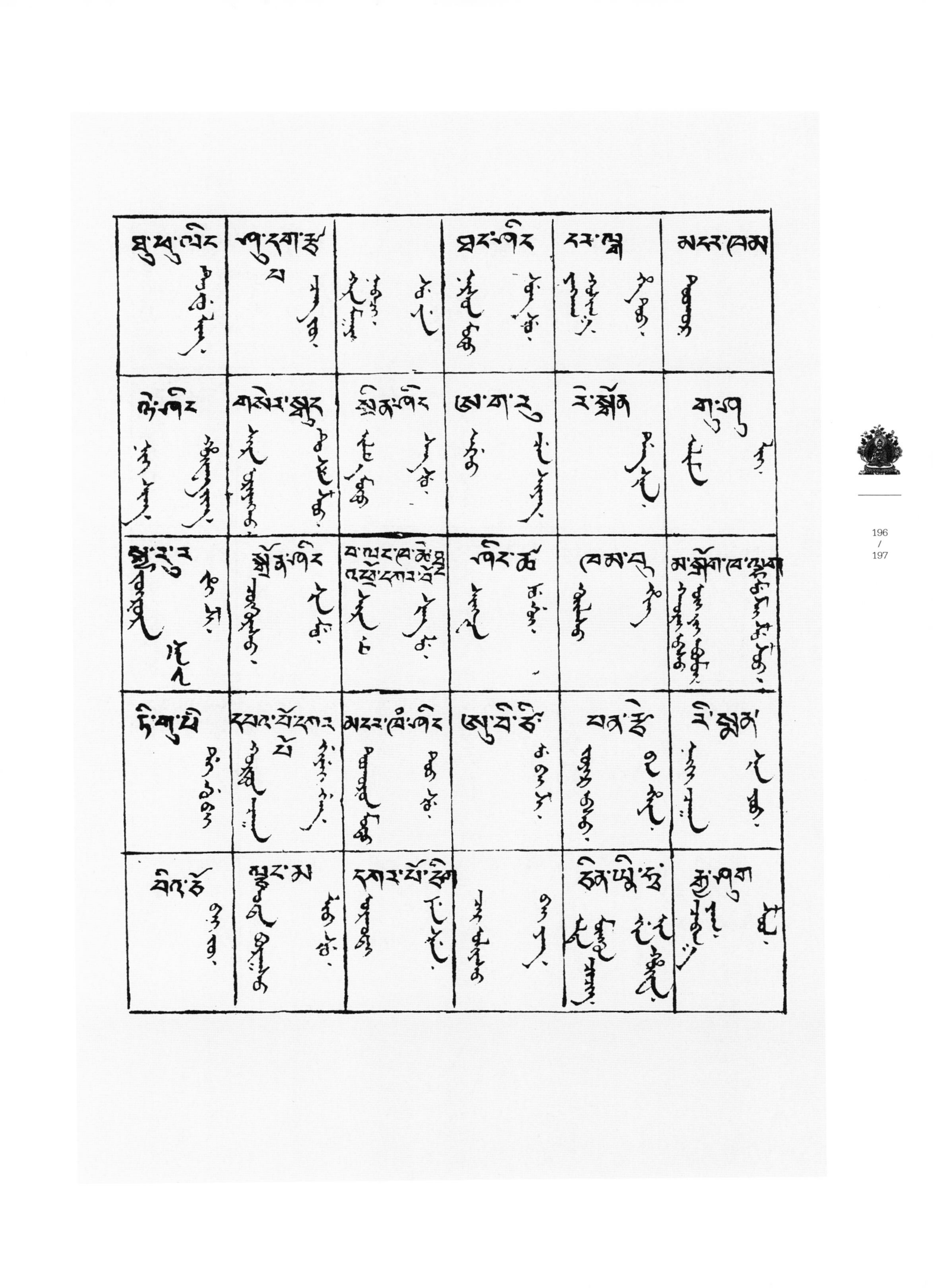

སྤུ་སྤུ་ལིང [illegible]	ཤུ་དག་རྩ་པ [illegible]	[illegible]	ཐང་ཤིང [illegible]	རར་ལྦ [illegible]	མདར་ཁེམ [illegible]
ཅེ་ཤིང [illegible]	གསེར་སྦུར [illegible]	སྨིན་ཤིང [illegible]	ཀྱེ་ག་རུ [illegible]	རེ་སྐོན [illegible]	ག་བུ [illegible]
སྐྱུ་རུ་ར [illegible]	སྨྲིན་ཤིང [illegible]	ཐ་ལྡང་ཁ་མི་ཐུ་འབྲེ་དཀར་ཐྲ [illegible]	ཤིང་ཚ [illegible]	ཁེམ་བུ [illegible]	མ་གྲོག་ཁེ་ལྕམ [illegible]
དི་ག་ཕི [illegible]	དཔའ་བོ་དཀར་པོ [illegible]	མདར་ཁྲེ་ཤིང [illegible]	ཨུ་བི་ཆེ [illegible]	བཙན་རྫེ [illegible]	རི་སྨན [illegible]
བིའུ་ཅོ [illegible]	སྤུར་མ [illegible]	དཀར་པོ་ཆིག [illegible]	[illegible]	ཙན་ཡུ་ཚ [illegible]	ཀྱི་ཤུག [illegible]

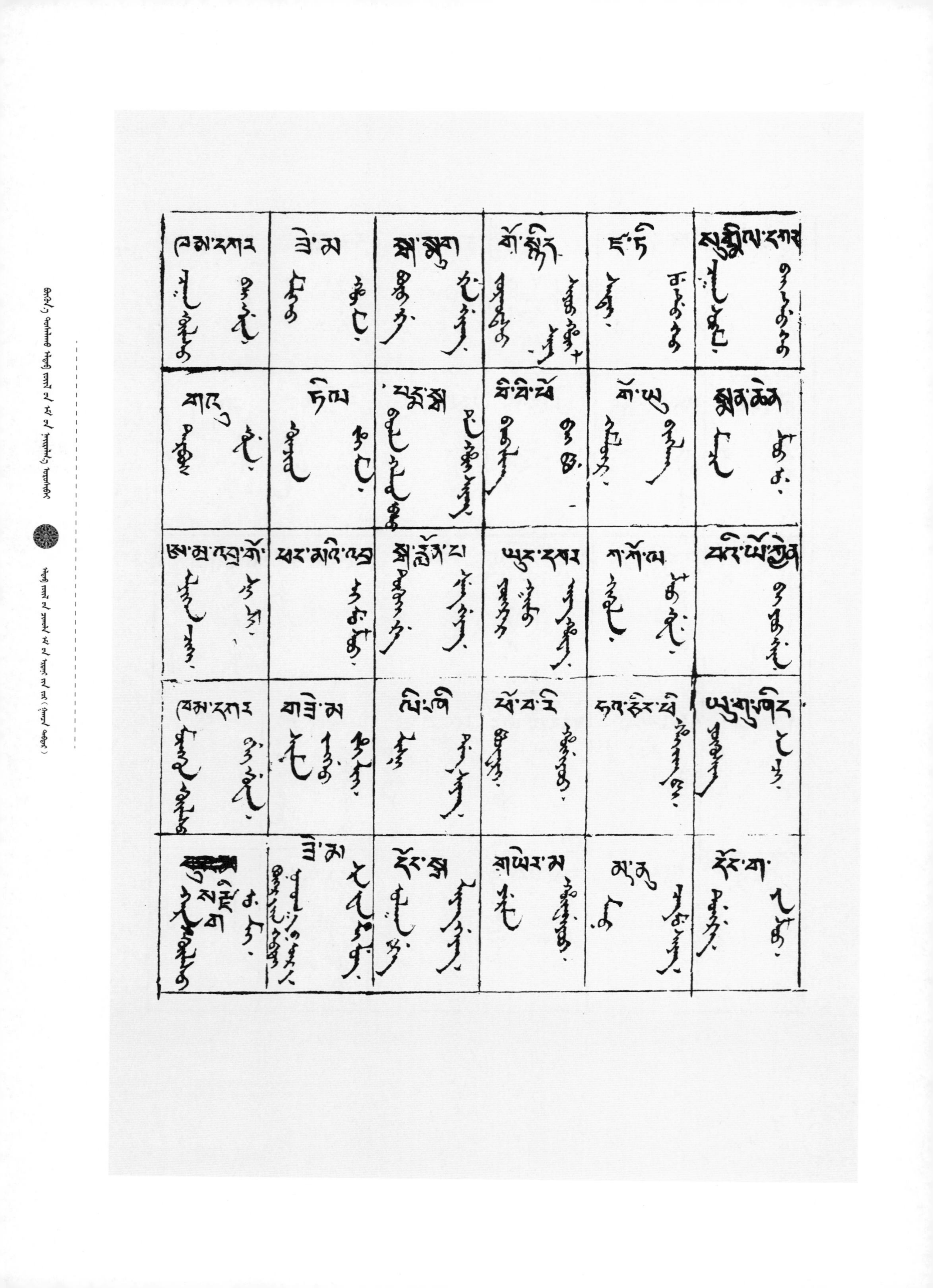

ཁམ་དཀར [illegible]	ཟེ་མ [illegible]	སྐྱ་སྐྱུག [illegible]	བོ་སྙིད [illegible]	ཛ་ཏི [illegible]	སུགྨེལ་དཀར [illegible]
ཀ་ཀོ [illegible]	ཏིལ [illegible]	ཙ་དུ་སྐྱ [illegible]	ཤི་ཕི་ཤོ [illegible]	ཀོ་ལ [illegible]	སྨན་ཆེན [illegible]
ཨ་ཤུ་འབྲུ་ཀོ [illegible]	ཕར་མའི་འབྲུ [illegible]	སྐྱ་རྩོད་པ [illegible]	ཡུར་དམར [illegible]	ཀ་ཀོ་ལ [illegible]	ཕར་ཡོ་གྲིན [illegible]
ཁེམ་དཀར [illegible]	གཟེ་མ [illegible]	ལི་ཤི [illegible]	ཕོ་བ་རི [illegible]	ཏག་ཆེར་བི [illegible]	ཡུ་གུ་ཤིང [illegible]
[illegible]	ཟེ་མ [illegible]	རྡོར་སྐྱ [illegible]	གཡེར་མ [illegible]	མ་ནུ [illegible]	རྡོར་ག [illegible]

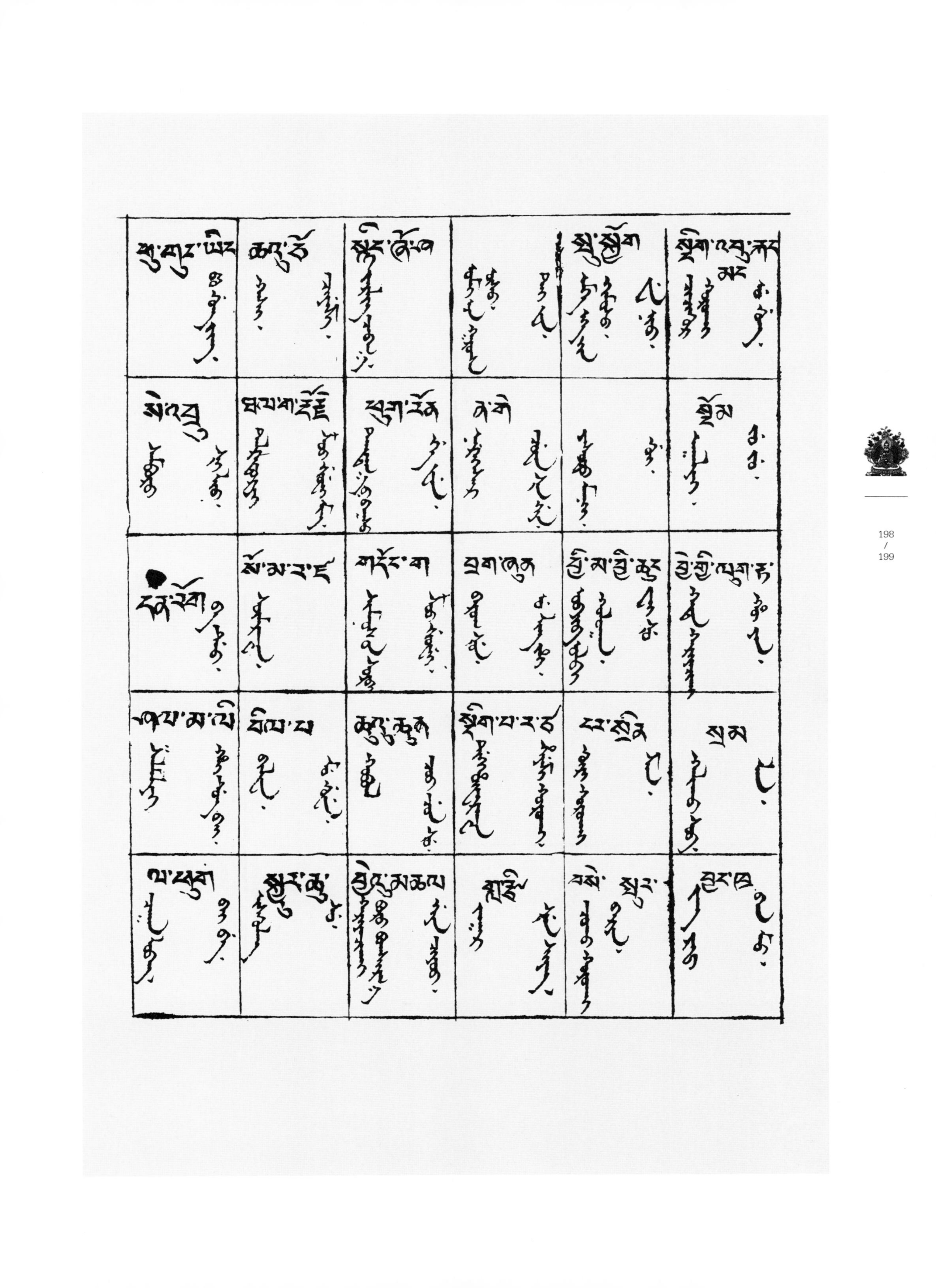

ཤུ་ཀུར་ཡིར [illegible]	ཆའུ་ཙེ [illegible]	སྙིང་ཞེ་བ [illegible]	[illegible]	སྤུ་སྒྲིག [illegible]	སྦྲིག་འབུ་ཁབ་མང [illegible]
མི་འབྲུ [illegible]	ཕལ་པག་ཧྲེ་ཧྲི [illegible]	སྤུག་རྩེན [illegible]	ཤ་ཁ [illegible]	[illegible]	སྒོམ [illegible]
དེའུ་རྩེག [illegible]	སོ་མ་ར་ཛ [illegible]	གདོང་ག [illegible]	བྲག་ཞུན [illegible]	བྱི་ས་བྱི་ཚུར [illegible]	བྱི་བྱི་ལུག་ཧ [illegible]
ཤལ་མ་ལི [illegible]	ཐིལ་བ [illegible]	ཆུ་རྒྱུན [illegible]	སྦྲིག་པ་ར་ཙ [illegible]	ངར་སྲིན [illegible]	སྤྲམ [illegible]
ལ་ཕུག [illegible]	སྨྱུག་ཆུ [illegible]	བྱེའུ་མཆལ [illegible]	སྐྱི་རྩི [illegible]	བསེ་སྤུར [illegible]	བྱིར་ཁྲ [illegible]

སྐྱལ་ཡ

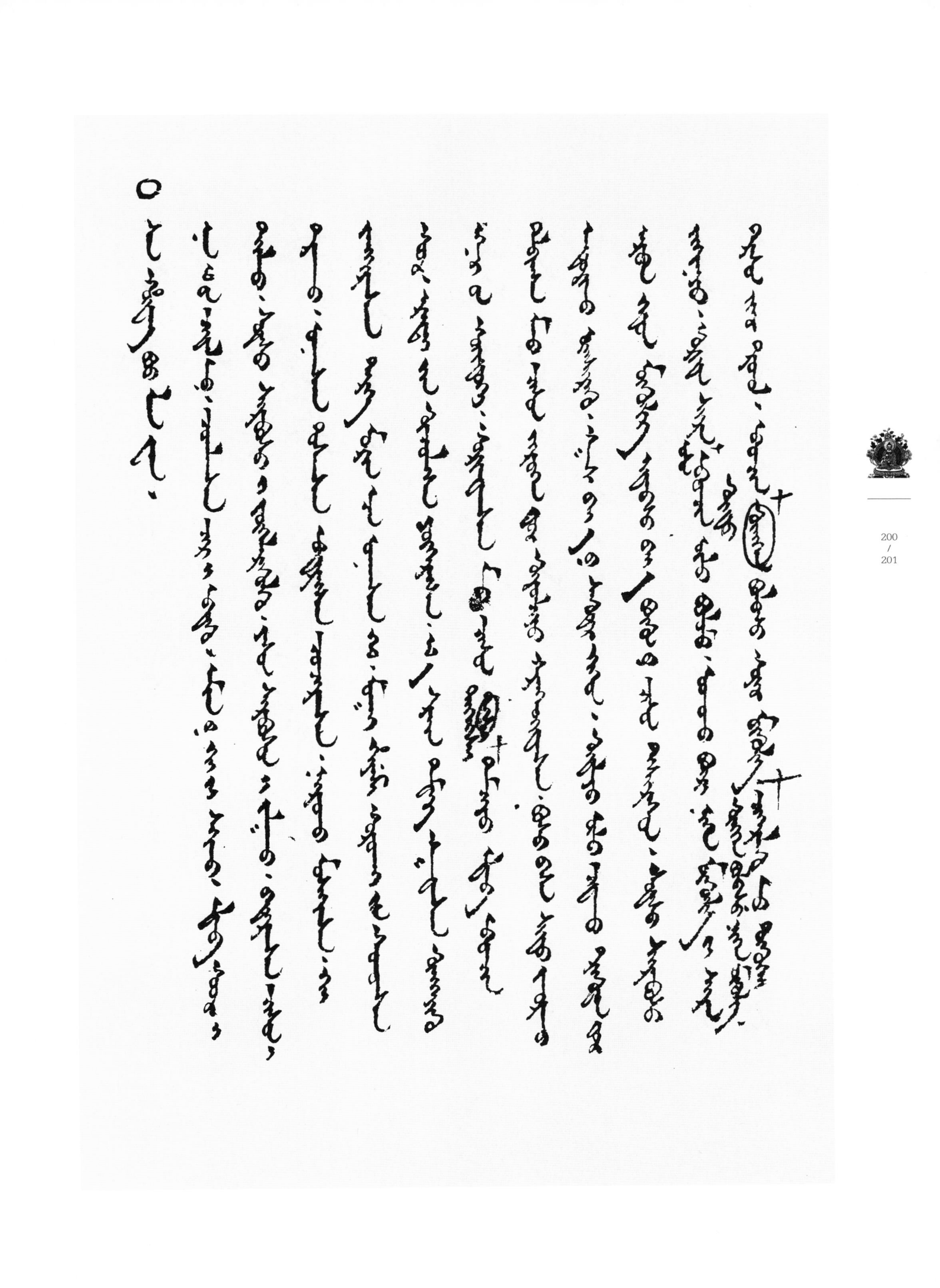

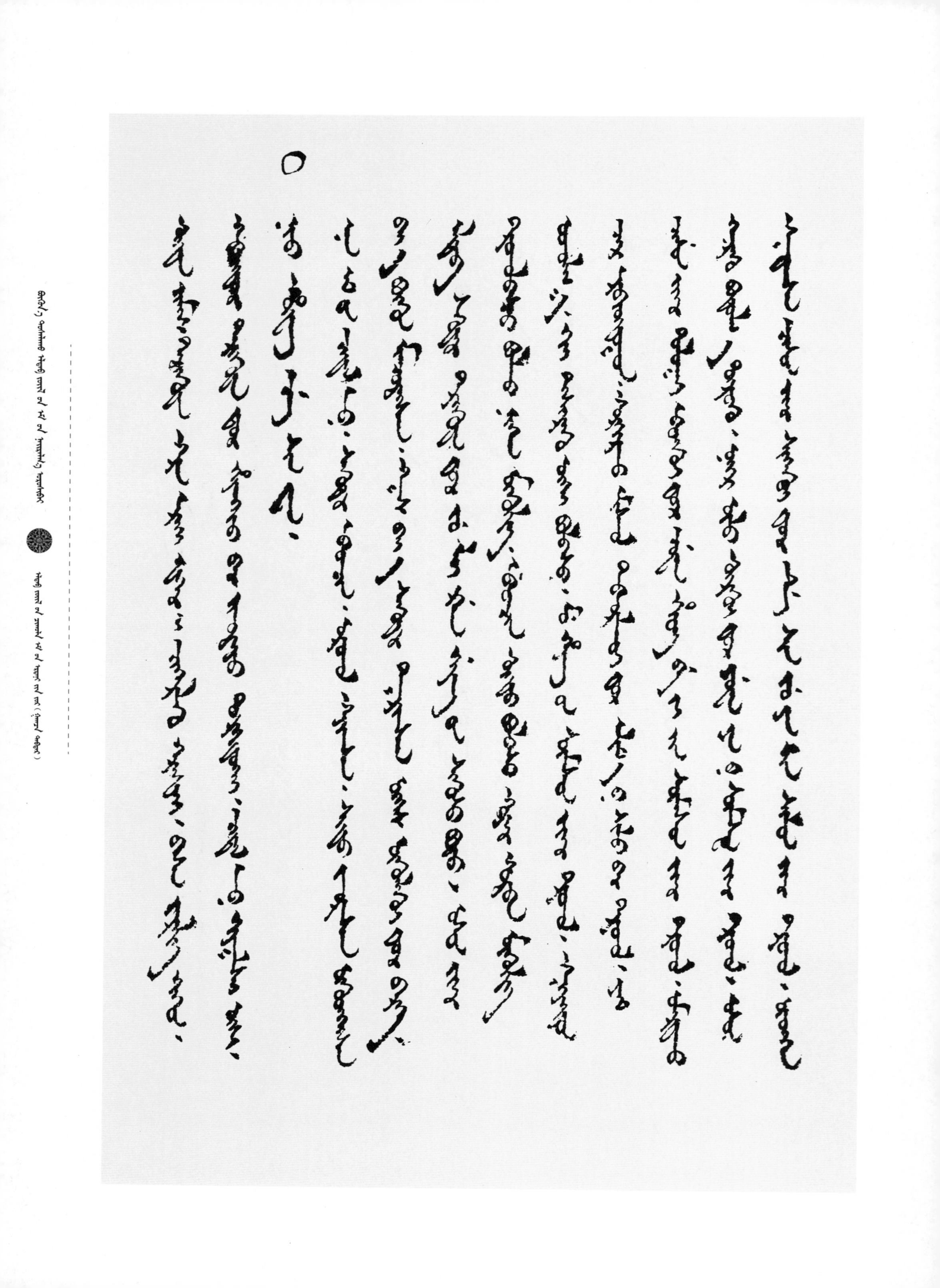

[illegible]

[illegible]

[illegible]

[illegible]

[illegible]

[illegible]

[illegible]

[illegible]

[illegible]

[illegible]

[illegible]

[illegible]

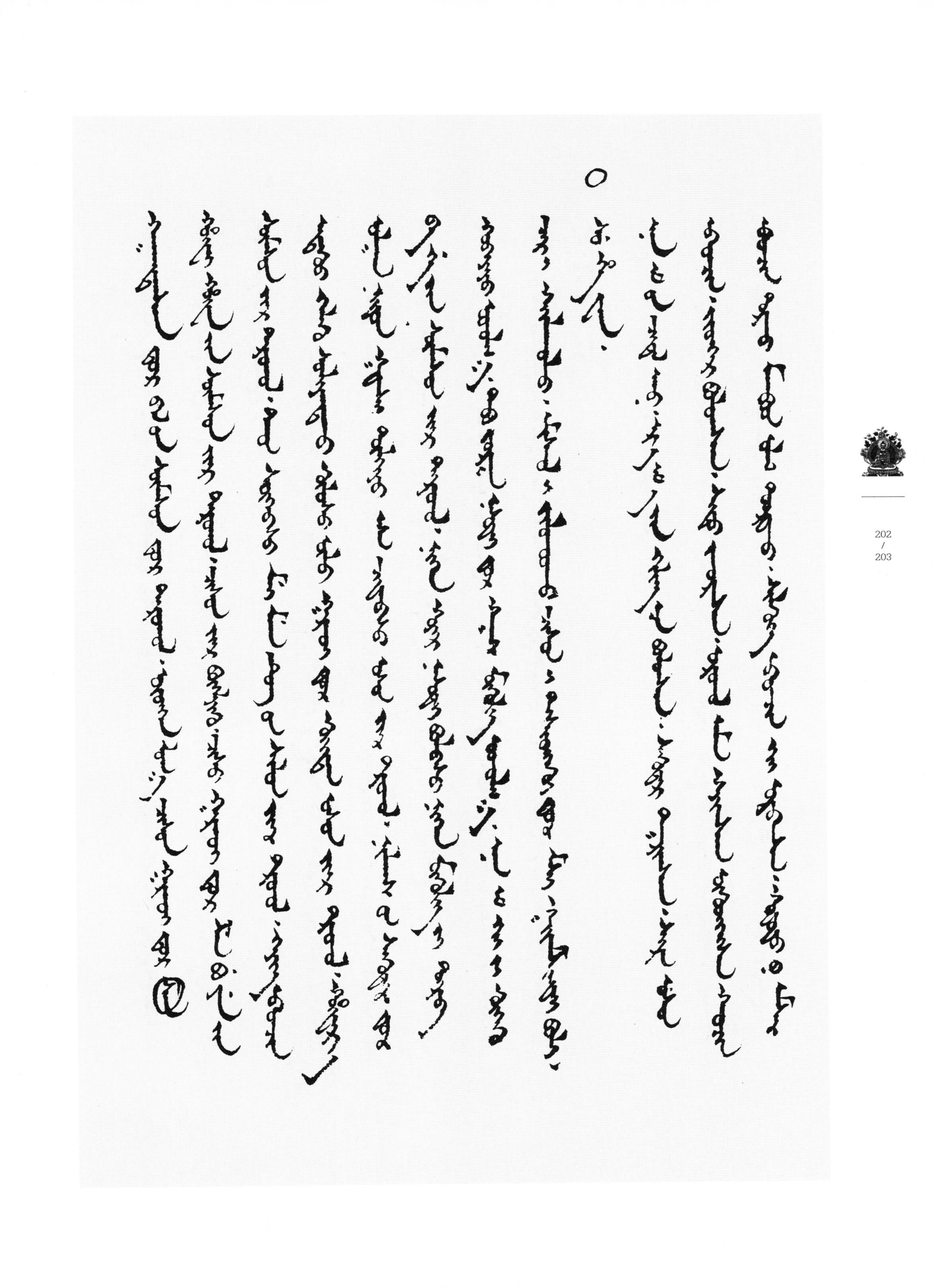

[illegible]

[illegible]

[illegible]

[illegible]

[illegible]

[illegible]

[illegible]

[illegible]

[illegible]

[illegible]

[illegible]

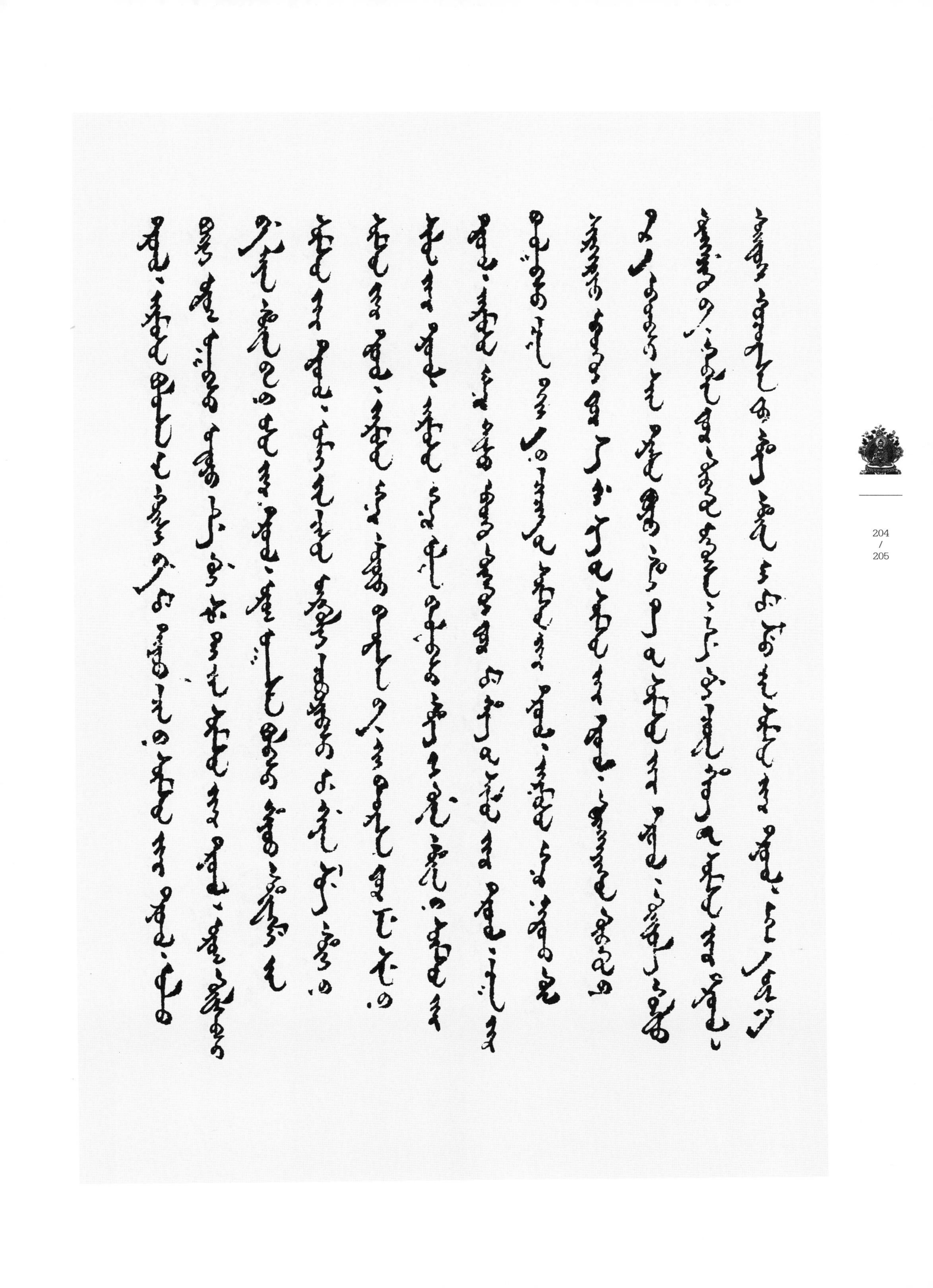

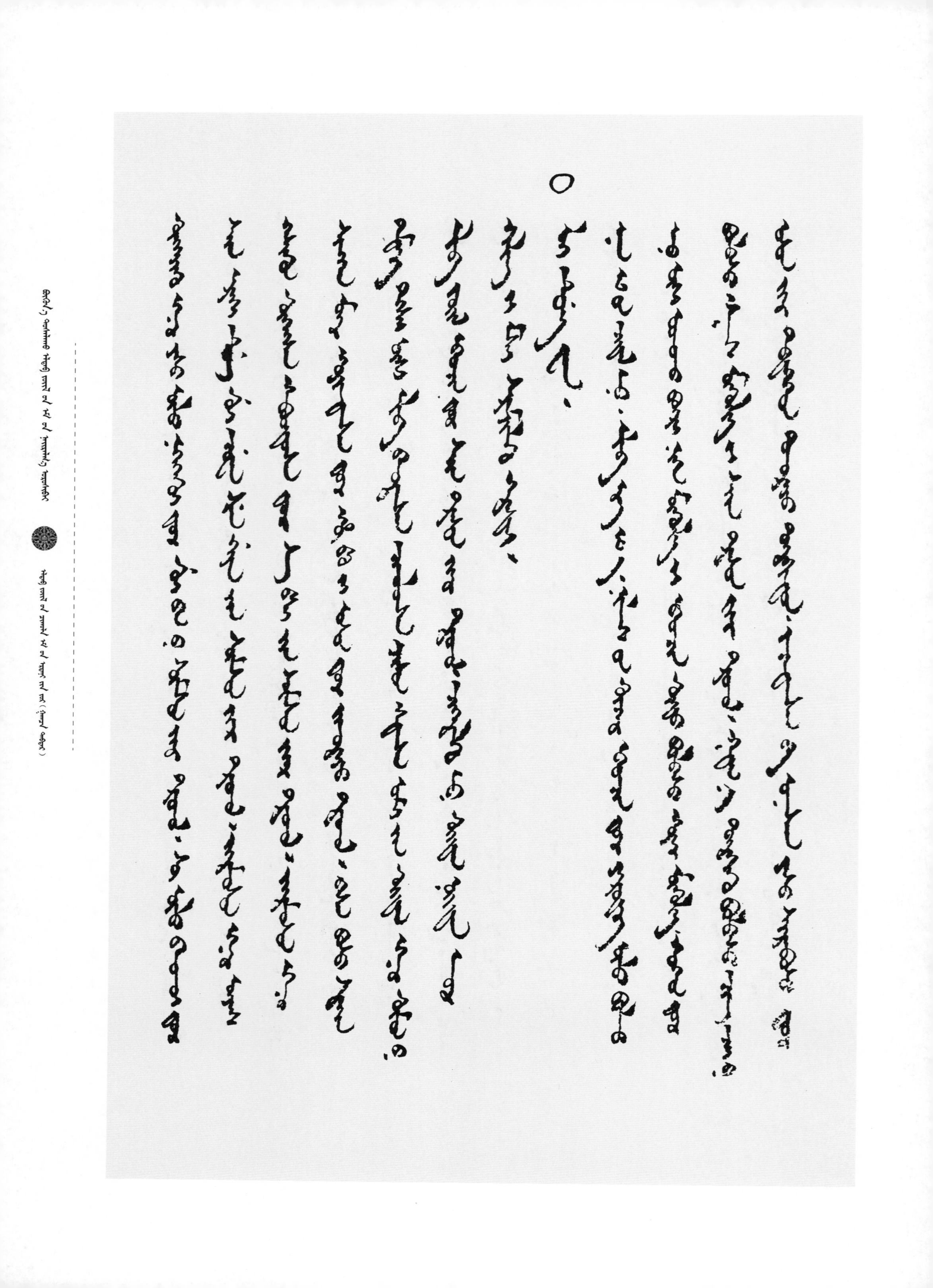

[illegible]

○ [illegible]

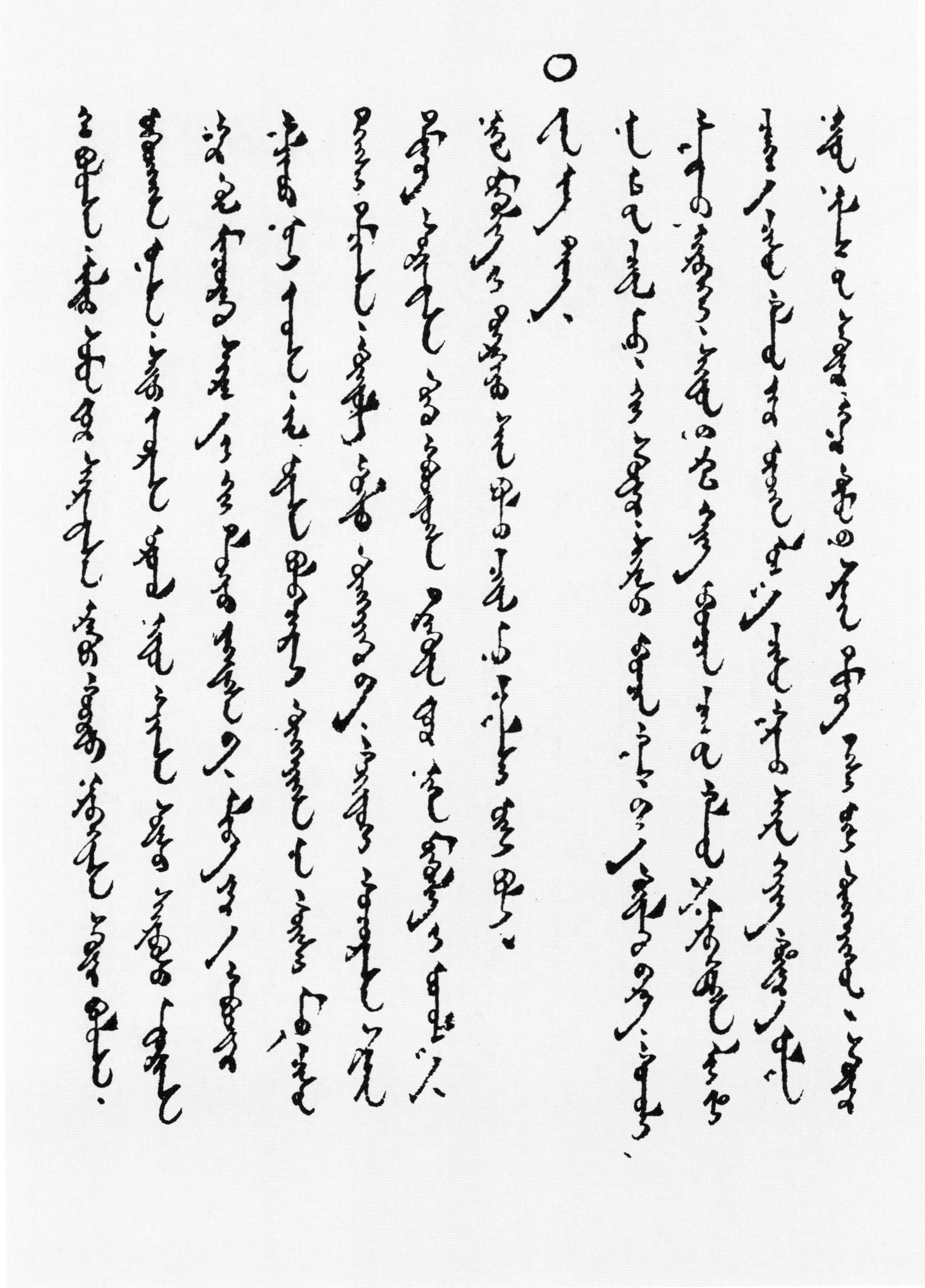

○

[illegible]

[illegible]

[illegible]

[illegible]

[illegible]

[illegible]

[illegible]

[illegible]

[illegible]

[illegible]

[illegible]

[illegible]

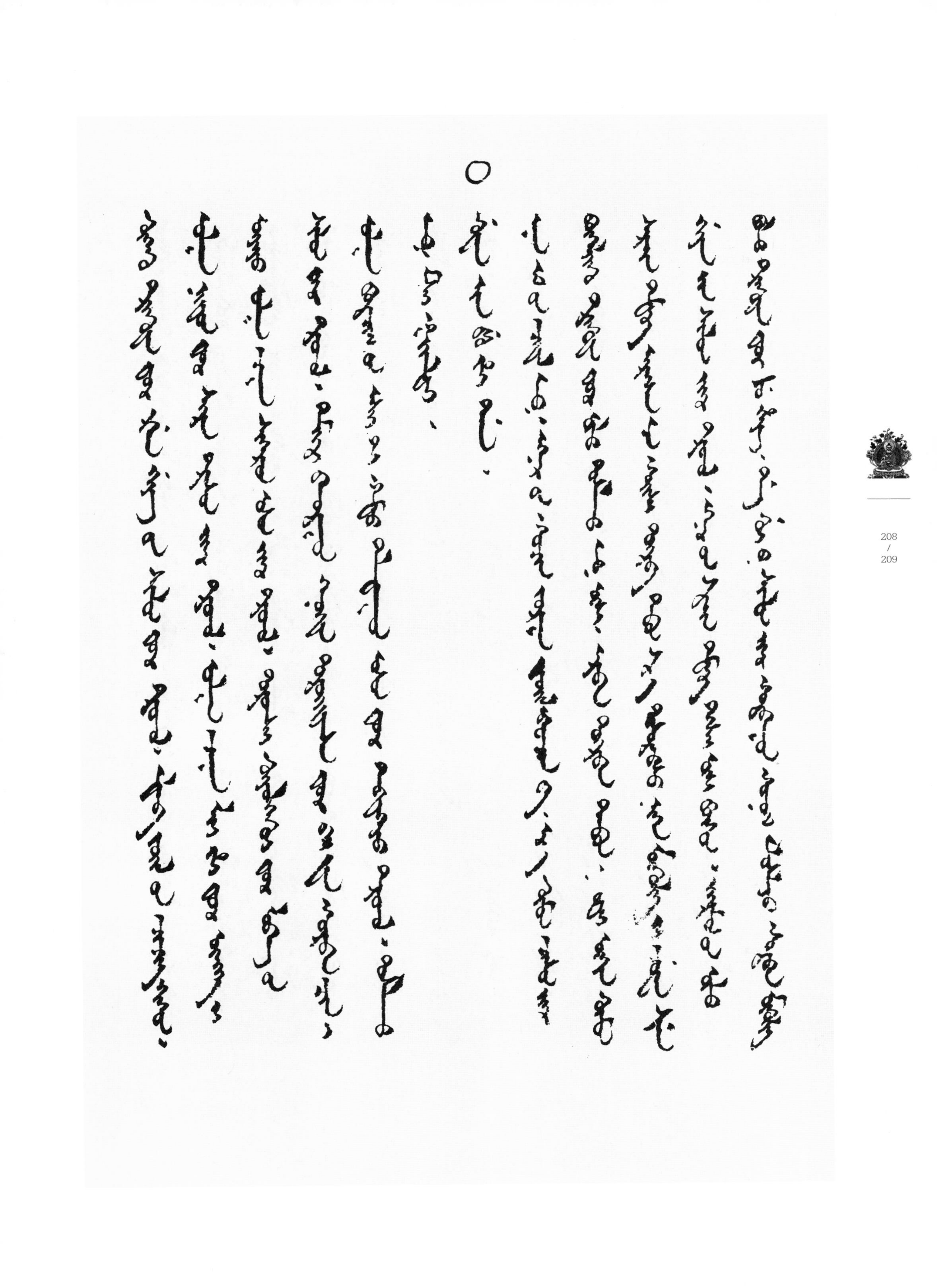

[illegible]

[illegible]

[illegible]

[illegible]

[illegible]

[illegible]

[illegible]

[illegible]

[illegible]

[illegible]

[illegible]

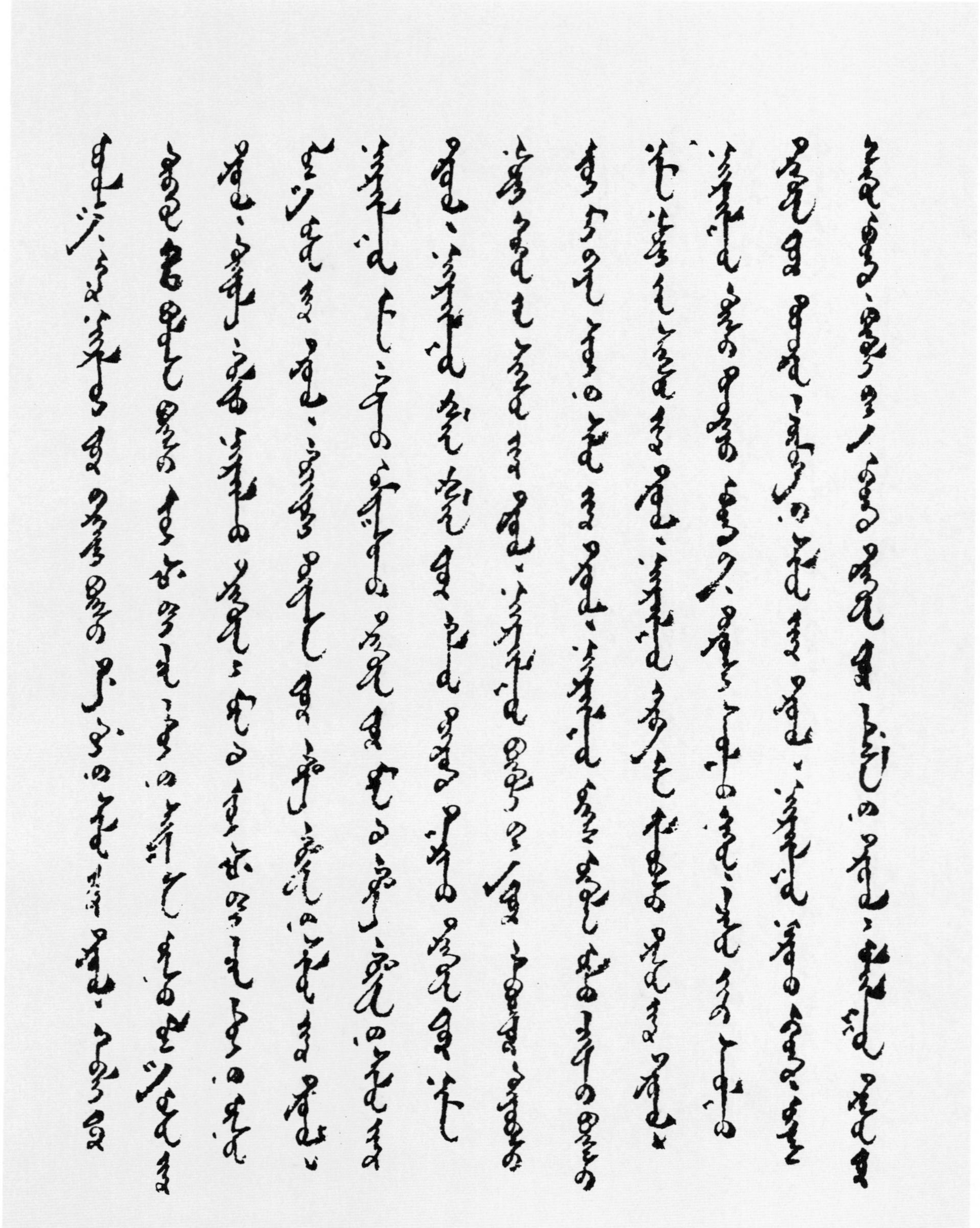

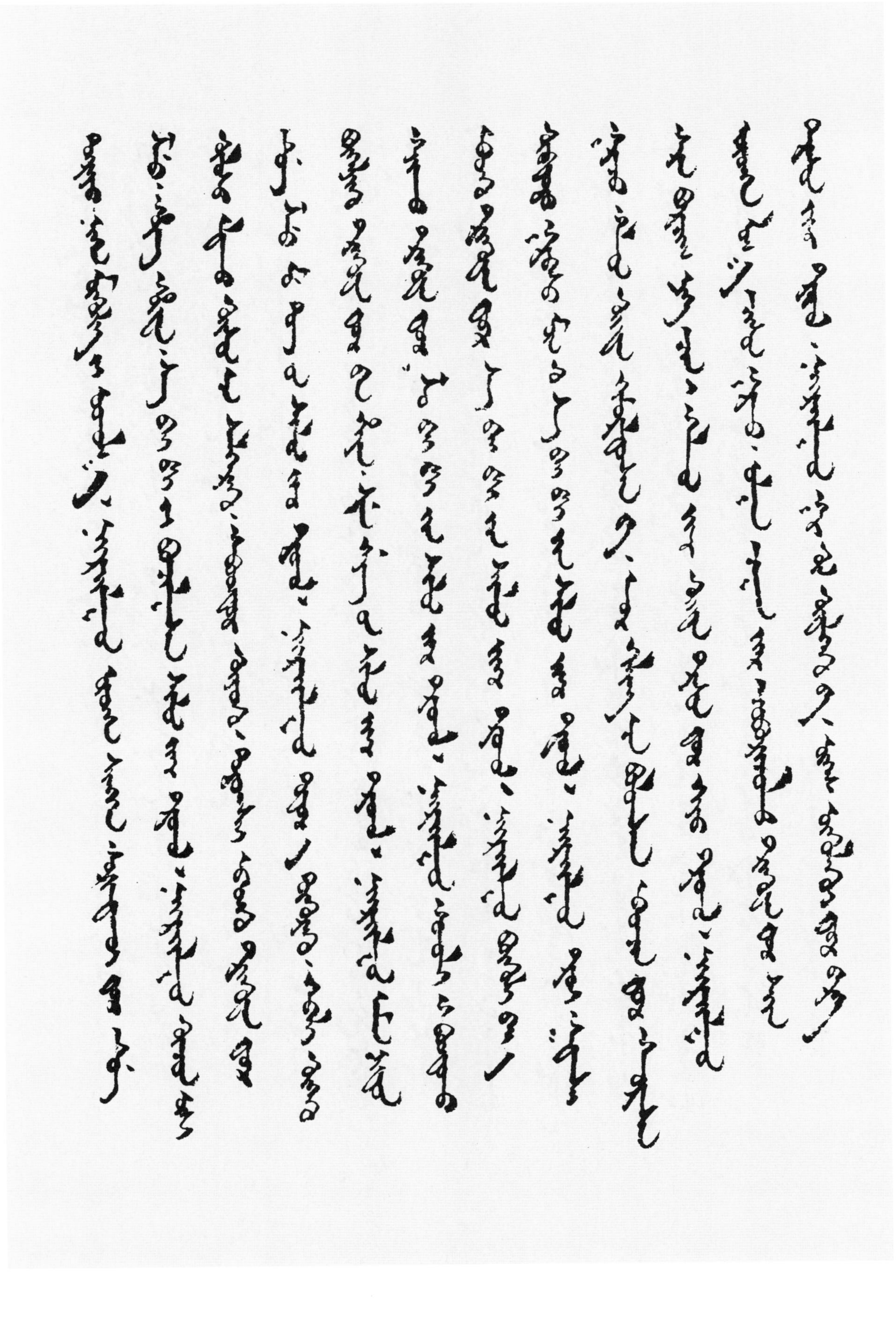

[illegible]
[illegible]
[illegible]
[illegible]
[illegible]
[illegible]
[illegible]
[illegible]
[illegible]
[illegible]
[illegible]
[illegible]
[illegible]

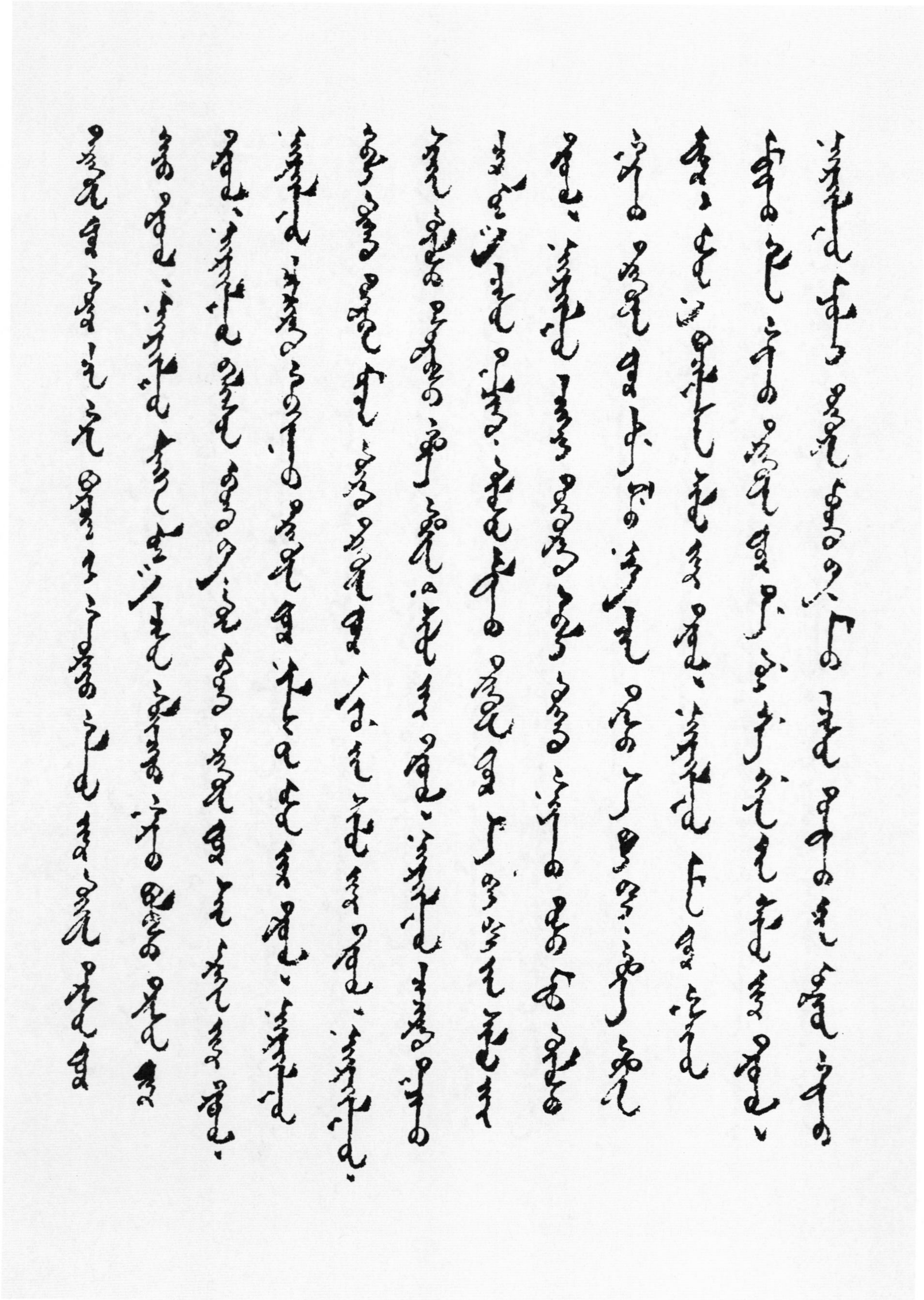

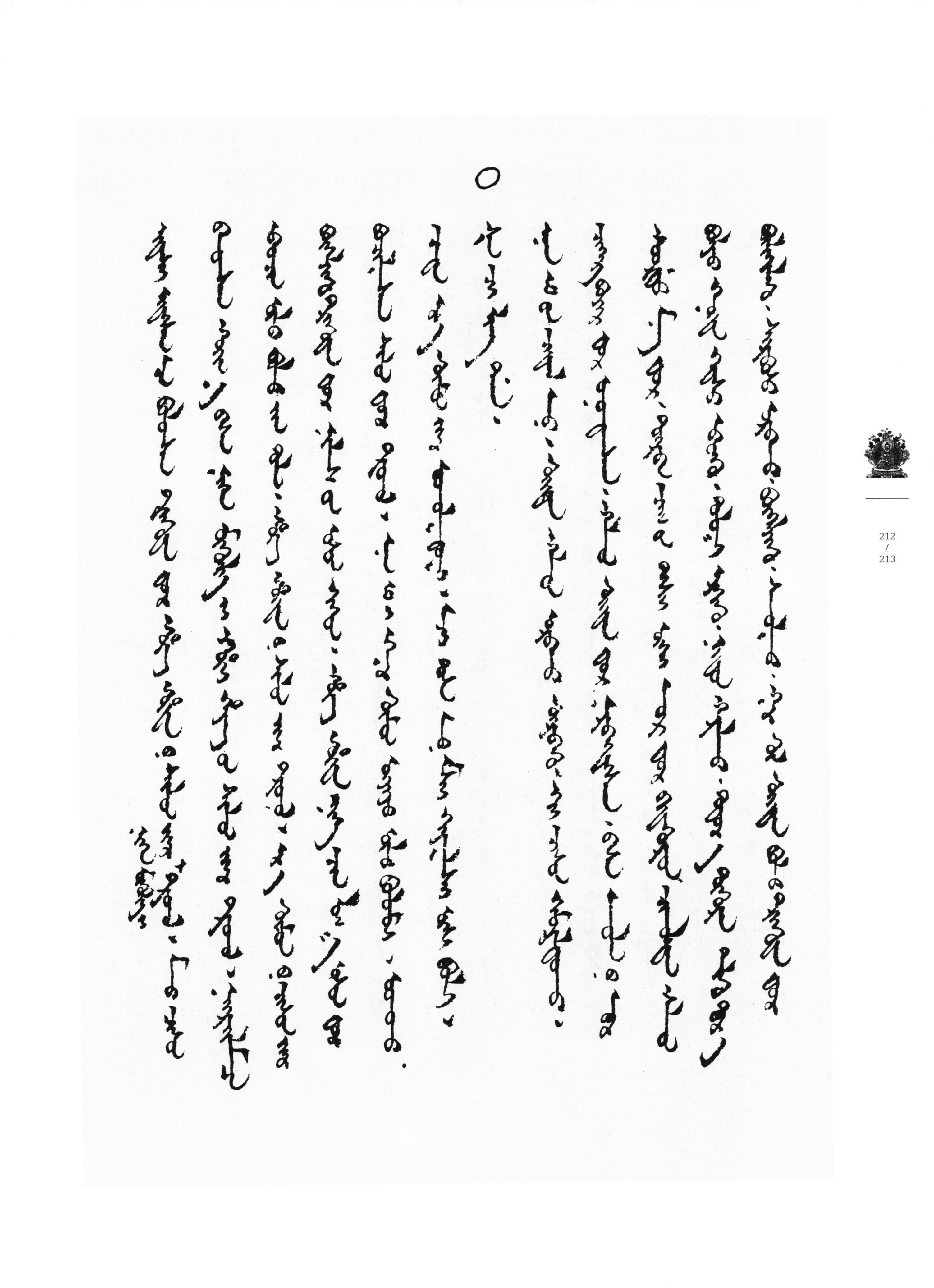

○

[illegible]

[illegible]

[illegible]

[illegible]

[illegible]

[illegible]

[illegible]

[illegible]

[illegible]

[illegible]

[illegible]

[illegible]

[illegible]

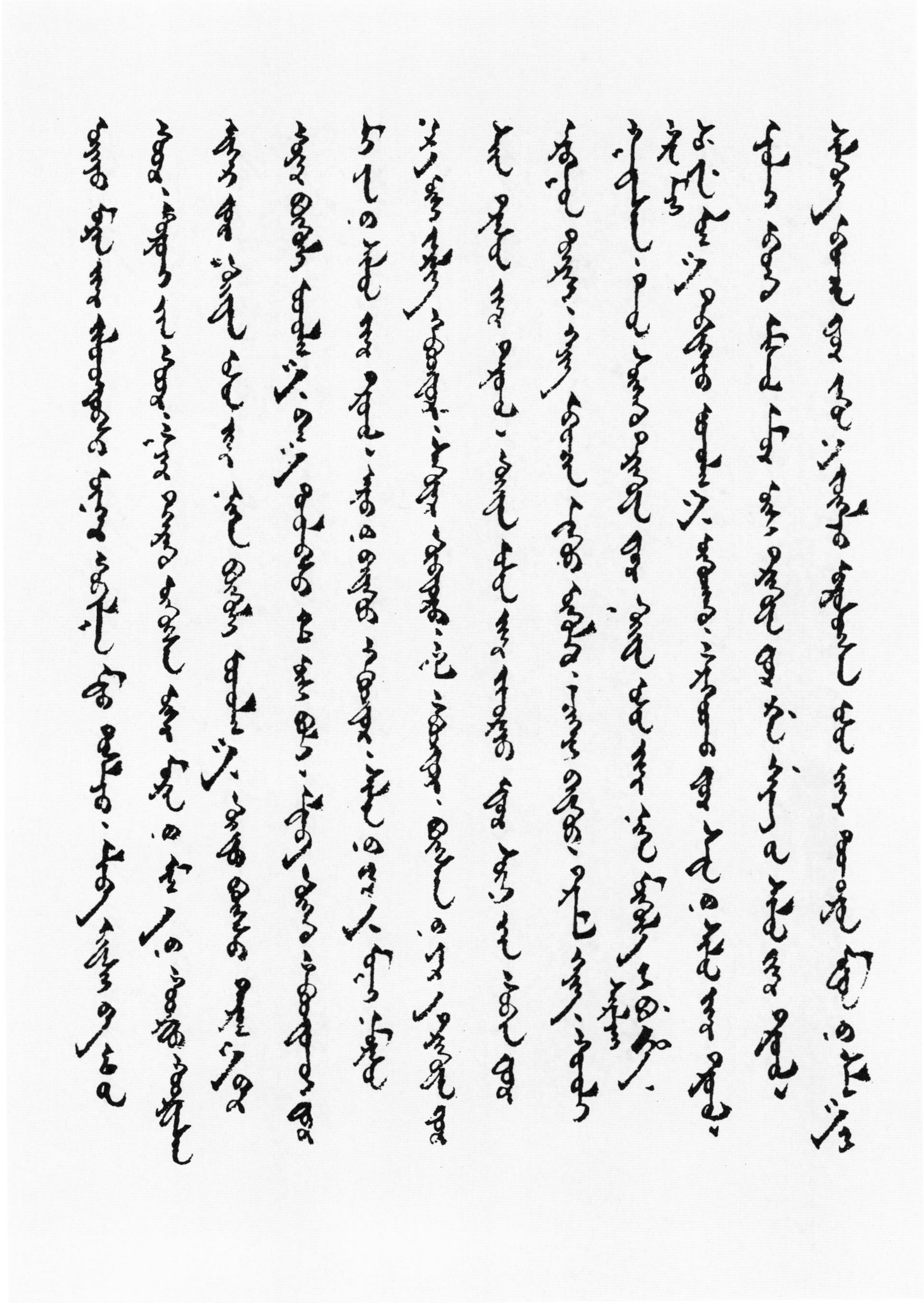

[illegible]

[illegible]

[illegible]

[illegible]

[illegible]

[illegible]

[illegible]

[illegible]

[illegible]

[illegible]

[illegible]

[illegible]

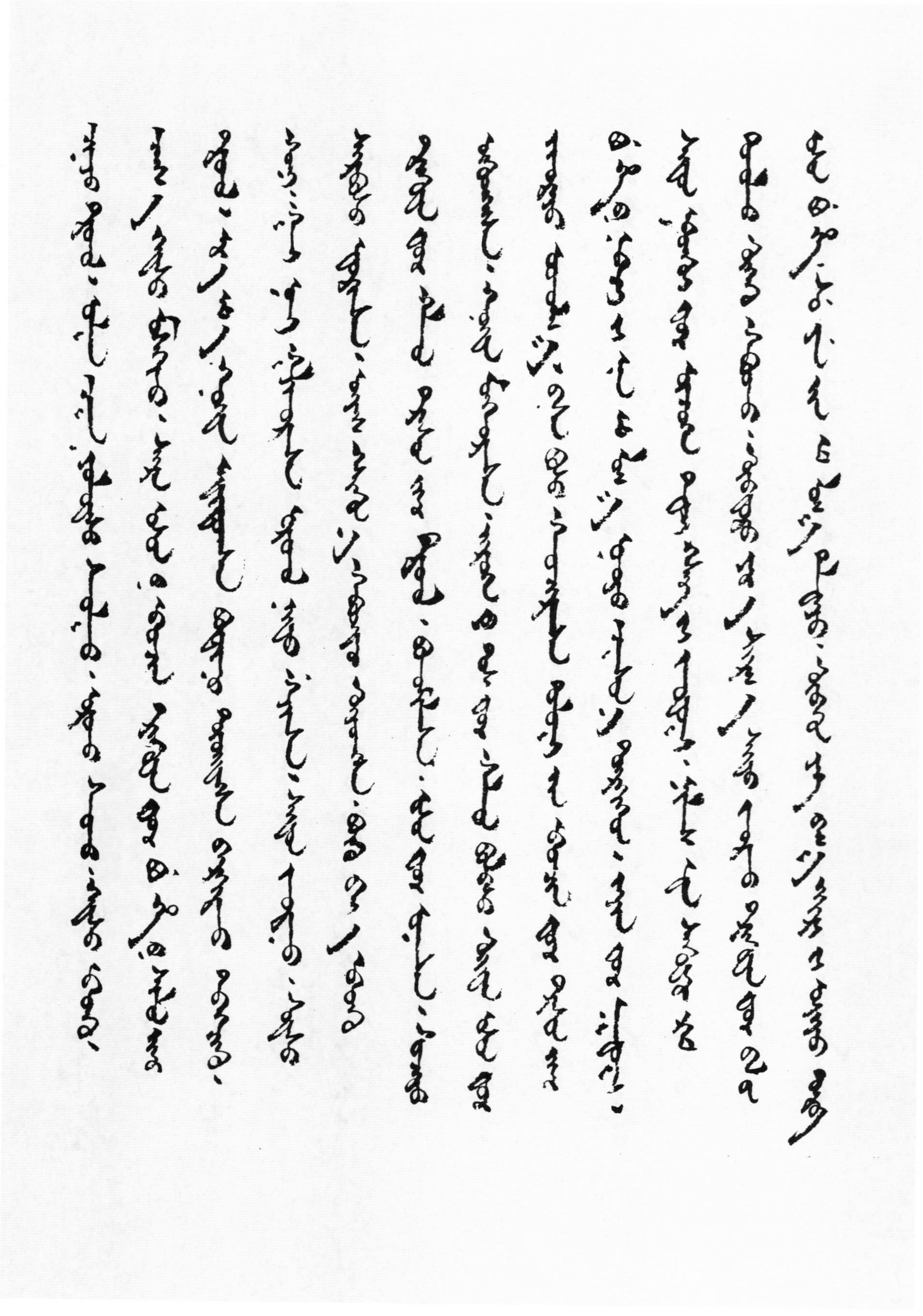

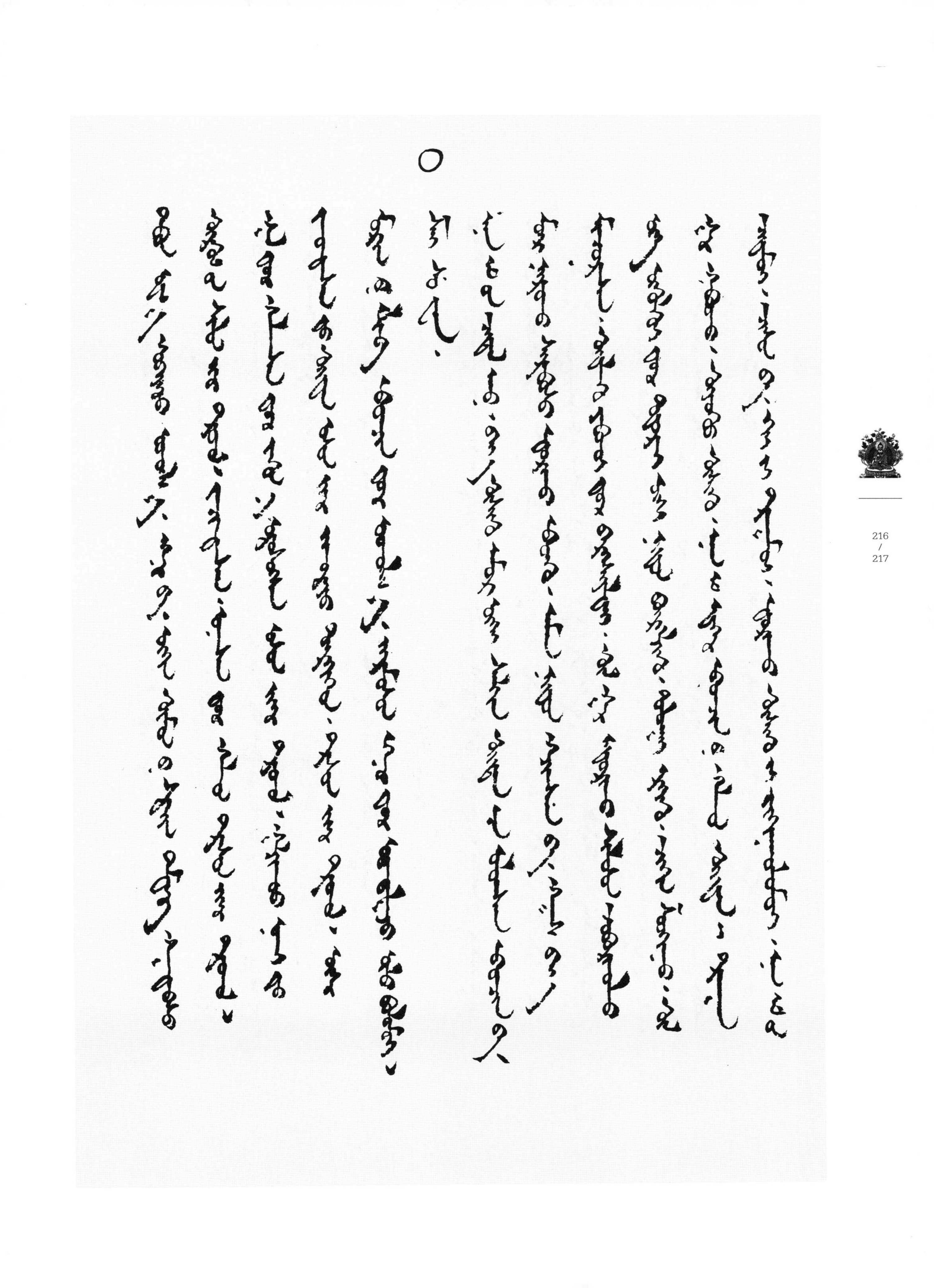

○

[illegible]

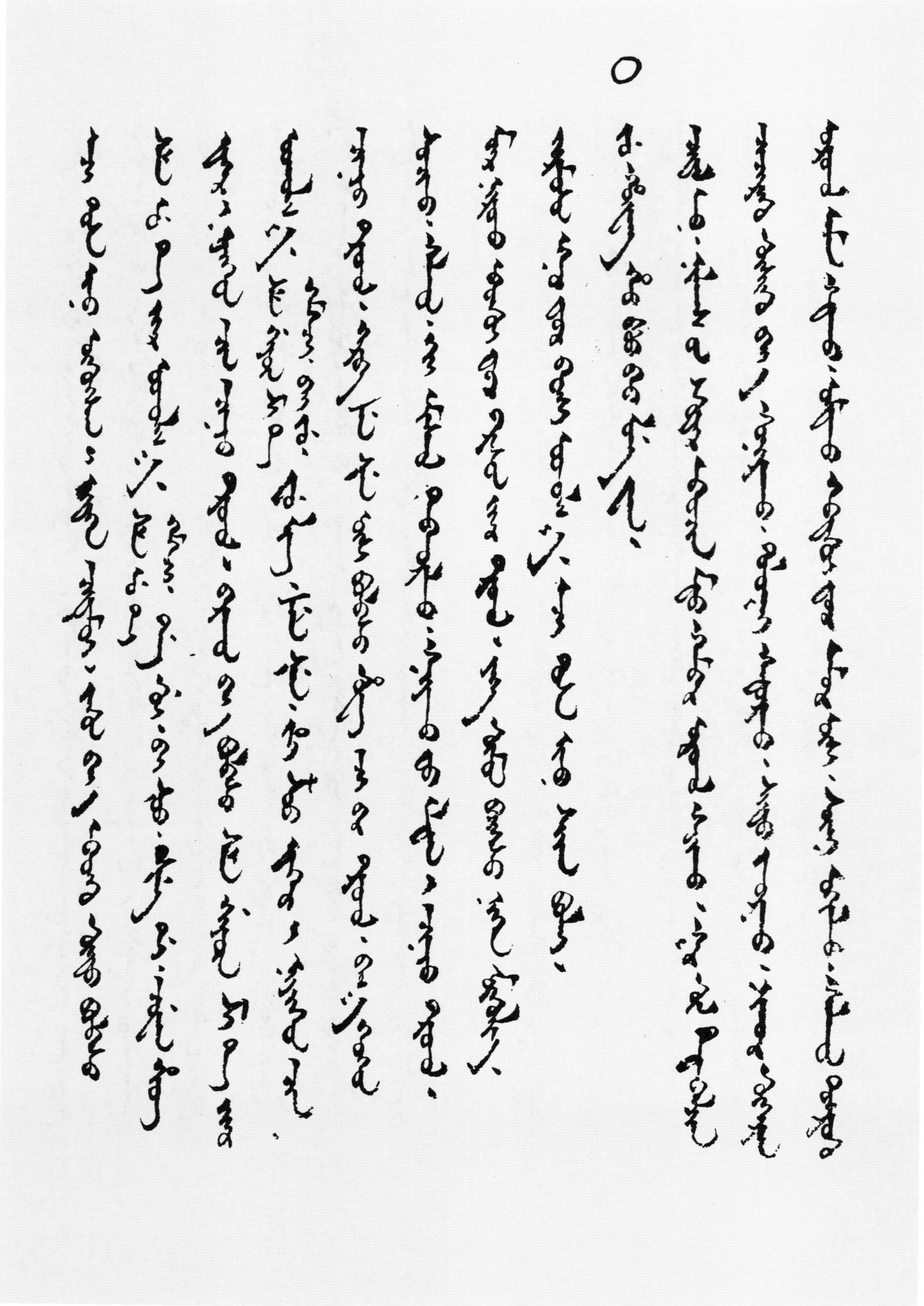

[illegible]

[illegible]

[illegible]

[illegible]

[illegible]

[illegible]

[illegible]

[illegible]

[illegible]

[illegible]

[illegible]

[illegible]

[illegible]

[illegible]

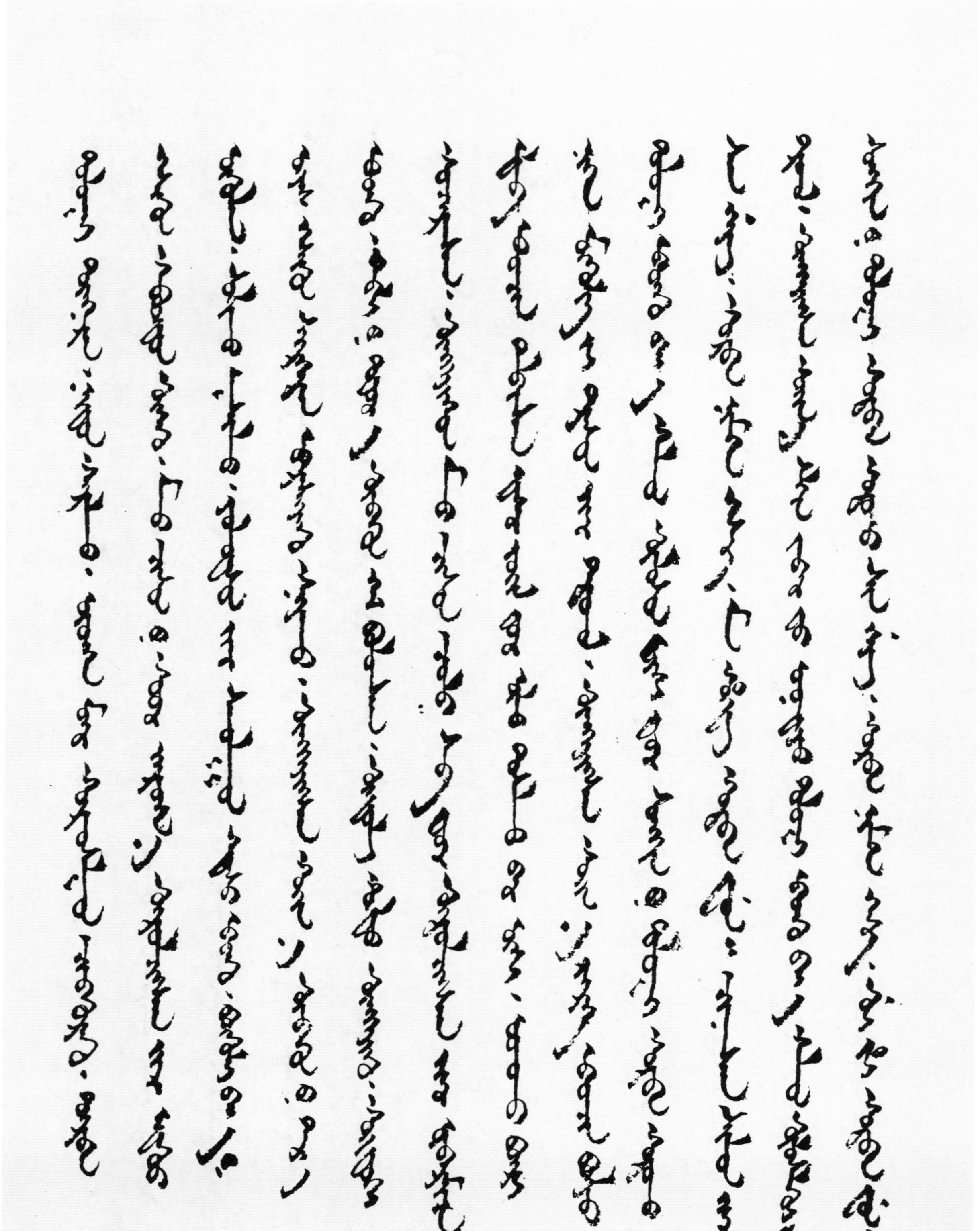

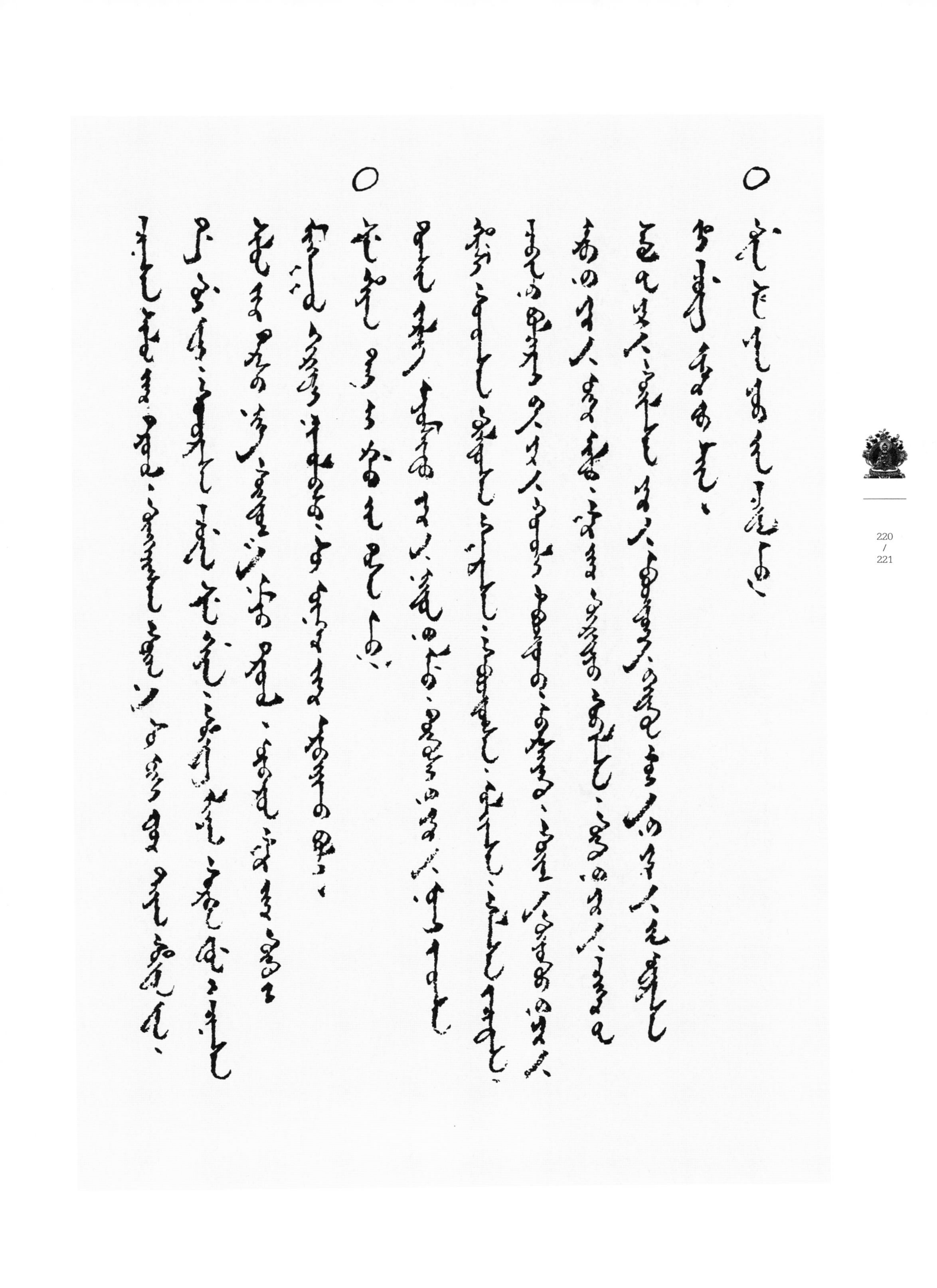

[illegible]

○ [illegible]

[illegible]

[illegible]

[illegible]

[illegible]

[illegible]

○ [illegible]

[illegible]

[illegible]

[illegible]

[illegible]

[illegible]

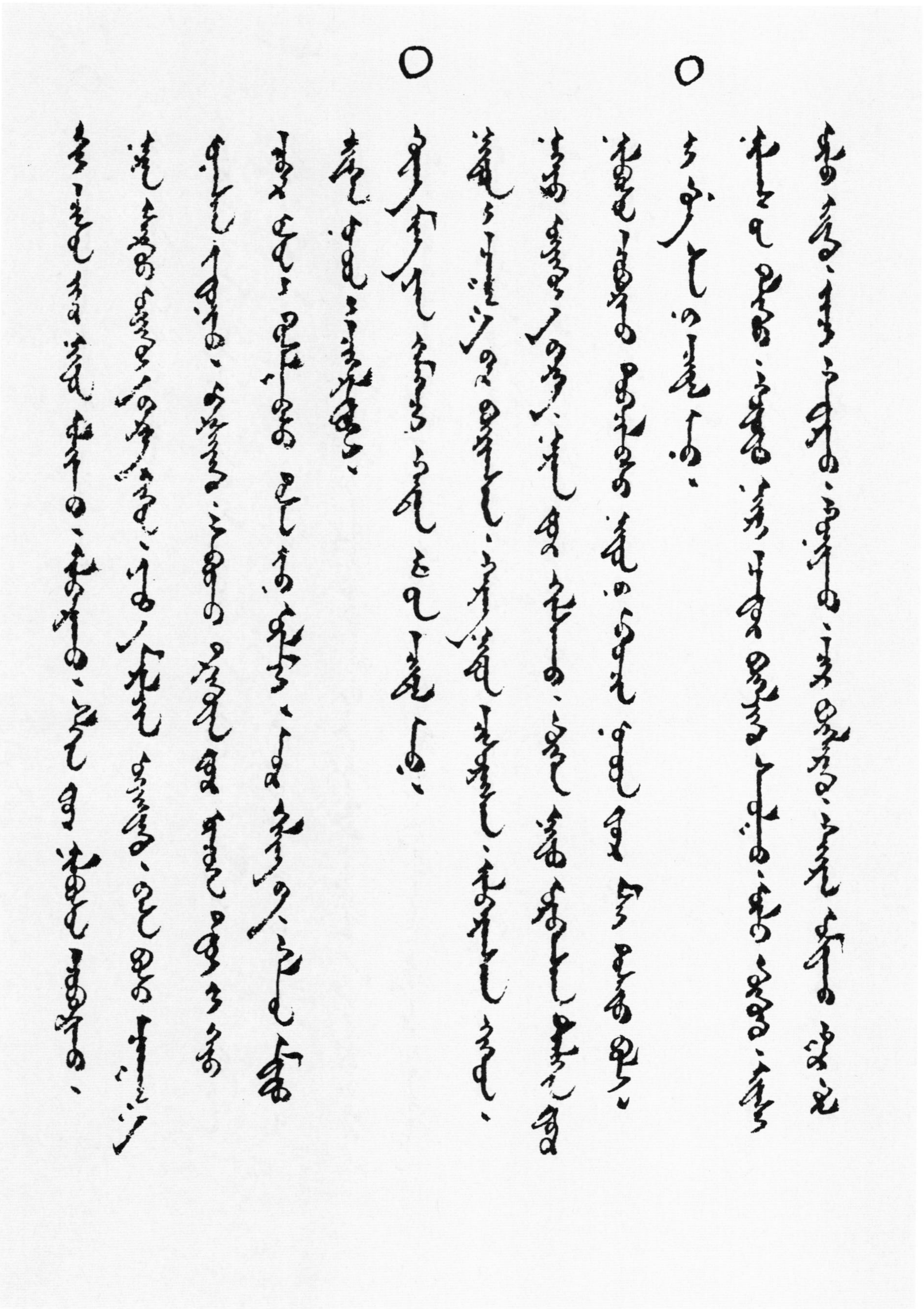

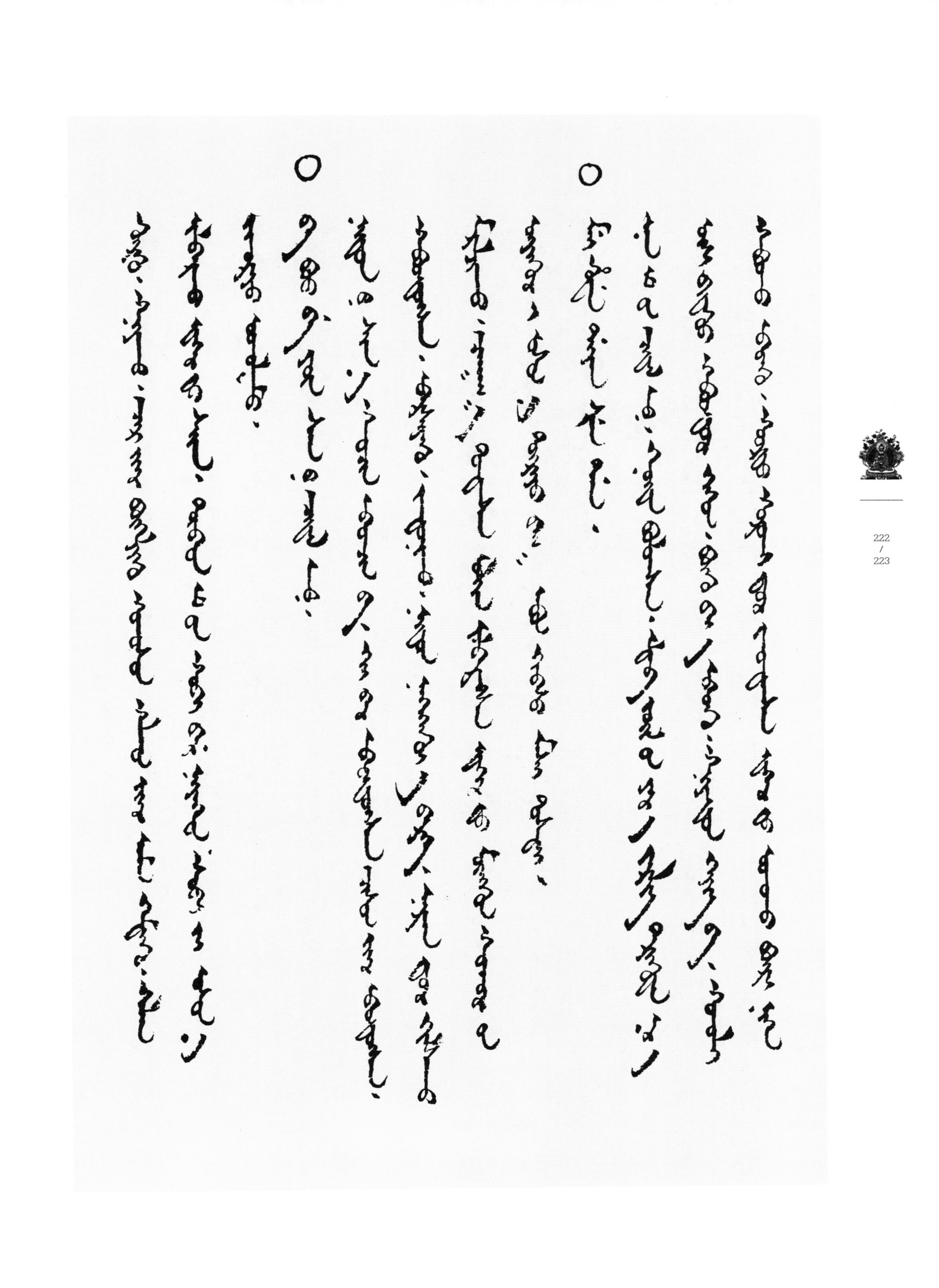

[illegible]

[illegible]

[illegible]

○ [illegible]

[illegible]

[illegible]

[illegible]

[illegible]

[illegible]

[illegible]

[illegible]

[illegible]

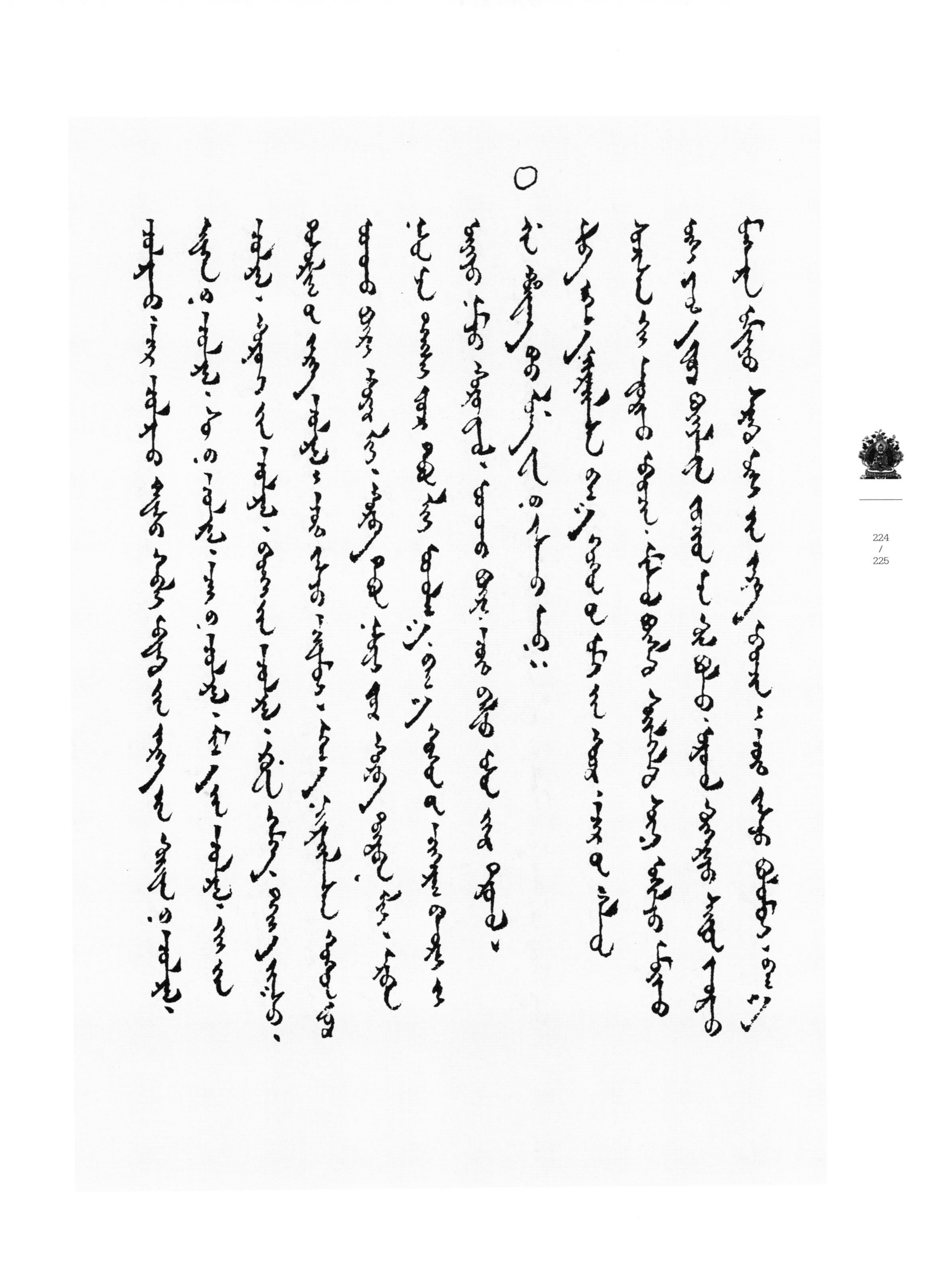

[illegible]

[illegible]
[illegible]
[illegible]
[illegible]
[illegible]
[illegible]
[illegible]
[illegible]
[illegible]
[illegible]
[illegible]

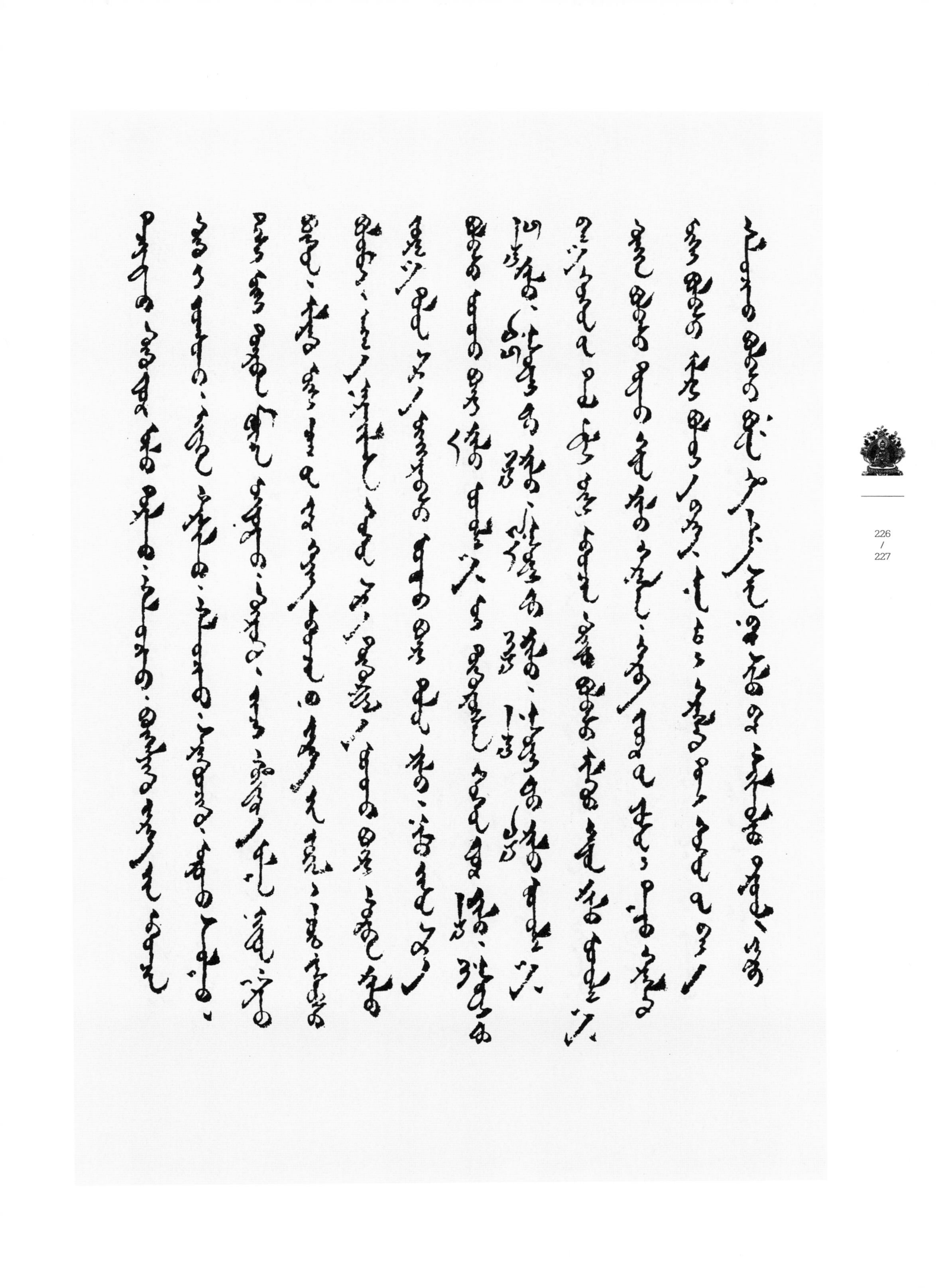

[illegible]
[illegible]
[illegible]
[illegible]
[illegible]
[illegible]
[illegible]
[illegible]

○ [illegible]

[illegible]
[illegible]
[illegible]

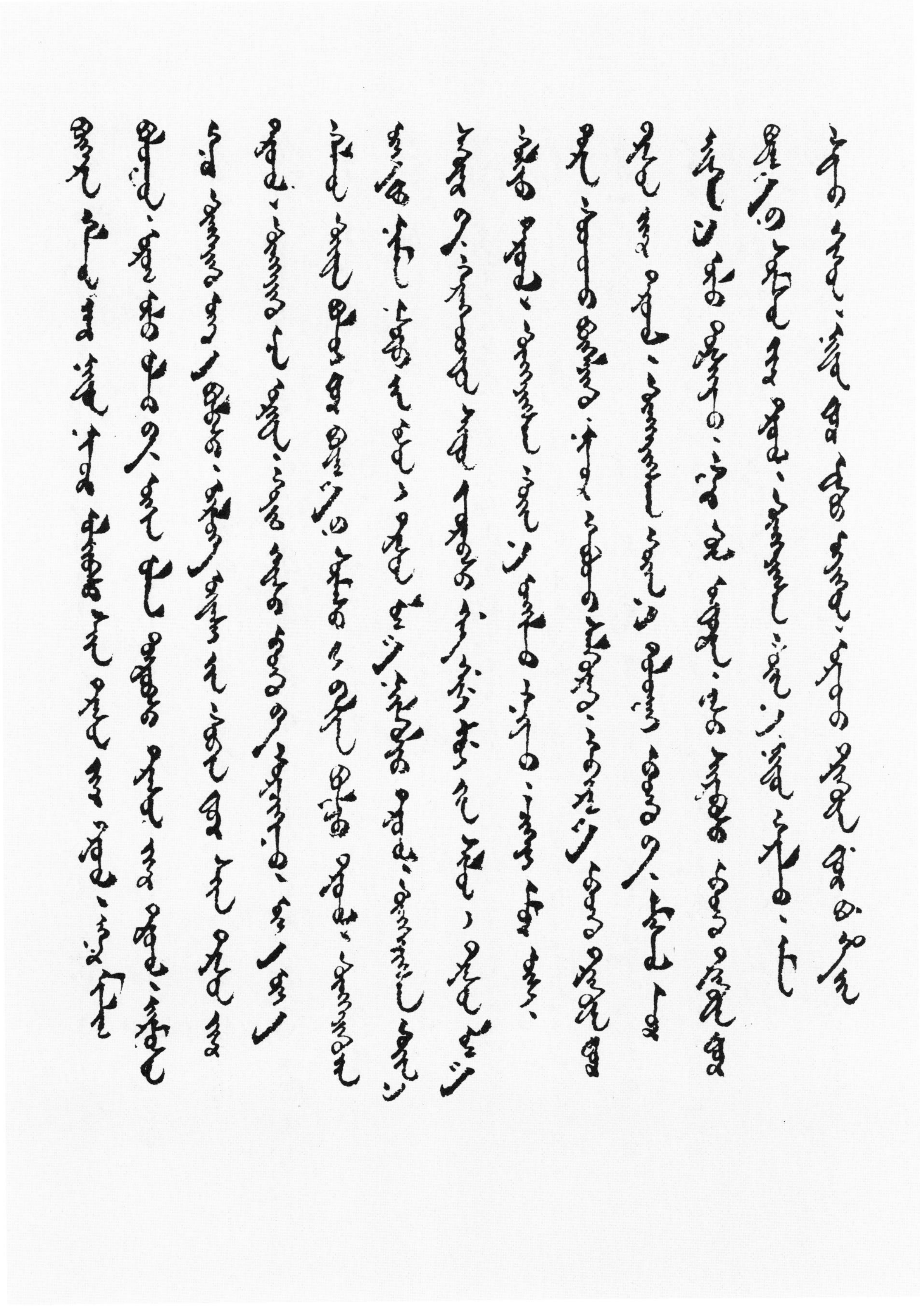

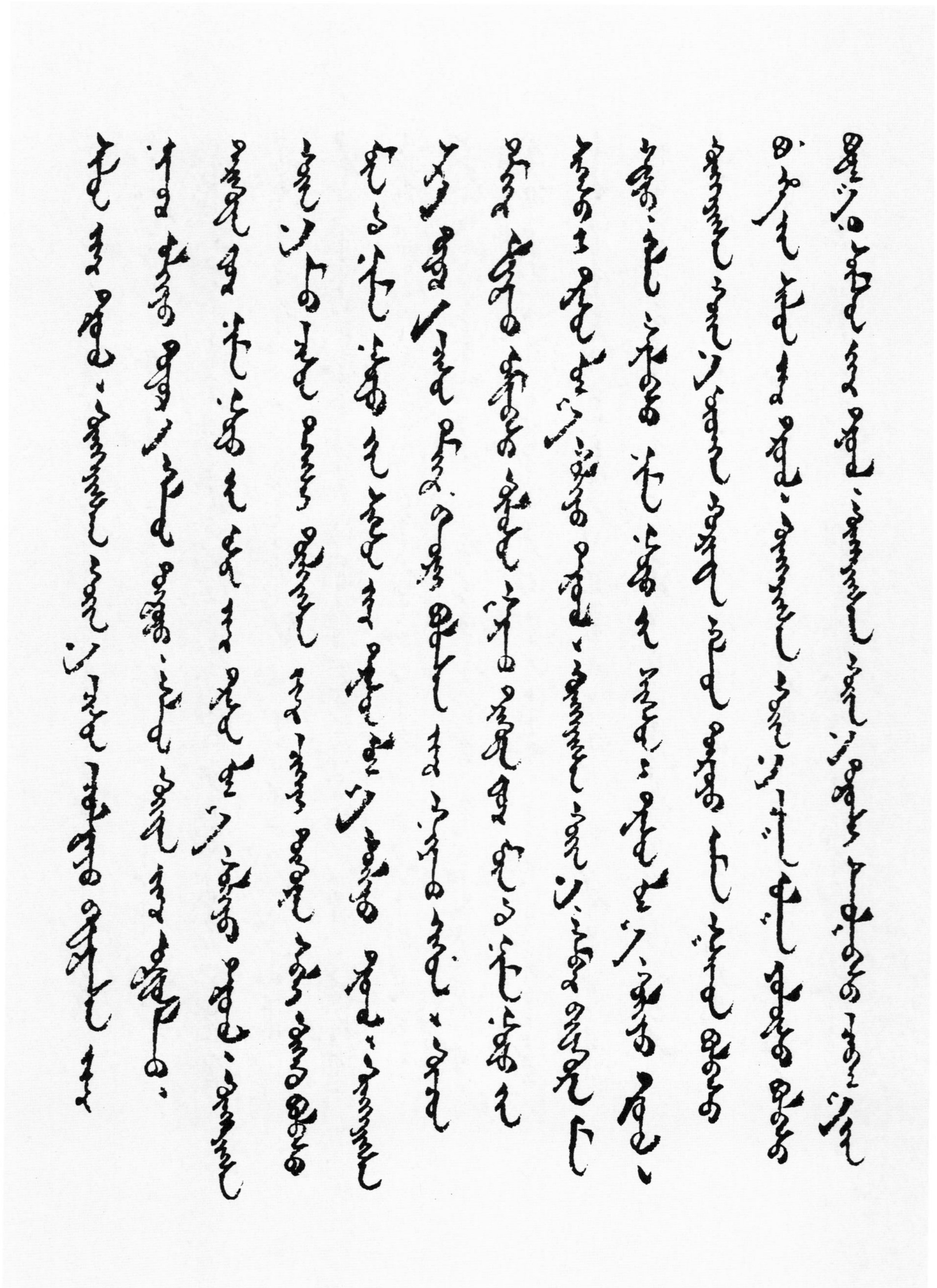

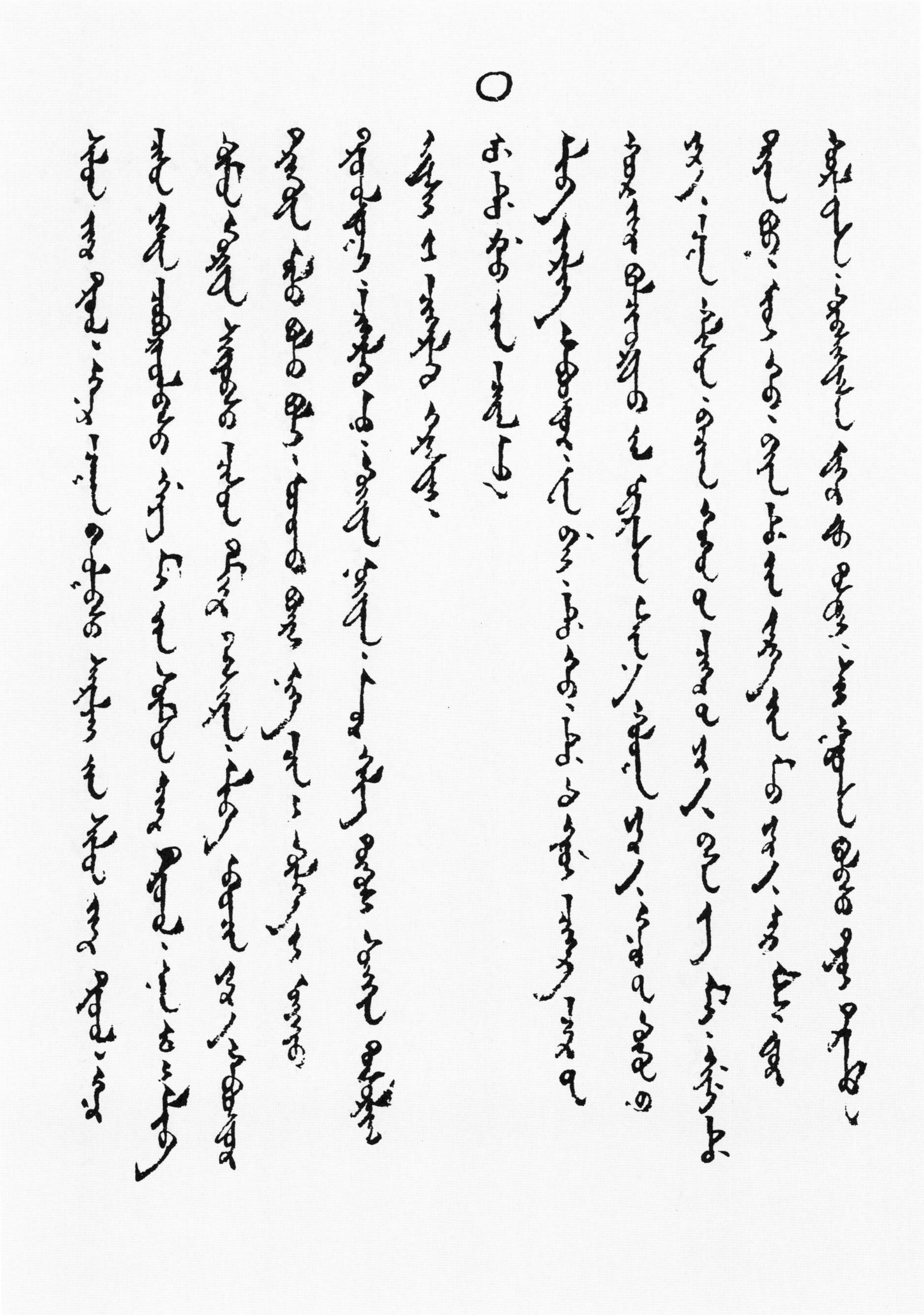

[illegible]

[illegible]

[illegible]

[illegible]

[illegible]

[illegible]

[illegible]

○ [illegible]

[illegible]

[illegible]

○ [illegible]

[illegible]

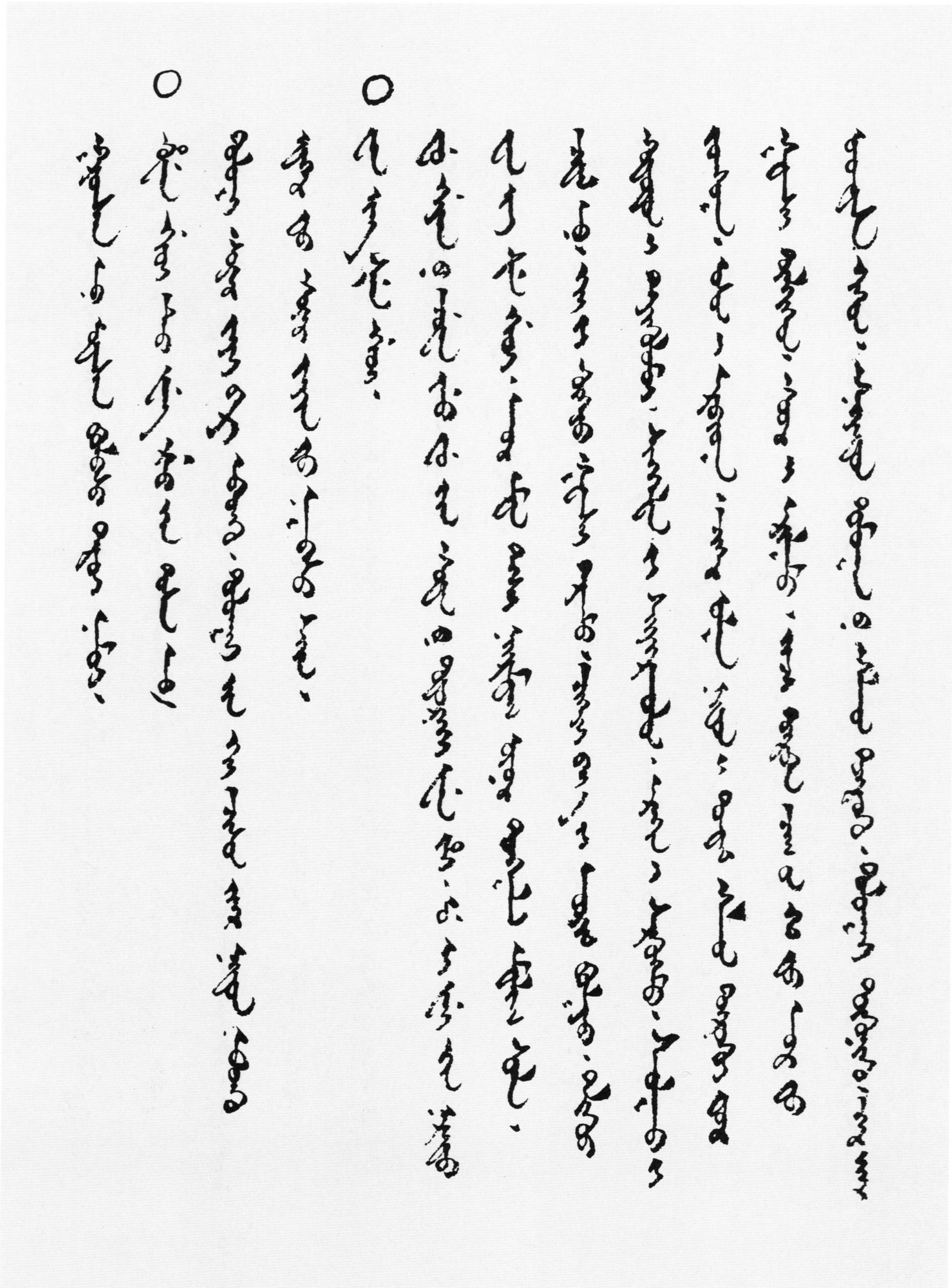

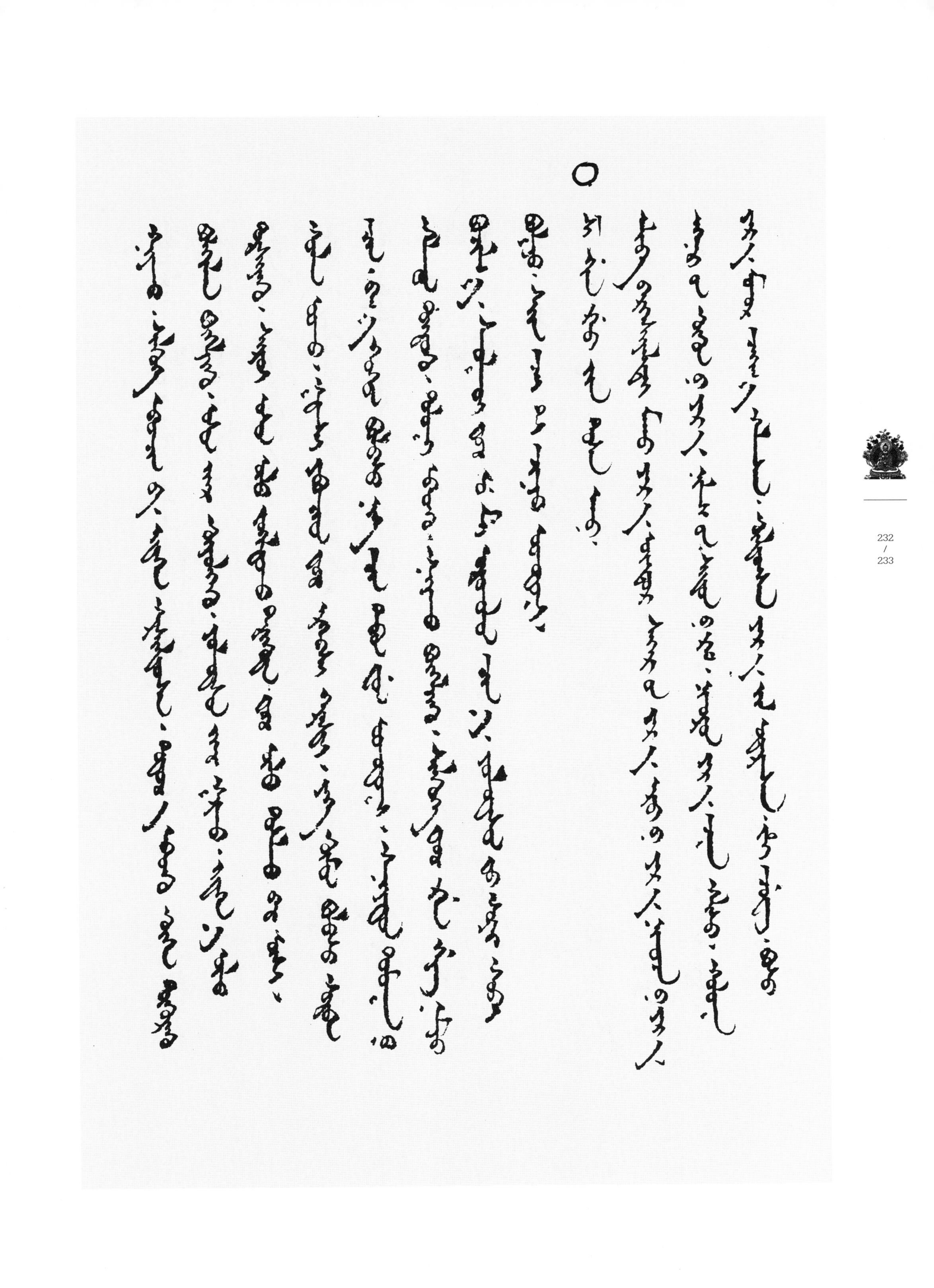

[illegible]

○ [illegible]

[illegible]

[illegible]

[illegible]

[illegible]

[illegible]

○ [illegible]

[illegible]

[illegible]

[illegible]

[illegible]

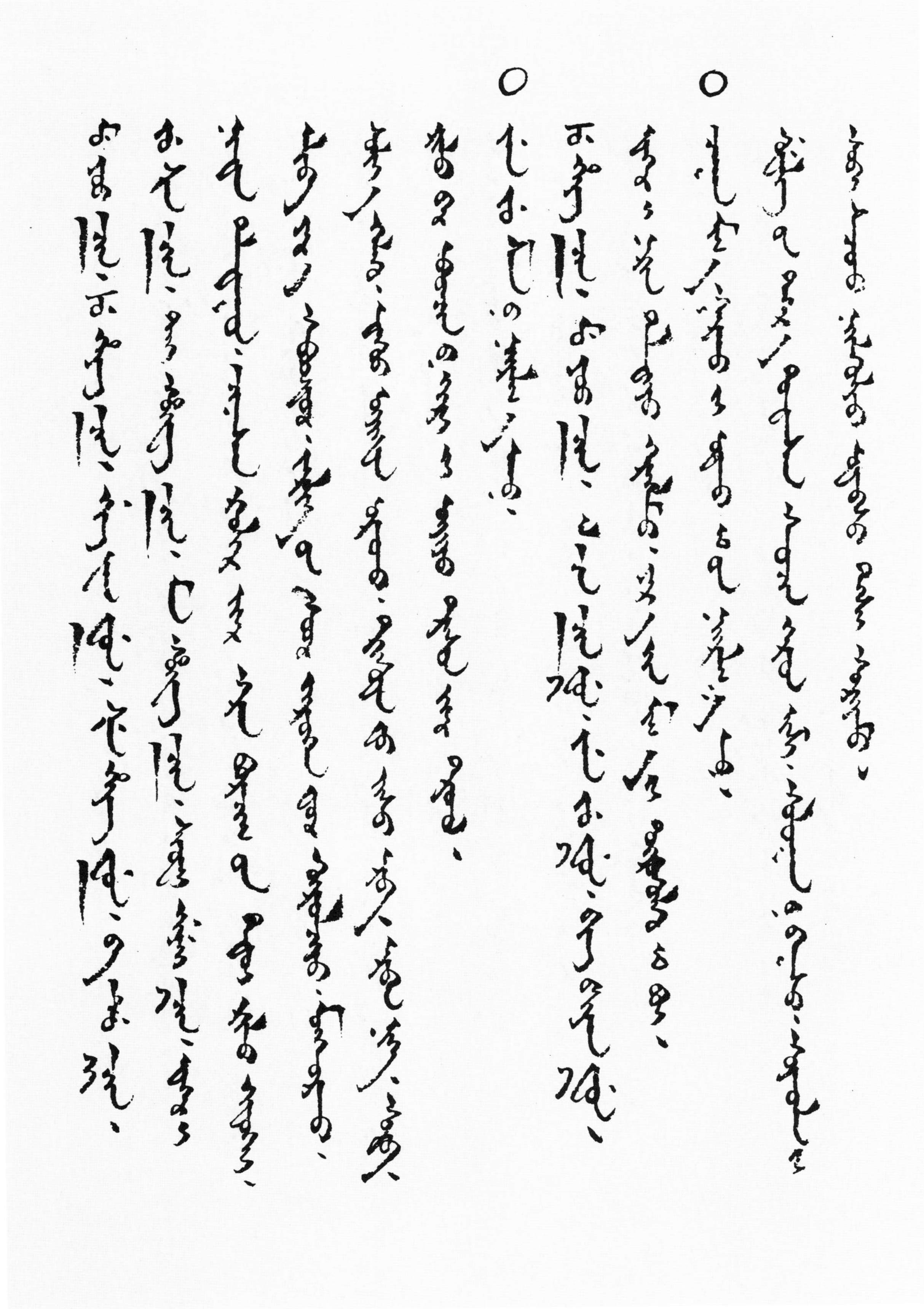

[illegible]

[illegible]

[illegible]

[illegible]

[illegible]

[illegible]

[illegible]

[illegible]

[illegible]

[illegible]

[illegible]

[illegible]

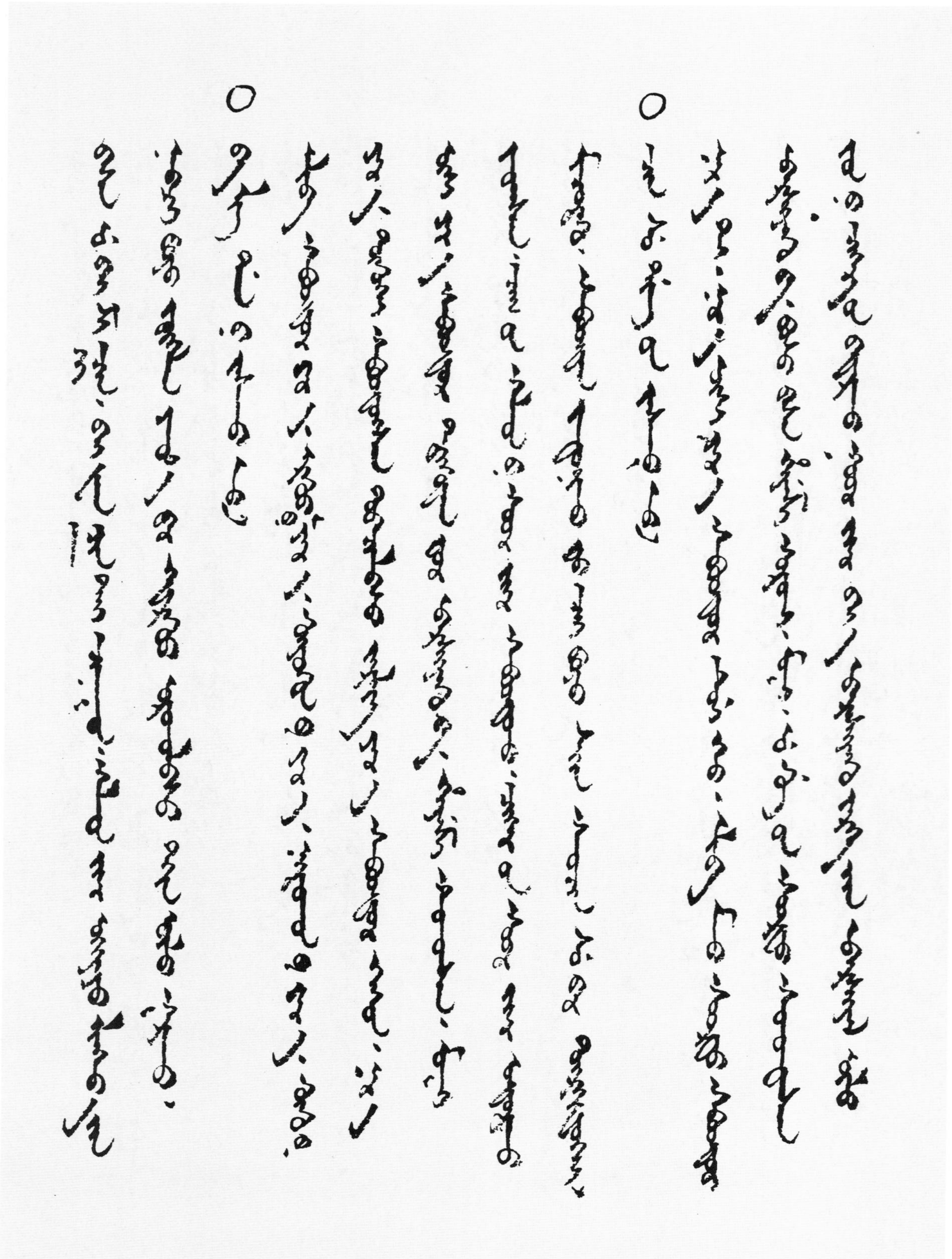

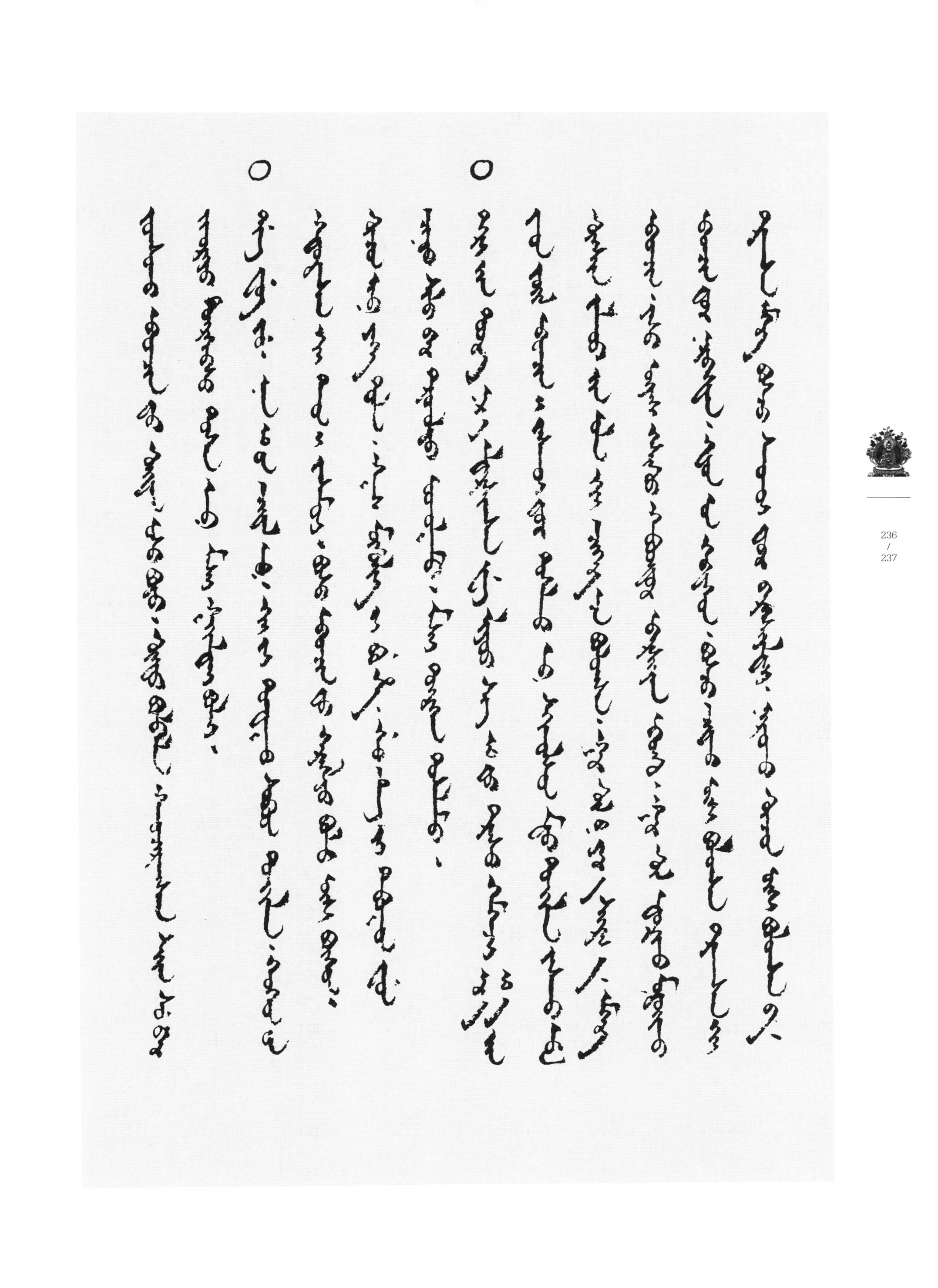

[illegible]

[illegible]
[illegible]
[illegible]
[illegible]
[illegible]
[illegible]
[illegible]
[illegible]
[illegible]
[illegible]
[illegible]
[illegible]

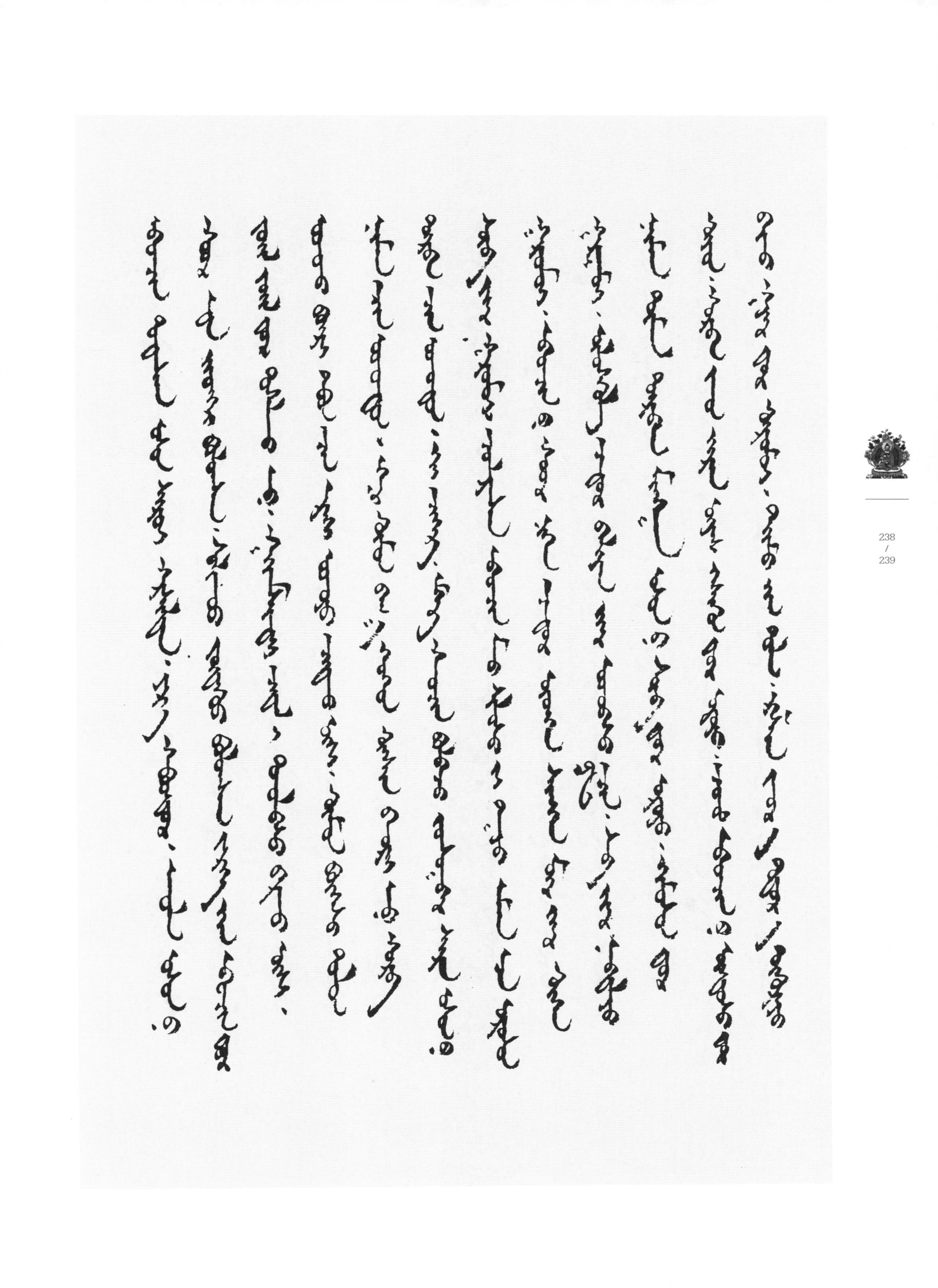

[illegible]

[illegible]
[illegible]
[illegible]
[illegible]
[illegible]
[illegible]
[illegible]
[illegible]
[illegible]
[illegible]
[illegible]
[illegible]

[illegible]
[illegible]
[illegible]
[illegible]
[illegible]
[illegible]
[illegible]
[illegible]
[illegible]
[illegible]
[illegible]
[illegible]

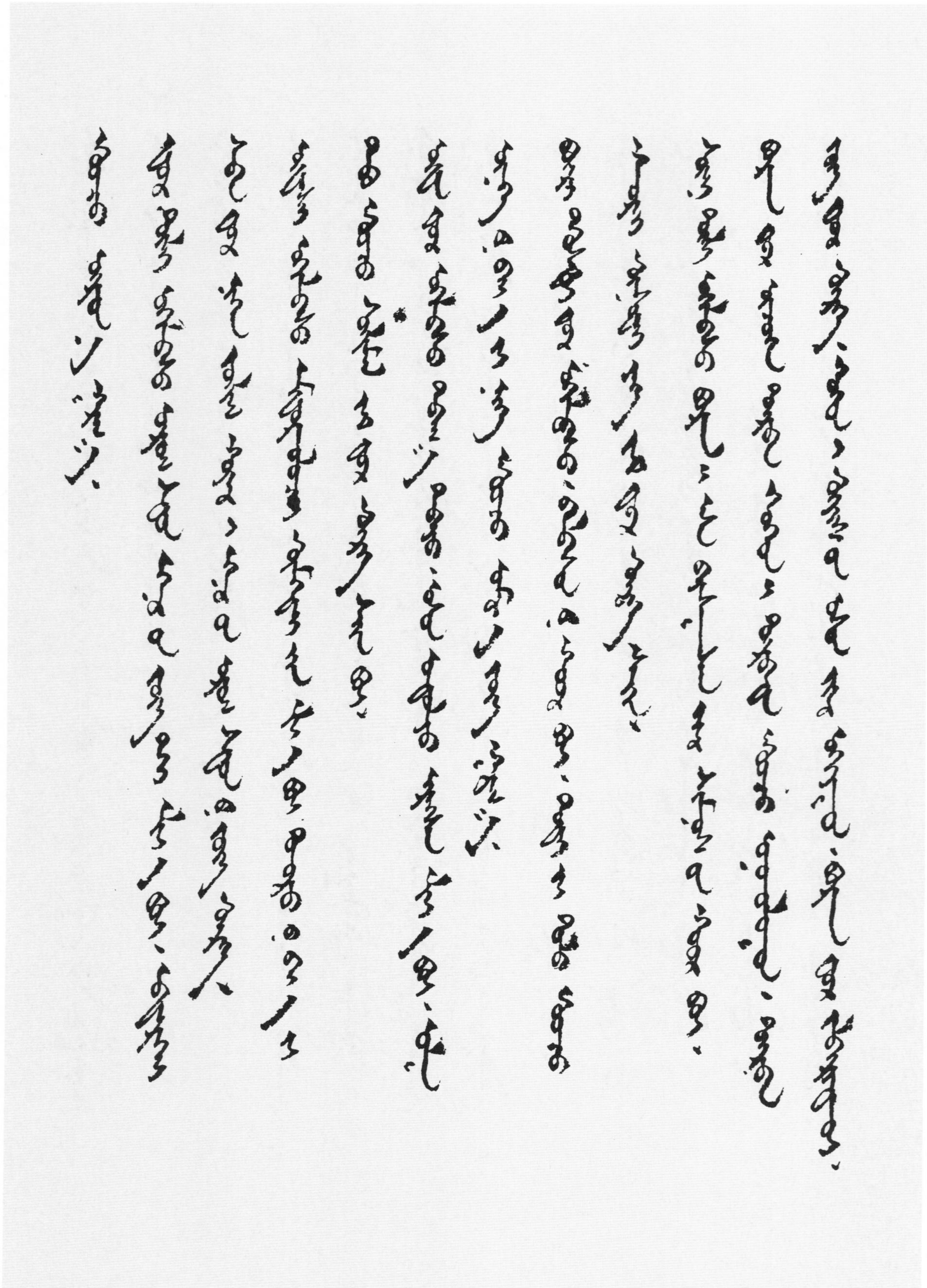

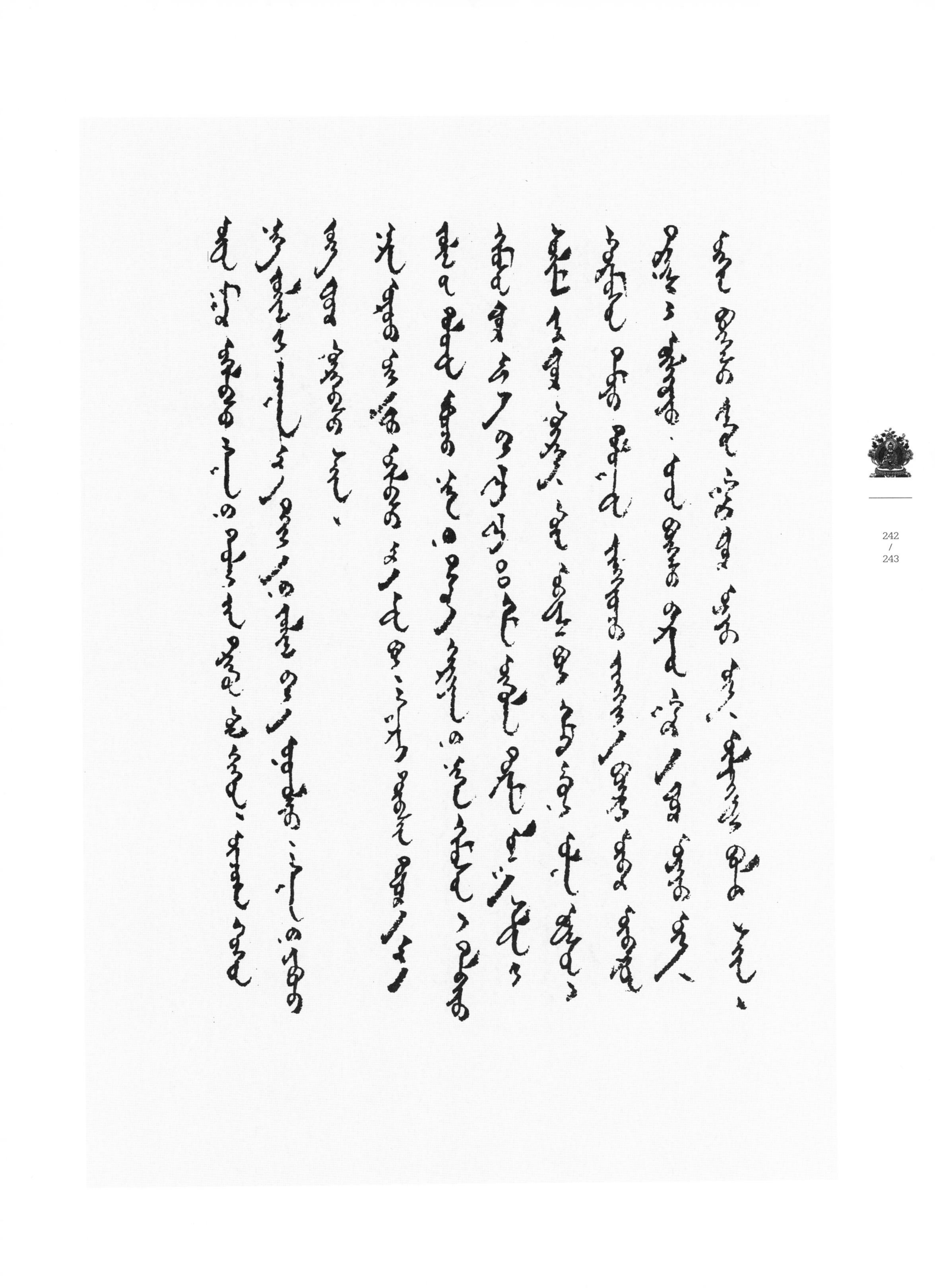

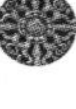

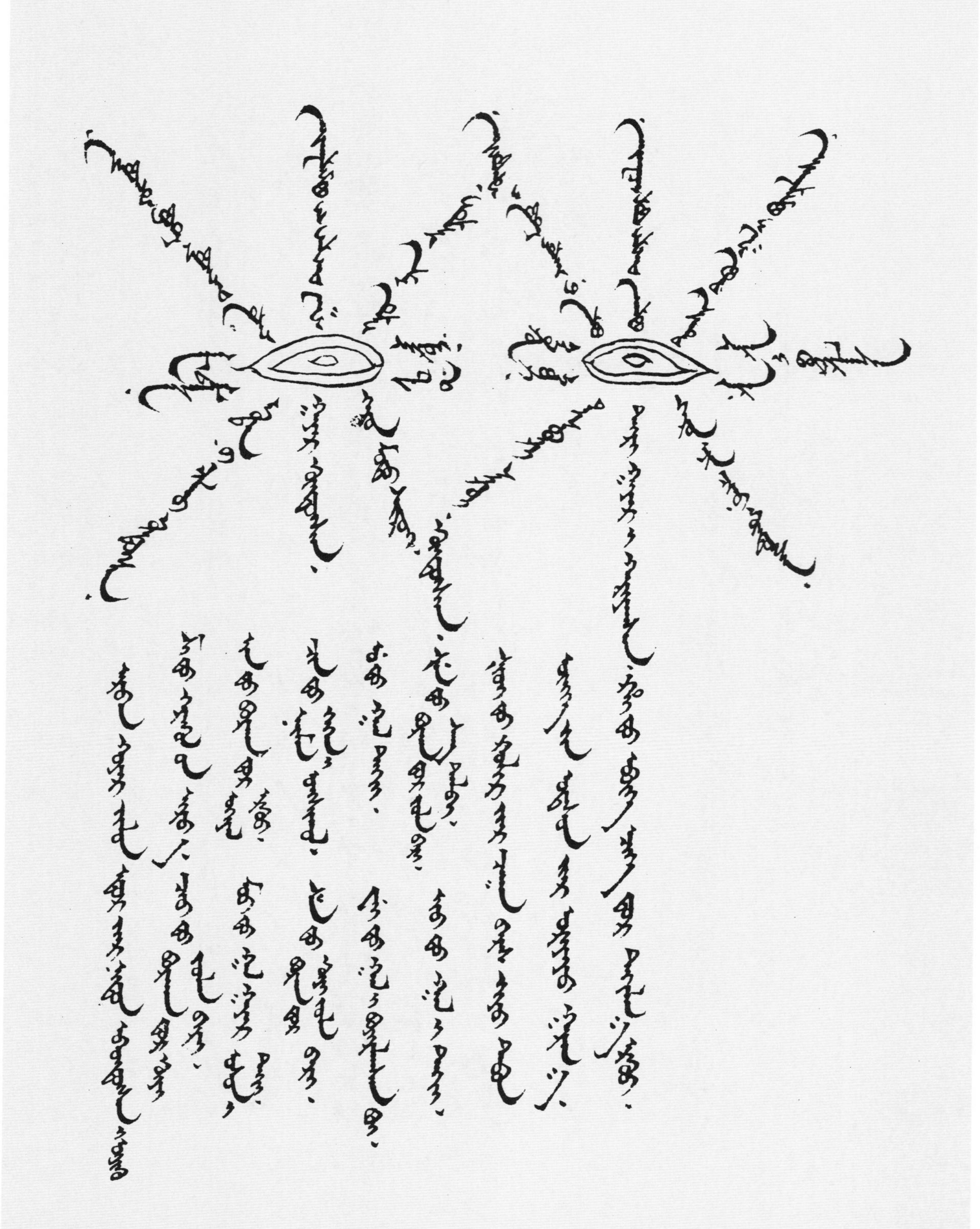

鬼

天 地

風

火

史

鬼

急急入条

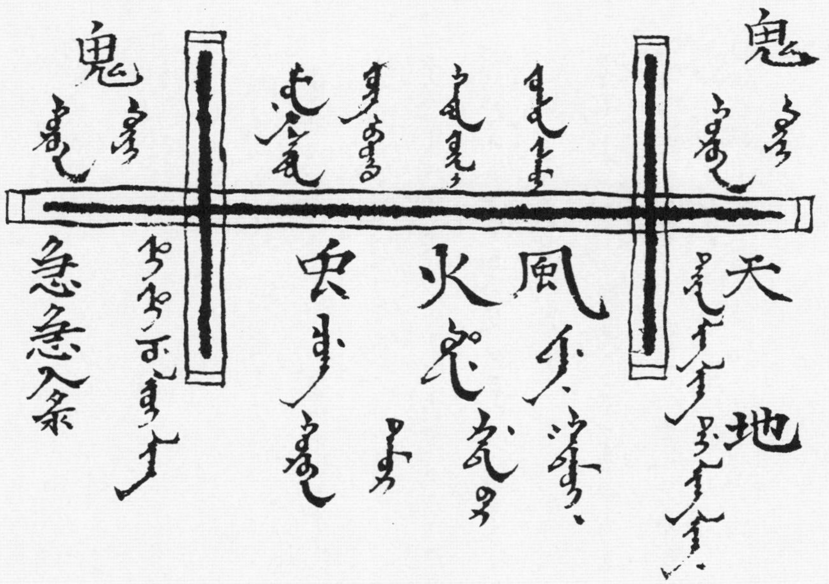

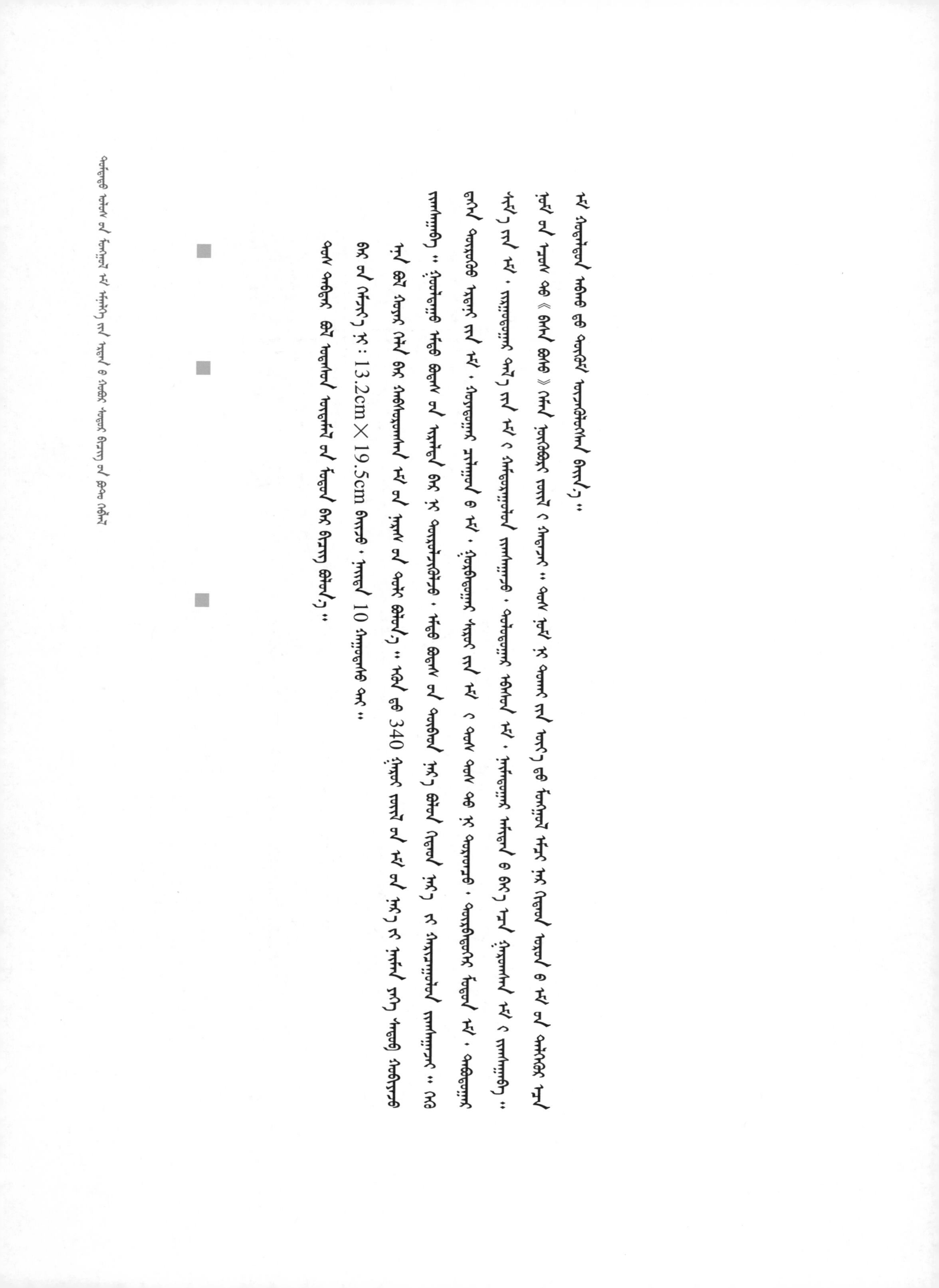

[illegible]

[illegible]

[illegible] 340 [illegible]

[illegible] : 13.2cm × 19.5cm [illegible] 10 [illegible]

[illegible]

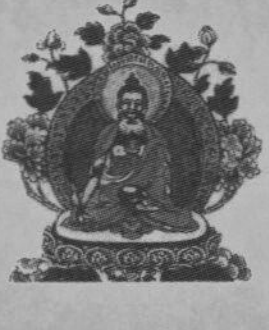

Mongolian, Tibetan and Chinese Names of Herbs

蒙、藏、汉合璧《番汉药名》

3

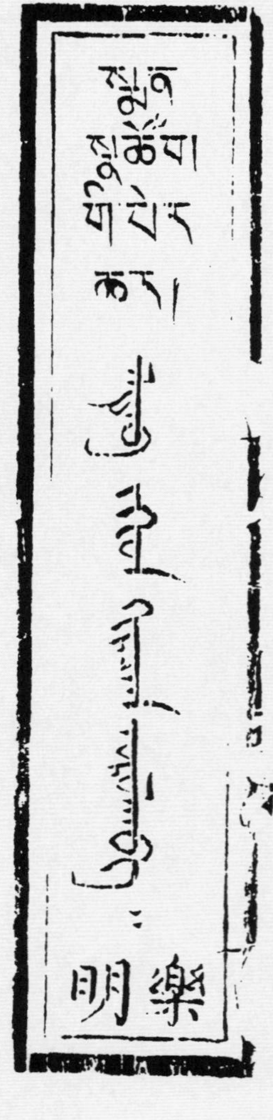

༄༅། །སངས་རྒྱས་སྨན་པའི་རྒྱལ་པོར་ཕྱག

འཚལ་ལ་འདིར་སྐྱབས་སུ་མཆིའོ། །དེ་ཡང་དཔོར་ཕྱོགས་སུ་ཚེ་འདི་རིག

ཀྱི་སྨོན་ནས་རང་གཞན་ཀྱི་དོན་ལ་མཐོན་པར་རབ་བརྩོན་པའི་སྐྱེས་རབ་ལ

མོ་ཆེས། ཅེ་སྨན་སོགས་པོ་ཁྲང་ཞིལ་ལེ་ནུ་ཅེ་ལ་རེས་ཀ་གེས། དེ་ཡག

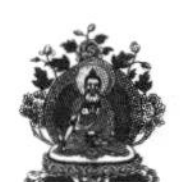

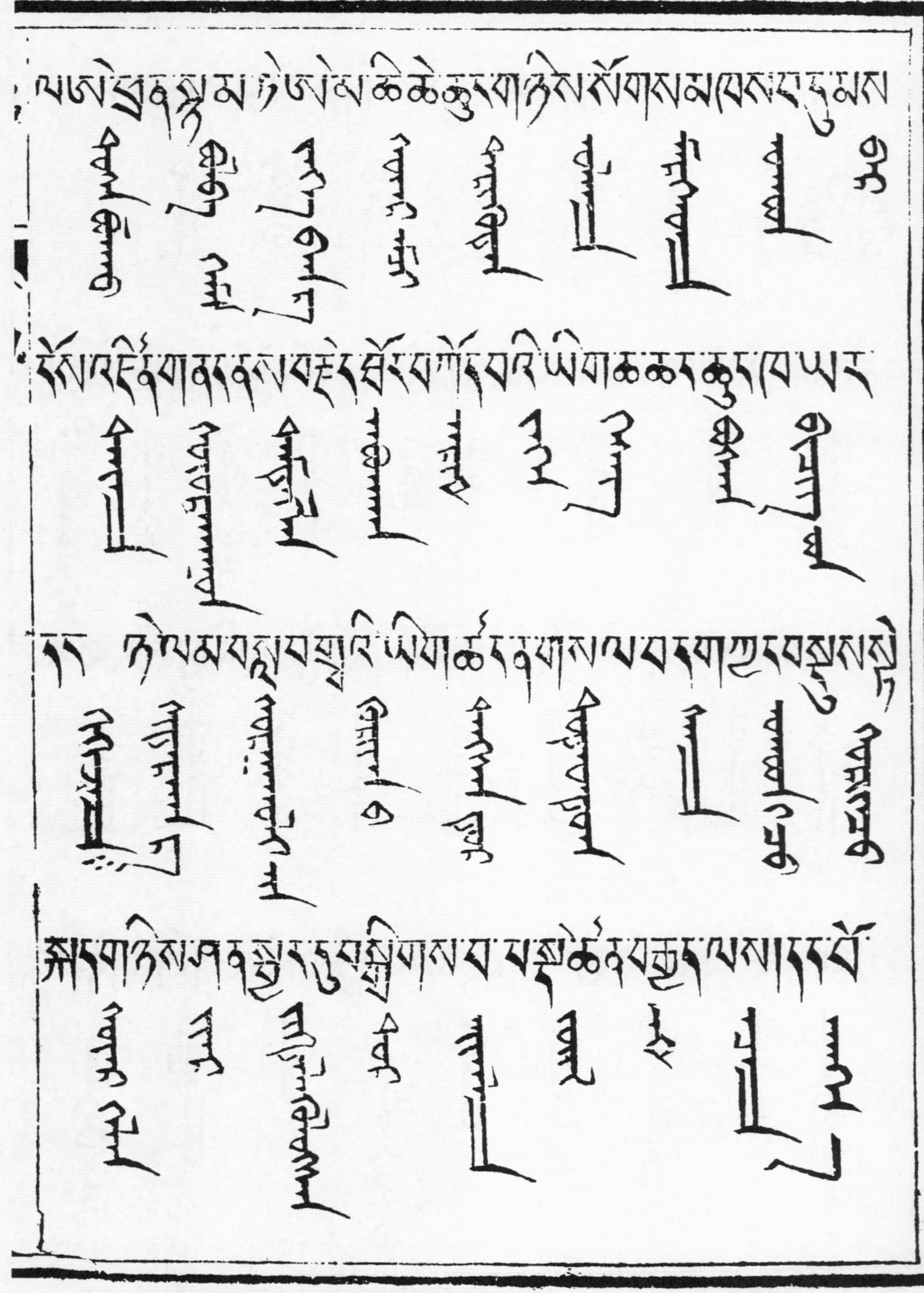

རིན་པོ་ཆེའི་སྐོར་ནི། གསེར། དངུལ། ཟངས། ལྕགས།

金 銀 銅 鐵

ཅིན ཡིན ཐུང ཐིཡེ

གཡུ། མུ་ཏིག ཉ་ཕྱིས། བྱུ་རུ། ཕྱི་རུ་ནག་པོ། དུང་། མུ་མེན།

松兒石 真珠 石決明 珊瑚 青琅玕 琸璖 青金石

ཤེལ། ཆུ་ཤེལ། སྤོས་ཤེལ། བཻ་ཌཱུ་རྱ། རྡོ་སྙིང་། ཨིནྡྲ་ནཱི་ལ།

真玻璃 水晶石 琥珀 真琉璃 瑪瑙 映青

པདྨ་ར་ག། མ་ར་ཀ་ཏ། ཕ་ལམ། ཀ་ཤེས་བརྗོད་སྐོར་ནི།

映紅 子母碌 金鋼石

སྨུག་པོ་སླ་ལ་རྒྱབ། གཉེར་ཤིག། །ཁབ་ལེན། །སྤང་ཚེ་དཀར་པོ། །

銀精石 ཡིན་ཅིང་ཤི

歃鉄石 ཧི་ཐེ་ཤི

爐甘石 ལུ་ཀན་ཤི

赤石脂 ཆི་ཤི་ཙི

無名異 ཝུ་མིང་ཡི

ལྷ་མ་སྤང་ཚེ་ད།

ཕྱང་ཚེར་ནག་པོ། མཆྲིར། ཐེམ་གོ། གསེར་རྡོ། དངུལ་རྡོ།

銀礦石 ཡིན་ཀུང་ཤི

金礦石 ཀིན་ཀུང་ཤི

石燕子 ཤི་ཡན་ཙི

雲母石 ཡུན་མུ་ཤི

礞石 མུང་ཤི

བ་ཁར་ལོ་རྩུ།

ཟངས་རྡོ། ལྕགས་རྡོ། གསེར་ཞེལ། དངུལ་ཞེལ། སྨུག་ཤེ། རྡོ་ཀླད།

腦石 ནའོ་ཤི

自然銅 ཙི་ཞན་ཐུང

玄精石 ཤྱན་ཅིང་ཤི

密陀僧 མི་ཐོ་སེང

鉄礦石 ཐེ་ཀུང་ཤི

銅礦石 ཐུང་ཀུང་ཤི

རྡོ་མཐིས། ལྡོང་རོས། བ་བླ། རྡོ་སོལ། བ་ཏྲུ། རྡོ་རྒྱུས། མཐིང་རྒྱུས།

馬起石 མ་ཆི་ཤི

陽起石 ཡང་ཆི་ཤི

石中乳 ཤི་ཅུང་གཞུ

煤 མེས

石黃 ཤི་ཧོང

雄黃 ཤུང་ཧོང

石中黃子 ཤི་ཅུང་ཧོང་ཙི

མཎྜུར་རྩི།

ཏི་རྐ་སེར་པོ། མཆལ་མགོ་ད། ཕག་ཐུ་མིག བཙག ཚ་ཚེར་ཞི། རྡོ་ཐལ།

花蕋石　窩鉛　朱砂　理石　長石　紅土　寒水石　石灰

ཏ་ལིག སྤྱང་ཚུར། གསུམ་པ་ལ་སྨན་ནི། གསེར་གྱི་བྱེ་མ།

滑石　銅青　海金沙

ལི་ཁྲི། ས་རྡོ། ཟེ་ཚྭ། ཡ་བ་ཀྵ་ར། རྒྱ་ལ་ཚྭ། མུ་ཟི་སེར་པོ།

黃丹　太一禹餘粮　火硝　芒硝　碱　硫黃

མུ་ཟི་ནག་པོ། ནག་མཚུར། སེར་མཚུར། དཀར་མཚུར། ཐིག་ཐལ།

硫青冬結石　黑礬　黃礬石　白礬　膽礬

རྡོ་ཏིག ཐག་ཟུན། མཚལ་ཡ། མཐིང་། ལ་སྨུག རྗེ་ང་། ཚོན་ལྗང་།

石花 ཤི་ཧྭ　五靈脂 ཨུ་ལིང་ཙི　銀朱 ཡིན་ཙུ　石青 ཤི་ཆིང་　泥皮 ནི་ཕི　兒茶 ཨེར་ཆ　石碌 ཤི་ལུ

ས་ཅིའི་དཀར་པོ། བཞི་བ་སེར་སྨན་ལ་བཅུ་སྨན་རྒྱ་ཀ་པ་ཐང་སྨན

官粉 ཀོན་ཧྥུན

རྣམས་གཞུང་ནས་སྨ་ཚན་གཅིག་ཏུ་བསྡུས་པ་ཡུང་དབང་རིགས་ཀྱི།

ཤེལ་གཟུར། མང་གཟུར། དངུལ་ཆུ། ཙན་དན་དཀར་པོ།

氷片 ཕིང་ཕཡན　朝腦 ཆའོ་ནའོ　水銀 ཧྲུའི་ཡིན　白檀香 པེ་ཐན་ཤང་

ཙནྡན་དམར་པོ། ཙནྡན་སྨུག་པོ། ཨ་ག་རུ། ཨ་ག་ར་ནག་པོ།

紫檀 ཙི་ཐན　降真香 ཅང་ཅིན་ཧྱང　速香 སུ་ཧྱང　沉香 ཆིན་ཧྱང

གི་ཝཾ། གུ་གུལ། གུར་གུམ། སུག་སྨེལ། སུག་སྨེལ། ཛཱ་ཏི།

牛黄 ཉིའུ་ཧྭང　石青 ཤི་ཀིང　紅花 ཧུང་ཧྭ　白荳蔻 པེ་ཏེའུ་ཁེའུ　益智仁 ཡི་ཚི་ཞིན　肉荳蔻 ཞུ་ཏེའུ་ཁེའུ

ལི་ཤི། ཀ་ཀོ་ལ། གླ་རྩི། [illegible] ཨུ་རྒྱལ། གསེར་དགུ།

丁香 ཏིང་ཧྱང　草菓 ཚའོ་ཀོ　麝香 ཤེ་ཧྱང　熊膽 [illegible]་ཏན　蜀葵子 ཤུ་ཁུའི་ཙི　使君子 ཤི་ཀྱུན་ཙི　金櫻子 ཀིན་ཡིང་ཙི

སྦྲེང་ཀར་སེ། སྦྲིན་ནག་པོ། ལ་ཕ་སྦྲུལ། སོ་མ་ར་ཛ། ཐལ་ཀ་རྡོ་རྗེ།

巨勝子 ཀྱུ་ཤིང་ཙི　雲南巨勝子 ཡུན་ནན་ཀྱུ་ཤིང་ཙི　蛇床子 ཤེ་ཁྭང་ཙི　線蔴子 སྱན་མ་ཙི　草决明 ཚའོ་ཅུ་མིང

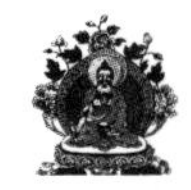

གསེར་གྱི་མེ་ཏོག	རྒྱ་མོ་འུར།	རྒྱུན་འབྲུམ།	རྒྱུན་འབྲུམ་དཀར་པོ།	
金絲沐鰲	雀地瓜	葡萄	白葡萄	

ཧུ་སུ།	ཧུར་སུ།	བསེ་ཡབ།	སེ་འབྲུ།	ན་ལེ་ཤམ།	པི་པི་ལིང་།
香菜子	慈梨膏	莫丹	酸李乾	石榴	胡椒 / 蓽撥

འཇམ་འབྲས།

སྒ་ནས།	སྒ་སྐྱ།	ཙི་ཏྲ་ཀ	ཤིང་ཚ།	ག་སྐྱེ།	ཤིང་ཀུན།	ཤུ་དག
姜	山柰	秦椒	官桂	建蓮子	阿魏	曼荊子

མ་ནུ།	ག་བྱི་ལ།	སྤོས་དཀར།	གུ་གུལ།	ཤ་ལ་ཁ།	རྒྱ་ཚྭ།
可瓜	番木鱉	芸香	奄巴香	沒藥	硇沙

རྒྱམ་ཚྭ། ཟླ་སྔོང་ཚྭ། ཁ་རུ་ཚྭ། བལ་ཚྭ། མདེ་ཚྭ། ཚ་ལ། སོ་ག་ཚྭ།

光明盐 ཀང་མིང་ཡན　黑盐 ཧེ་ཡན　红盐 ཧུང་ཡན　灰盐 ཧུའི་ཡན　皮硝 ཕི་ཤའོ　硼砂 ཕུང་ཤ　青盐 ཆིང་ཡན

ལན་ཚྭ། ཨ་རུ་ར། རྒྱ་ཨ་རུ་ར། བ་རུ་ར། སྐྱུ་རུ་ར། སྐྱེར་ཤོག

碱盐 ཅན་ཡན　诃子 ཧོ་ཙི　橄榄 ཀན་ལན　川楝 ཁྲོན་ལྷན　山查 ཤན་ཙ　达酸枣 ཏྭན་སོན་ཙའོ　广酸枣 ཀང་སོན་ཙའོ

མ་ཁལ་མ་ཞོ་ལ། ཀླུ་གོང་ཞོ་ལ། ཨ་འབྲས། སྨྱུ་འབྲས། འབྲ་གོ

荳鬼见愁 ཏོའུ་ཀུས་ཅན་ཚོའུ　黑大荳蔻 ཏས་ཏ་ཏོའུ　木腰子 ཧྲུ་ཡའོ་ཙི　榧实 ཧྥི་ཤི　龙眼 ལུང་ཡན　石莲子 ཤི་ལྷན་ཙི　楔枣 ཐེན་ཙའོ

མ་ནུ། སུ་ཀྲར་སྨུ་ལ། རུ་རྟ། ཡུ་གང་། ཤུ་དག་དཀར་པོ། ཆུ་ཤུག་གོ

青木香 ཆིང་མུ་ཤང　川广木香 ཁྲོན་ཀང་མུ་ཤང　广木香 ཀང་མུ་ཤང　姜黄 ཅང་ཧོང　白芷 པེ་ཙི　白菖蒲 པེ་ཚང་ཕུ　石菖蒲 ཤི་ཚང་ཕུ

བུ་ཤེལ་ཅི། ལྕང་སྤྱེར། དབའ་པོ་ལག་པོ། སྐྱ་རུ་ཚེན། བོང་ང་དཀར་པོ།

射ཤེ 干ཀན　鈎ཀེའུ 藤ཐེང　鬱ཡུས 金ཀིན　草ཚའོ 烏ཝུ　麥མེས 冬ཏུང

ཤི་ཚྭ་ལྷུབ་པོ།

བོང་ང་དམར་པོ། ཤིང་མངར། སླེ་ཏྲེས། ཀཎྚ་ཀ་རི། ག་ཞྲི། ཏིག་ཏ།

川ཆོན 烏ཝུ　甘ཀན 草ཚའོ　君ཀྱུན 參ཤིན　真ཅིན 朱ཀྲུ 干ཀན　蒔ཤི 蘿ལོ 干ཀན　蒲པུ 盤པན 枝ཀྲི　肉ཞུ 蒂ཏི 桂ཀུས 干ཀན

ཐ་ལ་ཁྲིག ཁ་ཤ་ཀ ཁ་ལེ་ཀ གཟེ་མ། གླ་སྒང་། སྤྲ་བ་ལེ། སྦྲུལ་ཤིང་།

紫ཙི 花ཧྭ 地ཏི 丁ཏིན　開ཁའེ 楊ཡང 花ཧྭ　木མུ 通ཐུང　草ཚའོ 河ཧོ 車ཆེ　附ཧྥུ 子ཙི　杜ཏུ 仲ཀྲུང　油ཡེའུ 松སུང

ཐང་ཤིང་། སྐྱེར་པ། སྐྱེར་ཤུན། ཙ་ཀྱ་ལྕེ་ར། མཚོ་མོ་ཤིང་། ཙོམ་བུ། ཙི་ཏྲུ།

榆ཡུས 松སུང　黄ཧོང 栢པེ　黄ཧོང 栢པེ 皮པི　紫ཙི 榆ཡུས　蘇སུ 木མུ　三སན 川ཆོན　山ཤན 杏ཧིན

...ཞོ། དན་ཁྲ། ཏེ་ཏེ་ག ཀ་ཀོ་ལ། ཏ་ཏིག སྐྱུག མོན་ཆ་ར།

蘿子 巴豆 蓖麻子 牙皂 葫蘆 五味子 臭裡子 象子

ཨ་ཀྲུས། མ་ནུ་རག ལ་ལ་མ་ཕི། སེ་ཏ། ཀྱུ་ལྦུ་རྩེ། གོ་ཡུ།

棟香 風茄子花 山茄子花 海桐皮 艾瓢 鈴蕩子 檳榔

ག་ཡུ་ཀྲུན་ཀྱུ་ཀས། ག་ཡེ་རམ། རྒྱ་མཚོའི་ལྦུ་བ། མ་ཏོག་ཏ་ལོ།

大腹皮 花椒 海漂硝 大蜀季花

མེ་ཏོག་ཁྲི་ཤི། རི་ནི་ཞོ་ཆེ་སྦུག ར་མཉེ། ས་ག་ར་མ་ཤི། སྒ་ནག་མར།

鷄冠花 碧澄茄 茅根 金箔 良姜

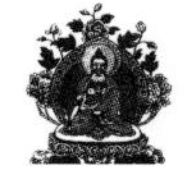

ཟྲ་ཀྲི། མེ་ཏོག་ཀ་ར་ལ། ཡ་ཐིམ། མ་མ་སྒོག་ལྕག ཡུ་ཀ་ཤིང་།

片子姜黄 ཕེན་ཙེ་ཅང་ཧོང་ 米壳 མི་ཁེ 鸦片 ཡ་ཕེན 木贼 མུ་ཙེ 三七 སན་ཚི 漆 ཚི

ཀ་ར་ཀྲུ་ར། བ་སྒྱ། ར་ལ་མོ་ས་ལི། ར་སྤུག སྒོག་ས་ཕེ་ལ།

青相子 ཆིང་ཤང་ཙེ 香绿 ཤང་ལུན 牛滕 ནིའུ་ཐིན 刘寄奴 ལིའུ་ཅི་ནུ 山慈姑 ཤན་ཚི་ཀུ

བ་དུར་བ་རྩི་སྨན་འདི། ཏོང་ལེན། སྤུར་རྩི་དབོ། ར་སྨོན། ཚི་སྐྱེ།

胡连 ཧུ་ལེན 老鹳筋 ལའོ་ཀོན་ཅིན 丹参 ཏན་ཤེན 葵花子 ཁུའེ་ཧྭ་ཙེ

འདི་བཙོ

ཐི་ཡང་ར། སྤོ་ལོ། སྤུག་རབ། བར་བ་ཆུར། ངང་པ་ཀ་ན། རྟ་ལྕགས།

卮子花 ཙི་ཙེ་ཧྭ 沙参 ཤ་ཤེན 桔梗 ཅེ་ཀིང 冬花 ཏུང་ཧྭ 葶苈 ཐིང་ལི 玉英叶 ཡུས་ཡིང

ཨ་བི་ལ། ཧྲུ་ག་ཤ ཀ་སྤྲུ་ག་གཞེར་འཛོམས། སྲོལ་སྔོན། གསེར་སྐུད།

百合根 པེ་ཧོ་ཀེན
山荳根 ཤན་ཏེའུ་ཀེན
番白草 ཧྥན་པེ་ཚའོ
旋覆花 ཧྱུན་ཧྥུ་ཧྭ
白頭翁 པེ་ཐེའུ་ཨུང
兔兒絲 ཐུ་ཨལ་སི

ལུག་རྫི་སྣ་ག་སོ། ཤིང་ཏོག་ཨ་མྲ། སེ་བའི་མེ་ཏོག ཨ་གྲོང་།

山躑躅 ཤན་ཅི་ཅུ
柿子 ཤི་ཙི
香蓋 ཧྱང་ཀའི
棘梅花 ཚི་མེས་ཧྭ
茵陳 ཨིན་ཚེན

ངང་ཀུན། སེ་ཀེ་ཏང་འབྲས་བུ། ཤུག་ཚེར། སྐྱེར་འབྲས། སེར་ཕྲེང་ཅན

當歸 ཏང་ཀུས
慈梅子 ཚི་མེས་ཙི
赤栢枝 ཆི་པེ་ཙི
构起子 ཀེའུ་ཆི་ཙི
商陸 ཤང་ལུ
當陸 ཏང་ལུ

ཨོ་རྟ་ངས

ལང་ཐང་ཙེ། རྡ་མ་འི་འབྲུ། རྟ་ལམ་མེ་ཏོག་སེར། སྤོང་ཀ་འི་པོ་ཆིག་སྦུག

浪蕩子 ལང་ཏང་ཙི
蘭花子 ལན་ཧྭ་ཙི
馬蘭蓬 མ་ལན་ཕང
人參 ཞིན་སེན

བ་རུ་བ་ཏ་རེ་རྩ་བ། རྡ་ཆའི་རྩ་བ། འདམ་བུ་ཀ་ར། འབྲི་ཏ་ས་འཛིན།

秦花根　秦椒根　南星　三稜草　地錦　雀卧蛋草

ཐུར་ལ་ཅེ་ཅེ། ཤུ་མོ་ཟ། སྨི་བའི་རྩ་བ། མེ་ཏོག་གེ་སར་ཆེན། སྦྲུག་སྐྱུར་དོ།

大黄荳　胡羅卜　貝母　金蓮花　覆盆子

ཤིང་སྤྲིན། སྤང་སྤོས། བ་ལ། སྦྲང་ཙི་སྨྱུག ལུག་མིག མཁའ་ད་བ།

山茶花　甘松　草鬼見愁　黄連　菊花　白蒿

ཙ་མ་ཁྲེས། ཏེ་རང་ལ། ཁུ་མཁན། ཚེར་ག་ཆེན། འབྲི་མོག སྐྱུ་བ།

鵞鳥食　管仲　石南　桃杷葉　紫草茸　茜草　子草　小蜀季花

ཧ་མེག བ་རྨ་འོ་འབྲུམ་བུ། སྤྲུ་དཀར། ཧི་ཏྲག མ་ཚེ་ལྷུ་མ།

淫羊草 ཡིན་ཡང་ཚའོ 益母草子 ཡི་མུ་ཚའོ་ཙི 茺蔚子 ཆུང་ཝེ་ཙི 老萱 ལའོ་ཧྭན 荊芥 ཅིང་ཅེས 麻黄 མ་ཧོང

སྦྲེག ལུག་རྒྱུན། ཤོ་མ་རྩ་བ། ས་འཛིག་དབྱི་མོང་། བ་ལུ། གོ་སྣོད།

猫兒眼 མའོ་ཨེལ་ཡན 旱蓮草 ཧན་ལྱན་ཚའོ 墨菜 མོ་ཚས 羌活 ཆང་ཧོ 烏梅 ཝུ་མེས 透骨草 ཐེའུ་གུ་ཚའོ 冬青子 ཏུང་ཆིང་ཙི 小茴香 ཞའོ་ཧུའི་ཤང

བ་ཙ་མ། དབང་ལག རྒྱ་ཤིང་། ཤ་ར། རྒྱ་མ་ཚ། རྒྱ་ཚ། དེ་ལྷག་པ།

車前子 ཆེ་ཆན་ཙི 仙人掌 ཤན་རིན་ཅང 離婁 ལི་ལུ 狼毒 ལང་ཏུ 大黄 ཏ་ཧོང 亞大黄 ཡ་ཏ་ཧོང 大戟 ཏ་ཅི

བསྒྲུབ

ཤུག། ཁེ་བ་། ར་མཉེ། ཨ་སོ་བྲུ། སྐྱུག སྒྲུབ་ལྒ སྒྲུབ་རྒྱ་ཚ།

玉竹 ཡུ་ཀྲུ 黄精 ཧོང་ཅིང 白芨 པེ་ཅི 百部 པེ་པུ 天門冬 ཐན་མན་ཏུང 蘄艾 ཆི་ཨའི 膏木 ཀའོ་མུ 獨活 ཏུ་ཧོ

ག་ཉེ་མ། མཐུན་ཤིང་། ཟུ་ག་ཙུ། ཁུར་མང་། རྒྱ་སྐྱུར། མེ་ཏོག་ཙ་ཙ་སུ་ཤེང་།

蒺藜 ཅི་ལི 食斛 ཤི་ཧུ 牛旁子 ནིའུ་ཕང་ཙི 蒲公英 ཕུ་ཀུང་ཡིང་ 馬茱 མ་སྒྲུ་ཙེའུ 細辛 ཤི་ཤིན

སྤུར་མོང་། ནགི་ཆི། ཆུ་ཆུ་ཙ། སྐྱེ་ཚེར། ཞི་མ་བ། སྒོག་པ་ཅིག་སྐྱེ།

蒿子 ཧའོ་ཙི 鵞不食 ཨོ་པུ་ཤི 地榆 ཏི་ཡུས 大小薊 ཏ་ཤའོ་ཀི 山豆根 ཤན་ཏེའུ་ཀེན 獨頭蒜 ཐུ་ཐེའུ་སྲན

བ་ར་སྤྲོ་མ་ནག་པོ། སྐྱུར་ཏི། བཅུད་པ་ཐོབ་ཚགས་ཡས་སྦྱང་

補骨脂 པུ་ཀུ་ཙི 橘餅 ཀྱུས་པིང་

ཝ་རི། བ་ས་ཏུ། ག་ཡེར། མ་སྒོ་ན་བུ། ཡ་ཚོ་ཞེ་ཤིག། སྦྲུལ་ཤ

犀角 སི་ཅའོ 鹿茸 ལུ་ཞུང་ 海巴豆 ཧའེ་པ་ཏེའུ 靈羊血 ལིང་ཡང་ཤུའེ 蛇肉 ཤེ་ཞུའུ

རྨ་བྱའི་ཤ། འབྲུག་རུས། སྟག་ཁྲི། ཆུ་རྟ། གངས་སྦལ། བ་ཀོ།

孔雀肉 ཁུང་ཆོ་ཞུ　龍骨 ལུང་ཀུ　大雲虎皃 ཏ་ཡུན་ཧུ་ཤེལ　海馬 ཧས་མ　雪蝦蟆 ཤུའེ་ཧ་མ　牛皮 ནེ་པི

གླང་པོ་ ནགི་ རྩེ་ཆུ་གྲིན་ཤིང་མོ། བྱ་མ་བྱི་ལི་སྒྲོ། སྦྲང་བ། སྡིག་སྲིན།

象皮 ཞང་པི　川山甲 ཆུན་ཤན་ཅཱ　卷柏 ཀྱུན་པེ　鼺鳥鼠羽 ལུས་ཉོ་ཤུས་ཡུ　斑猫虫 པན་མོ་ཆུང　螃蟹 པང་ཧྲེ

ཆུ་སྲིན་ཁྲག　དབྱར་རྩྭ་དགུན་འབུ། ཚ་རྡོ། སྦལ་དུག དབང་ལོ།

血竭 ཧྲུའི་ཅེ　夏草冬虫 ཧྲ་ཚའོ་ཏུང་ཆུང　鲜苔 ཤ་ཏ　蟾蜍 ཆན་ཆུ　腹中寶 ཧྥུ་ཅུང་པའོ

གཞན་ཡང་ཤིང་དཀར་རྩེ་སོ། ཡུངས་དཀར། ཡུངས་ནག ཙུང་མ།

芽茶 ཡ་ཆ　白芥子 པེ་ཅེས་ཙེ　芥菜子 ཅེ་ཚས་ཙེ　饅徑 མན་ཅིང

སྦྲ་ཚིལ། སྦྲང་སོས། སྦྲང་རྩི། སྦྲང་དཀར། ཤེལ་ཀར། ཧྲེ་མ་ཀར།

沙糖 ཧྲ་ཐང
冰糖 པིང་ཐང
白蜂蜜 པེ་ཧྥུང་མི
蜂蜜 ཧྥུང་མི
生蜂蜜 ཤེང་ཧྥུང་མི
黃蠟 ཧོང་ལ

བུ་རམ། ནས། སོབ། གྲོ། འབྲས། ཁྲེ། བྲ་བོ། ཏིལ་དཀར། ཟར་མ།

胡蔴 ཧུ་མ
白芝蔴 པེ་ཙི་མ
喬麥 ཆའོ་མས
小米子 ཤའོ་མི་ཙི
粳米 ཅིང་མི
小麥 ཤའོ་མས
大麥 ཏ་མས
青料 ཆིང་ལེའོ
黑糖 ཧེ་ཐང

ཏིལ་ནག སྲན་ཆུང། སྲན་གྲུག། མོན་སྲན། མ་ཤ ལ་ཕུག

蘿卜乾 ལོ་པོ་ཀན
大黃荳 ཏ་ཧོང་ཏེའུ
赤小荳 ཆི་ཤའོ་ཏེའུ
蠶荳 ཚན་ཏེའུ
豌荳 ཝན་ཏེའུ
黑芝蔴 ཧེ་ཙི་མ

སྒ་གསེར། ཆང་ཕབ། ཏིལ་ཁུ། ཁ་ཆེ་གུར་གུམ། དཀྱུར་ཚོན་

梵紅花 ཧྥན་ཧོང་ཧྭ།
蔴合油 མ་ཧོ་ཡིའུ
酒麯 ཅིའུ་ཆུས
閩姜 མིན་ཅང

ག་སུམ་བརྒྱ་བཞི་བཅུ་ཡོད་པ་ལས། ལ་ལ་ཡུལ་ཕྱོགས་ཀྱིས་དབྱེ་བ་ན་སམ

ཁ་དོག་པོད་སྨུག་ནང་མི་འདྲ་ཡང་དངོས་སུ་མི་འགལ་བ་དང་། འགའ་ཞིག

རྡོས་རྣམ་མི་གཅིག་ཀྱང་རོ་ནུས་འདྲ་ཧེ་ས་ཀྱི་དཔྱད་གཞིས་ཚབ་དུ་རུང་

འཛོག་པ་དག་ཡོད་མོད་ཀྱིས། འབྲེལ་མེད་ཐུག་སྤྲུག་རྒྱུ་བཞག་བསྡོད

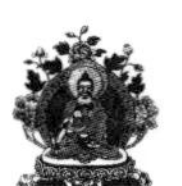

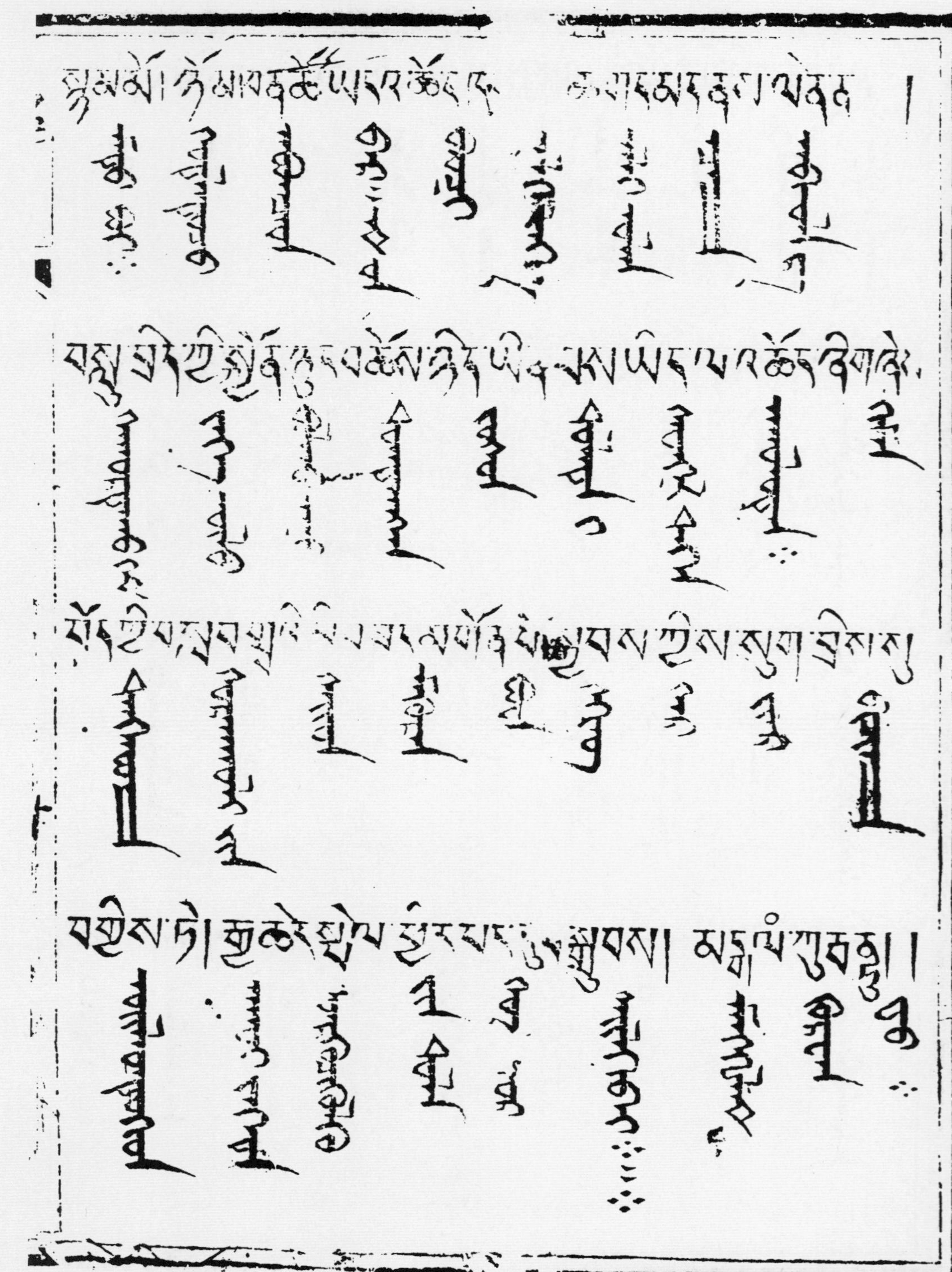

ᠣᠷᠣᠨ ᠤᠳᠤᠮ ᠪᠠᠷ ᠰᠢᠯᠢᠭᠳᠡᠭᠰᠡᠨ ᠬᠡᠪᠯᠡᠯ ᠦᠨ ᠡᠷᠲᠡᠨ ᠨᠣᠮ ᠪᠣᠯᠤᠨ᠎ᠠ ::

ᠳᠡᠪᠲᠡᠷ ᠦᠨ ᠬᠡᠮᠵᠢᠶ᠎ᠡ ᠨᠢ : 25.5cm×11.4cm ᠪᠣᠯᠤᠭᠰᠠᠨ᠂ ᠨᠢᠭᠤᠷ 24 ᠬᠤᠳᠠᠰᠤᠲᠠᠢ ᠪᠠᠢᠨ᠎ᠠ ::

ᠣᠷᠣᠨ ᠰᠤᠳᠤᠯᠭᠠ ᠪᠠ ᠬᠡᠪ ᠦᠨ ᠰᠢᠨᠵᠢᠯᠡᠭᠡ ᠶᠢ ᠬᠡᠯᠡᠪᠡᠯ᠂ ᠮᠣᠩᠭᠣᠯ ᠪᠢᠴᠢᠭ ᠦᠨ ᠬᠡᠪᠯᠡᠭᠰᠡᠨ ᠨᠣᠮ ᠪᠣᠯᠤᠨ᠎ᠠ :: ᠬᠡᠪ ᠦᠨ ᠵᠢᠷᠤᠭ ᠢ ᠬᠠᠳᠠᠭᠠᠯᠠᠭᠰᠠᠨ ᠪᠣᠯᠤᠨ᠎ᠠ᠂ ᠪᠠᠷᠢᠮᠲᠠ ᠶᠢᠨ ᠬᠡᠪ ᠦᠨ ᠳᠡᠭᠡᠷ᠎ᠡ ᠪᠠᠷᠢᠮᠲᠠᠯᠠᠭᠰᠠᠨ ᠪᠣᠯᠤᠨ᠎ᠠ ::

4

药方

Prescriptions

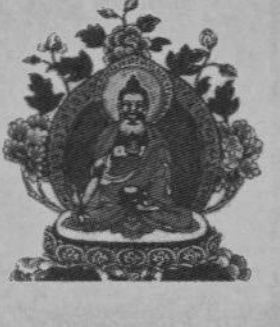

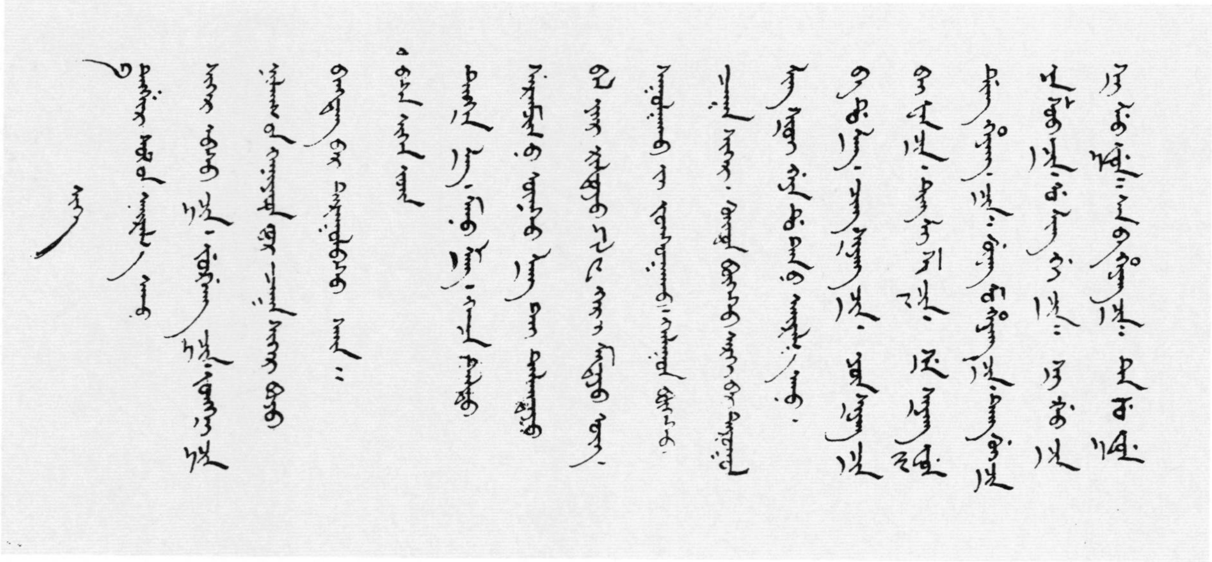

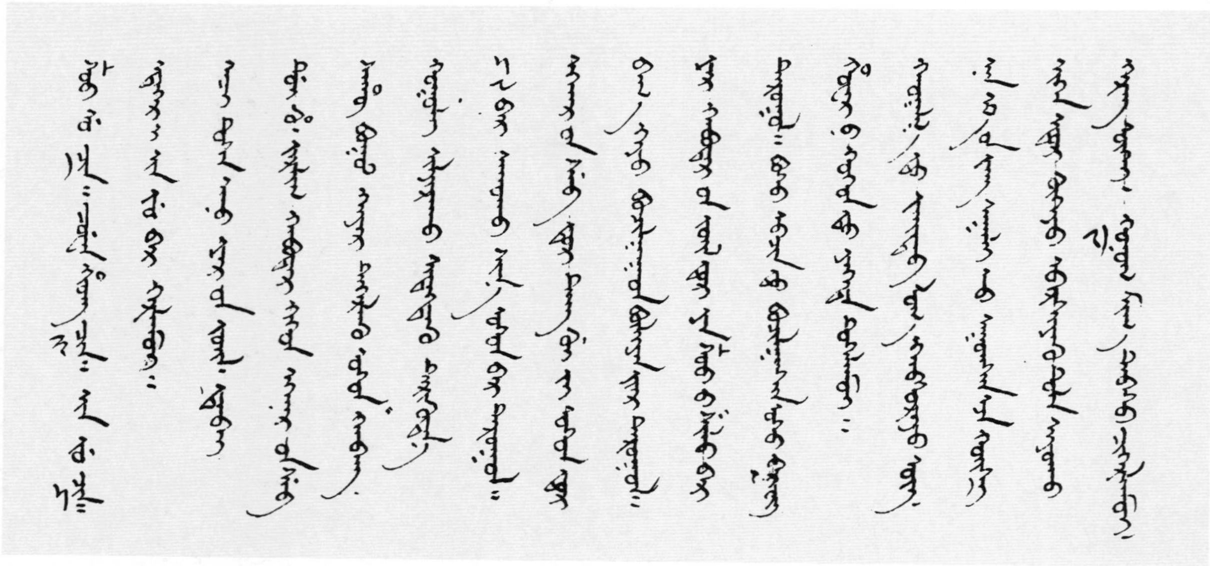

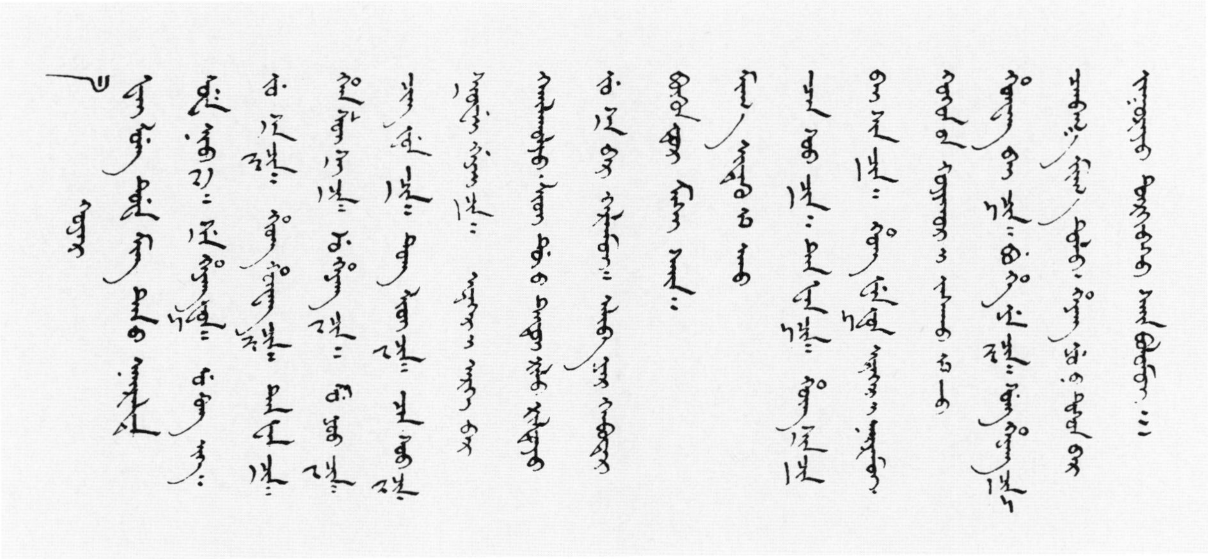

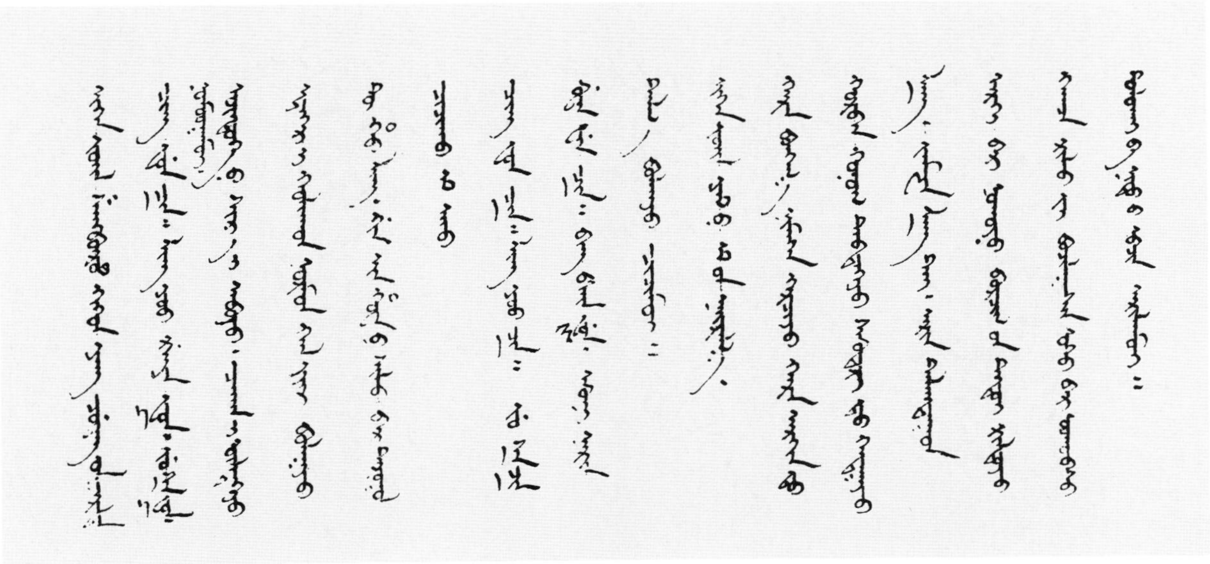

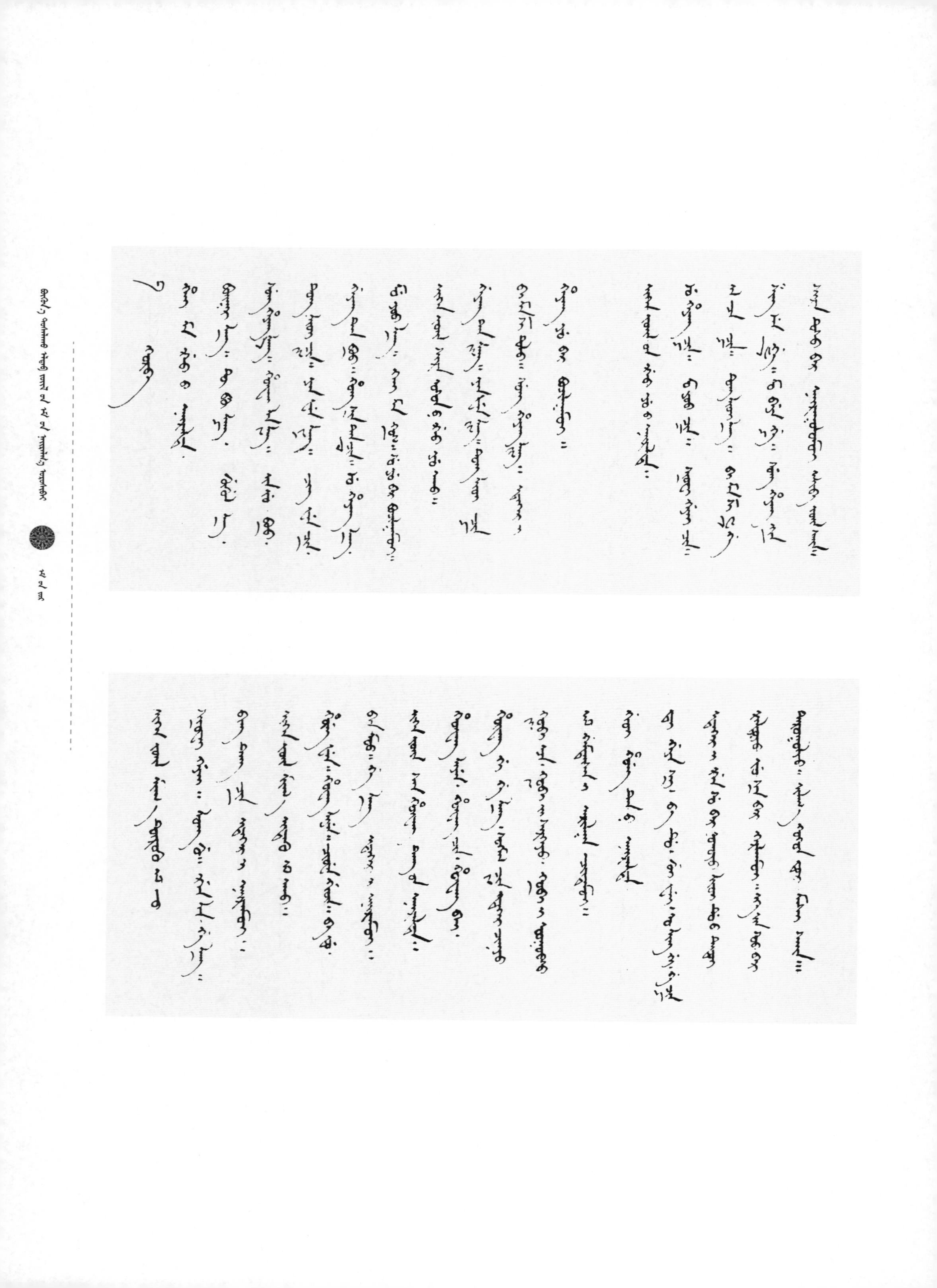

[illegible]

[illegible]

[illegible]

[illegible]

[illegible]

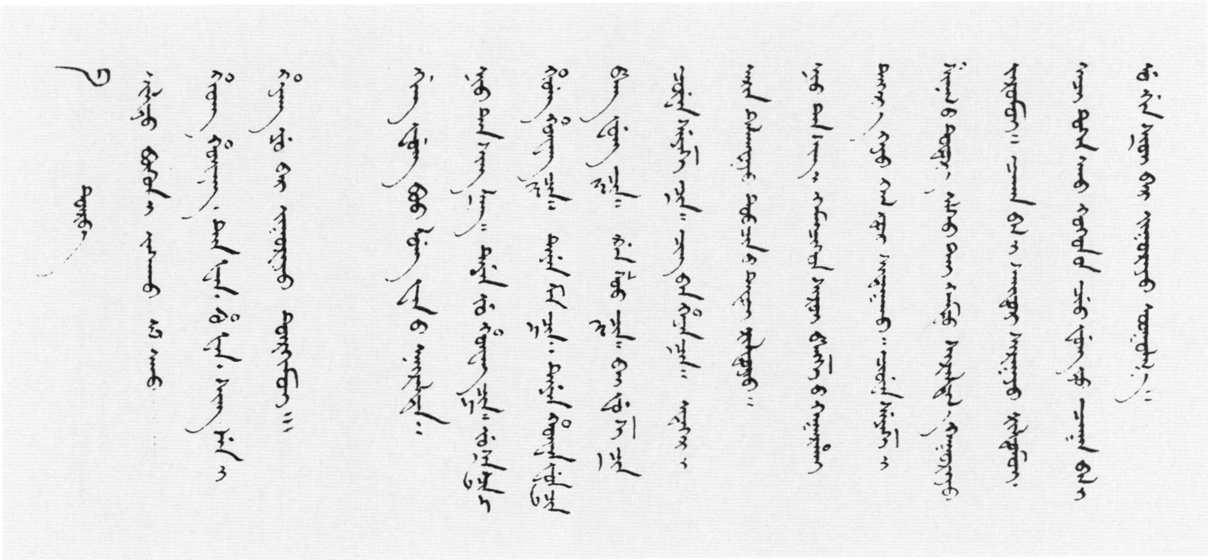

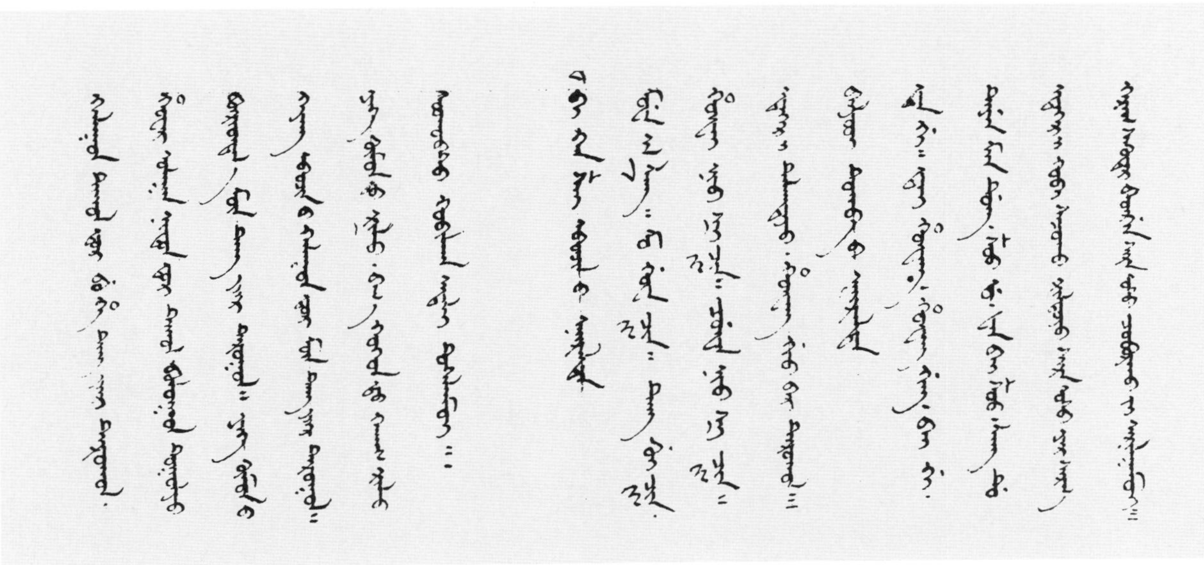

[illegible]

[illegible]

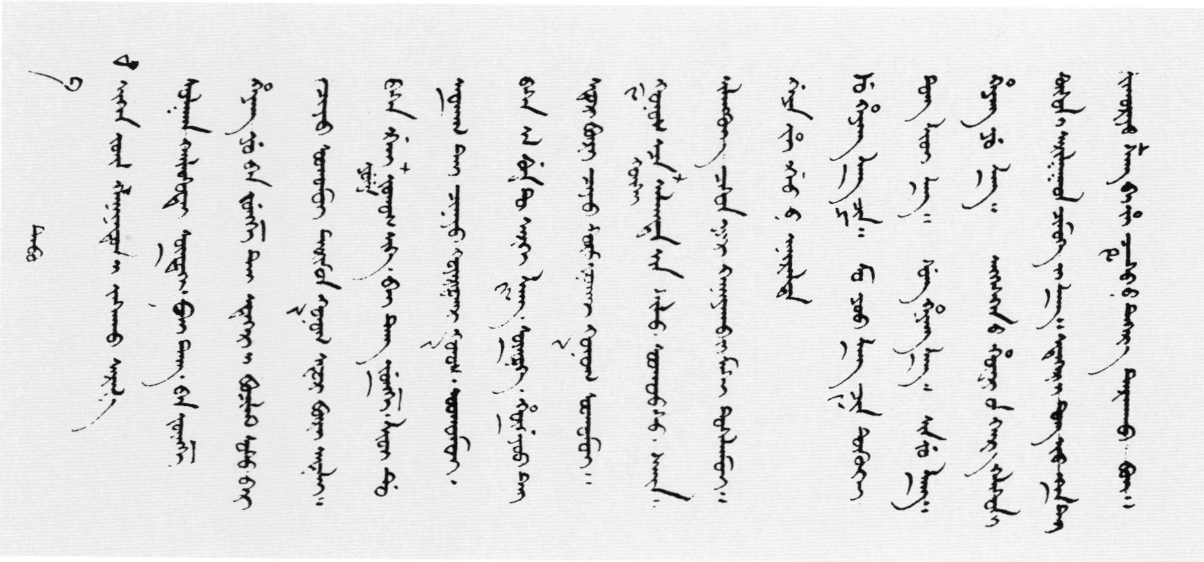

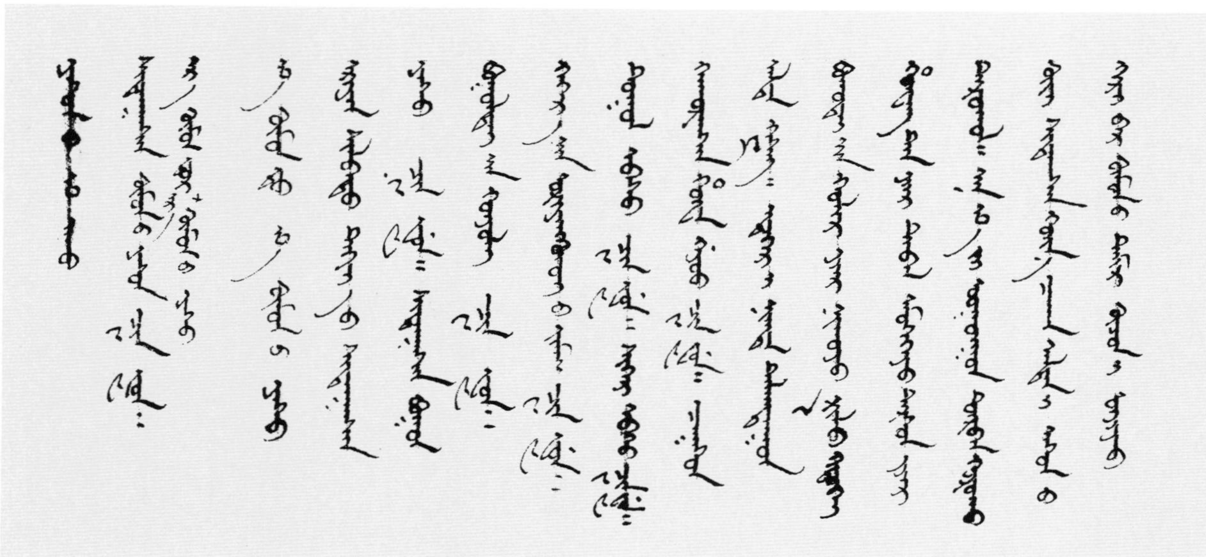

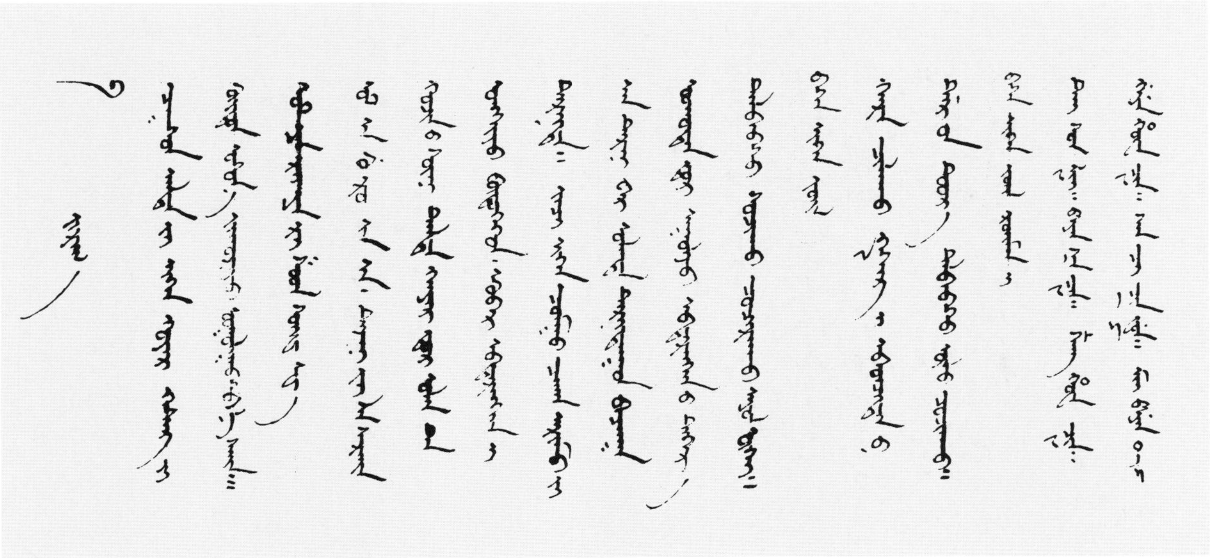

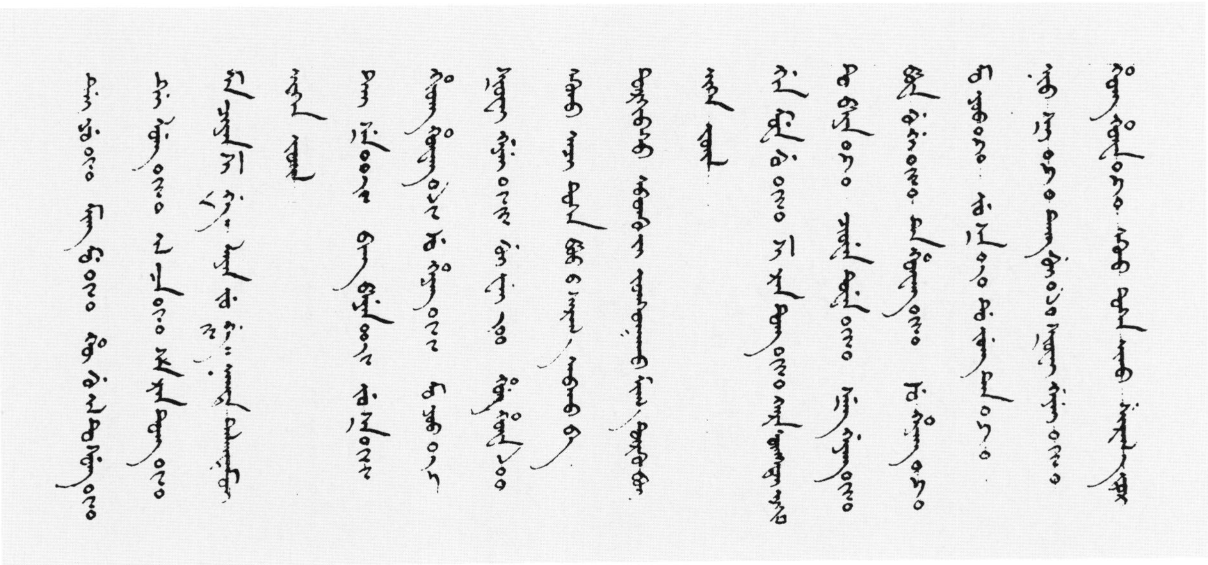

[illegible]

[illegible]

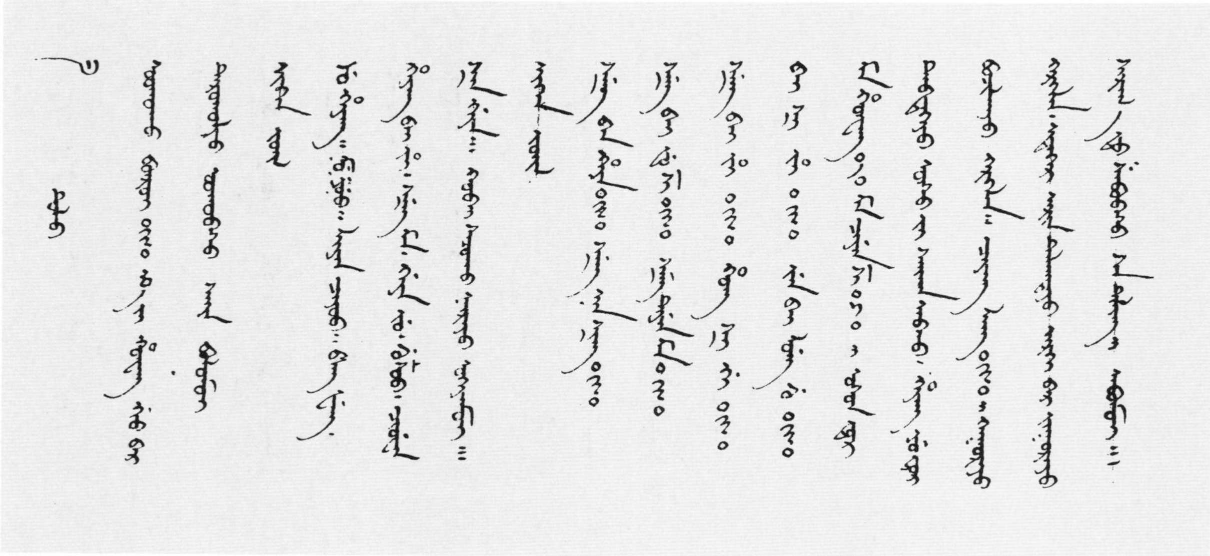

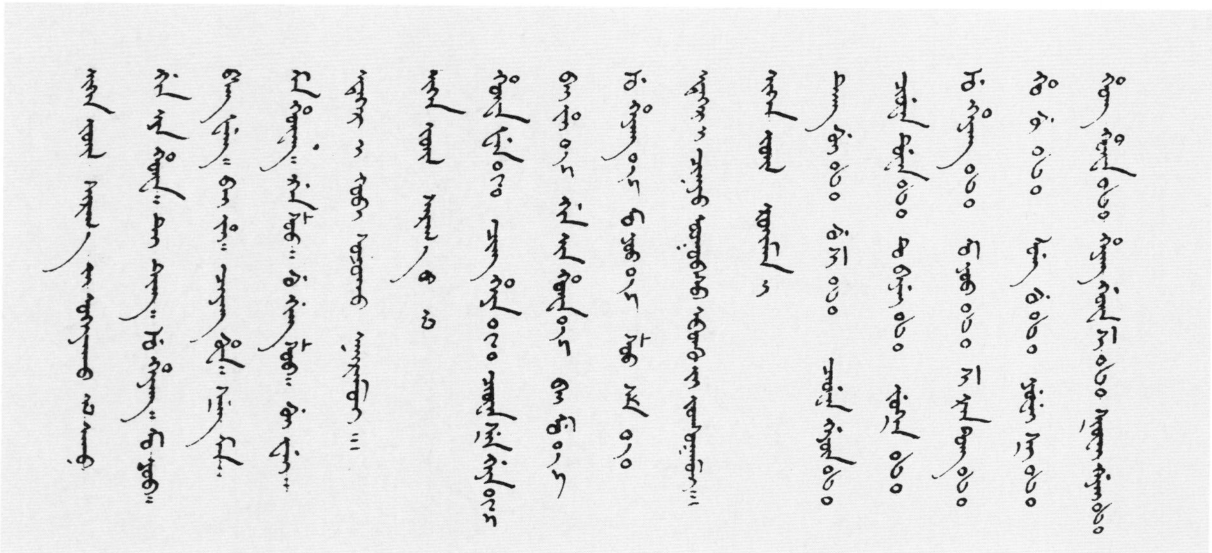

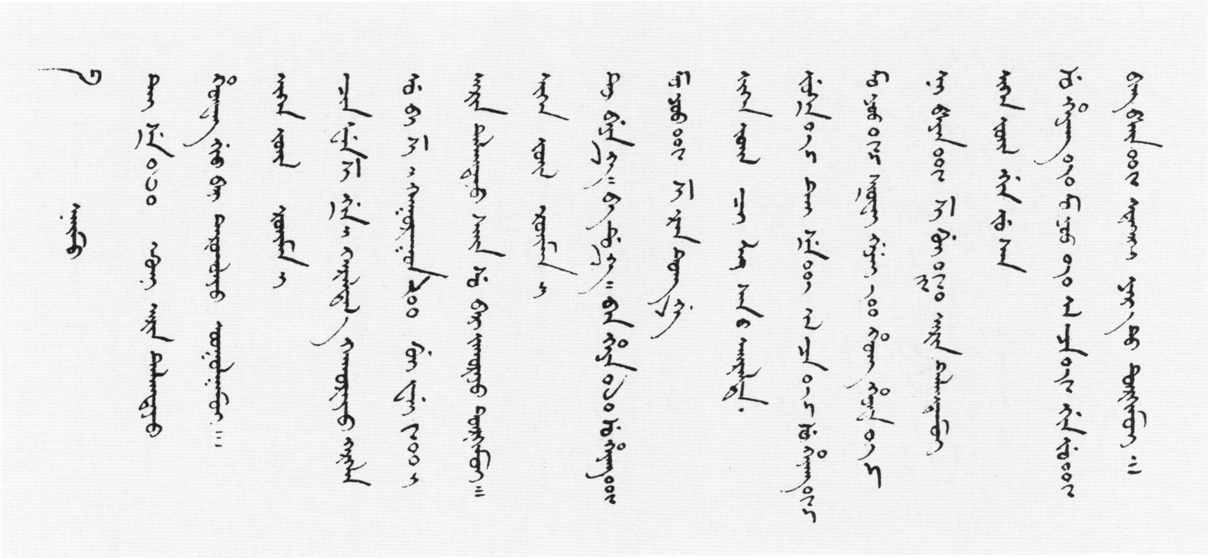

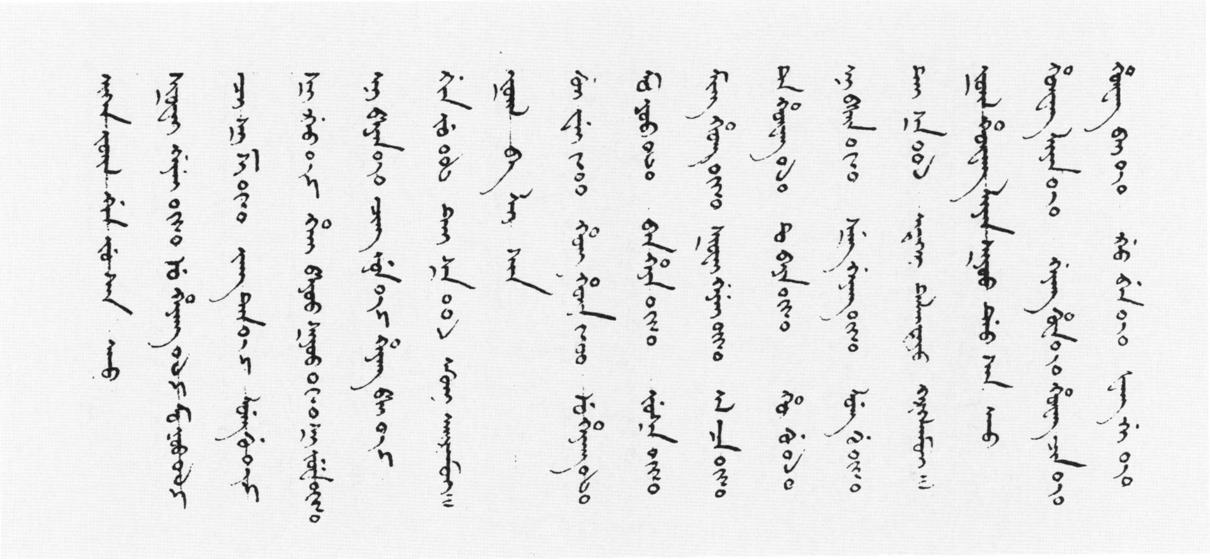

[illegible]

[illegible]

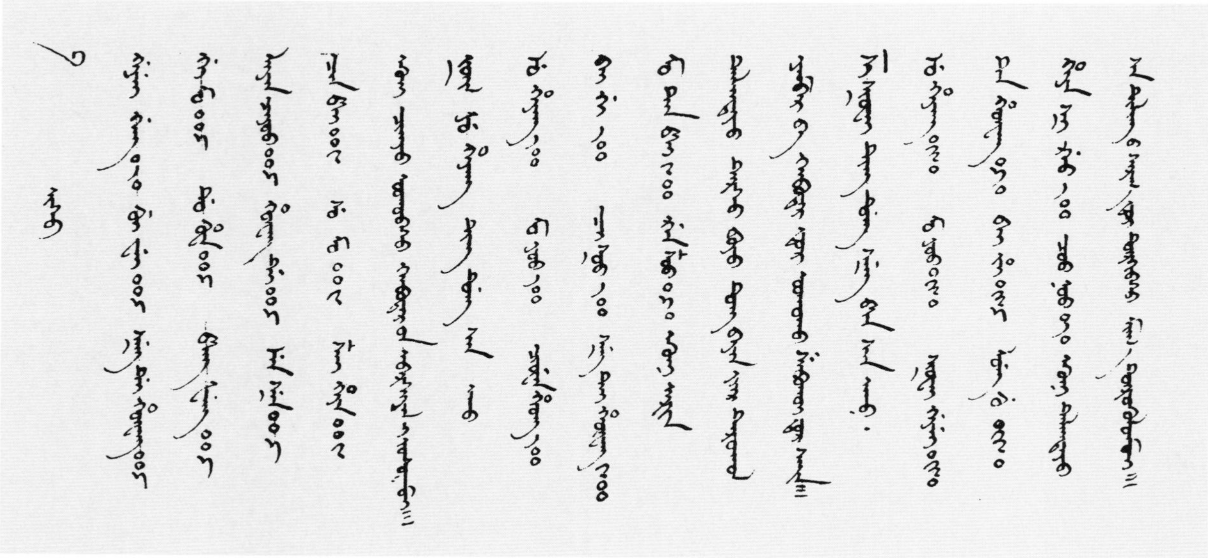

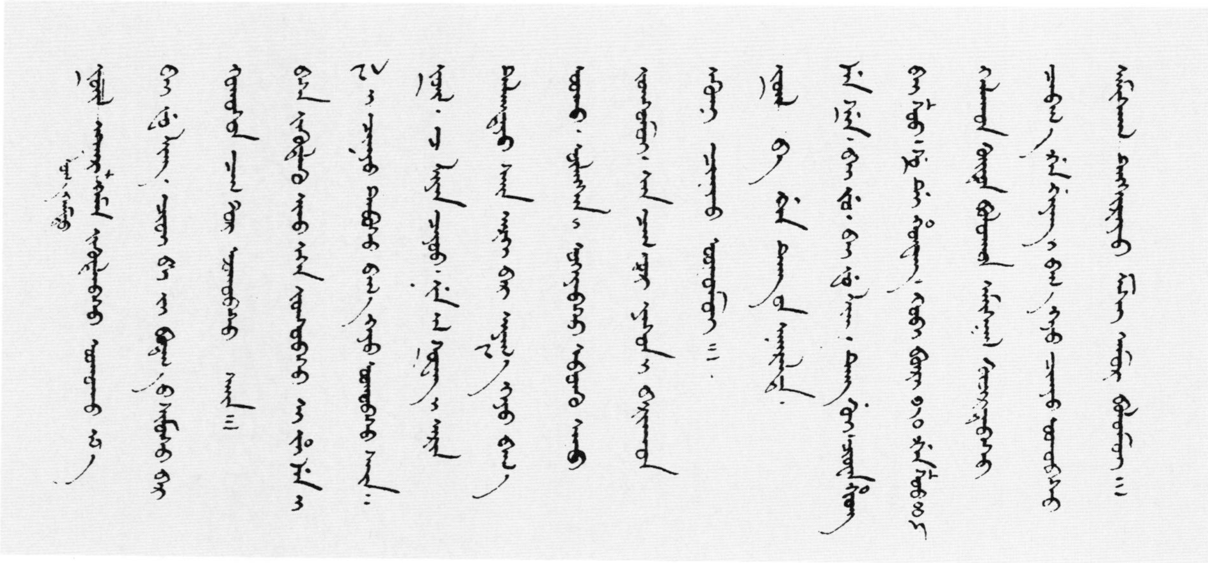

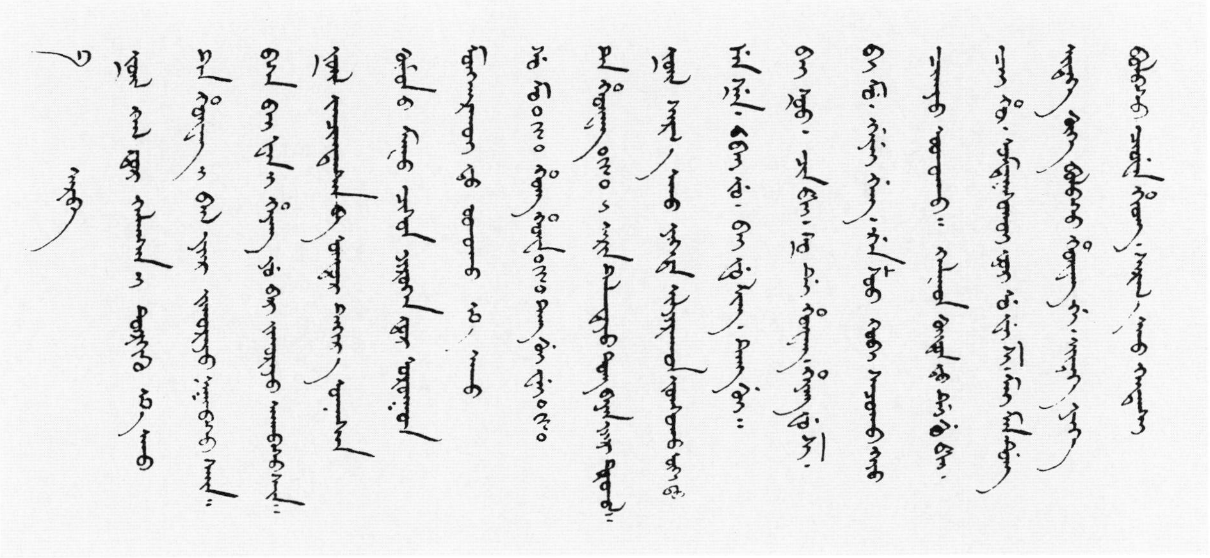

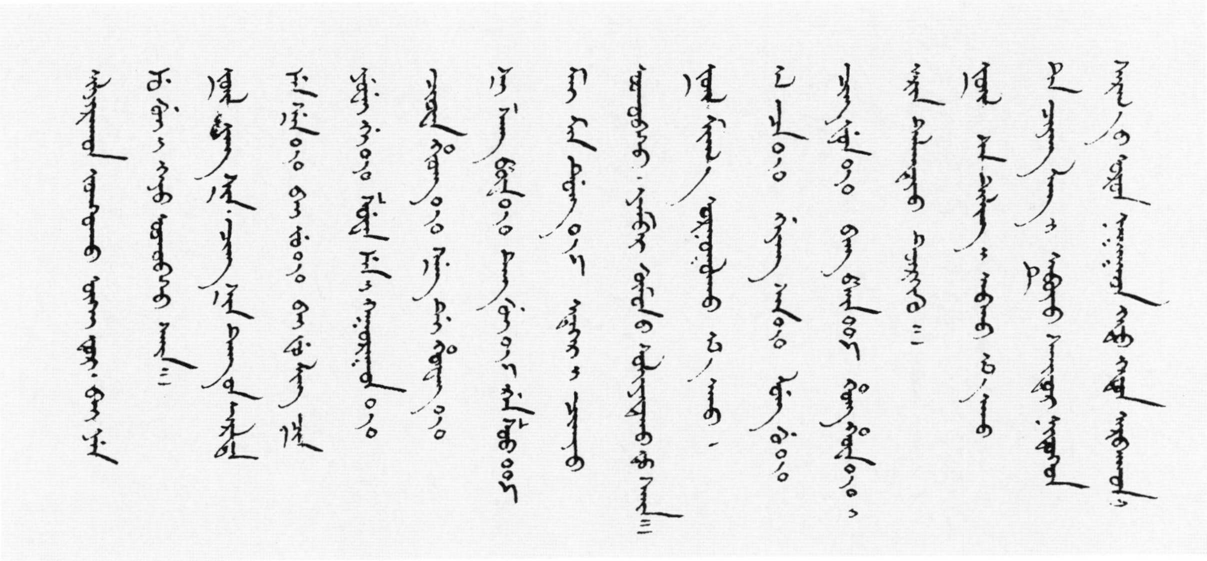

[illegible]

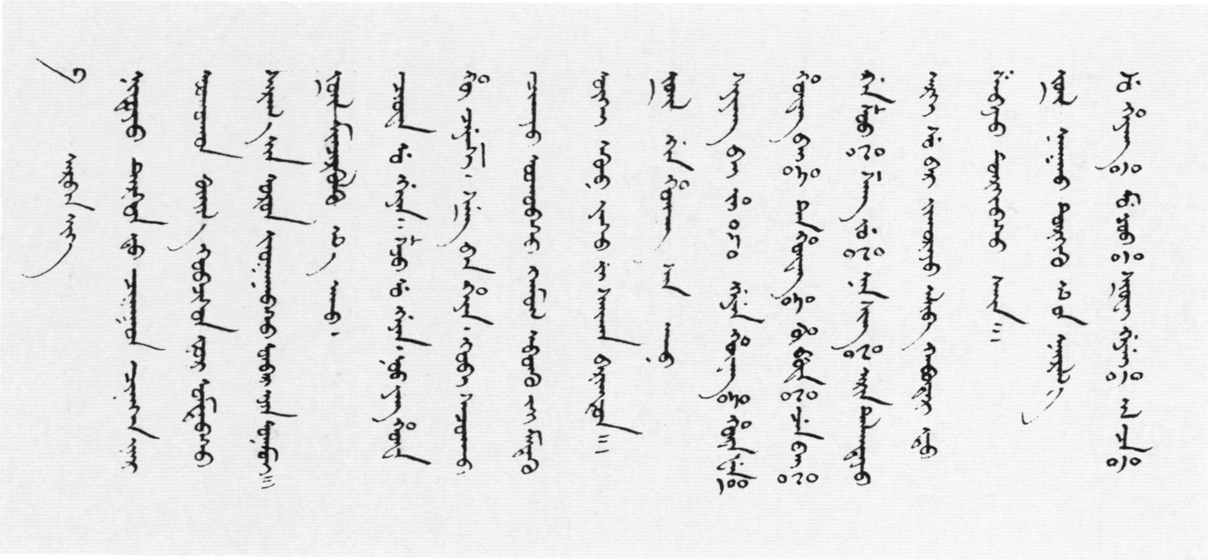

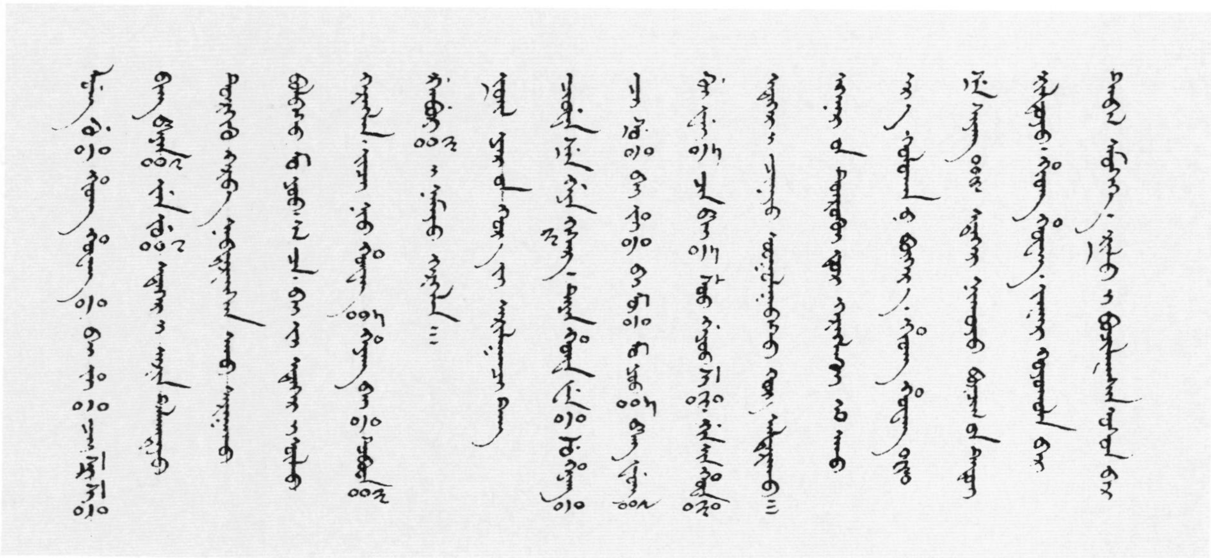

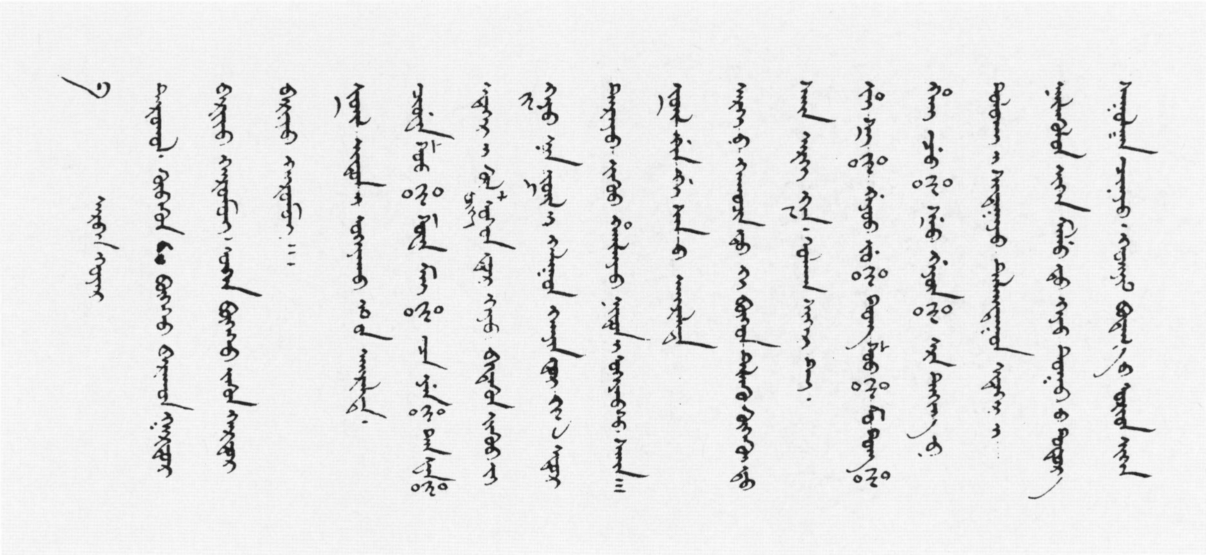

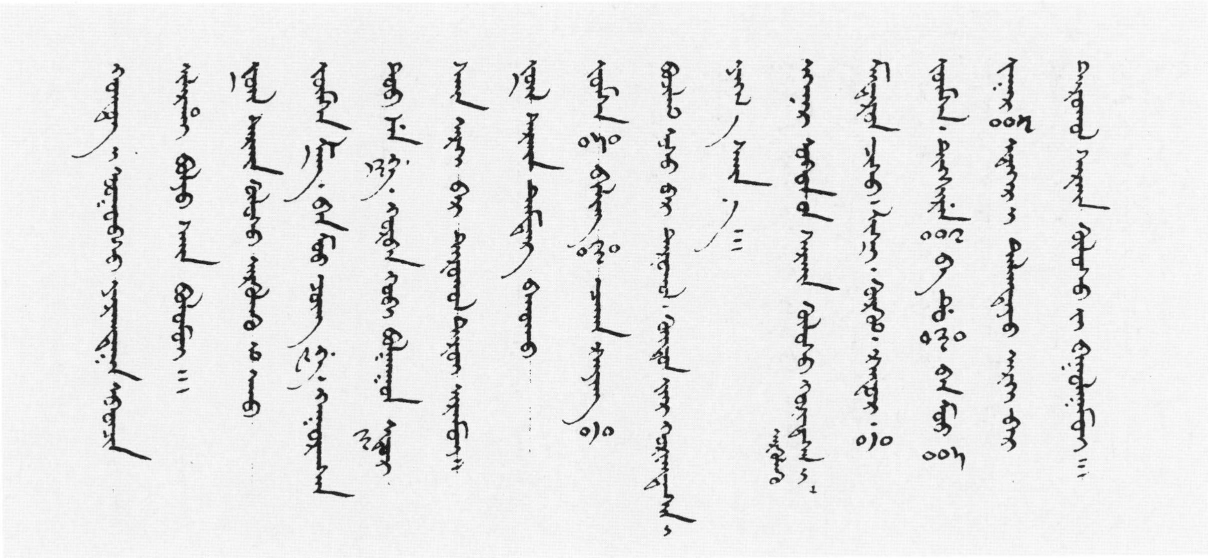

[illegible]

[illegible]

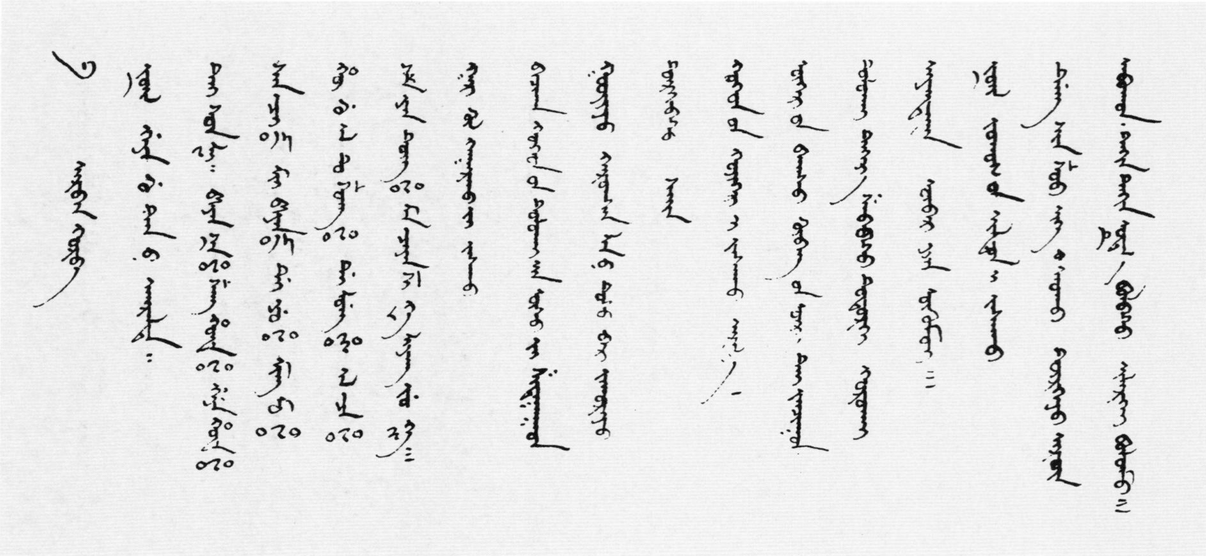

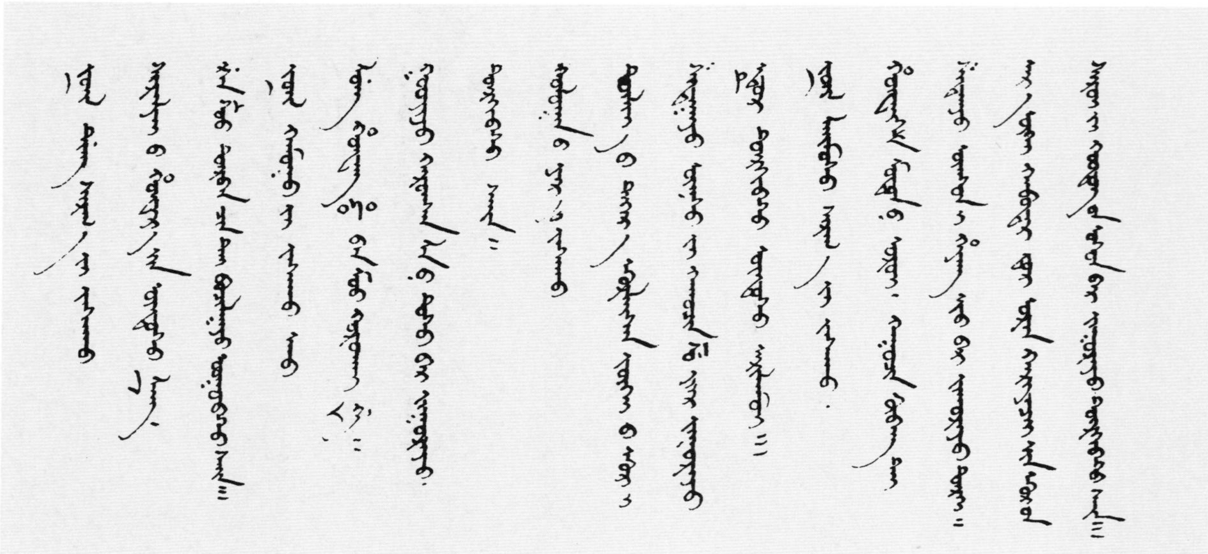

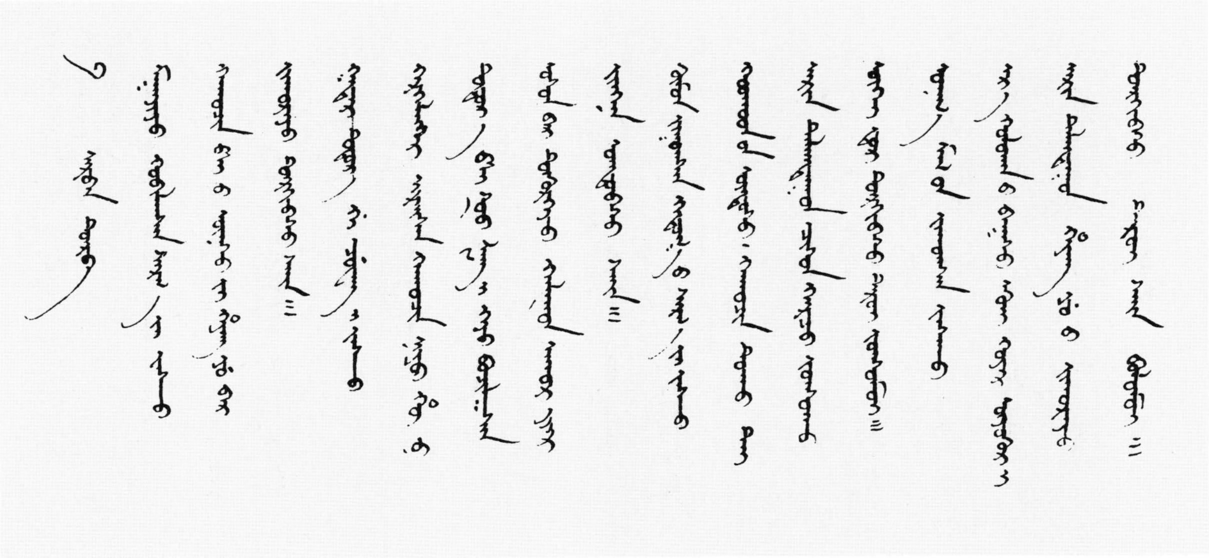

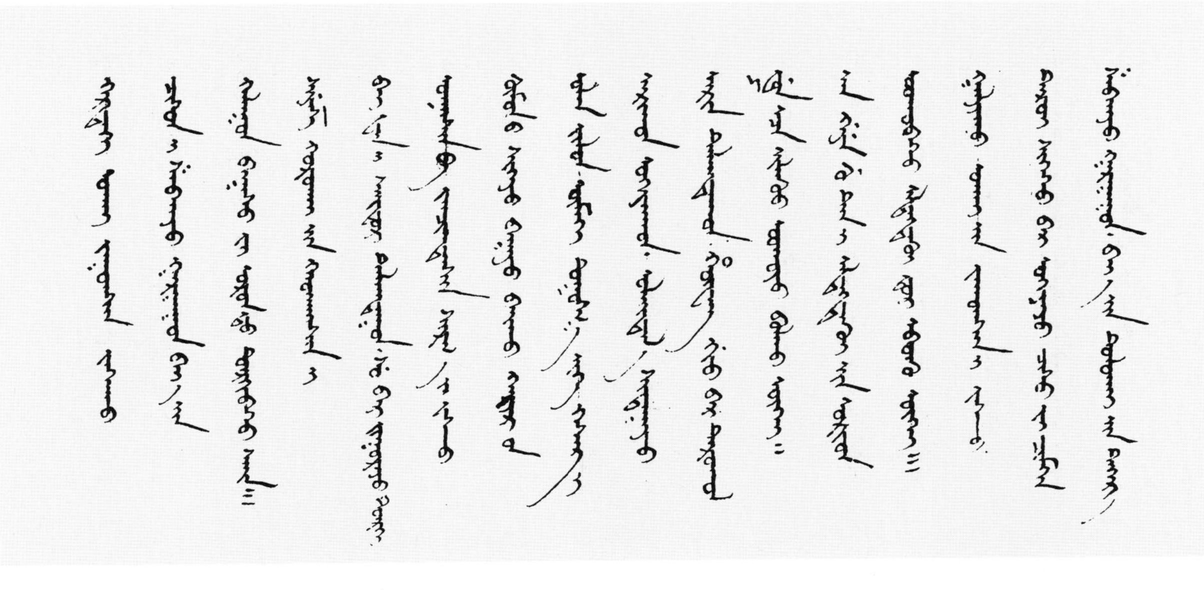

[illegible]

[illegible]

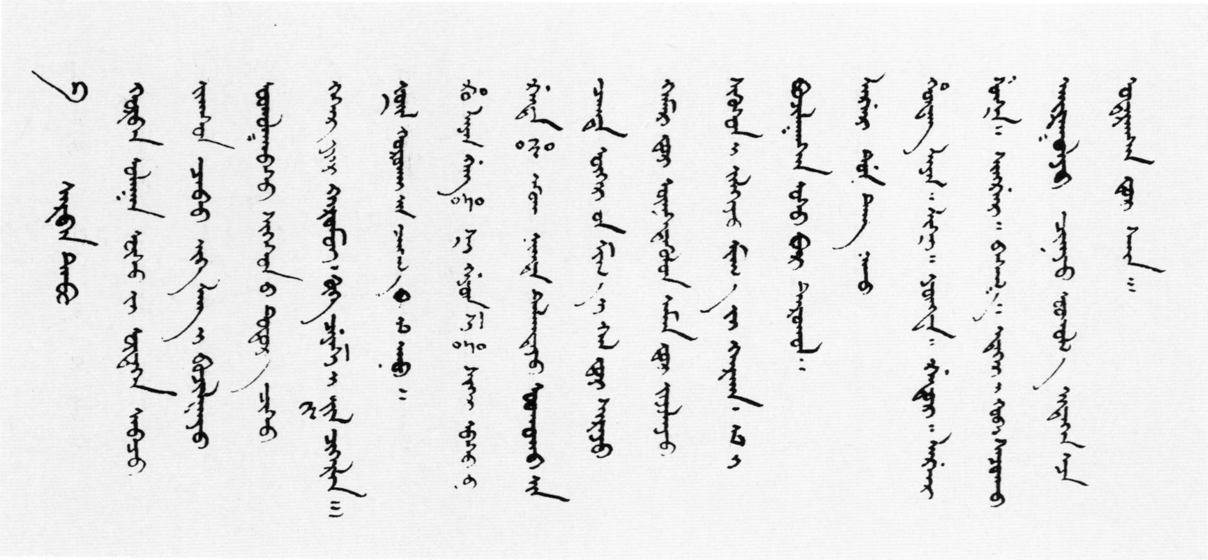

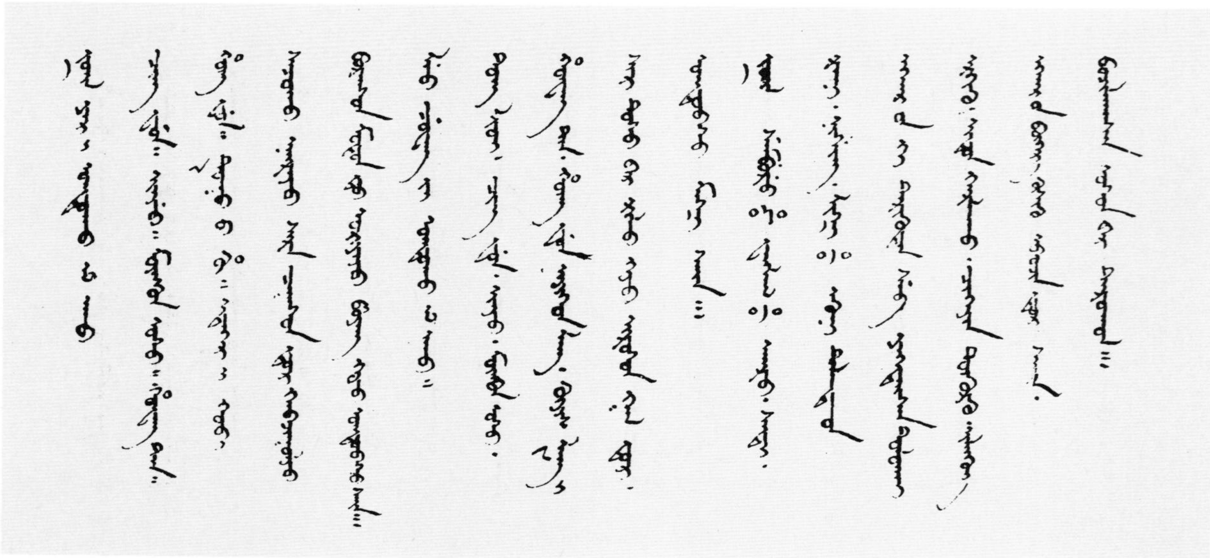

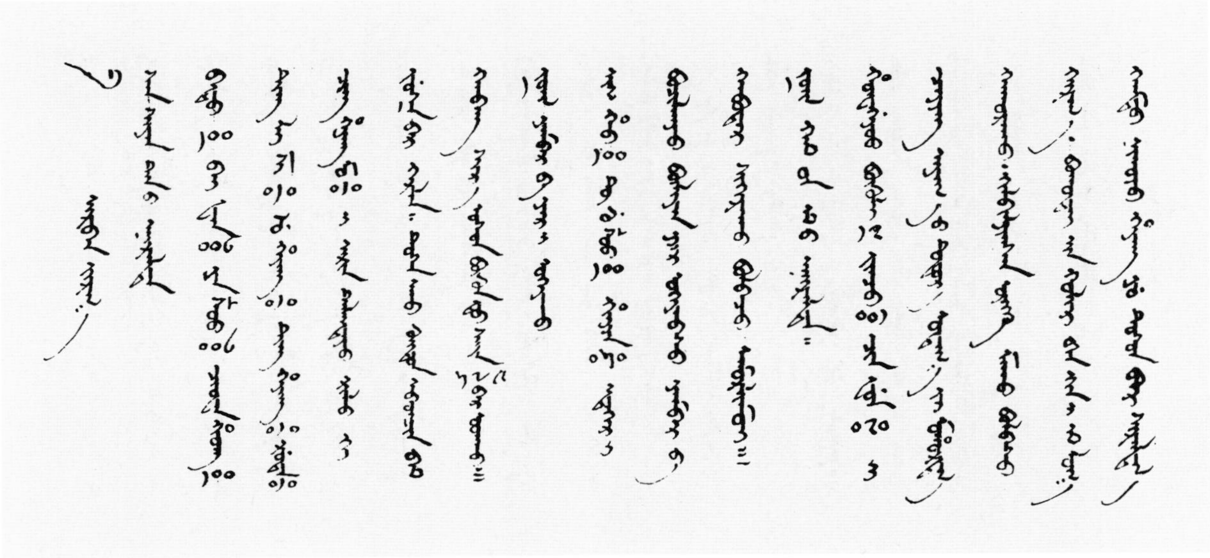

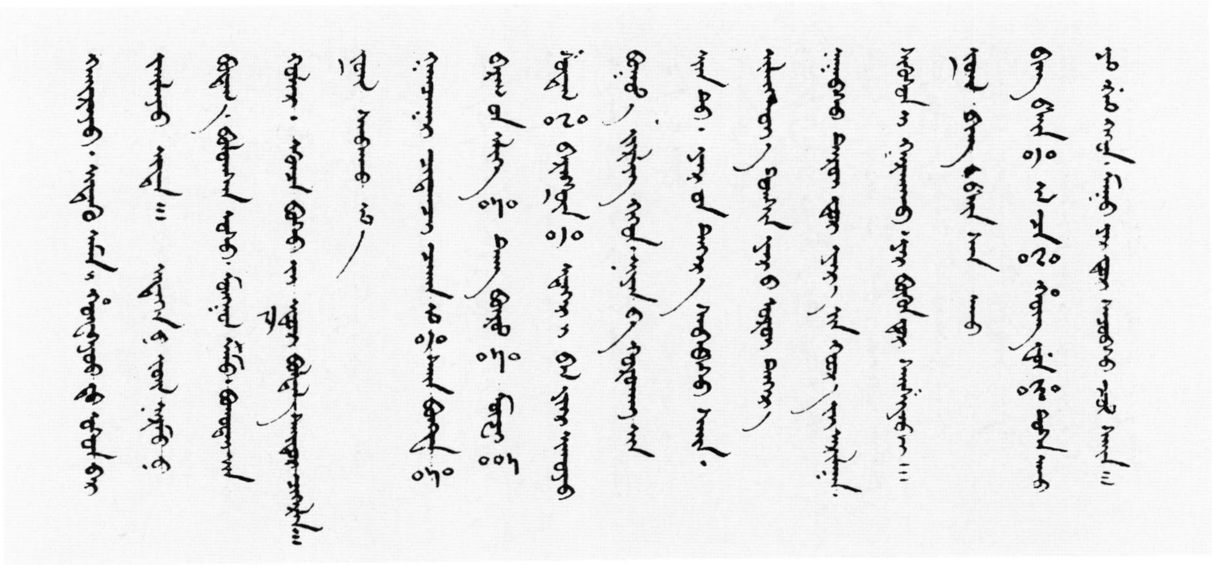

[illegible]

[illegible]

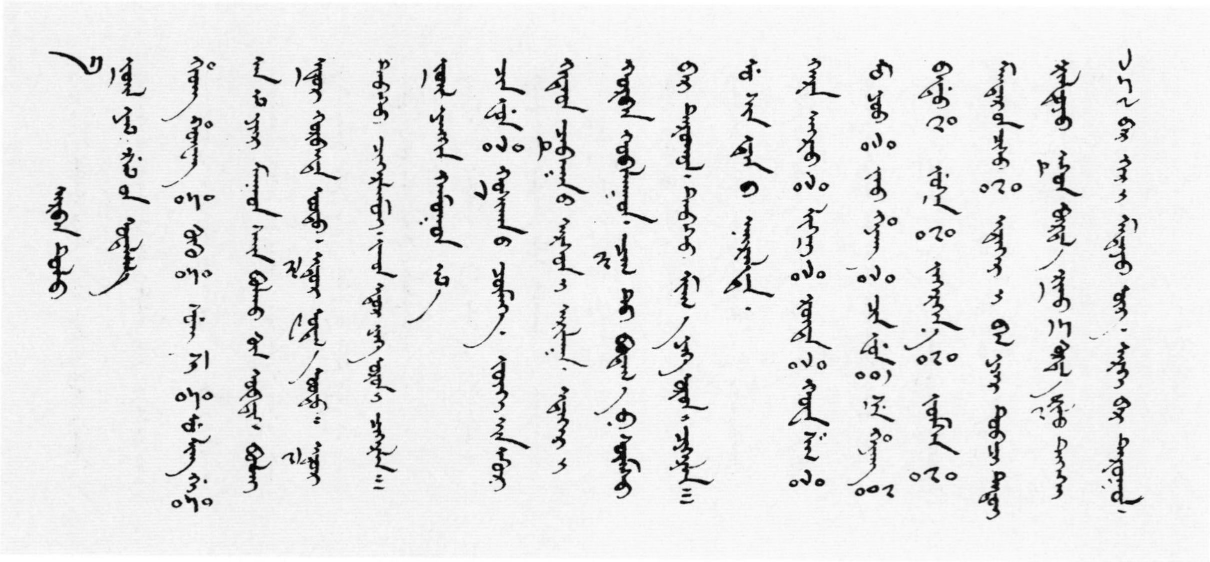

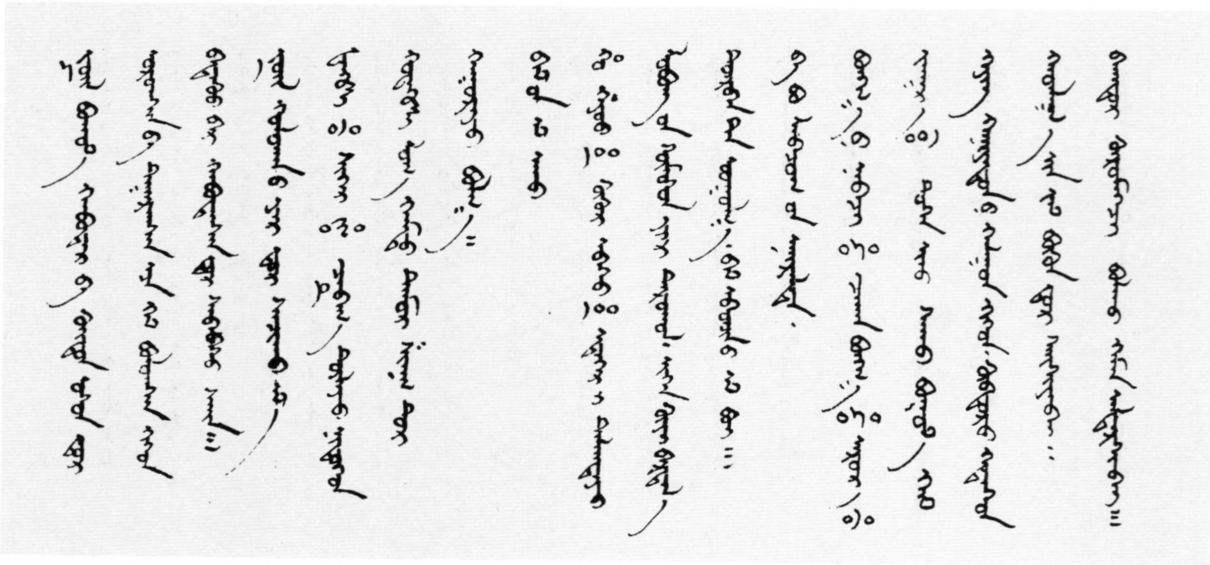

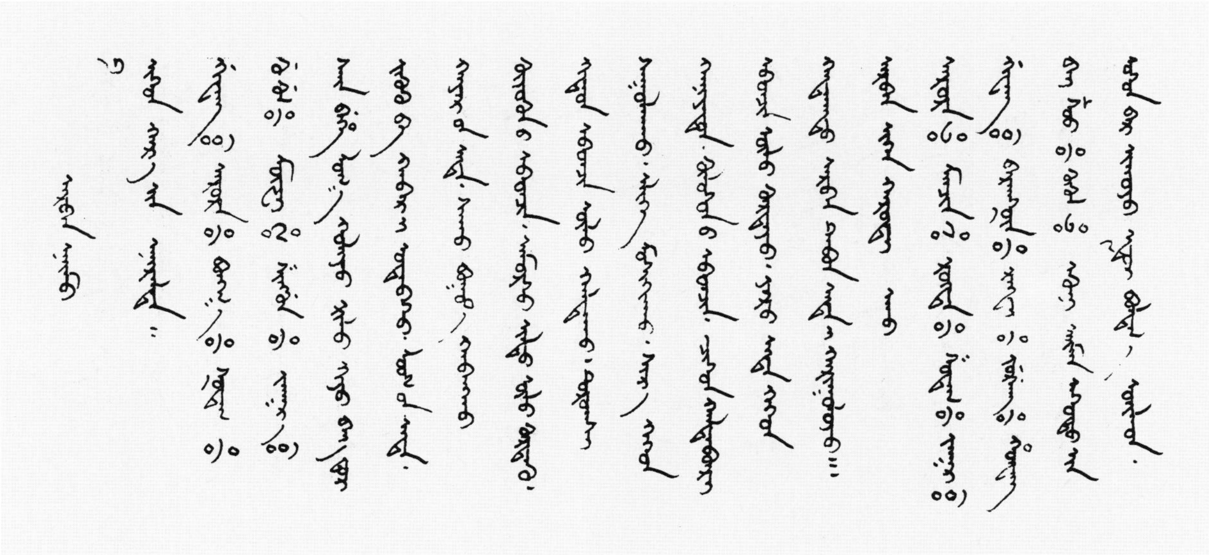

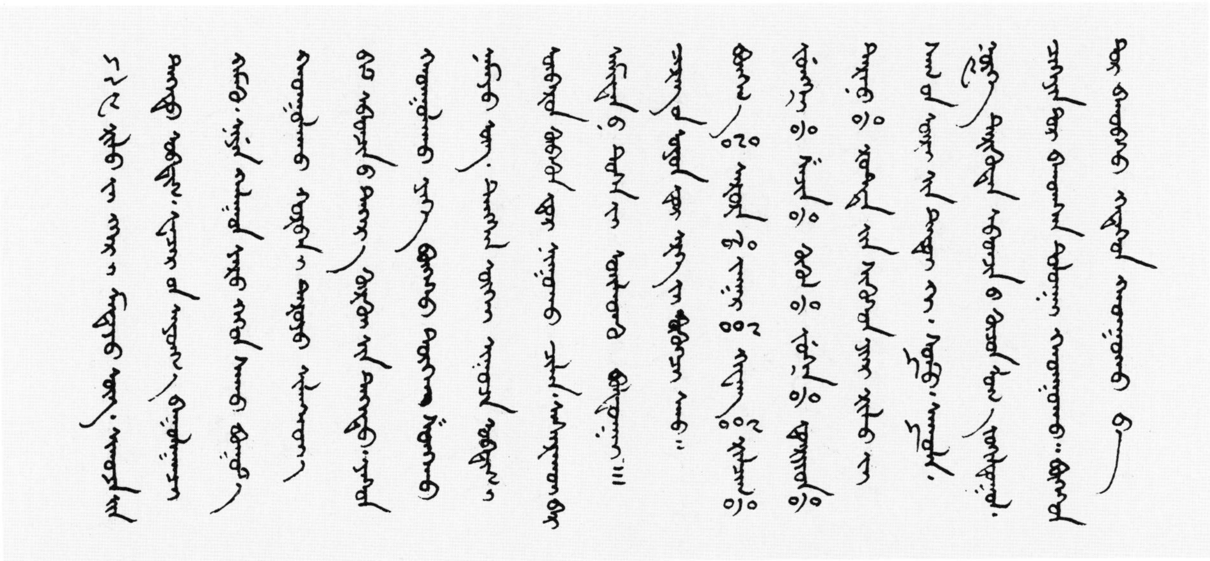

[illegible]

[illegible]

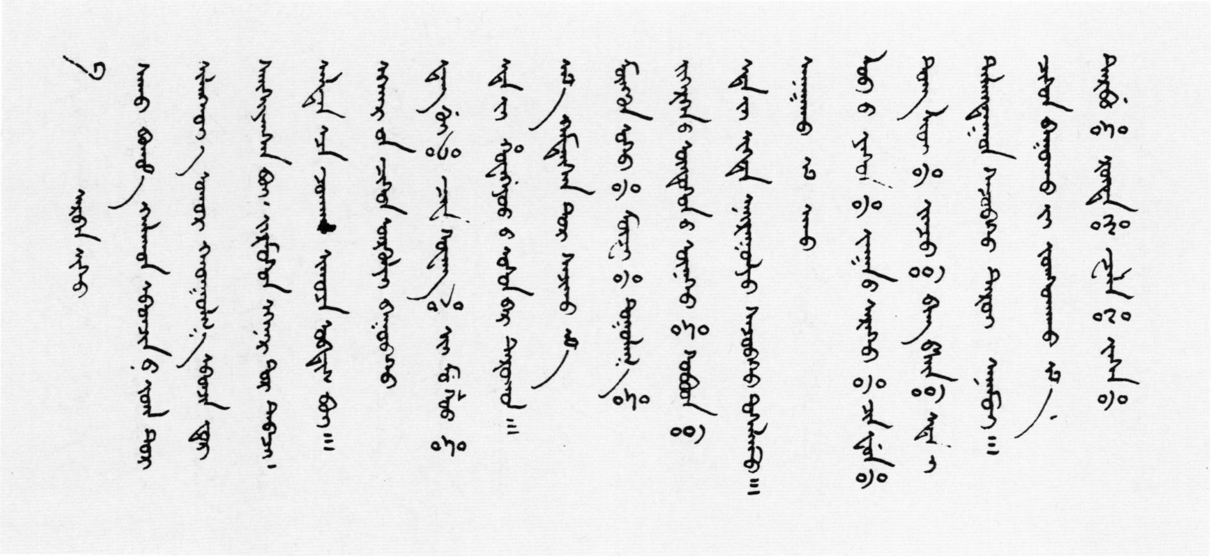

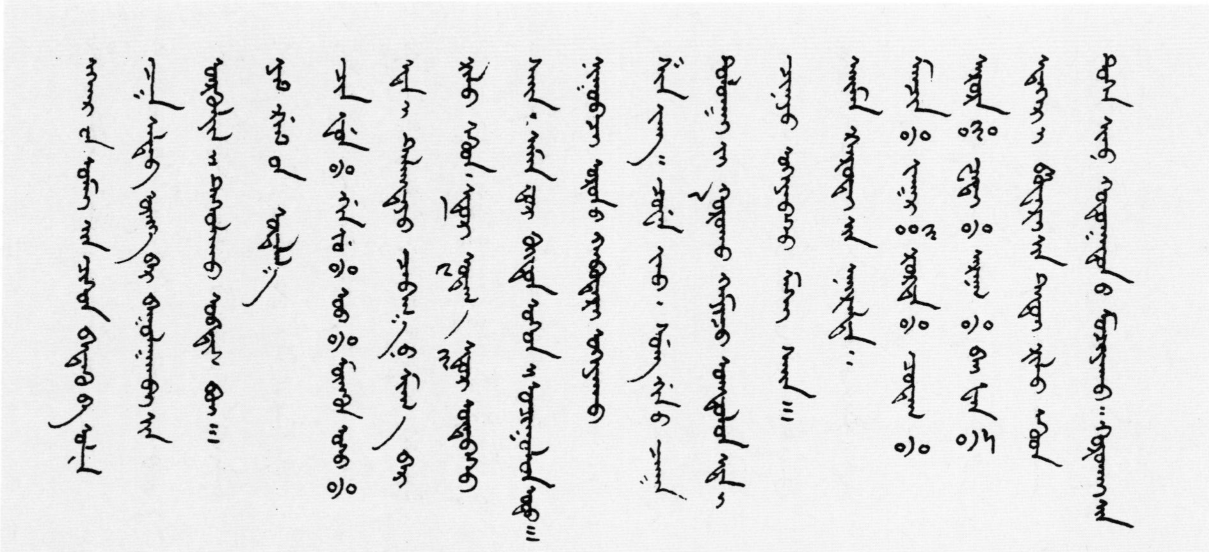

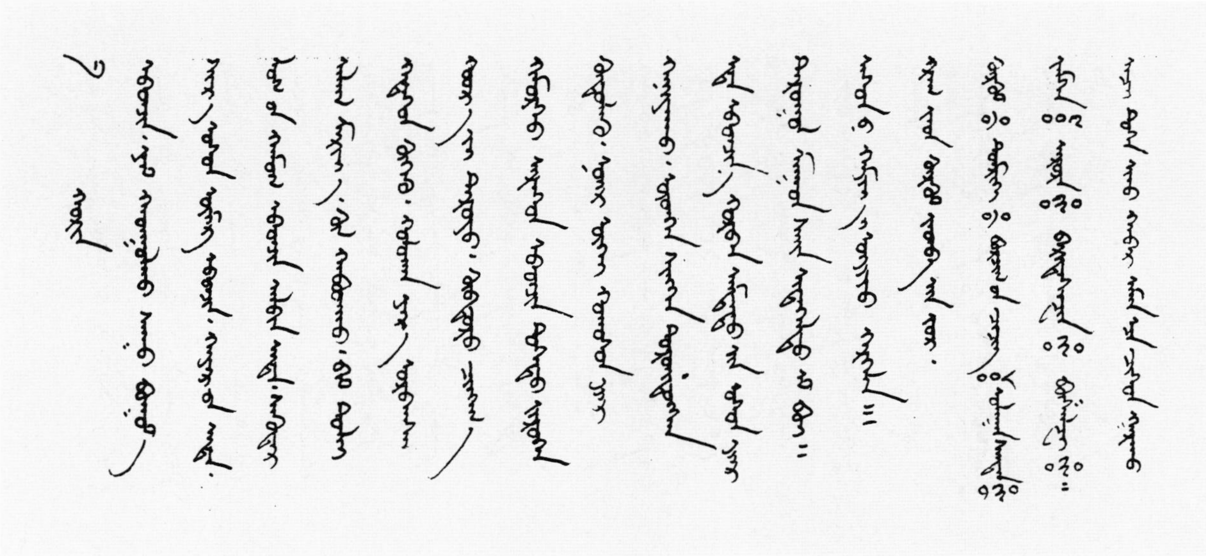

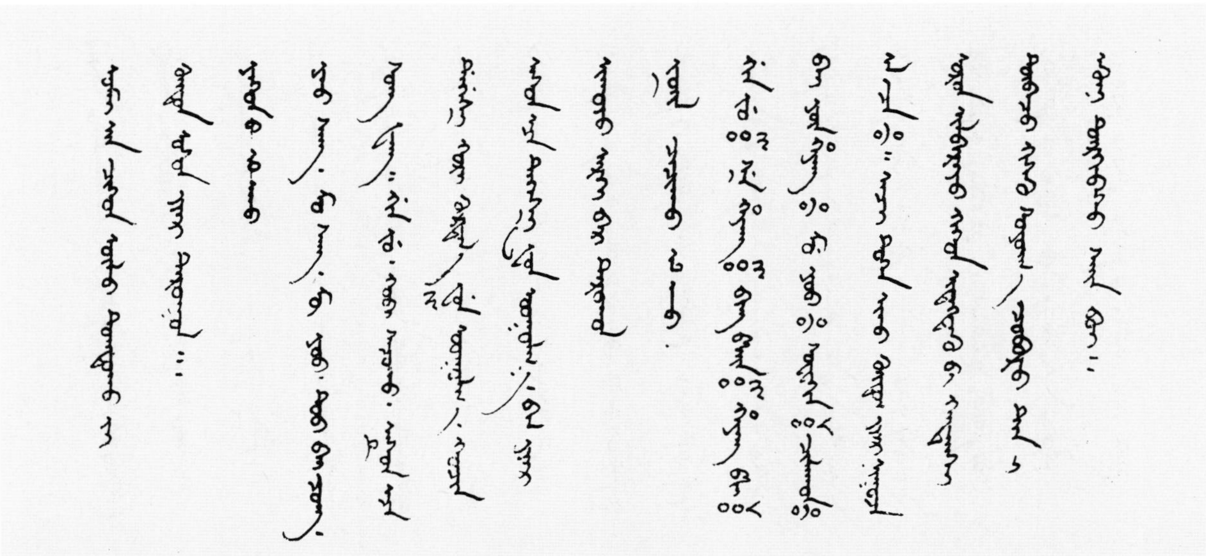

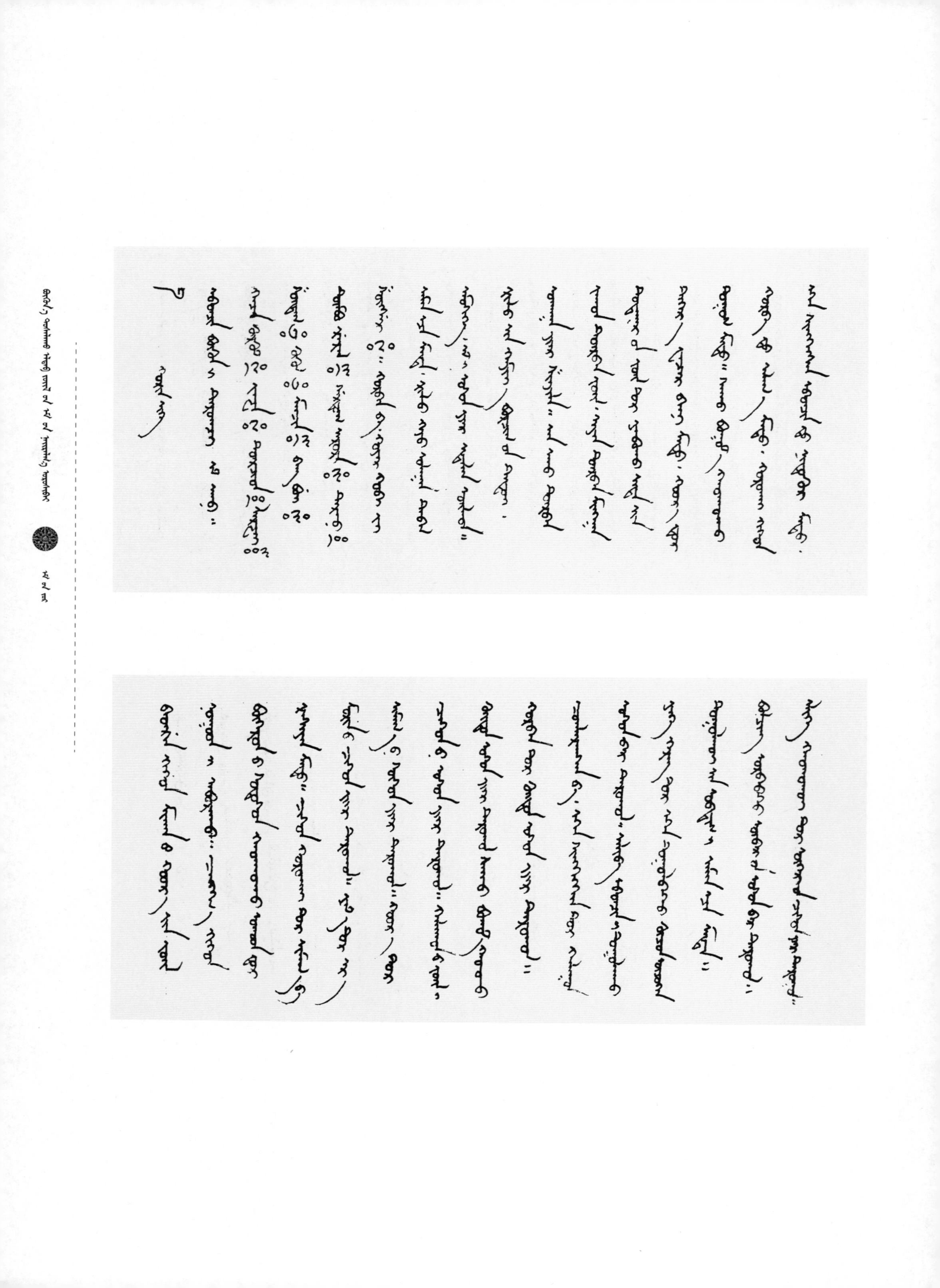

[illegible]

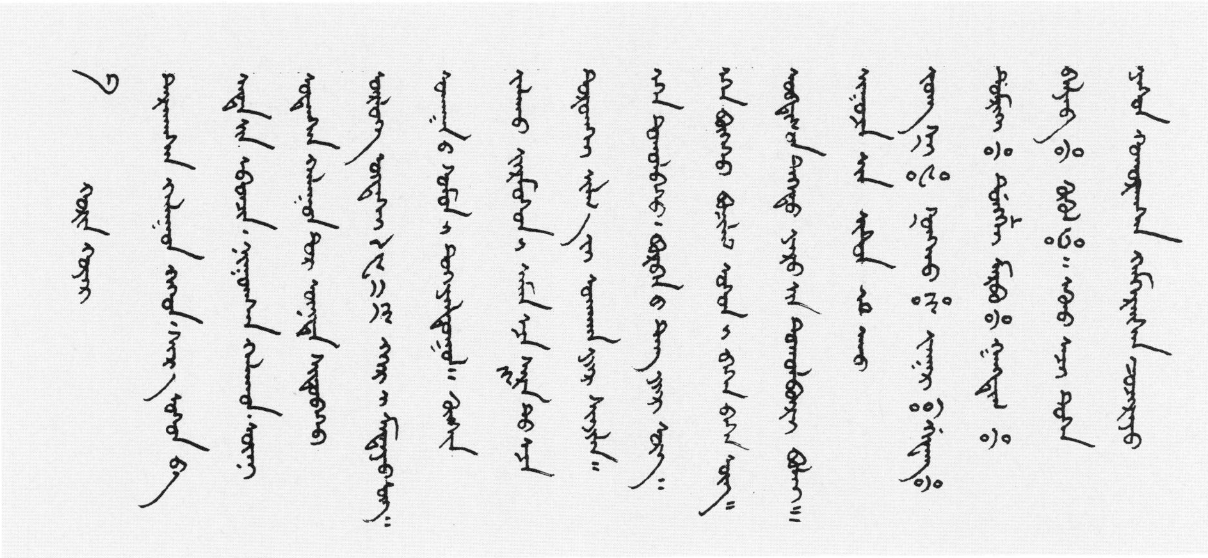

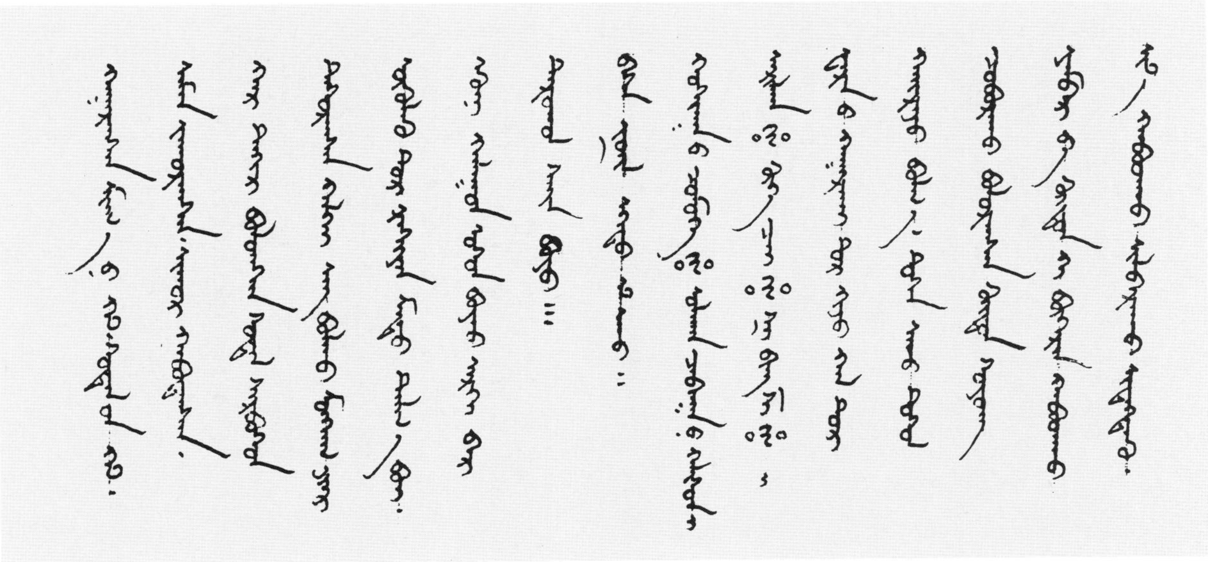

[illegible] ::
[illegible]
[illegible]
[illegible]
[illegible]
[illegible]
[illegible]

[illegible] ::
[illegible]
[illegible]
[illegible] ::
[illegible] ::
[illegible]
[illegible]
[illegible]

[illegible]
[illegible]
[illegible]
[illegible]

[illegible] ::
[illegible]
[illegible]
[illegible]
[illegible]
[illegible]
[illegible]
[illegible]
[illegible]
[illegible]
[illegible]
[illegible]
[illegible]

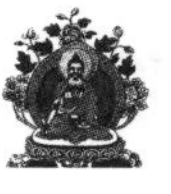

ᠮᠣᠳᠣᠨ ᠬᠡᠪᠯᠡᠯ ᠪᠡᠷ ᠰᠢᠷᠦᠭᠦᠯᠦᠨ ᠬᠡᠪᠯᠡᠭᠰᠡᠨ ᠤᠨ ᠬᠡᠪᠯᠡᠯ ᠨᠣᠮ ᠤᠨ ᠳᠤᠭᠤᠢ ᠬᠡᠪᠯᠡᠯ ᠪᠣᠯᠤᠨ᠎ᠠ ::

ᠨᠣᠮ ᠤᠨ ᠬᠡᠮᠵᠢᠶ᠎ᠡ ᠨᠢ: 23cm×21.5cm ᠪᠣᠯᠤᠨ᠎ᠠ · ᠨᠡᠢᠲᠡ 17 ᠨᠢᠭᠤᠷ ᠲᠠᠢ ::

ᠨᠢᠭᠡ ᠬᠡᠰᠡᠭ ᠤᠨ ᠬᠡᠪᠯᠡᠯ ᠳᠦ ᠪᠠᠭᠲᠠᠭᠰᠠᠨ ᠬᠡᠯᠡ ᠪᠡᠷ ᠪᠢᠴᠢᠭ ᠤᠨ ᠬᠡᠯᠪᠡᠷᠢ ᠶᠢᠨ ᠠᠷᠭ᠎ᠠ ᠵᠢᠷᠤᠮ ᠢ ᠲᠣᠳᠣᠷᠬᠠᠢᠯᠠᠨ ᠪᠠᠢᠭ᠎ᠠ ᠪᠣᠯᠬᠤ ᠳᠤ ᠨᠣᠮ ᠤᠨ ᠬᠡᠪᠯᠡᠯ ᠦᠨ ᠬᠣᠶᠠᠷ ᠨᠢᠭᠤᠷ
ᠪᠦᠷᠢᠳᠦ 17 ᠨᠢᠭᠤᠷ :: ᠬᠣᠶᠠᠷ ᠬᠡᠰᠡᠭ ᠲᠦ ᠬᠤᠪᠢᠶᠠᠷᠢᠯᠠᠨ ᠲᠣᠭᠲᠠᠭᠰᠠᠨ ᠨᠣᠮ ᠪᠣᠯᠤᠨ᠎ᠠ :: ᠳᠤᠷᠠᠳᠤᠭᠳᠠᠭᠰᠠᠨ ᠣᠨ ᠤ 1915 ᠣᠨ ᠤ ᠬᠣᠶᠠᠷ ᠰᠠᠷ᠎ᠠ ᠶᠢᠨ ᠰᠢᠨ᠎ᠡ ᠶᠢᠨ ᠬᠡᠪᠯᠡᠯ
ᠪᠢᠴᠢᠭ ᠬᠡᠪᠯᠡᠯ ᠪᠣᠯᠤᠨ᠎ᠠ ::

ᠲᠣᠭᠲᠠᠭᠰᠠᠨ ᠬᠡᠪᠯᠡᠯ ᠦᠨ ᠪᠢᠴᠢᠭ ᠦᠨ ᠬᠠᠷᠢᠴᠠᠭ᠎ᠠ ᠶᠢᠨ ᠬᠡᠯᠪᠡᠷᠢ : ᠬᠡᠰᠡᠭ ᠦᠨ ᠲᠣᠭᠠ ᠨᠢ ᠨᠢᠭᠡ · ᠨᠡᠢᠲᠡ ᠪᠦᠲᠦᠭᠡᠯ ᠤᠨ ᠲᠣᠭᠠ ᠨᠢ ᠬᠣᠶᠠᠷ ᠲᠤ ᠲᠣᠭᠲᠠᠭᠰᠠᠨ ᠬᠡᠪᠯᠡᠯ ᠦᠨ ᠨᠣᠮ
ᠬᠡᠯᠡᠨ ᠦ 97 ᠨᠢᠭᠤᠷ ᠲᠠᠢ ᠪᠠᠢᠭ᠎ᠠ ᠨᠡᠢᠲᠡ ᠨᠣᠮ ᠤᠨ ᠬᠡᠪᠯᠡᠯ ᠦᠨ ᠲᠣᠭᠲᠠᠭᠰᠠᠨ ᠪᠣᠯᠤᠨ᠎ᠠ :: ᠨᠢᠭᠡ ᠰᠠᠷ᠎ᠠ ᠶᠢᠨ ᠬᠡᠪᠯᠡᠯ ᠦᠨ ᠬᠦᠮᠦᠨ ᠪᠠᠢᠭ᠎ᠠ
ᠨᠡᠢᠲᠡᠯᠡᠭᠰᠡᠨ ᠦ ᠪᠢᠴᠢᠭ ᠬᠡᠯᠡᠨ ᠪᠣᠯᠤᠨ ᠬᠠᠳᠠᠭᠠᠯᠠᠭᠳᠠᠭᠰᠠᠨ ᠨᠢ ᠬᠣᠶᠠᠷ ᠪᠣᠯᠤᠨ᠎ᠠ :: ᠣᠨ ᠤ ᠬᠡᠪᠯᠡᠯ ᠦᠨ ᠲᠣᠭᠠ ᠨᠢ ᠬᠡᠪᠯᠡᠯ ᠦᠨ ᠨᠣᠮ ᠤᠨ ᠬᠡᠰᠡᠭ ᠨᠢ
ᠰᠤᠷᠭᠠᠯ ᠤᠨ ᠬᠡᠪᠯᠡᠯ ᠦᠨ ᠪᠢᠴᠢᠭ ᠬᠤᠪᠢᠶᠠᠷᠢᠯᠠᠭᠰᠠᠨ ᠨᠣᠮ ᠤᠨ ᠲᠣᠭᠲᠠᠭᠰᠠᠨ ᠬᠡᠯᠡ ᠶᠢᠨ ᠬᠡᠪᠯᠡᠭᠰᠡᠨ ᠦ ᠪᠢᠴᠢᠭ ᠰᠤᠷᠭᠠᠯ ᠪᠠᠢᠭᠰᠠᠨ ::

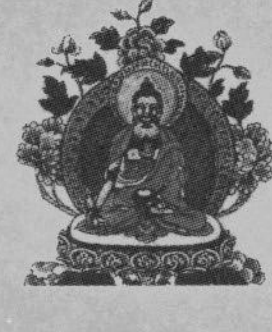

Encyclopedia of Treatment of Smallpox, Measles and Other Diseases in Children

小儿天花麻疹诸病治法大全

5

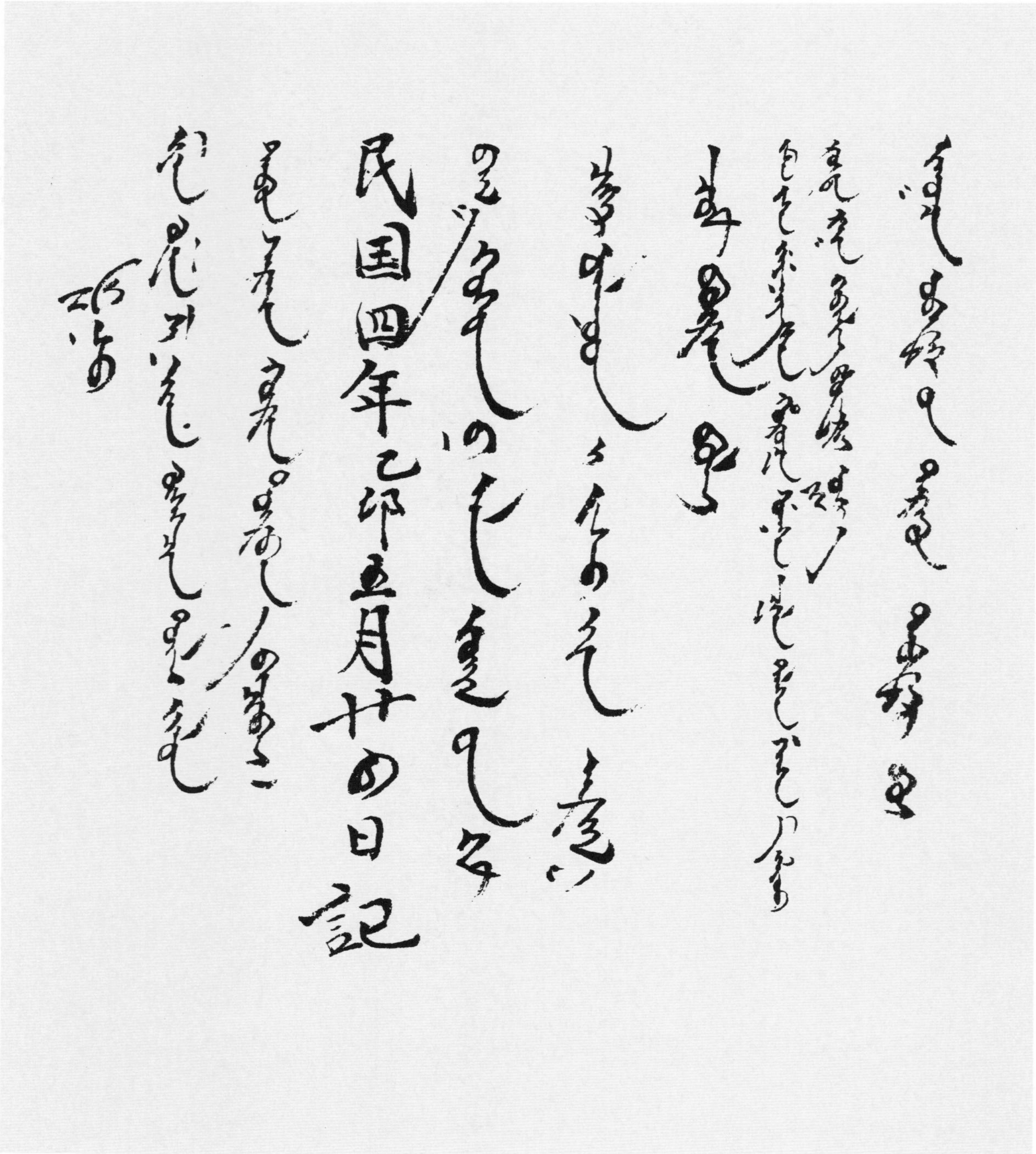

民国四年乙卯五月廿四日記

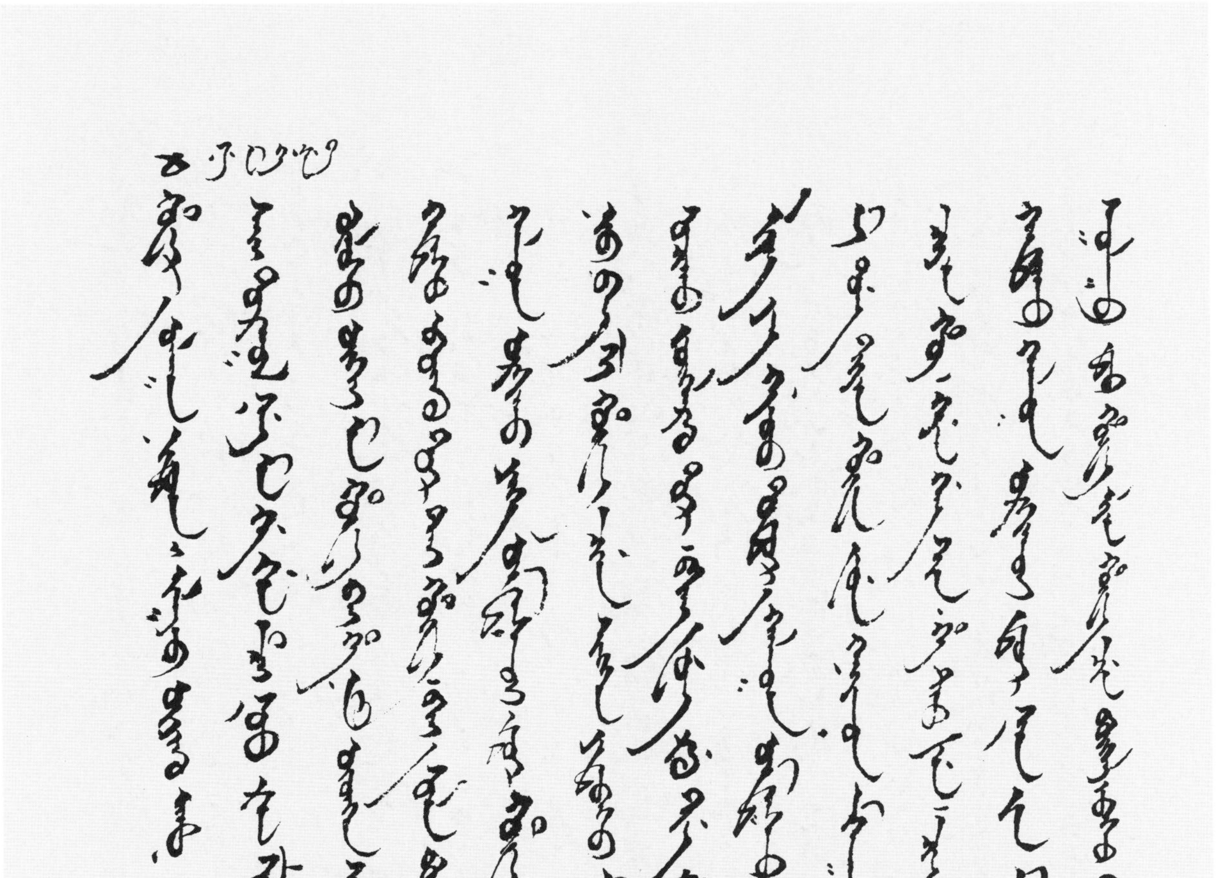

[illegible]

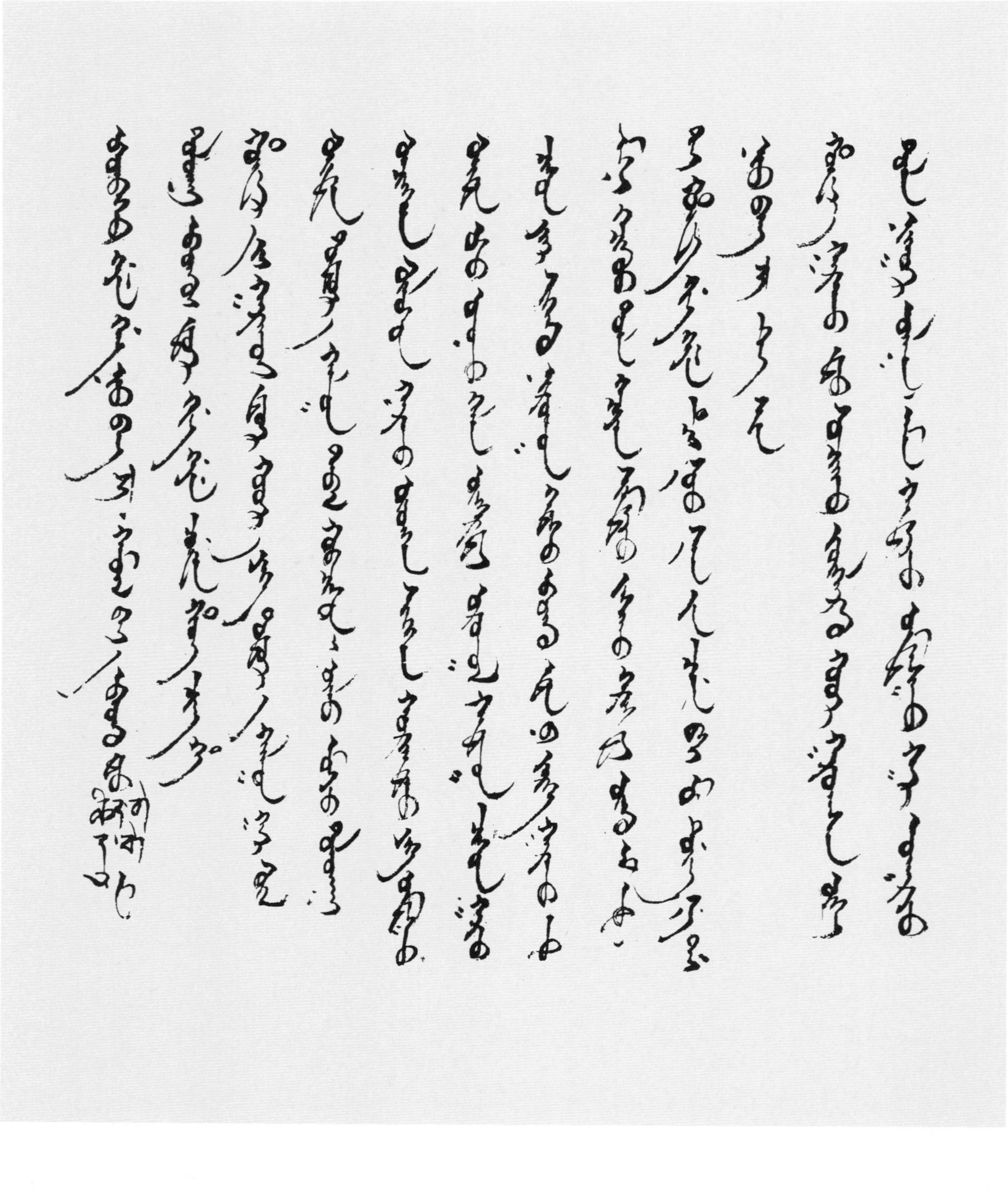

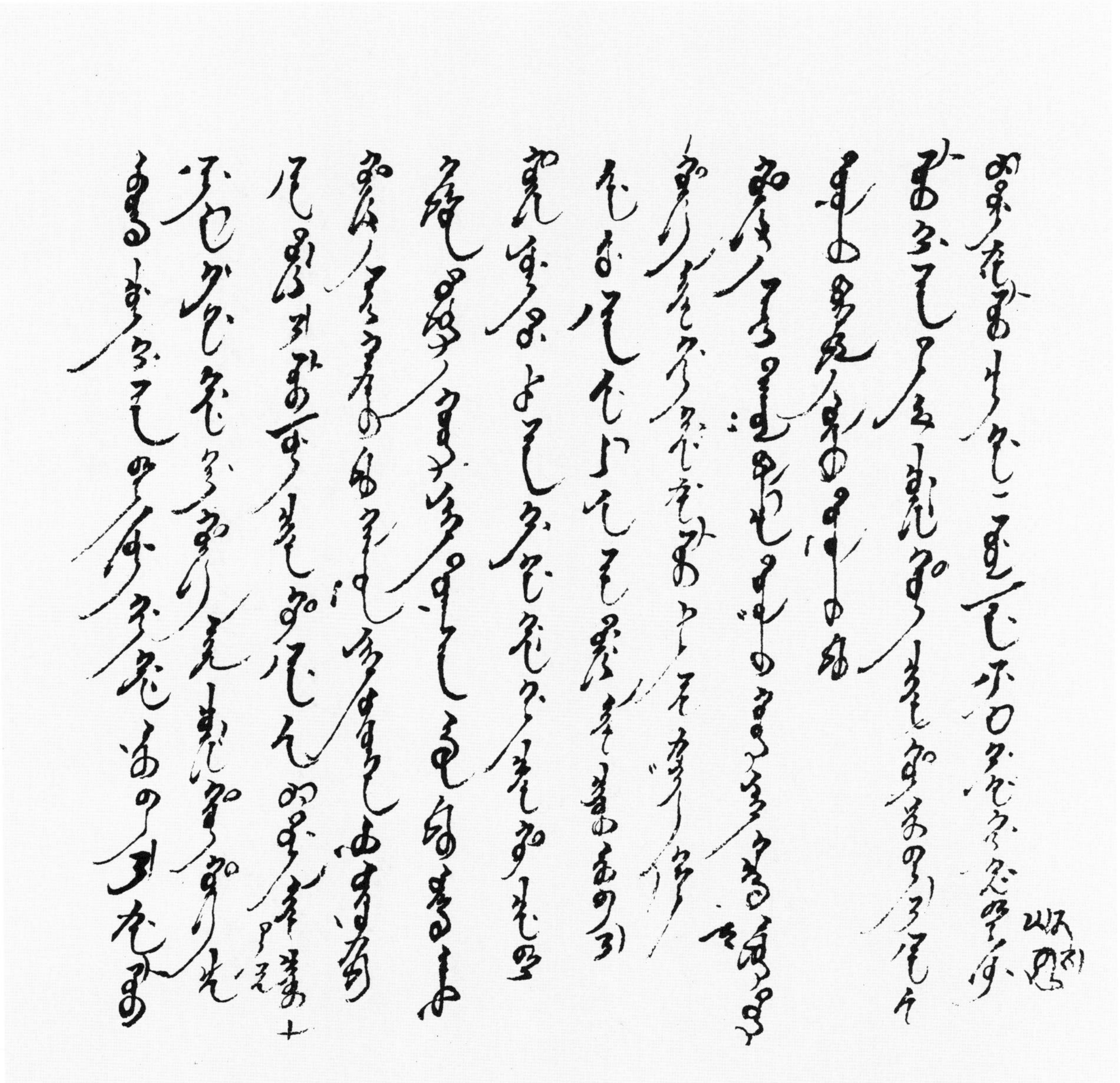

[illegible]

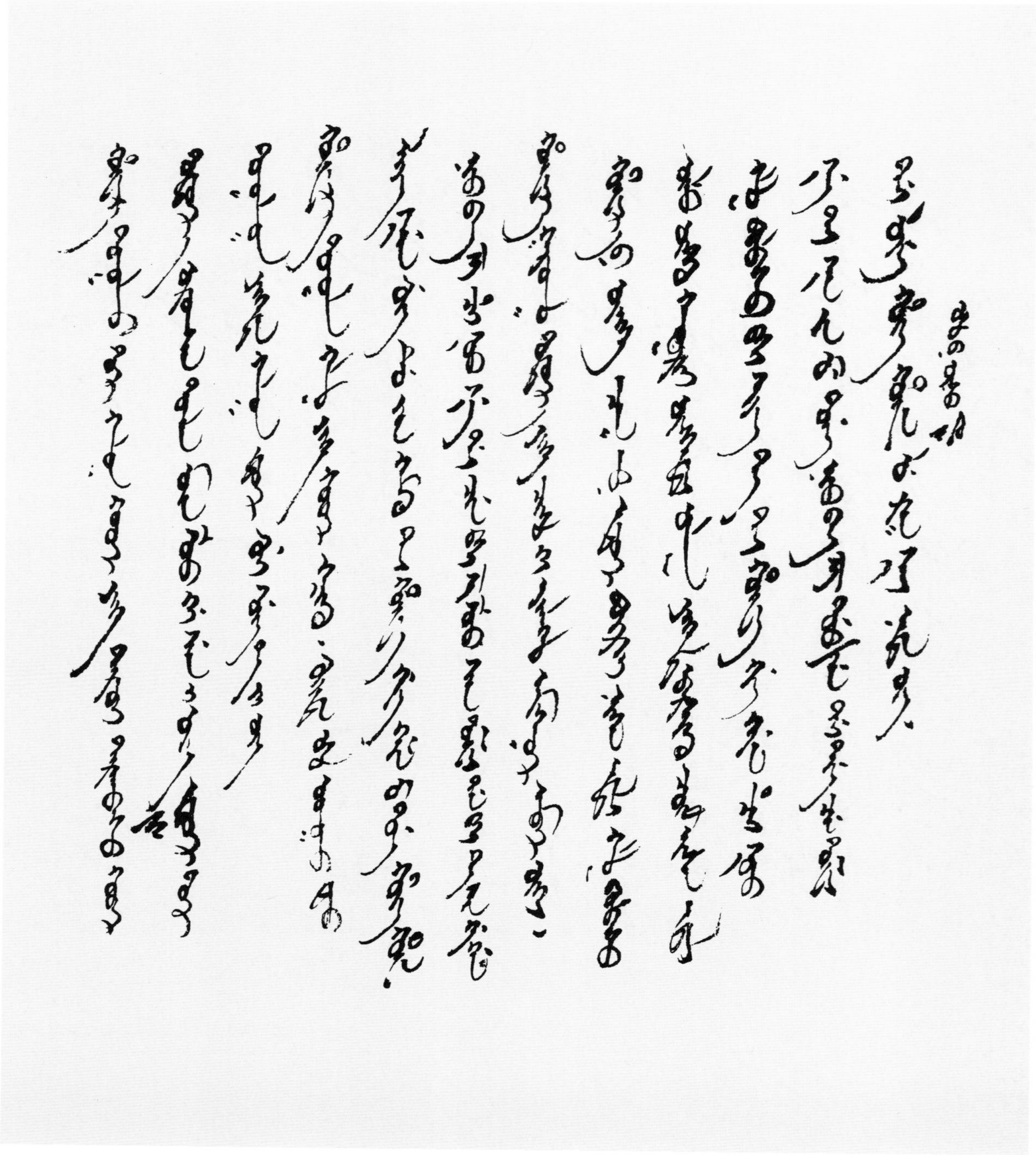

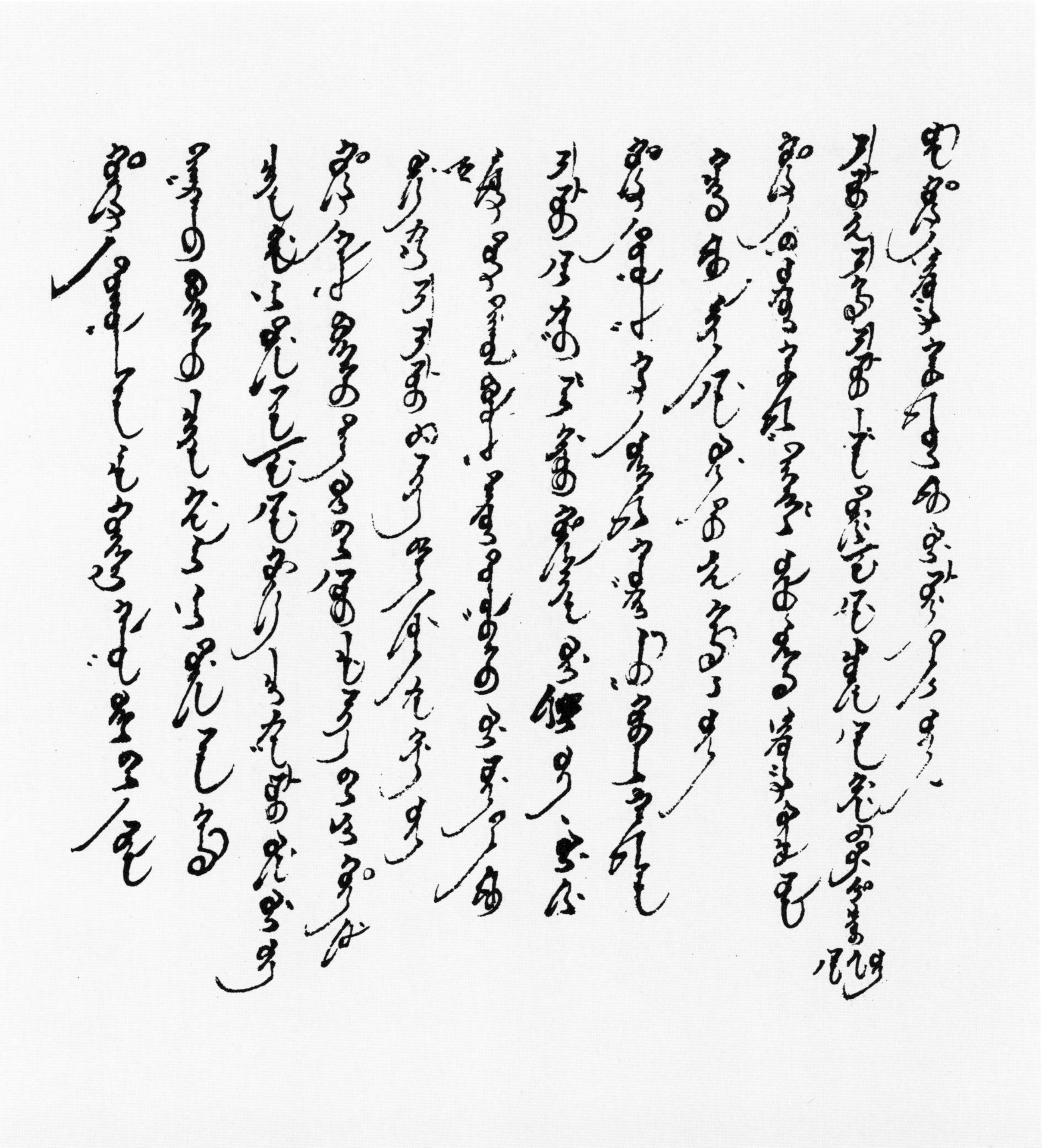

[illegible]

[illegible]

[illegible]

[illegible]

[illegible]

[illegible]

[illegible]

[illegible]

[illegible]

[illegible]

[illegible]

[illegible]

[illegible]

[illegible]

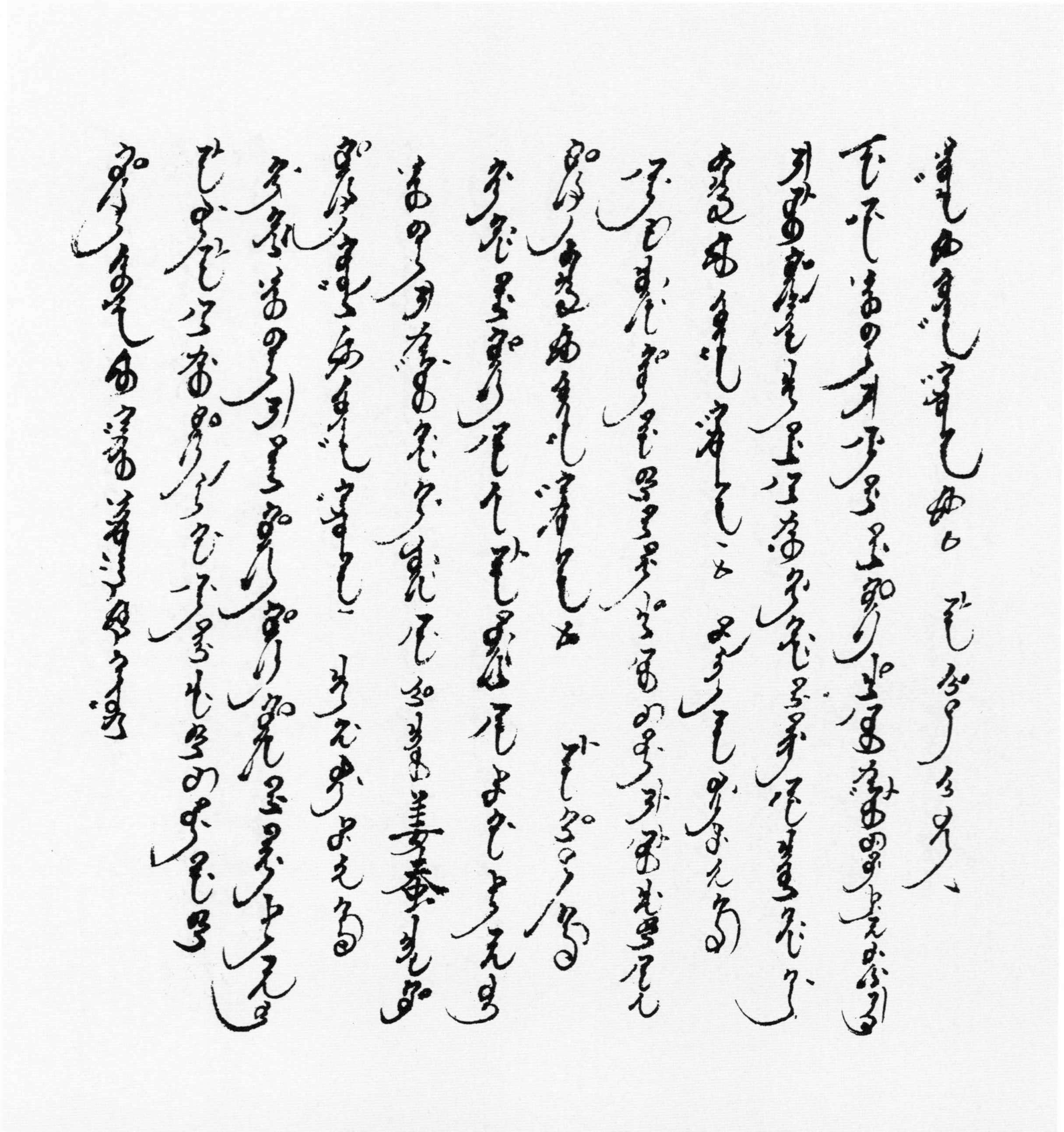

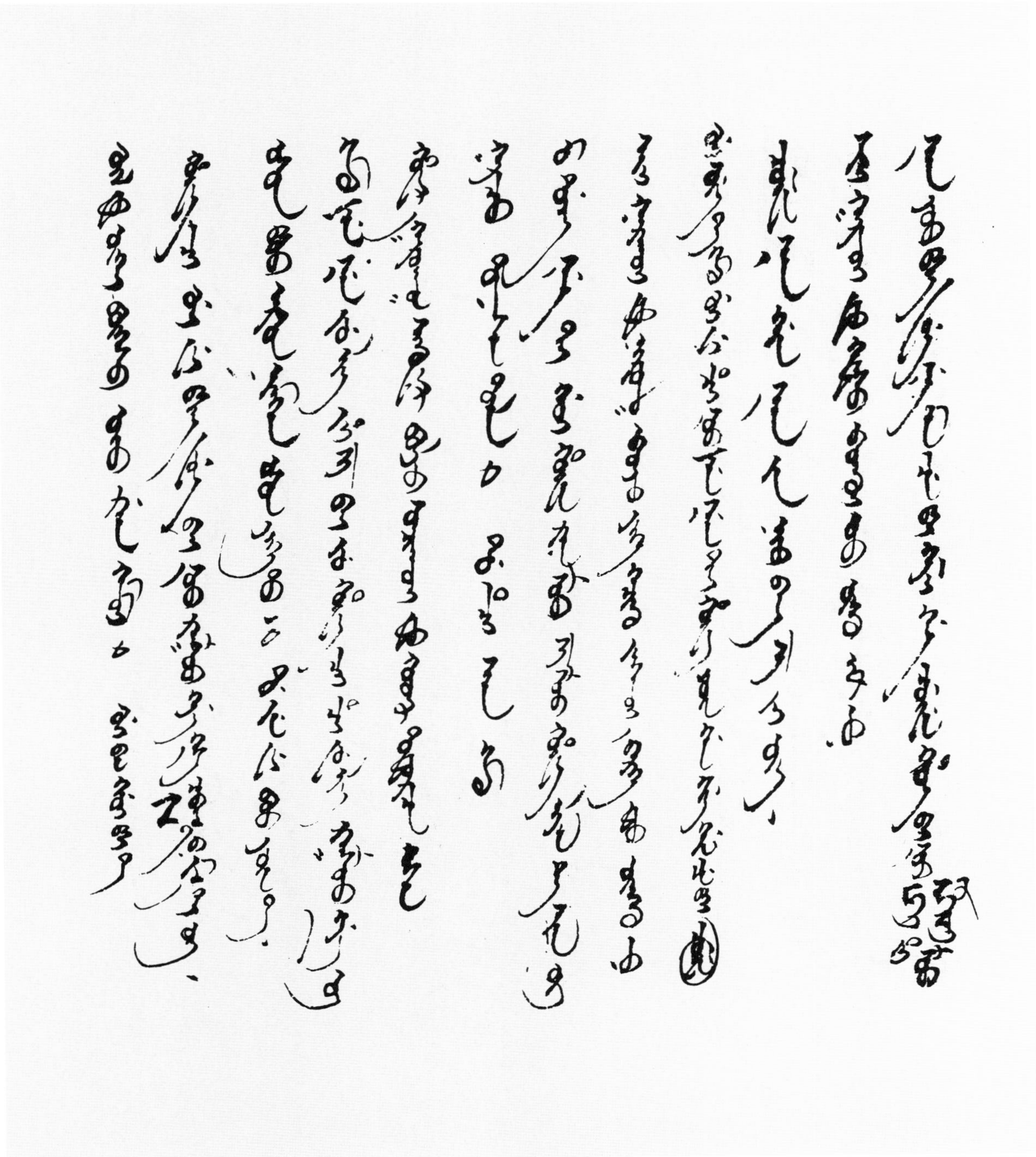

[illegible]

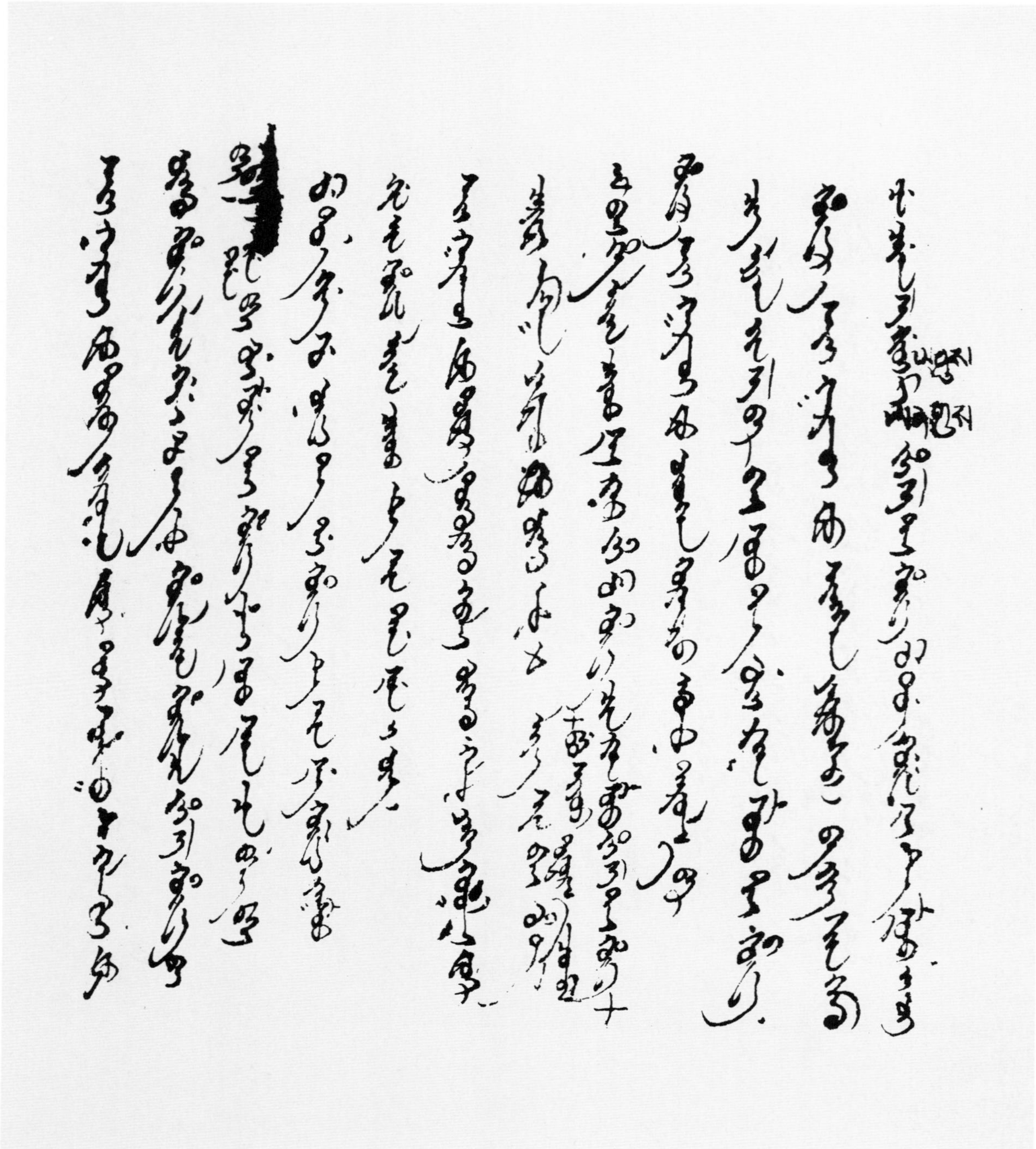

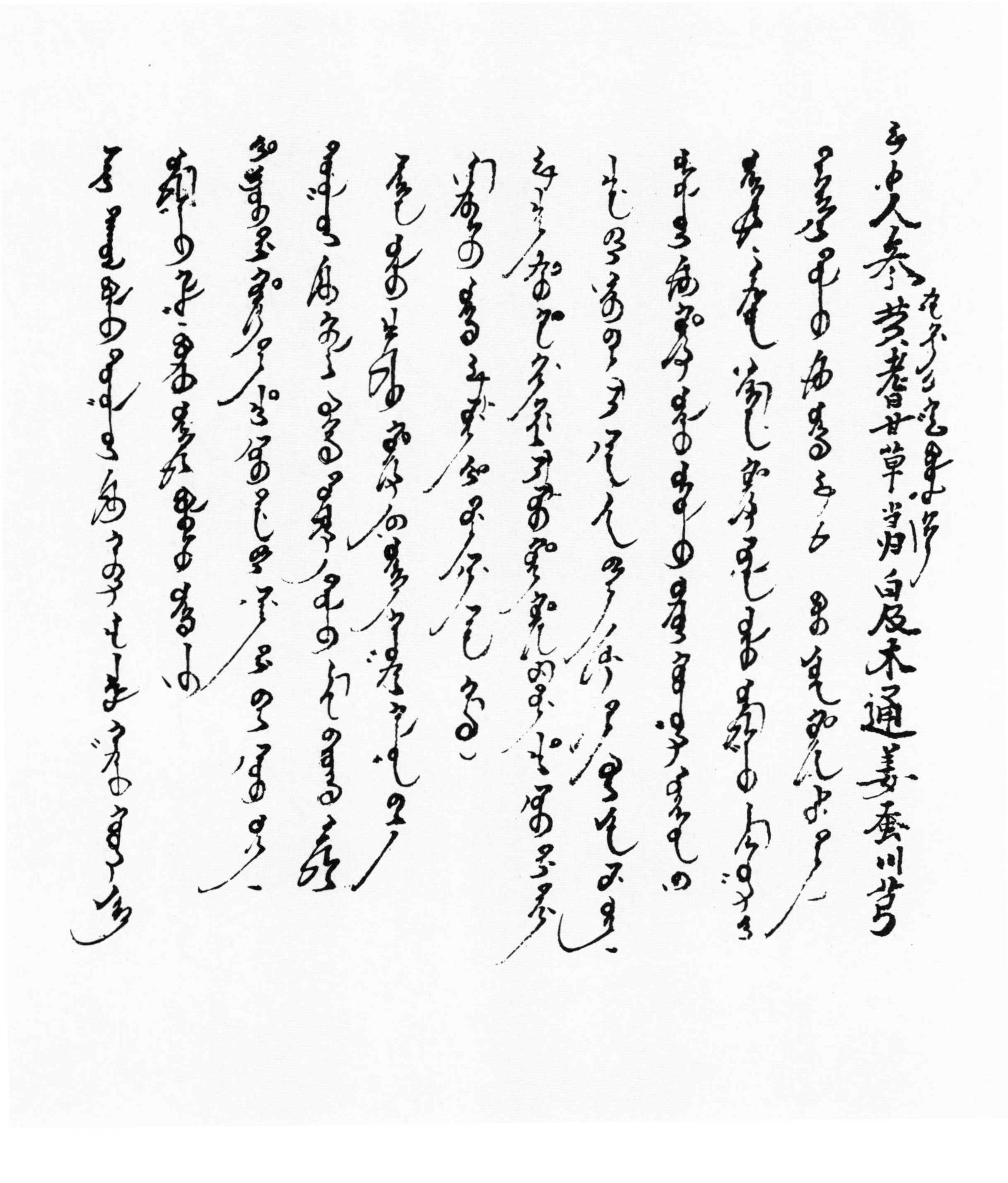

人参 黄耆 甘草 当归 白及 木通 姜蚕 川芎

人参当归黄芩甘草白及川芎防风紫草茸木贼山香紅花桔梗

桔梗白及防风人参紅花

麻連子牛仿子升麻黄芩川芎連石

当归川芎赤芍生地紅花紫草黃耆黃連太黃

人參黃耆紫草茸前胡牛防子

甘草白芍生地

陳皮半夏木通巴葉甘草米葉[illegible]十 赤茯苓

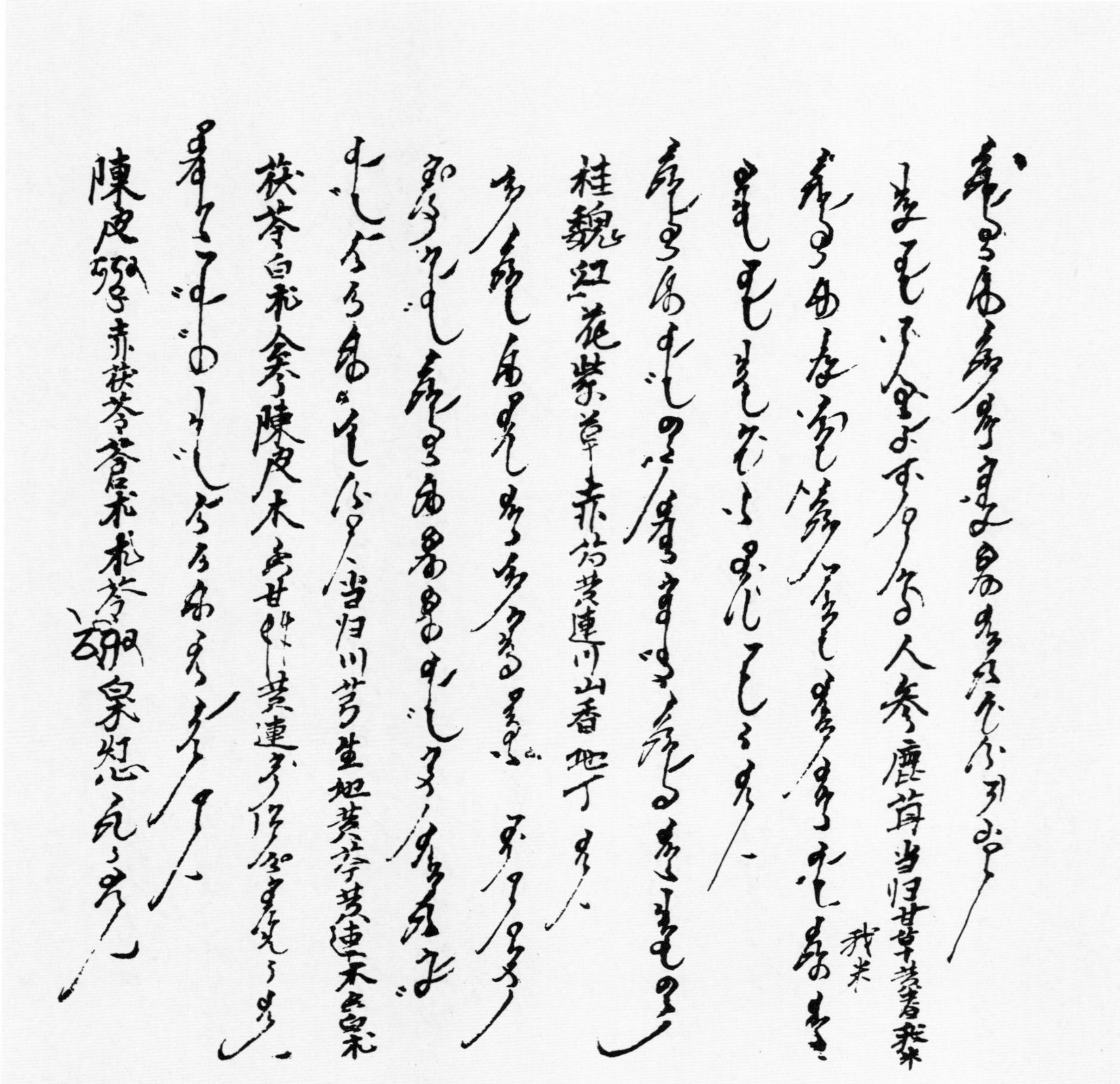

[illegible] 人参 鹿茸 当归 甘草 黄耆 莪术 [illegible]

[illegible]

[illegible]

[illegible]

[illegible]

桂[illegible] 红花 紫草 赤芍 黄連 川山香 地丁 [illegible]

[illegible]

[illegible]

[illegible] 當归 川芎 生地 黄芩 黄連 木香 白术

茯苓 白术 人参 陳皮 木香 甘草 黄連 [illegible]

[illegible]

陳皮 [illegible] 赤茯苓 蒼术 [illegible] [illegible]

[illegible] 青代赤芍连翘木通

[illegible]

[illegible]

[illegible]

[illegible]

[illegible]

[illegible]

白术人参升麻赤芍陈皮当归甘草

[illegible] 苍术大黄人参 [illegible]

[illegible]

[illegible]

[illegible]

生地当归川芎白芍连翘紫草葛根 [illegible]

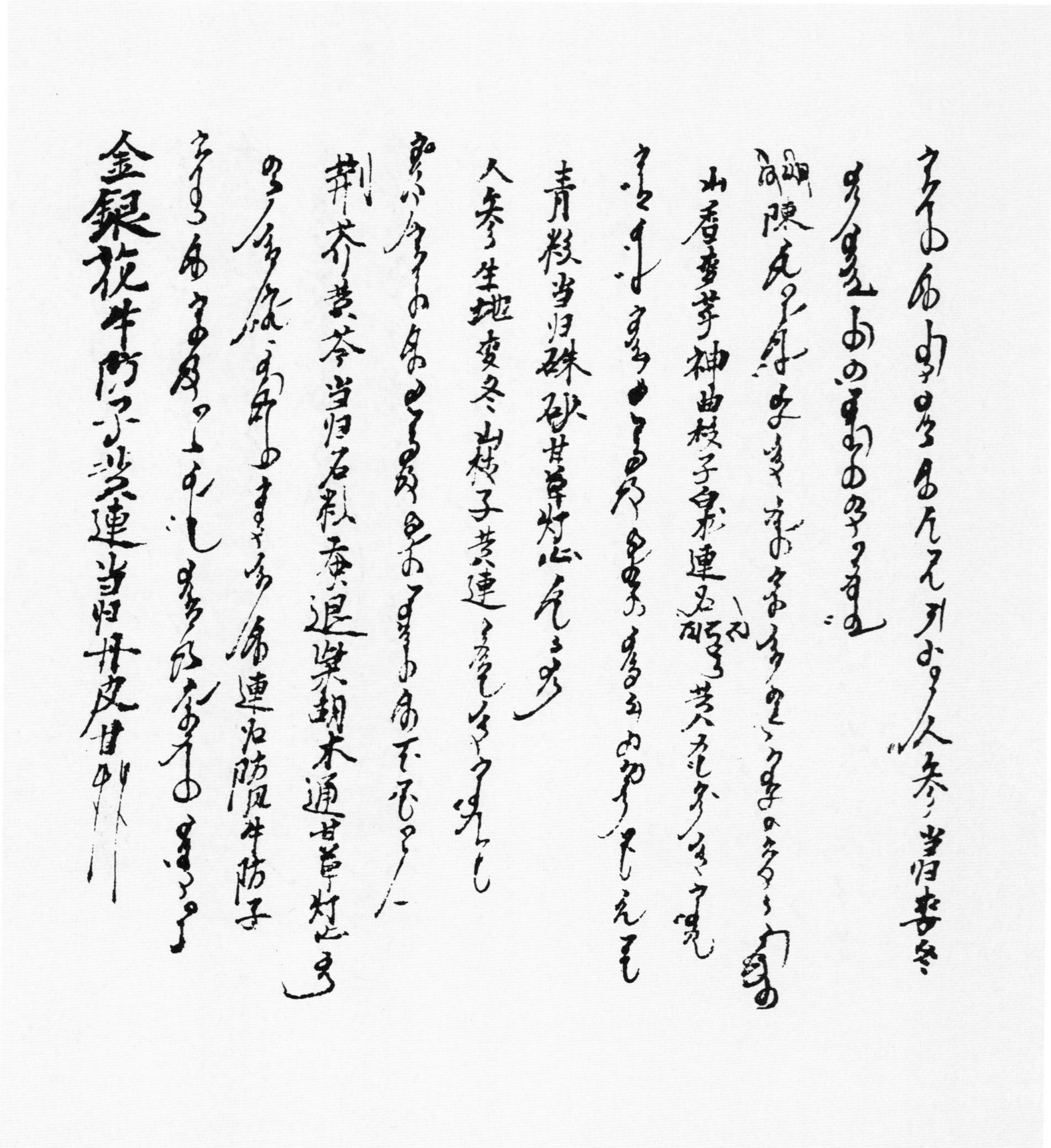

金銀花 牛蒡子 連翹 當歸 丹皮 甘草

連 防風 牛蒡子

荆芥 黄芩 當歸 石斛 蚕 退 柴胡 木通 甘草 灯心

人參 生地 麦冬 山梔子 黄連

青黛 當歸 硃砂 甘草 灯心

山查 麦芽 神曲 枳子 連 黄

陳皮

人參 當歸 麦冬

当归 生地 丹皮 紅花 連翹 白芨 黄連 甘草 灯心

地骨皮 桑白皮

麦冬 陳皮 半夏 茯苓 白芍 甘草

人参 五味子

枝子 白芍

黄芩生地連召牛防子荆芥防風金銀花甘草十[illegible]

甘草金銀花木通 … 六服皮連召九 …

荆芥防風赤芍生地

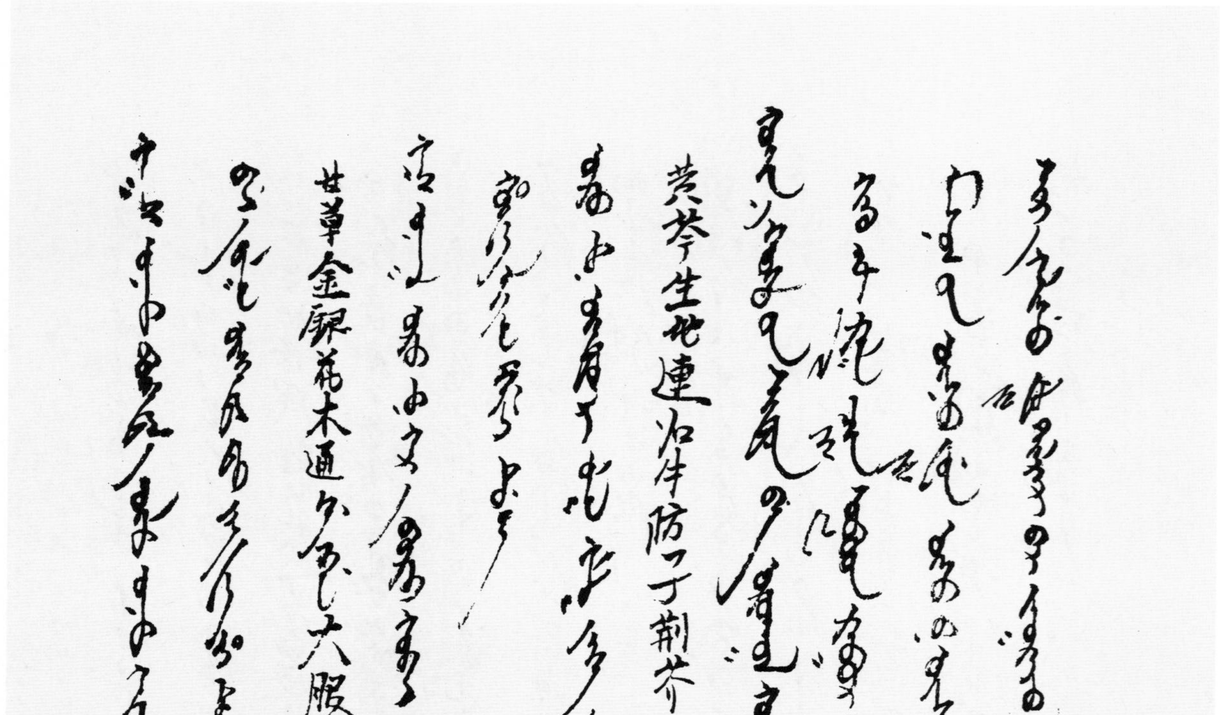

防风

天术黄 射虫 雄黄 甘草 牛黄 天麻

硃砂 保龍丸 胆星

天化粉 甘草

胆南星 天术黄 硃砂 天麻 防风

雄黄 聚命丹

[illegible]

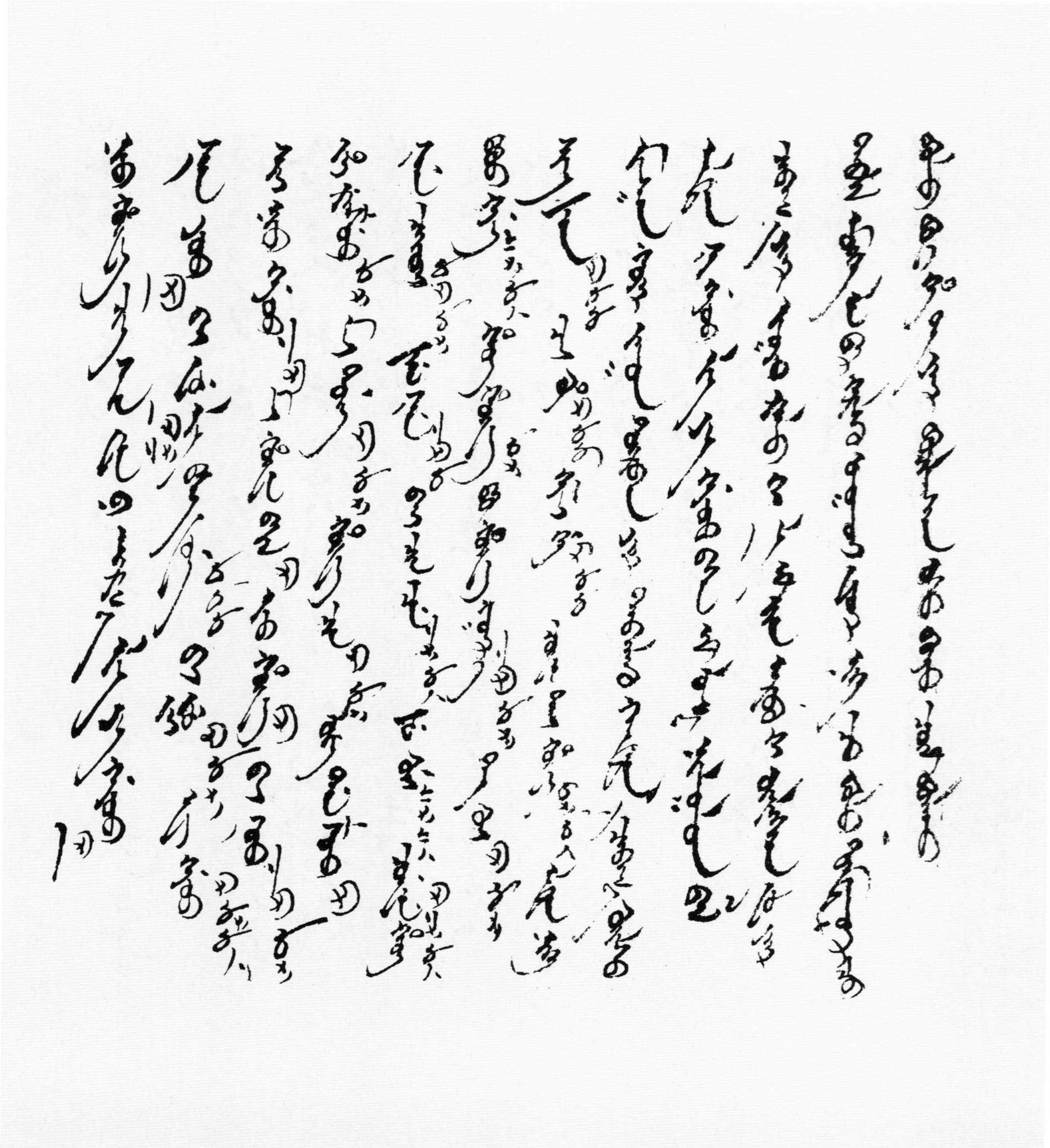

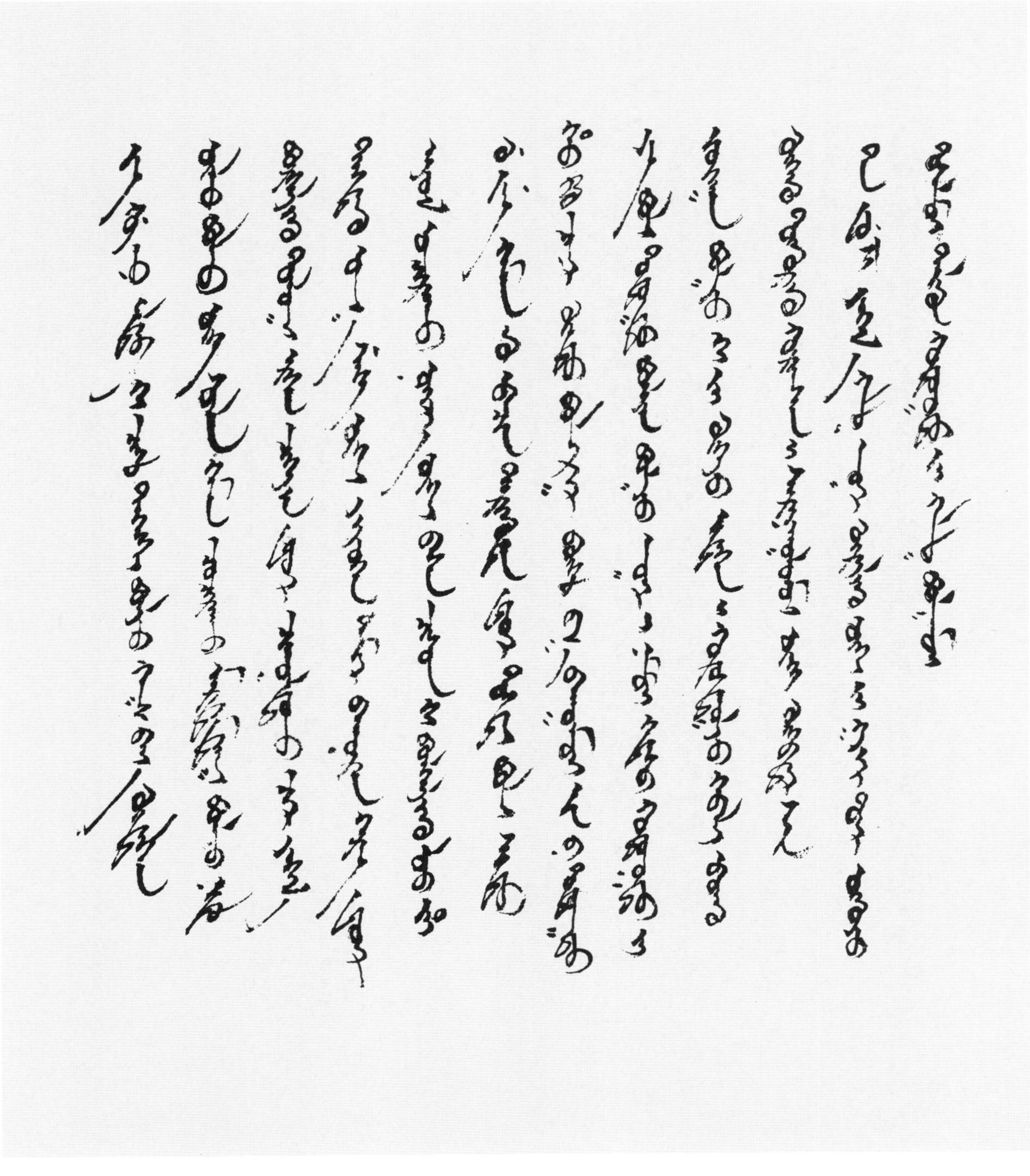

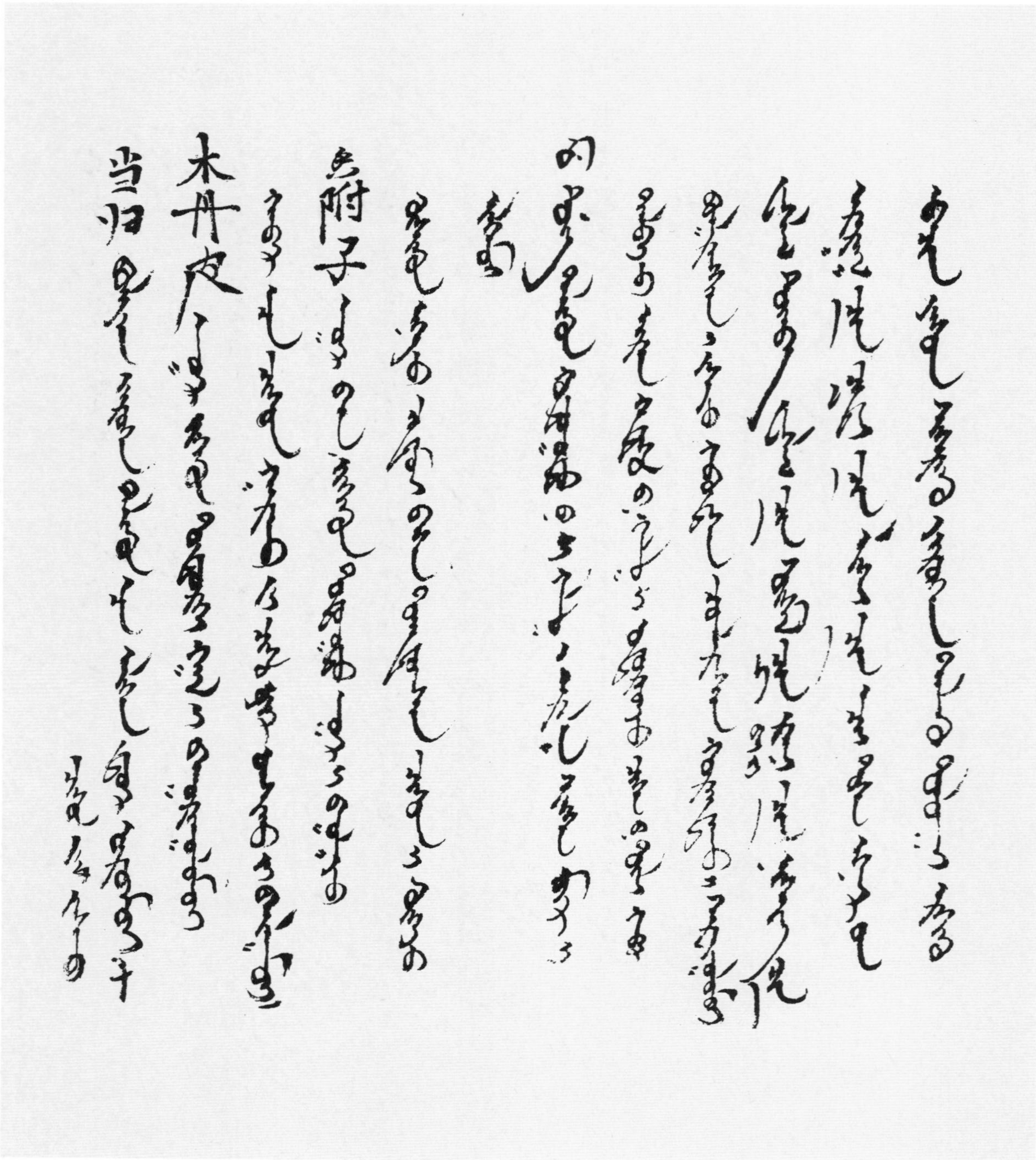

附子

木丹皮

当归

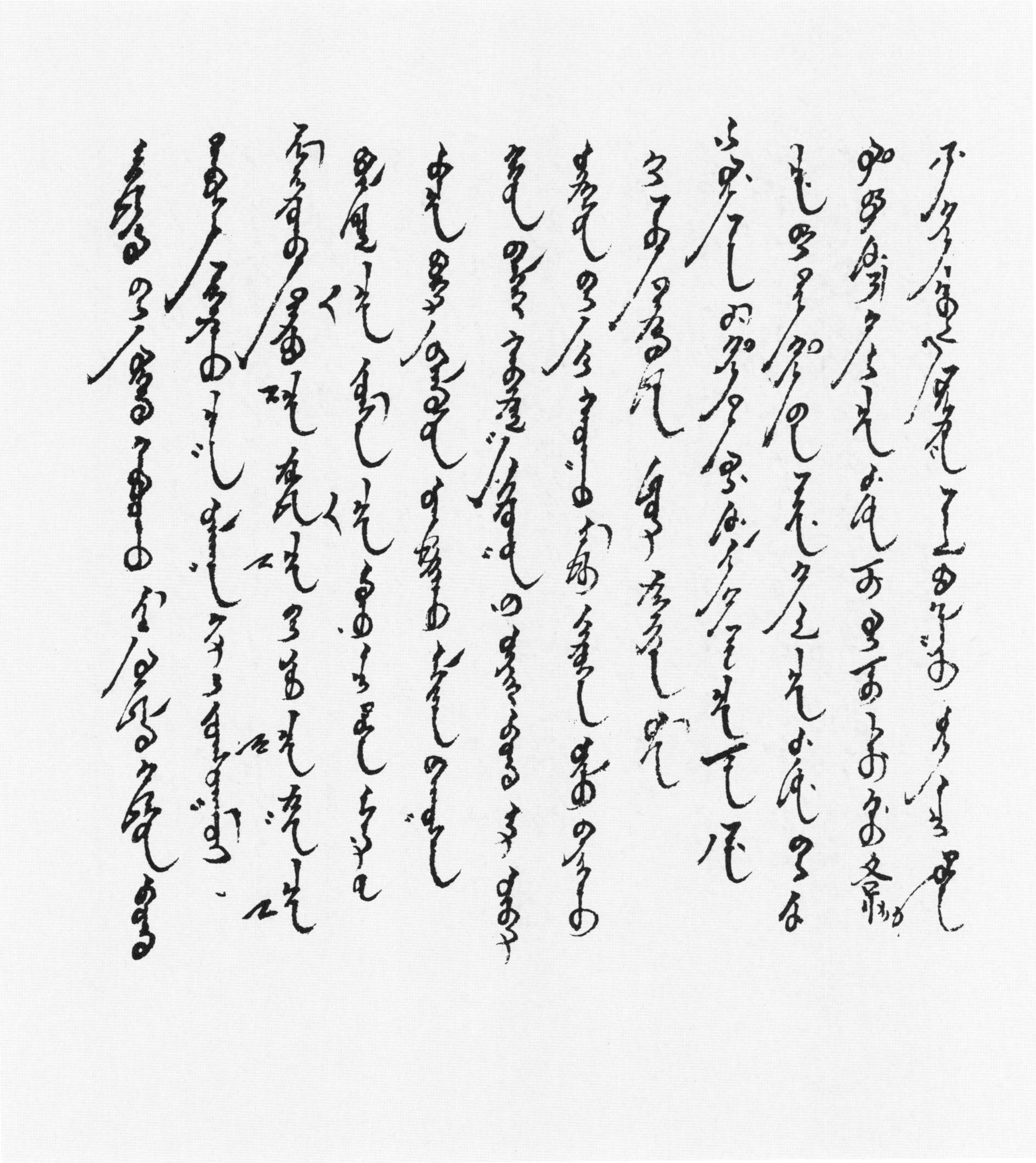

[illegible]

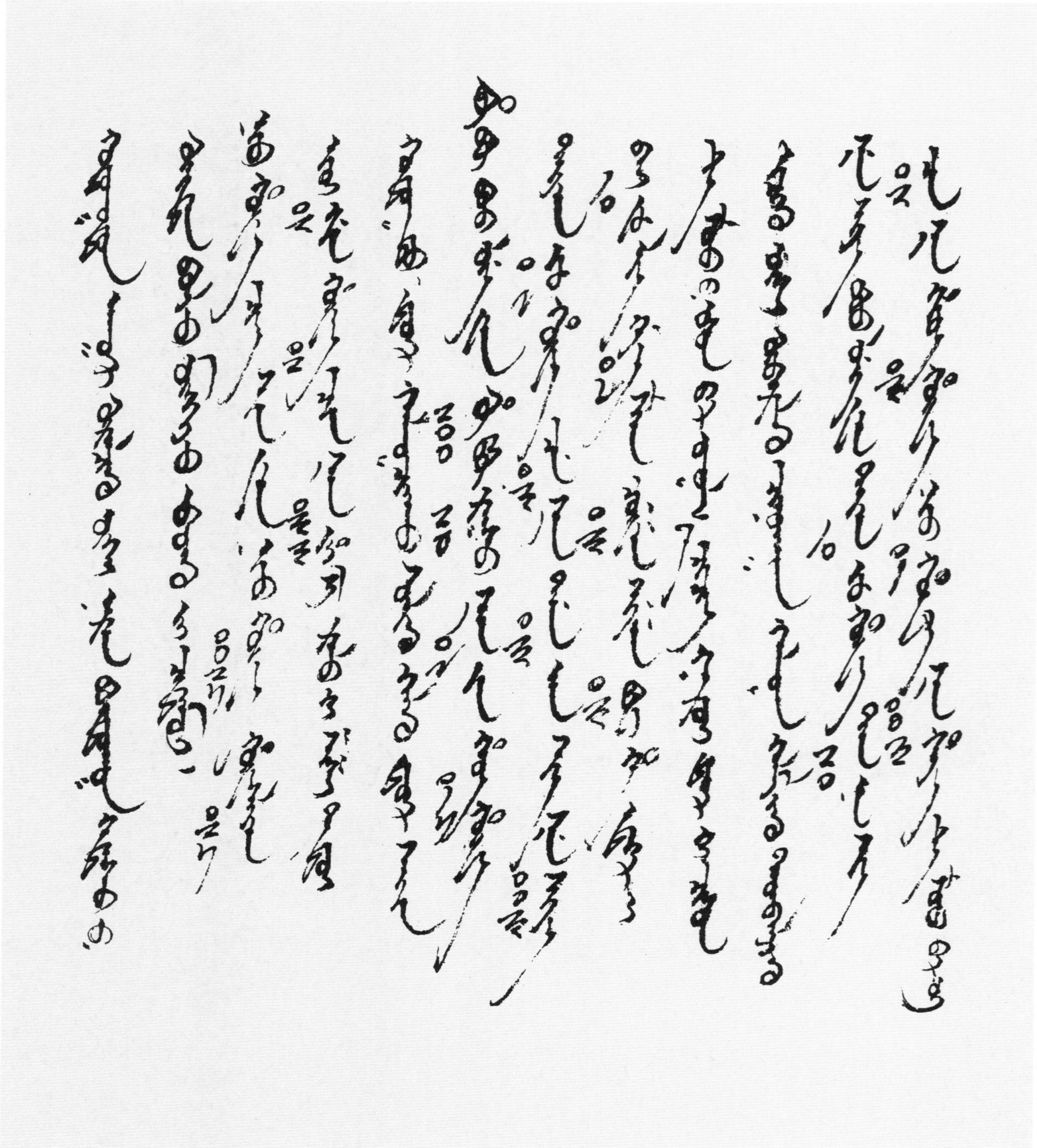

各卜引生姜外用防风

各卜

各卜

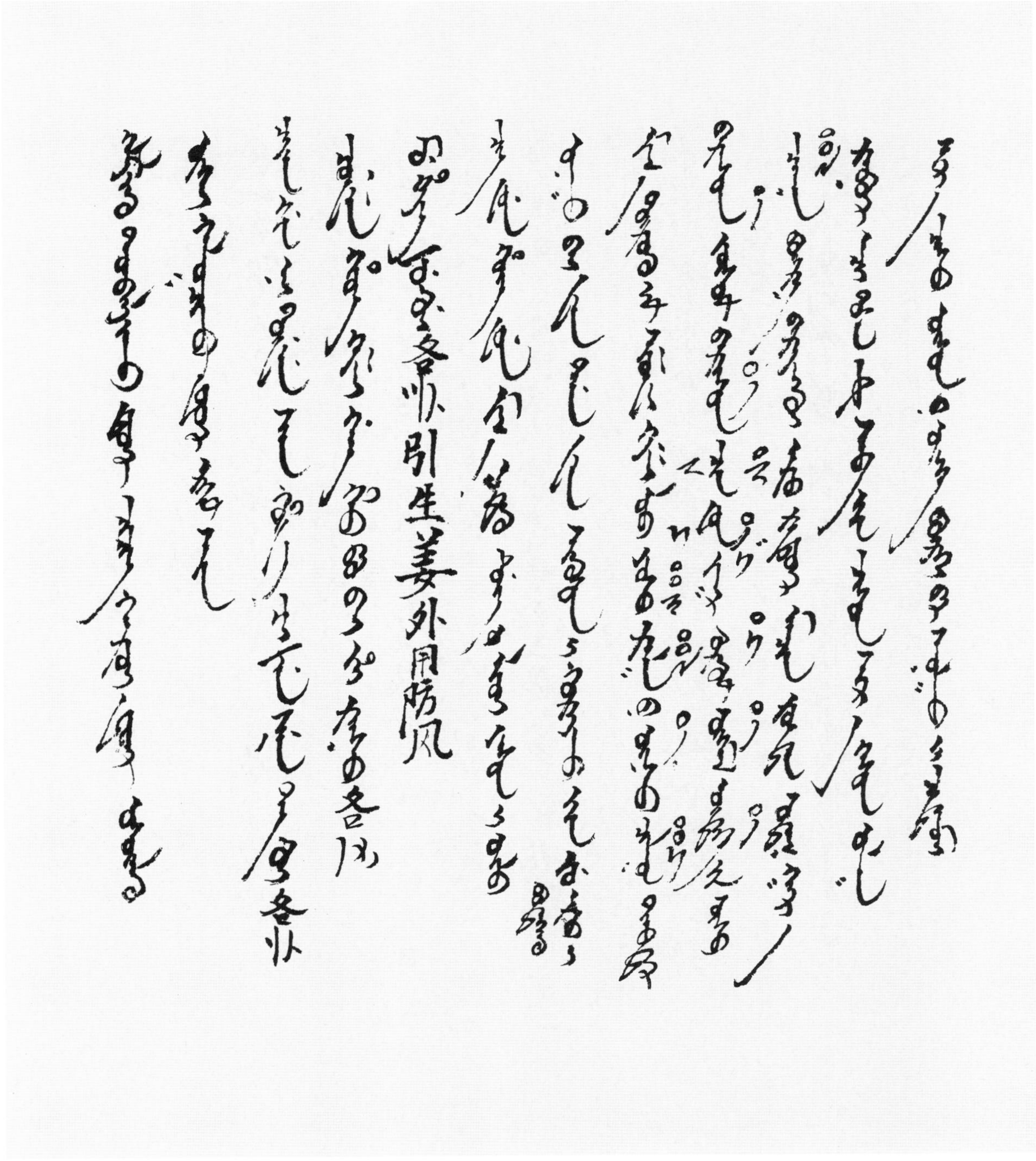

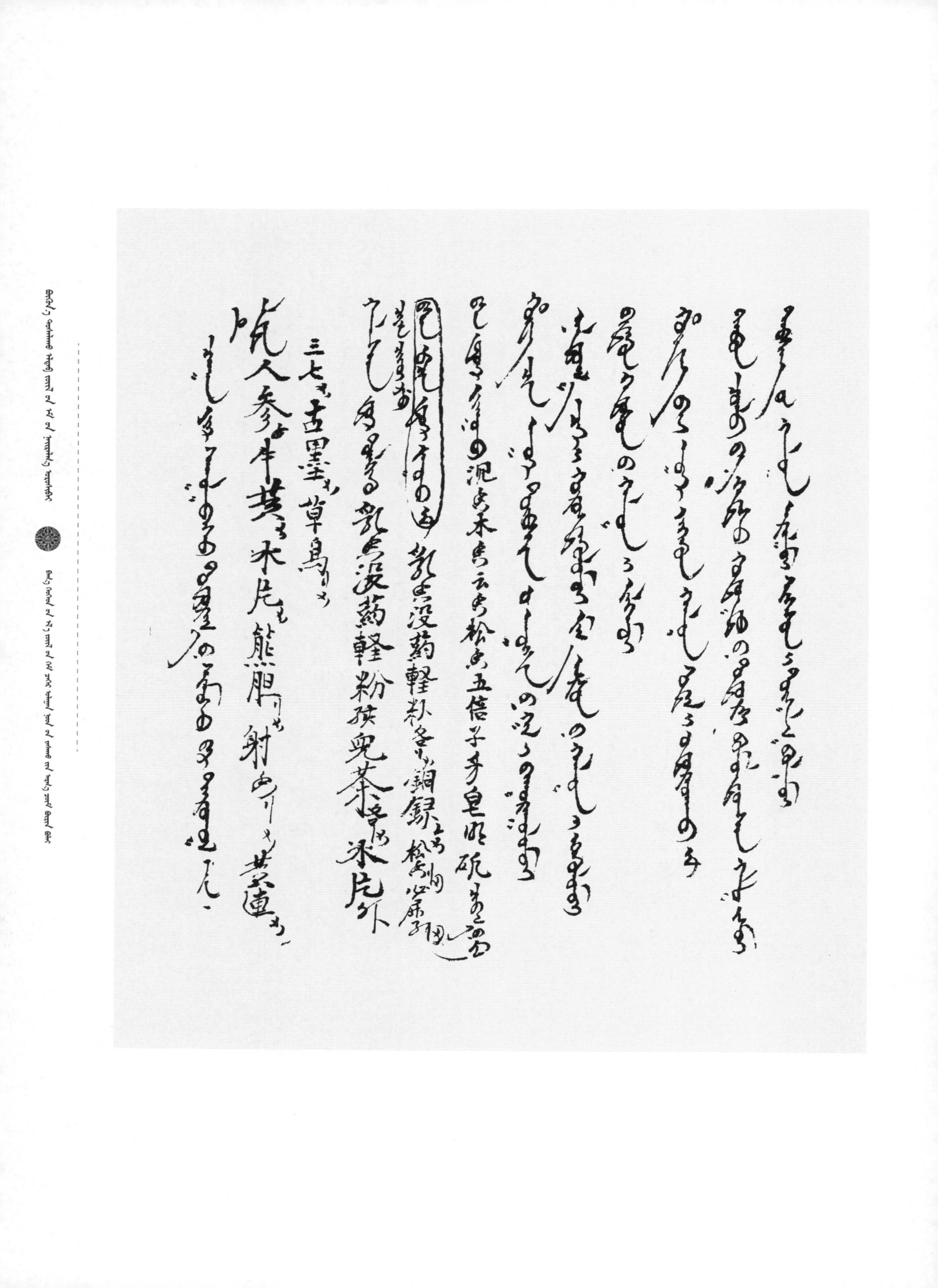

[illegible]

[illegible] 人参 [illegible] 牛黄 [illegible] 冰片 [illegible] 熊胆 [illegible] 射 [illegible] 黄連 [illegible]

三七 [illegible] 古墨 [illegible] 草烏 [illegible]

[illegible] 乳 [illegible] 没藥 輕粉 茯 兒茶 [illegible] 冰片 外

[illegible] 乳 [illegible] 没藥 輕粉 各 [illegible] 銅録 [illegible] 松 [illegible] 必麻子 [illegible]

[illegible] 泥 [illegible] 木 [illegible] 云 [illegible] 松 [illegible] 五倍子 [illegible] 皂 [illegible] 矾 [illegible]

[illegible]

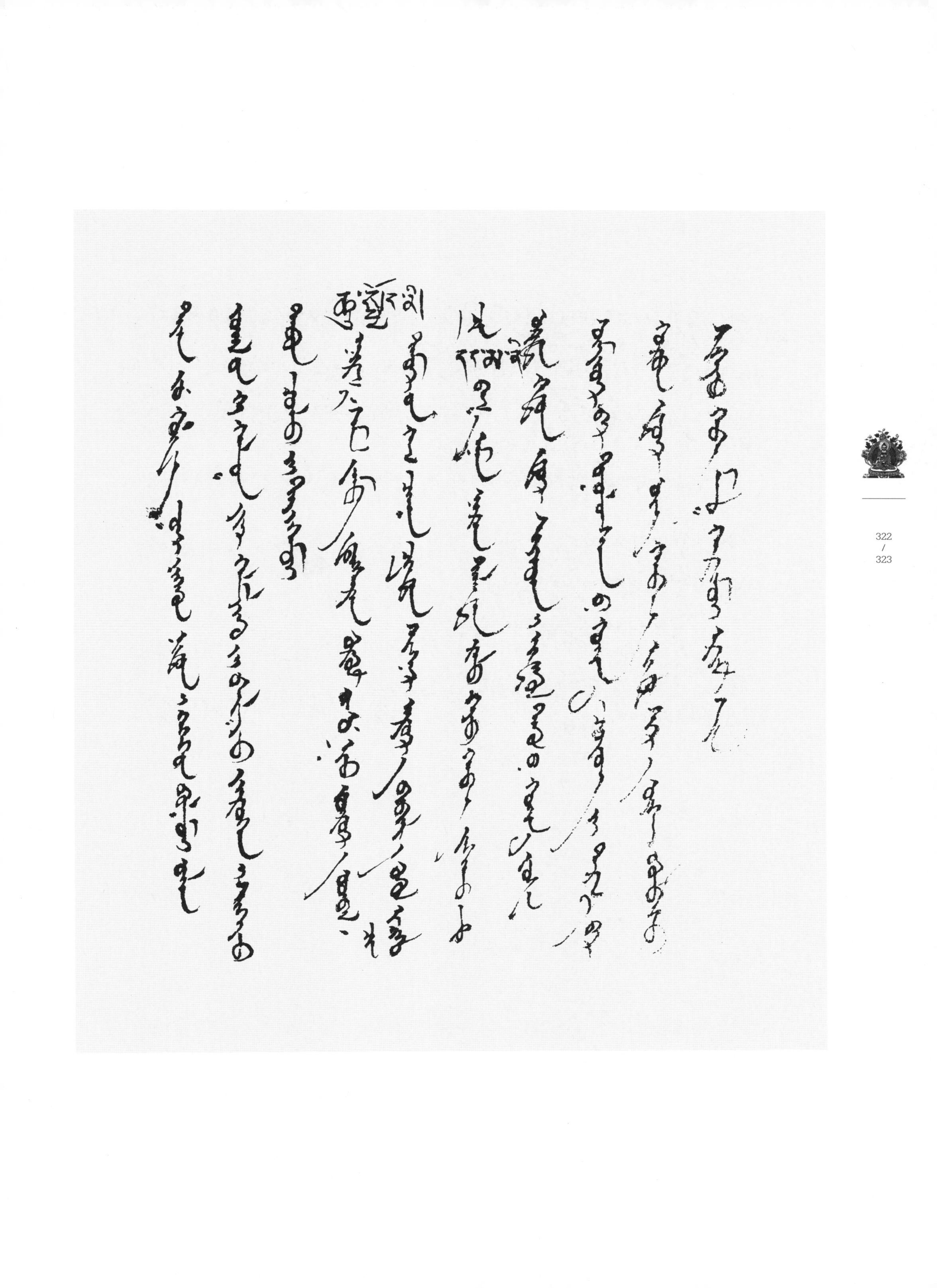

ཀྱཻ། ༄ མཁྱེན་ནོ༔ སློབ་དཔོན༔ པདྨ་ཐོད་ཕྲེང་རྩལ༔ ཆོས་དཀར་དམར༔ ཡེ་ཤེས་གཉིས༔ རྡོ་རྗེ༔

ཞལ་ལ་གཉེན་ཐེ༔ སེམས་མེད༔ ཟེར་བ་ཡི༔ ཨོ་རྒྱན་པ་ལ༔ ཐུགས་ཀ༔ ཀེ་སྲི༔ སི་གང་ངུ༔ འགྲུས་བུ་མ་གསུམ

སྲུང་སྲུང༔ ཀར ‖ ཀྱཻ་ སྤྲུལ་སྐུའི་ཉེར་ལྔ་ཡི་ སྤྲུལ་ཆེན་དཀར༔ ཚོགས་གཉིས་ལ༔

བློ་བཟང་རྒྱ་མཚོ་འཆི་མེད་སྐྱབས།།

ཨར་དབང༔ པ་ལི་ཀ༔ སྐྱེ་སྤྲོ་ཚ༔ འབྲུག་ད༔ ཀུན་ཀ་རི༔ འབྲས་བུ་སེམས༔ ངེས་ཀུ༔ ངང་ལས༔

འབྱུང་པོ་དང༔ པད་ཀ༔ ཀུན་འདུས༔ ཤེར་མར༔ སྤྲོ་ལོ༔ ཀྱི་སྐྱོ༔ པར་ཀར༔།། གར་རྒྱུད་ཚ་སེར

ལྗོངས་ལ་རྟ་ད་ བཀྲ་ཤིས་ པར་ཀར་སྒྲུབ་བུ་བཀུར ཀར་ཅིག་ངང

ཀྱཻ། །ཨོ་སྤྲོད༔ མཁས་ཉུ༔ ཀ་སྲི༔ ཧ་བུ༔ འབྱུང་དག༔ ཨོ་རྒྱན་པ་ལ༔ ཀ་སྲུད༔ ཀུན་བུ་བུམ༔ ཚེ་རིང༔

ཏོམ་ཀྱི༔ རེ་ར་ཀ༔ ཞལ་གཉེན་ཐེ༔ སེམས་ར༔ པད་ཀ༔ ཞལ་ཀ༔ ཤེར་མར༔ ཏ་བྲ་ཝཛྲ་ཏྲུ

བློ་བཟང་མཆོག་ལོག་གསོལ་བ་དེས།།

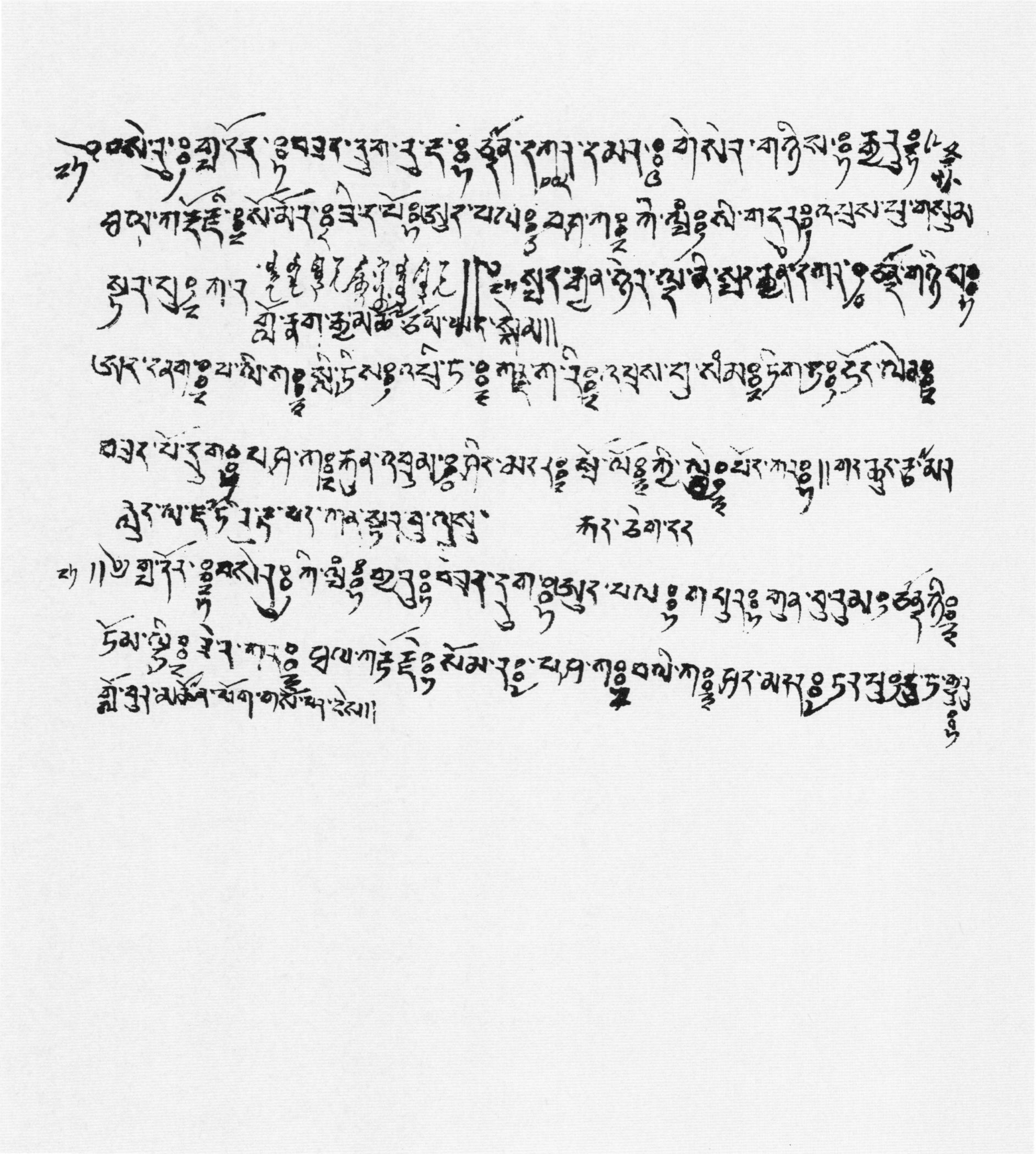

輕粉 銅 錫 松香 黑砒 胆礬 細末

杏仁 個 見茶 香油 茶

珍珠 三金 豆 廿粒 早晚二付 麥日用完

治楊梅輕粉 大黃 杏仁 紅花 桃仁

龍骨 半 青鹽 水丸 吉豆大

治淋症如神 牡蠣 煅 白茯苓 五味子

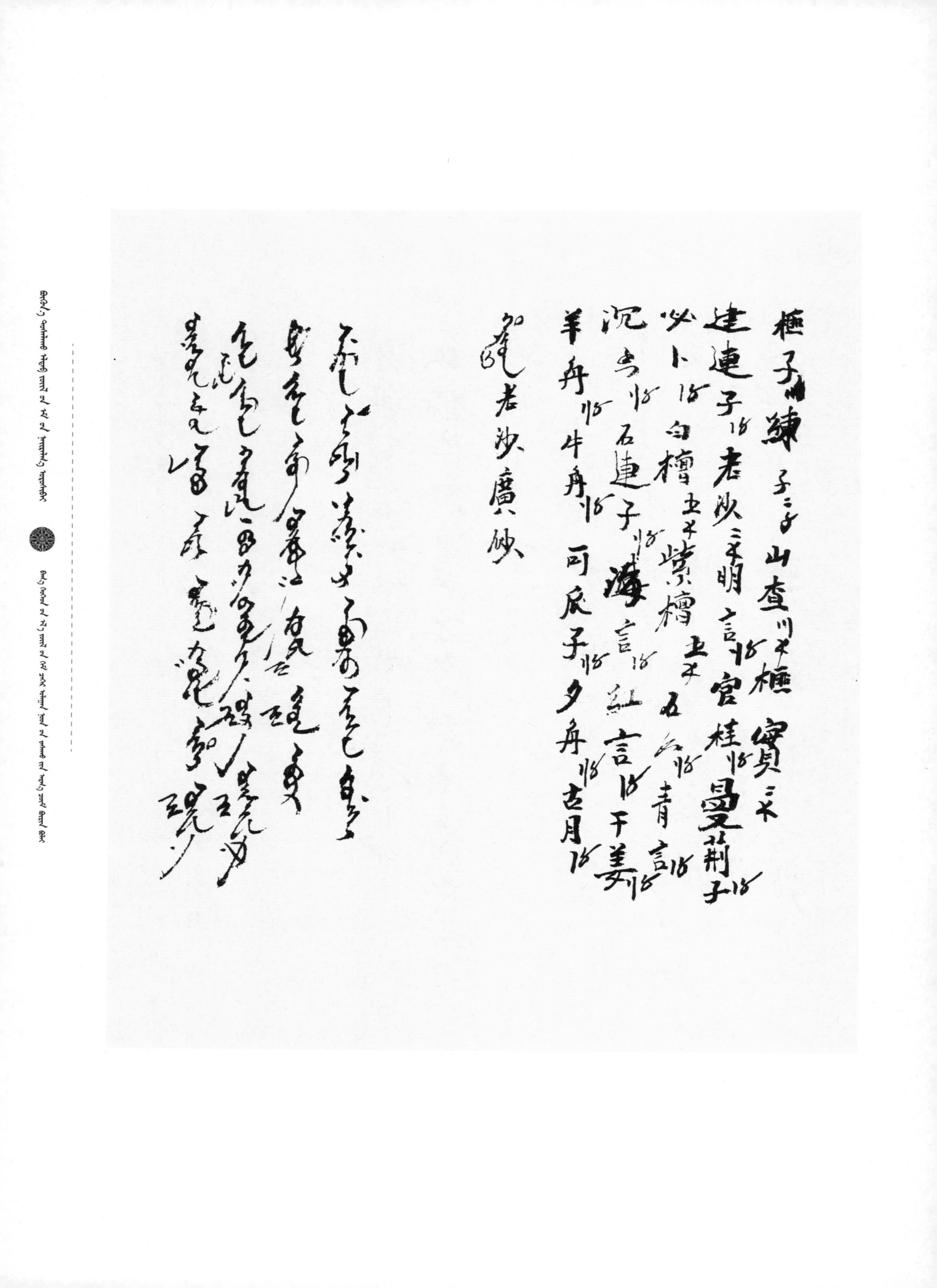

榧子川練子二千山查川千榧寶二卜
建蓮子一钱老沙三千明言一钱官桂一钱曼荊子一钱
必卜一钱白檀土千紫檀土千石言一钱青言一钱
沉香一钱石蓮子一钱海言一钱紅言一钱干姜一钱
羊舟一钱牛舟一钱可辰子一钱夕舟一钱古月一钱
加老沙廣砂

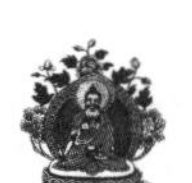

ལོ་སོགས་ཞིབ་གི་ནང༌།། ཀུན་འདོམས་ཀྱུང་ཡང་ཞིབ་མཐེར་ཚགས་པ་བགྱིབ།།

ཞིབ་བར་ཀྲུག་དུ་འབབ་བའི་བཀྲུབ་ཏྲི་ཡིན།། སྦྲུམ་བཀྱིག་བའི་ཉེན་ཚེན་ལྷ་ལེམ་ཡིན།།

གཞེར་ལ་མ་སྦྲུབ་ལ་ཚེ་པོའི་སྦྱོར་ག་མཐའ་ཡིན།། མར་སྤུམ

སྦྱོར་བདམ་ ཡིན

ཚེས་སོར་ཀྲམ་ཚེ

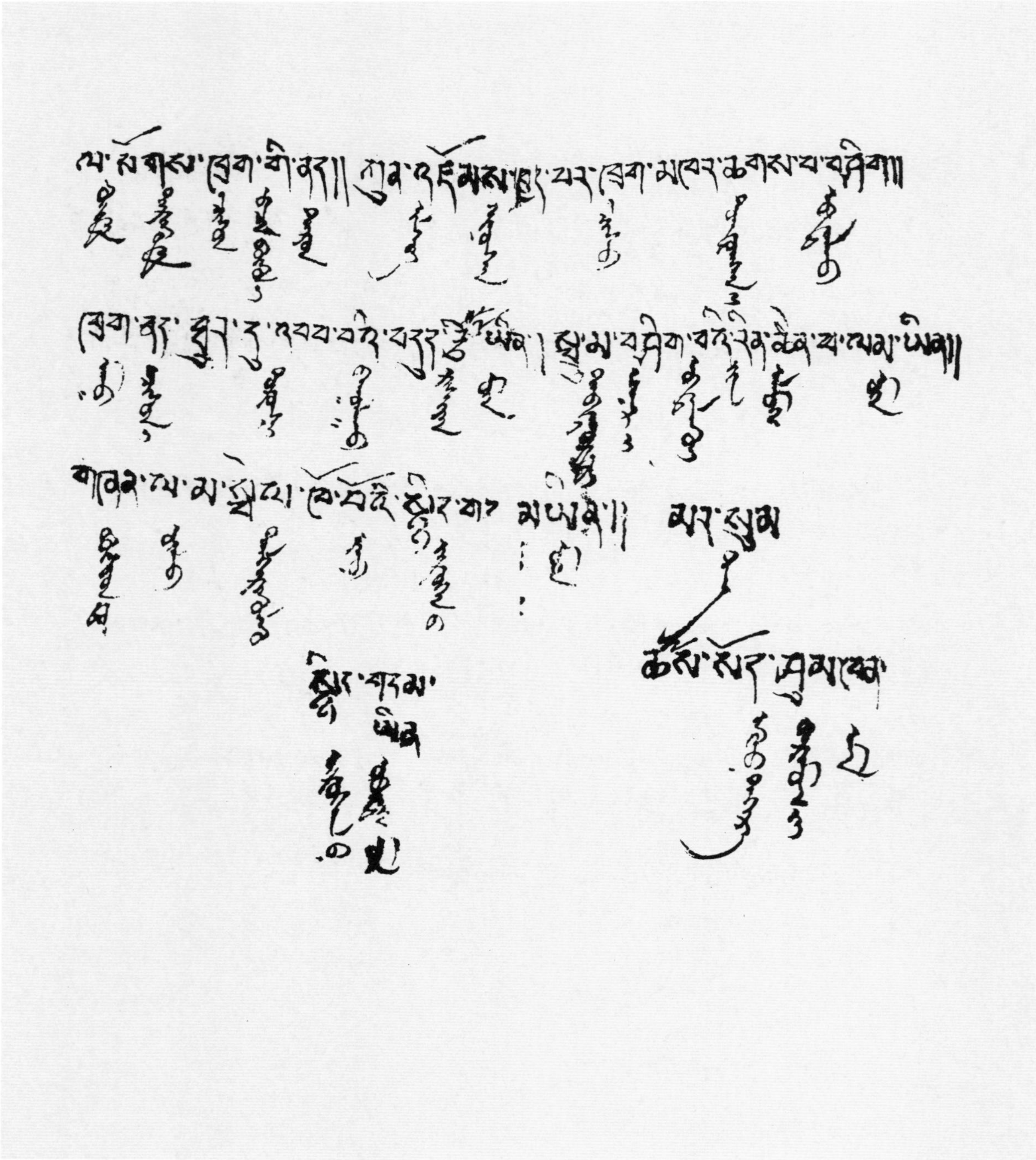

ᠲᠤᠰ ᠨᠣᠮ ᠢ ᠮᠣᠳᠤᠨ ᠬᠡᠪ ᠦᠨ ᠡᠬᠢ ᠪᠢᠴᠢᠭᠰᠡᠨ ᠨᠣᠮ ᠪᠣᠯᠤᠨ᠎ᠠ ::

ᠬᠡᠪ ᠦᠨ ᠬᠡᠮᠵᠢᠶ᠎ᠡ ᠨᠢ : 23cm×23.5cm ᠪᠣᠯᠤᠨ᠎ᠠ · ᠨᠡᠢᠲᠡ 18 ᠨᠢᠭᠤᠷ ᠲᠠᠢ ::

ᠲᠤᠰ ᠰᠤᠳᠤᠷ ᠢ 《 ᠭᠠᠩᠵᠤᠤᠷ ᠭᠠᠨᠵᠤᠤᠷ ᠤ ᠳᠠᠷᠤᠭᠠᠯ ᠬᠠᠷᠢᠶᠠᠯᠠ 》 ᠲᠠᠢ ᠰᠦᠮ ᠤᠨ ᠪᠣᠳᠤᠭᠠᠯ ᠢ ᠬᠠᠷᠢᠴᠠᠭᠤᠯᠤᠯ ᠤᠨ ᠵᠠᠭᠤᠷ ᠤᠨ ᠬᠡᠪᠯᠡᠯ ᠪᠣᠯᠤᠨ᠎ᠠ :: ᠲᠤᠰ 《 ᠭᠠᠩᠵᠤᠤᠷ
ᠭᠠᠩᠵᠤᠤᠷ ᠤ ᠳᠠᠷᠤᠭᠠᠯ ᠬᠠᠷᠢᠶᠠᠯᠠ 》 ᠲᠠᠢ 《 ᠬᠠᠷᠢ ᠶᠢᠨ ᠬᠠᠷᠢᠶᠠᠯᠠ 》 ᠲᠠᠢ ᠰᠣᠨᠢᠷᠬᠠᠭᠤᠯᠤᠯ ᠪᠠᠢᠳᠠᠯ ᠪᠠᠢᠬᠤ 《 ᠰᠦᠮ ᠤᠨ ᠪᠣᠳᠤᠭᠠᠯ ᠤᠨ ᠬᠠᠷᠢᠴᠠᠭᠤᠯᠤᠯ ᠪᠠᠢᠳᠠᠯ 》 ᠤᠨ ᠮᠣᠩᠭᠣᠯ ᠪᠢᠴᠢᠭ ᠦᠨ ᠨᠣᠮ
ᠪᠣᠯᠤᠨ᠎ᠠ :: ᠳᠠᠭᠠᠨ ᠭᠤᠷᠪᠠᠨ ᠪᠠᠢᠭ᠎ᠠ ᠢ ᠬᠠᠮᠲᠤ ᠬᠠᠷᠢᠴᠠᠭᠤᠯᠪᠠ · ᠰᠦᠮ ᠤᠨ ᠬᠠᠷᠢᠶᠠᠯᠠ ᠬᠠᠷᠢᠴᠠᠭᠤᠯᠤᠯ ᠪᠠᠢᠨ᠎ᠠ :: ᠲᠤᠰ ᠮᠣᠩᠭᠣᠯ ᠪᠢᠴᠢᠭ ᠦᠨ ᠨᠣᠮ ᠲᠠᠢ ᠬᠠᠮᠲᠤ ᠪᠠᠢᠳᠠᠭ ·
ᠪᠠᠷ ᠲᠠᠢ ᠬᠠᠮᠲᠤ ᠲᠦ ᠬᠡᠪᠯᠡᠯ ᠰᠦᠮ ᠤᠨ ᠪᠣᠳᠤᠭᠠᠯ ᠢ ᠰᠣᠨᠢᠷᠬᠠᠭᠤᠯᠤᠯ ᠲᠤ ᠬᠠᠮᠢᠶᠠᠷᠤᠯᠠᠭᠰᠠᠨ ᠬᠡᠪᠯᠡᠯ ᠬᠠᠮᠲᠤ ᠤᠨ ᠭᠠᠨᠵᠤᠤᠷᠯᠠᠭᠰᠠᠨ ᠪᠠᠷᠢᠭᠰᠠᠨ ᠲᠤ ᠬᠠᠷᠢᠶᠠᠯᠠᠭᠰᠠᠨ ::

6

四部医典（药效部分）

Efficiency of the Drug in Rgyud bzhi

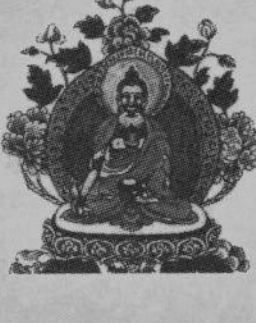

[illegible]
[illegible]
[illegible]
[illegible]
[illegible]
[illegible]
[illegible]
[illegible]
[illegible]
[illegible]
[illegible]
[illegible]

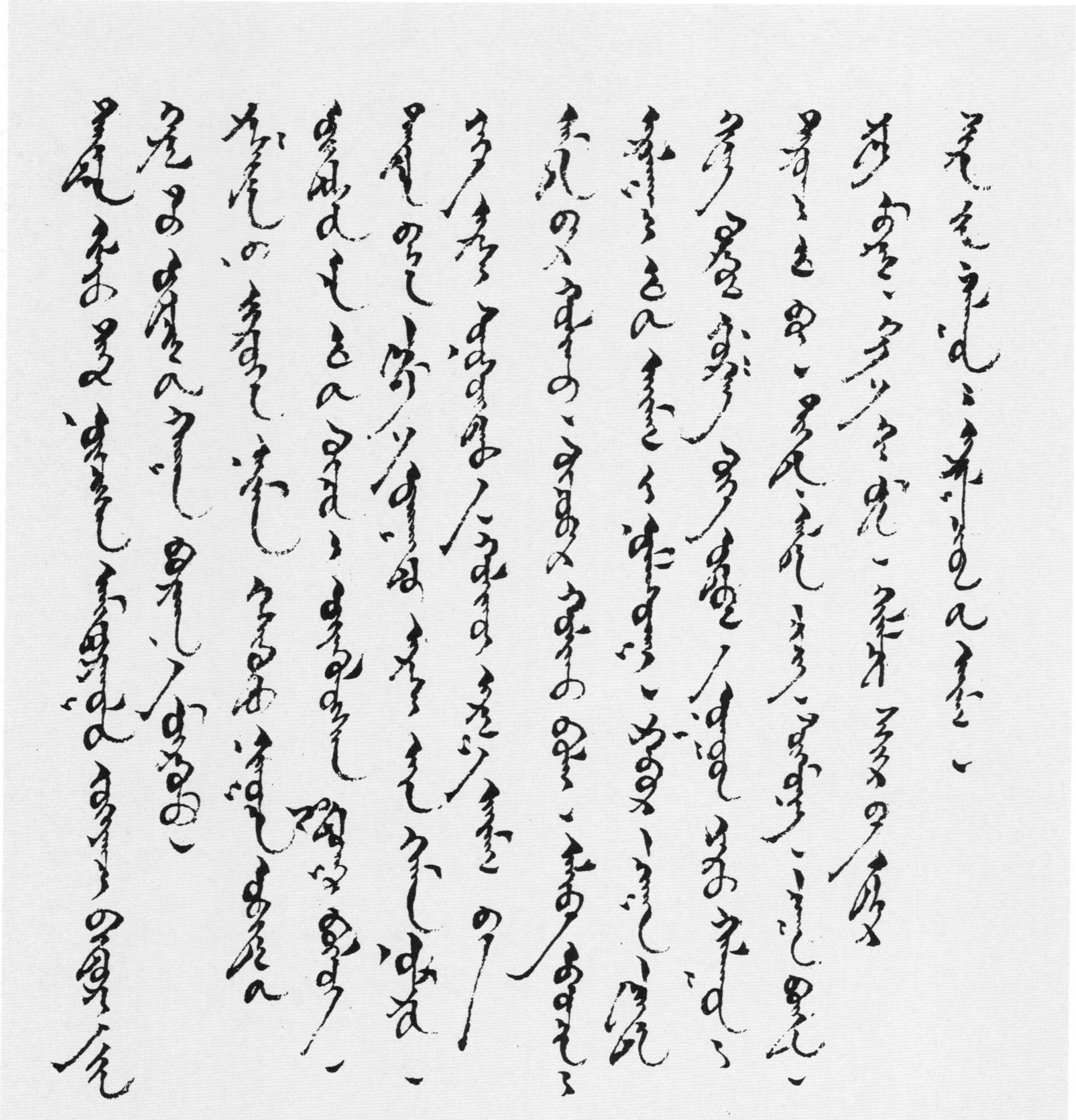

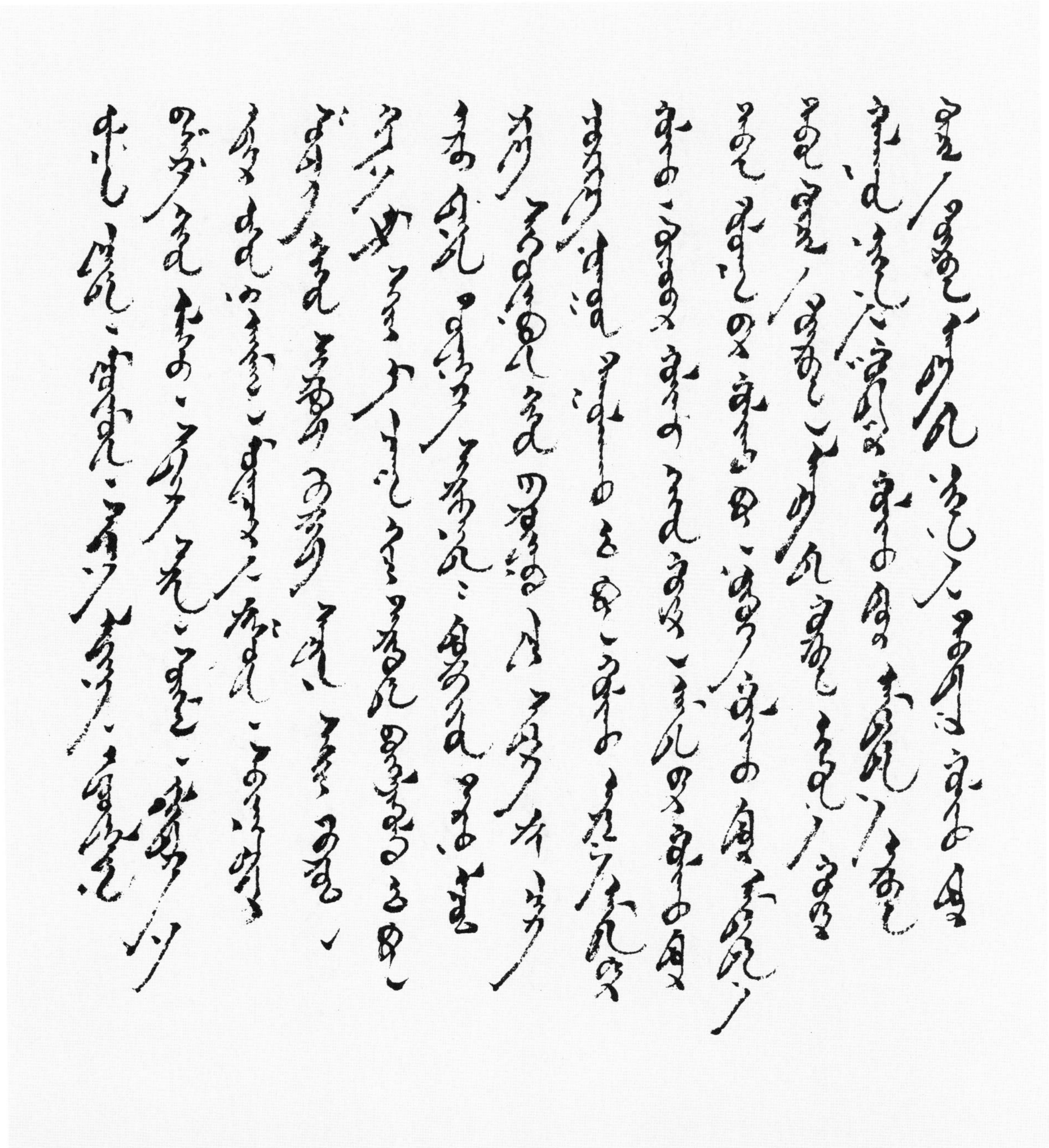

[illegible]
[illegible]
[illegible]
[illegible]
[illegible]
[illegible]
[illegible]
[illegible]
[illegible]
[illegible]
[illegible]

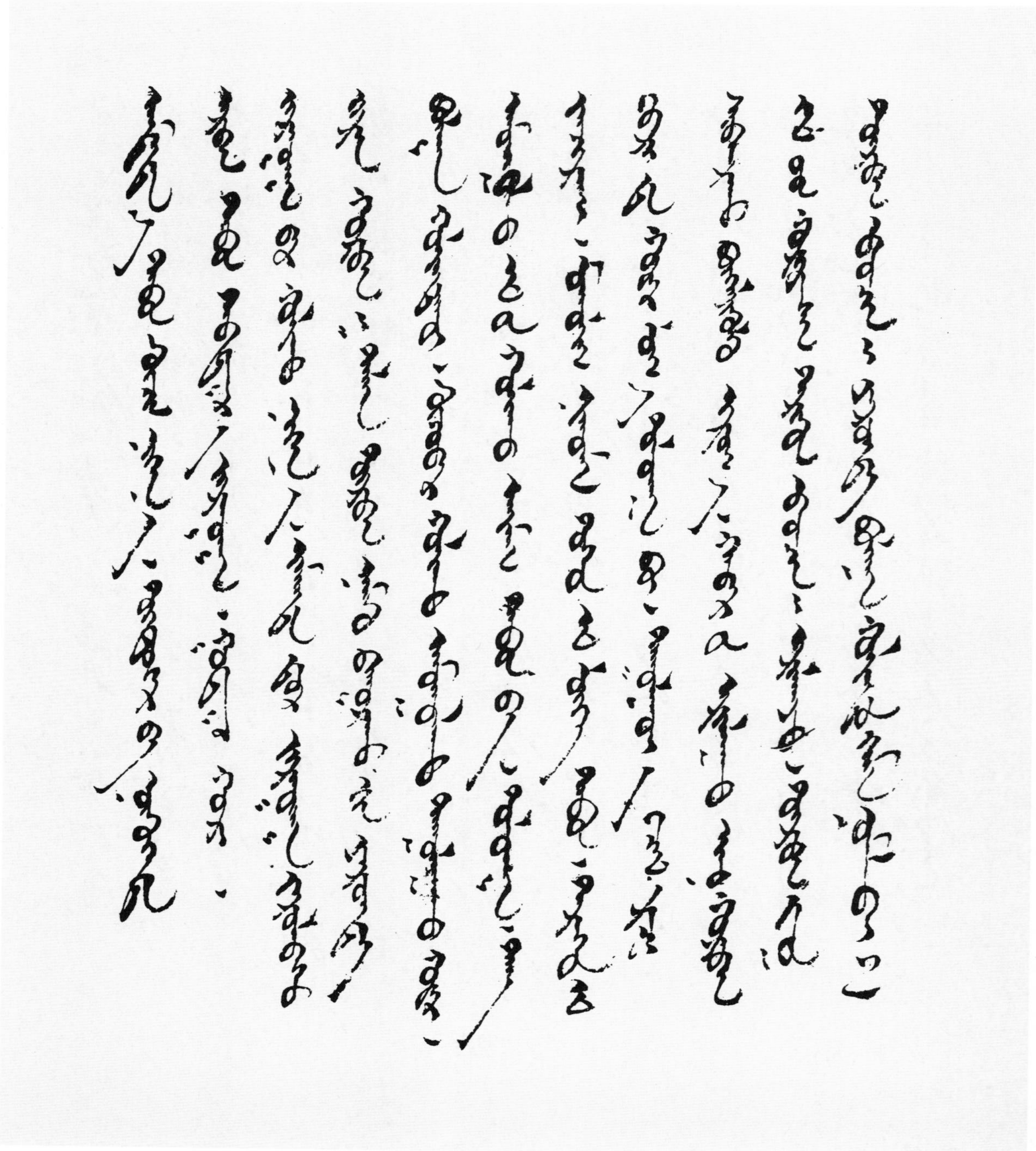

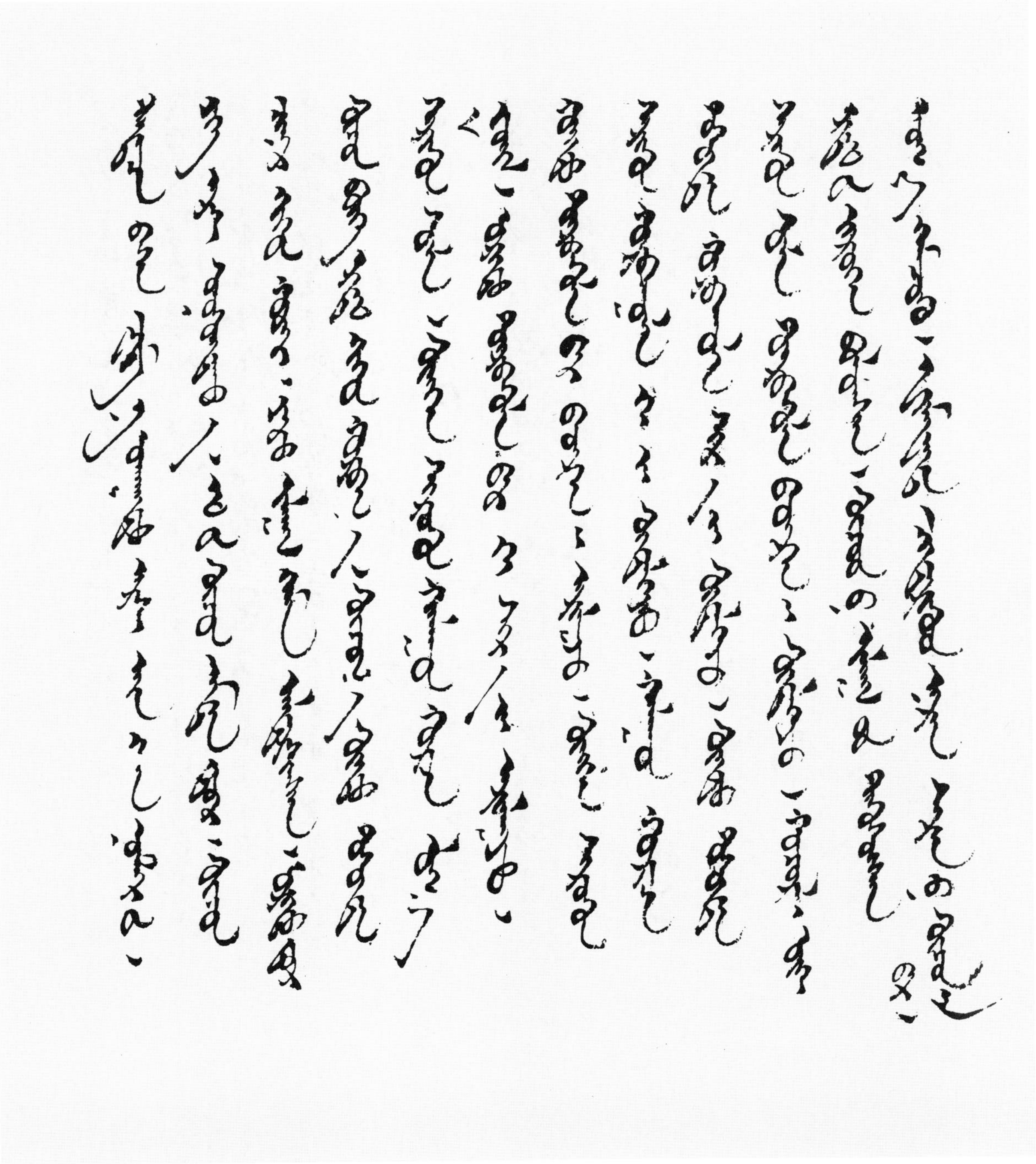

[illegible]

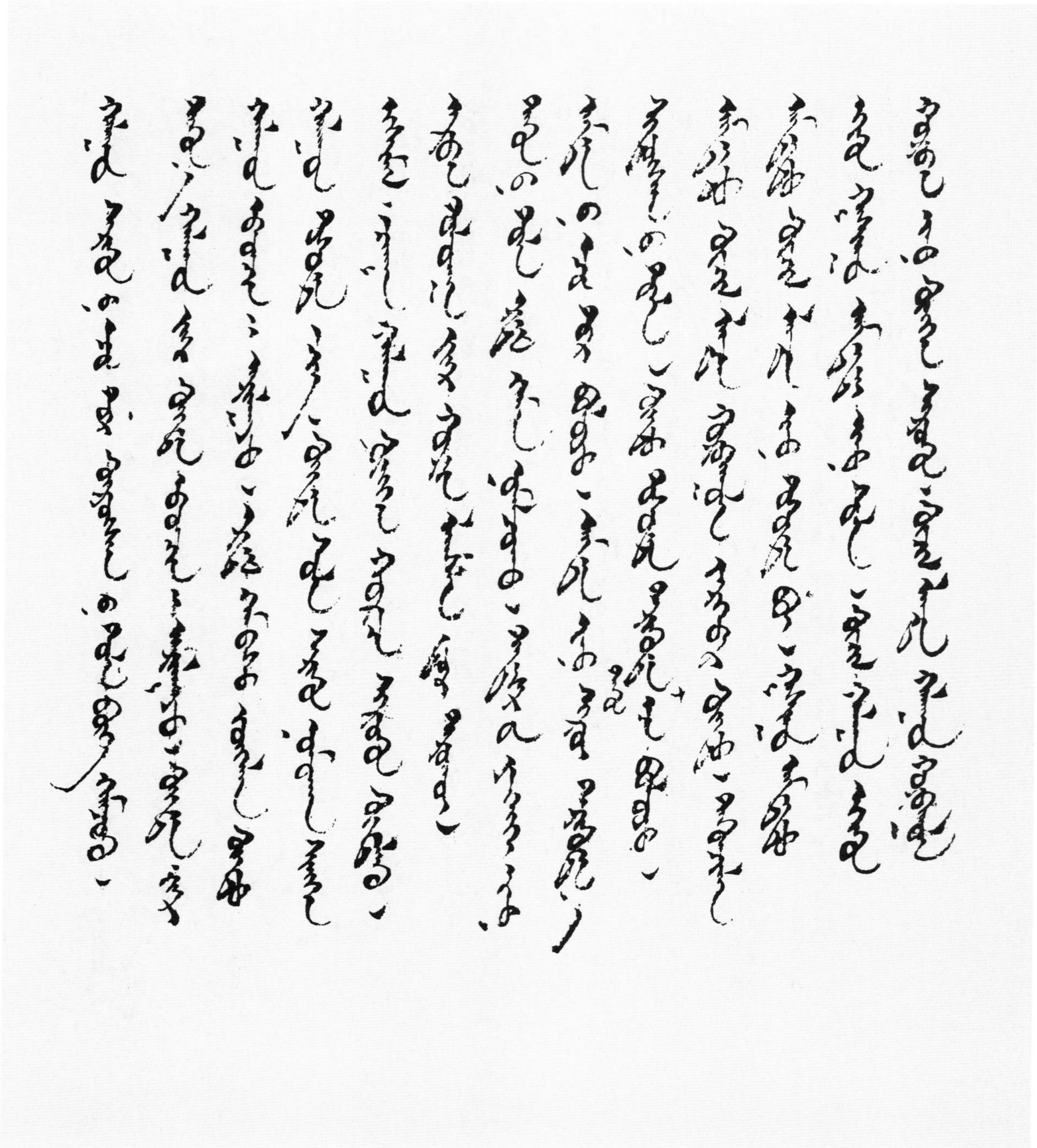

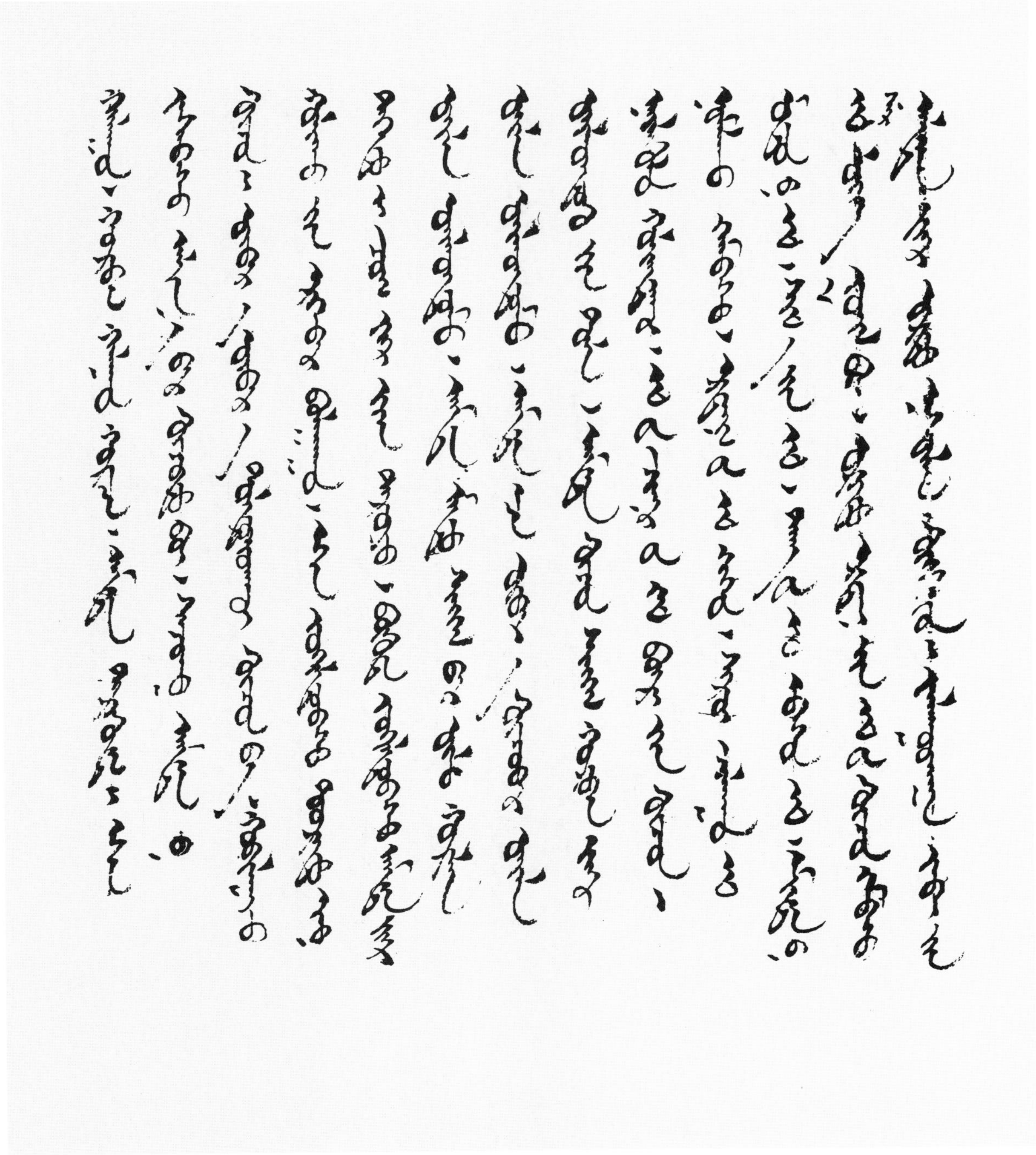

[illegible]

[illegible]
[illegible]
[illegible]
[illegible]
[illegible]
[illegible]
[illegible]
[illegible]
[illegible]
[illegible]
[illegible]
[illegible]
[illegible]
[illegible]

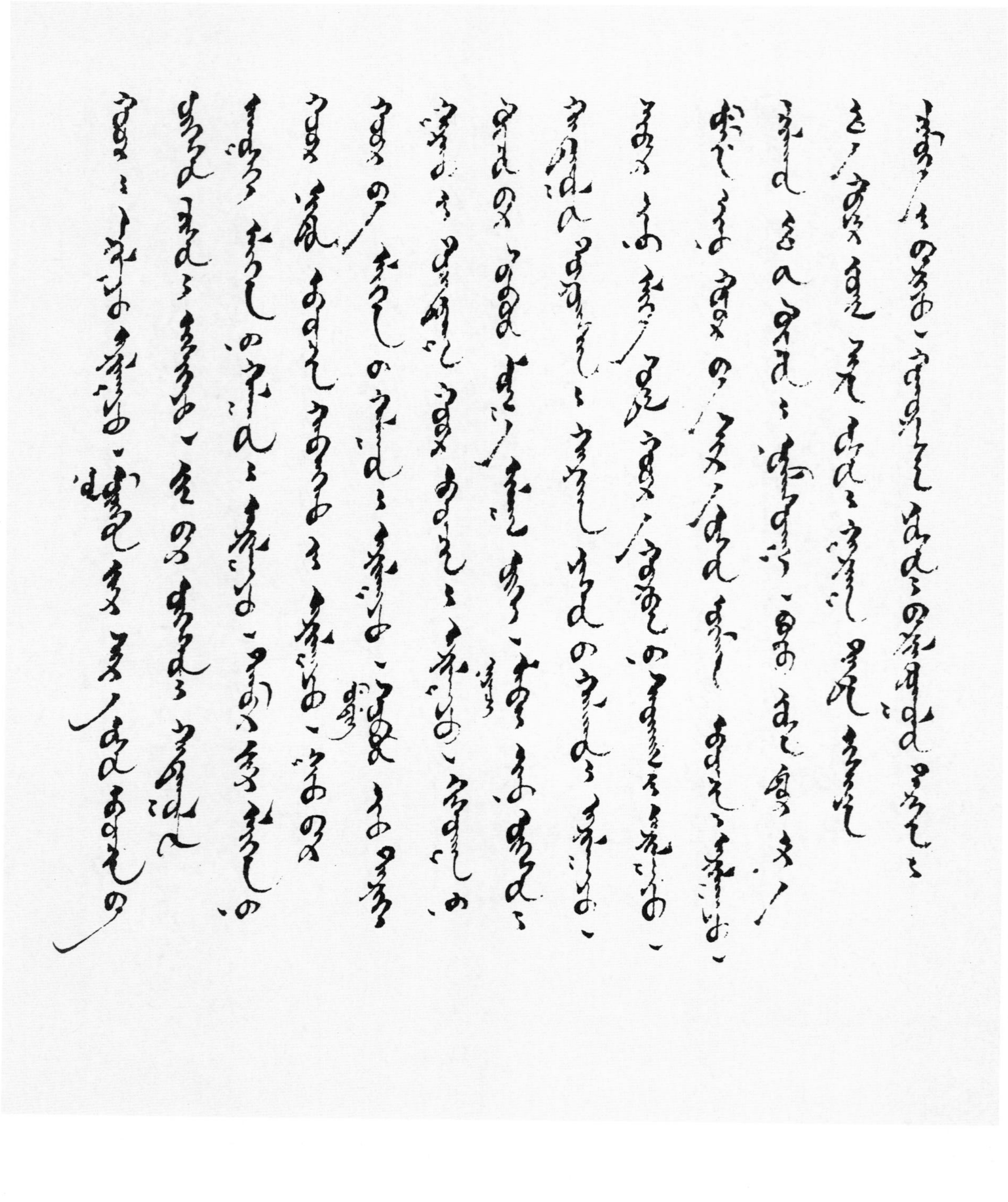

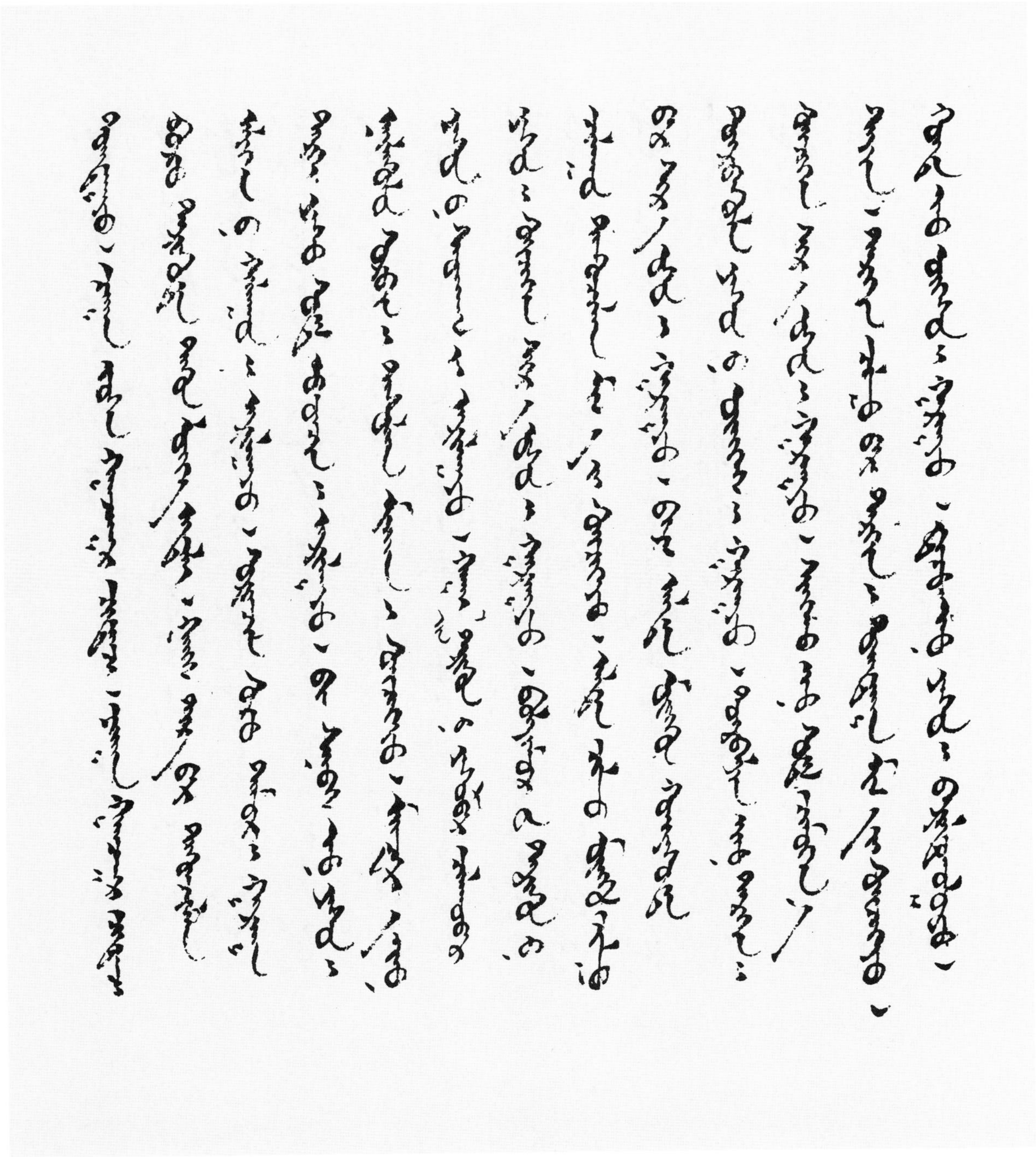

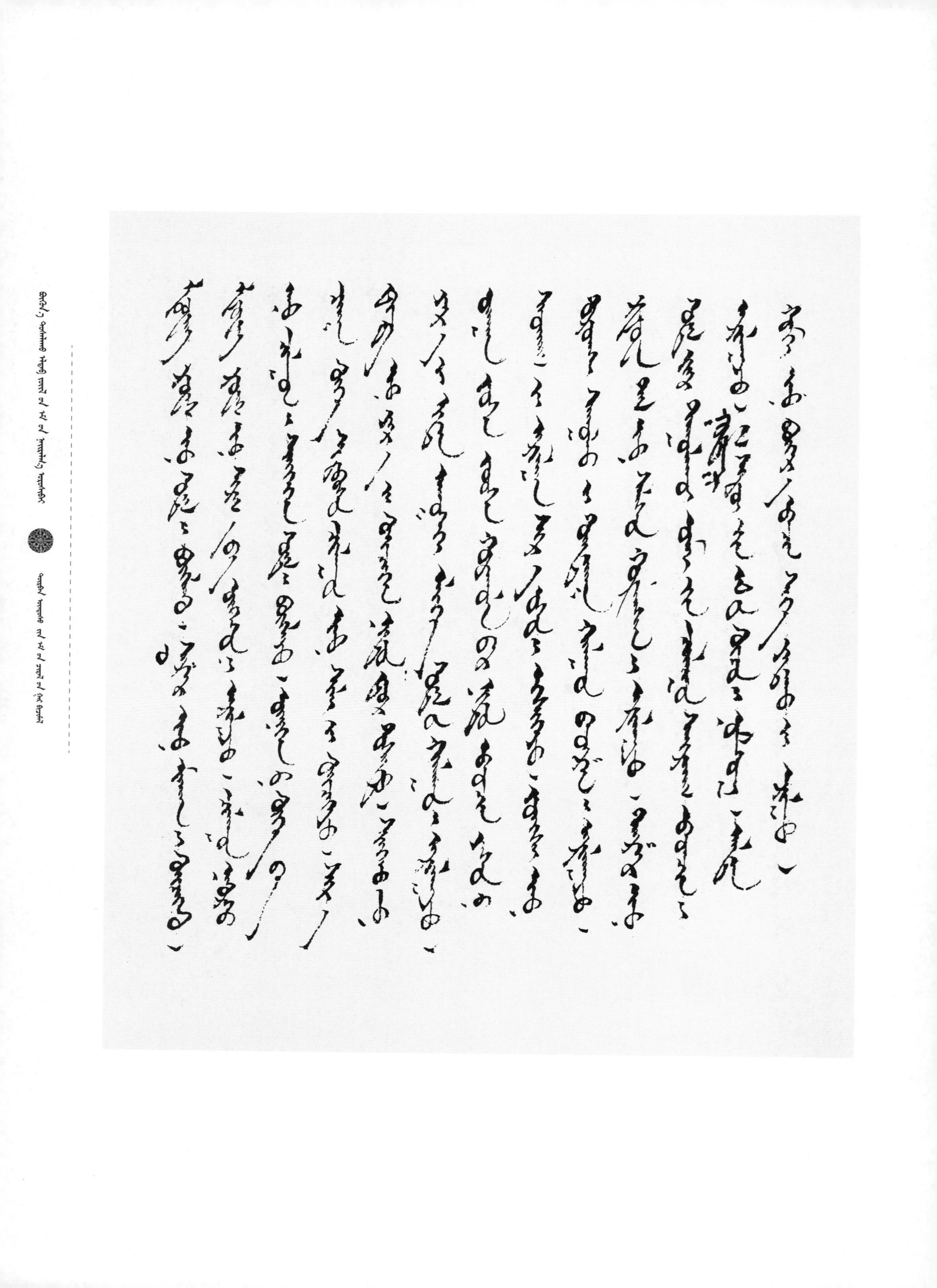

[illegible]

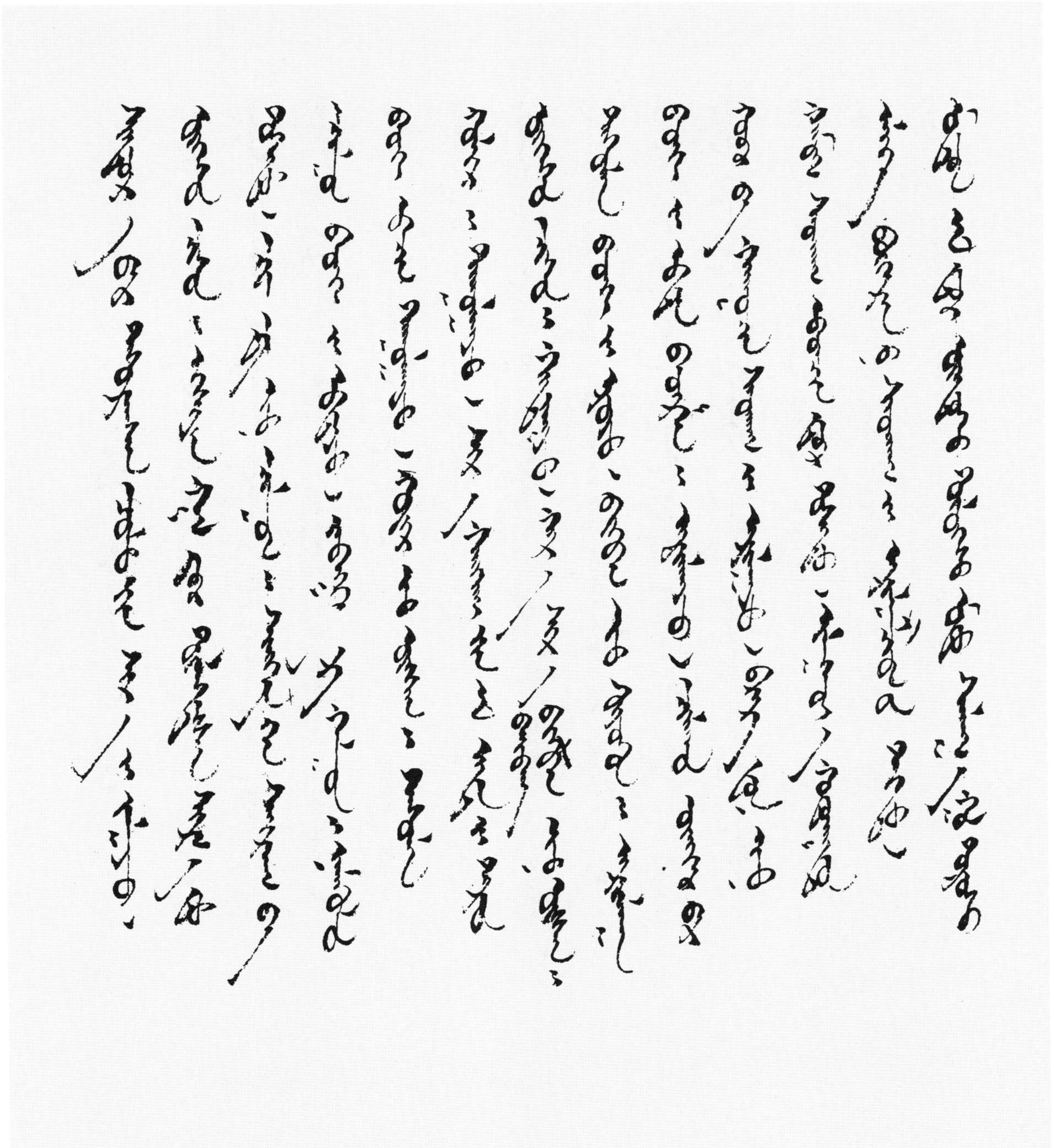

[illegible]

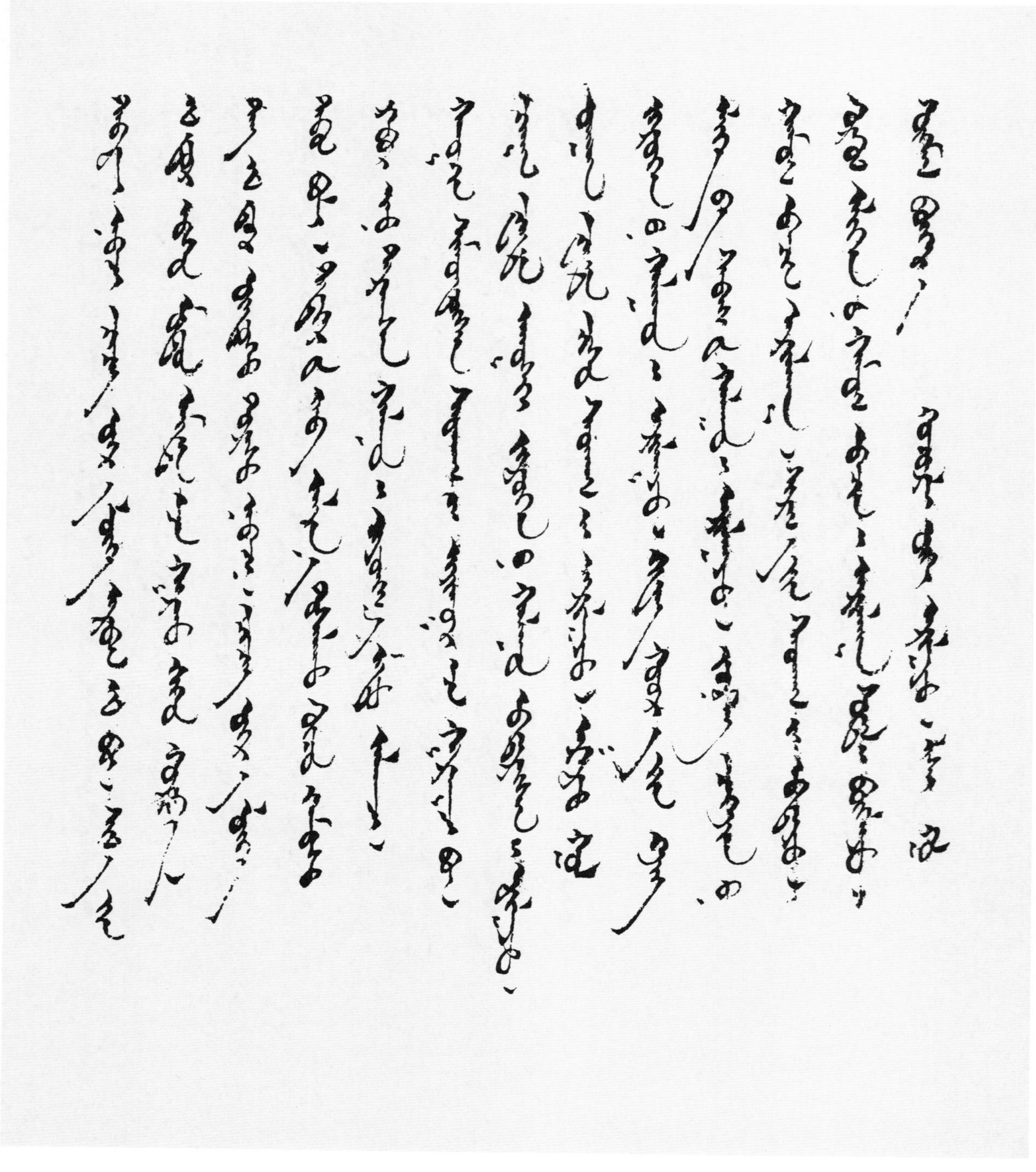

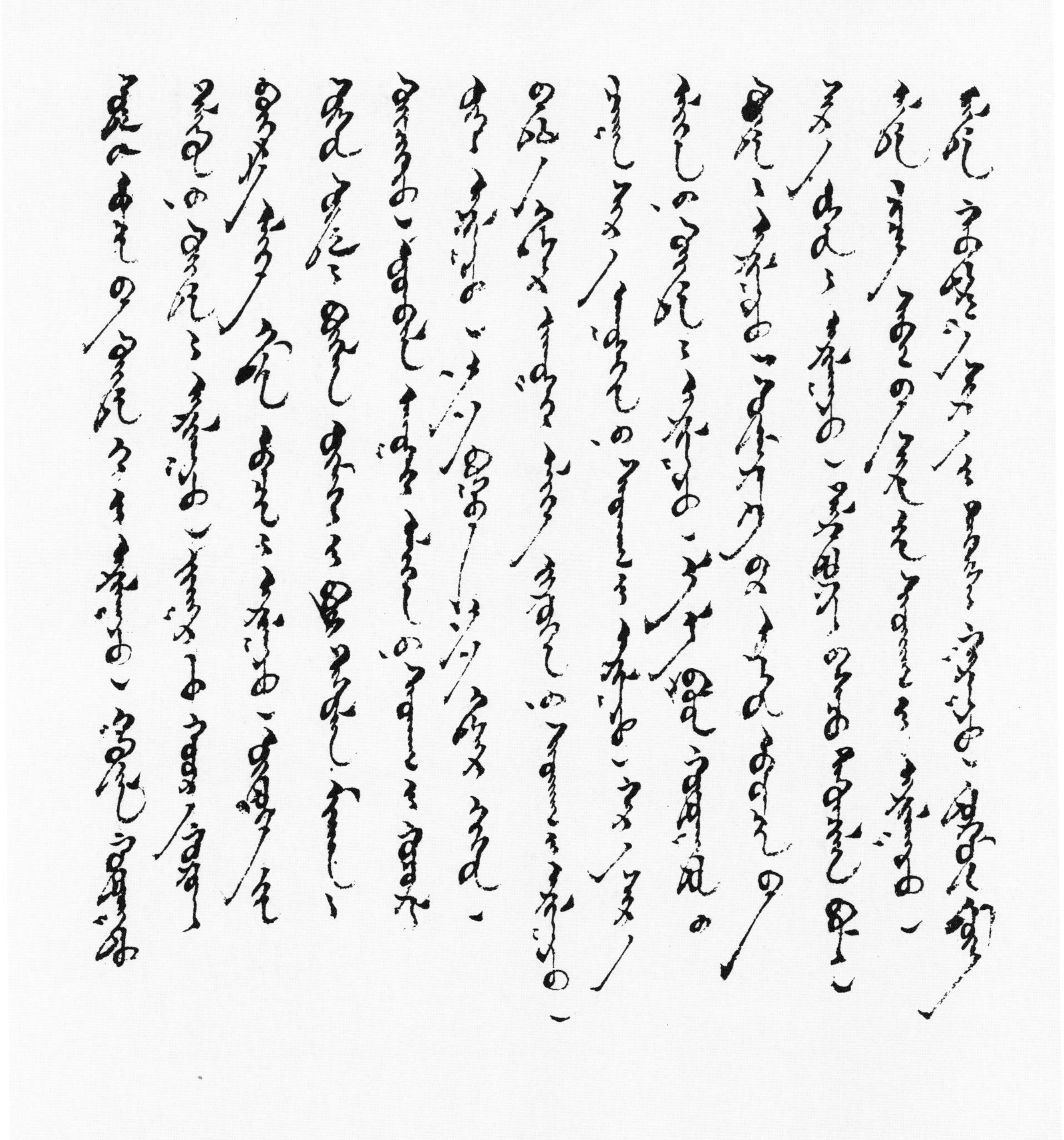

[illegible]
[illegible]
[illegible]
[illegible]
[illegible]
[illegible]
[illegible]
[illegible]
[illegible]
[illegible]
[illegible]
[illegible]
[illegible]

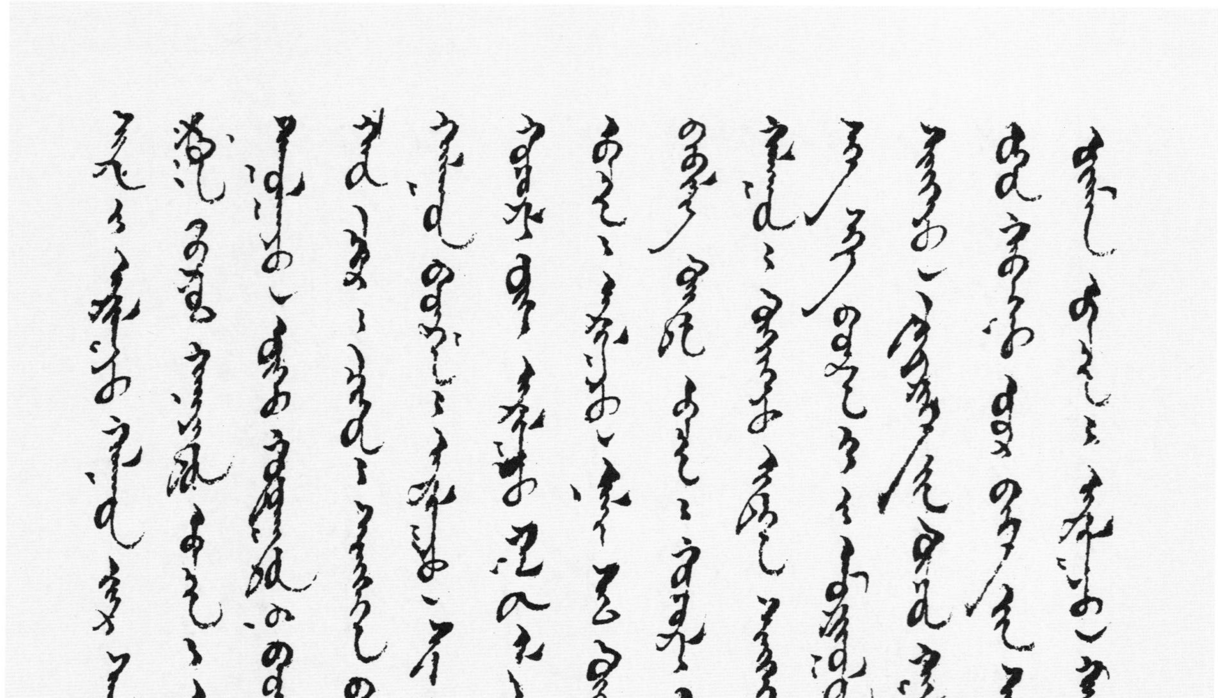

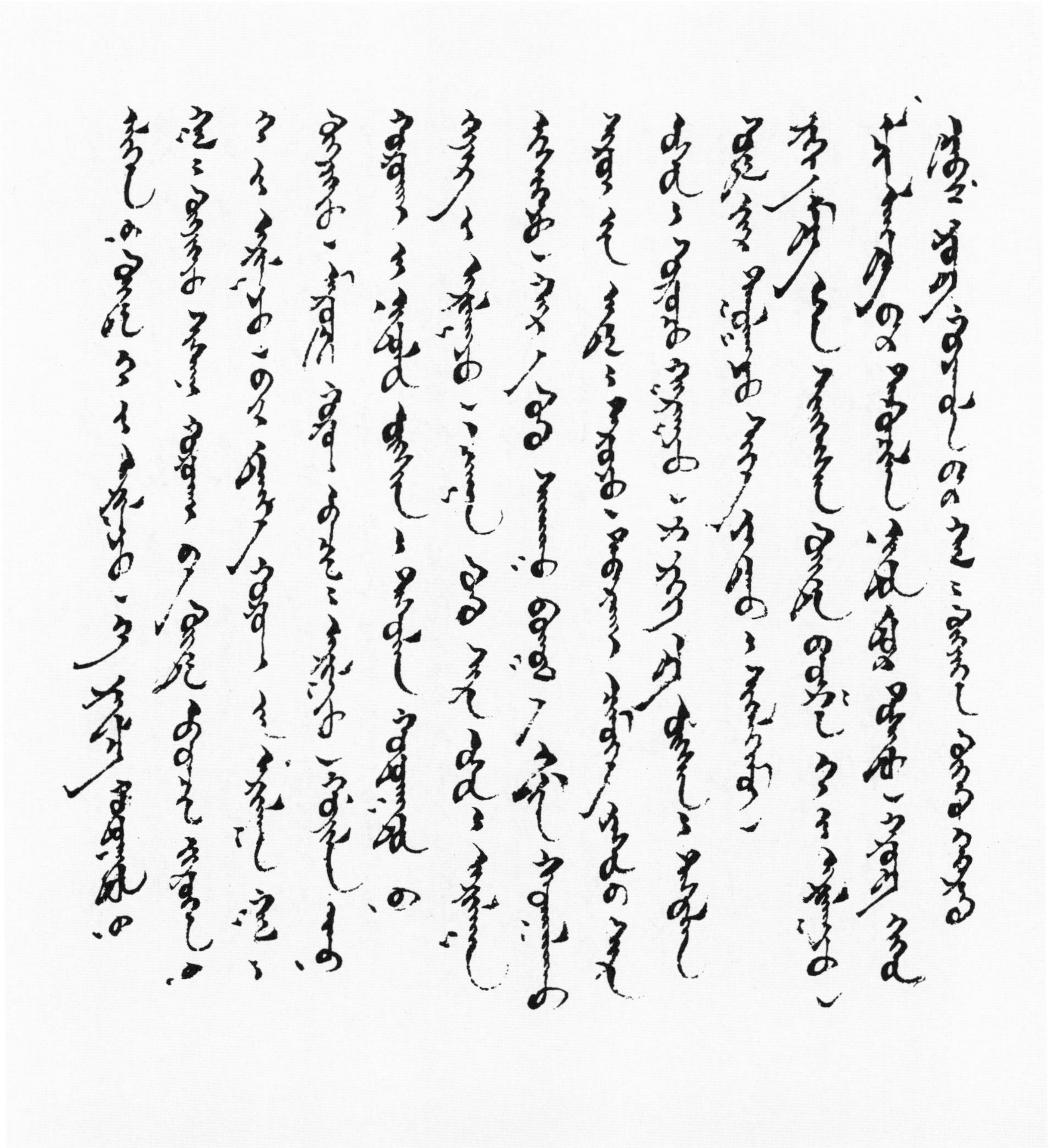

[illegible]

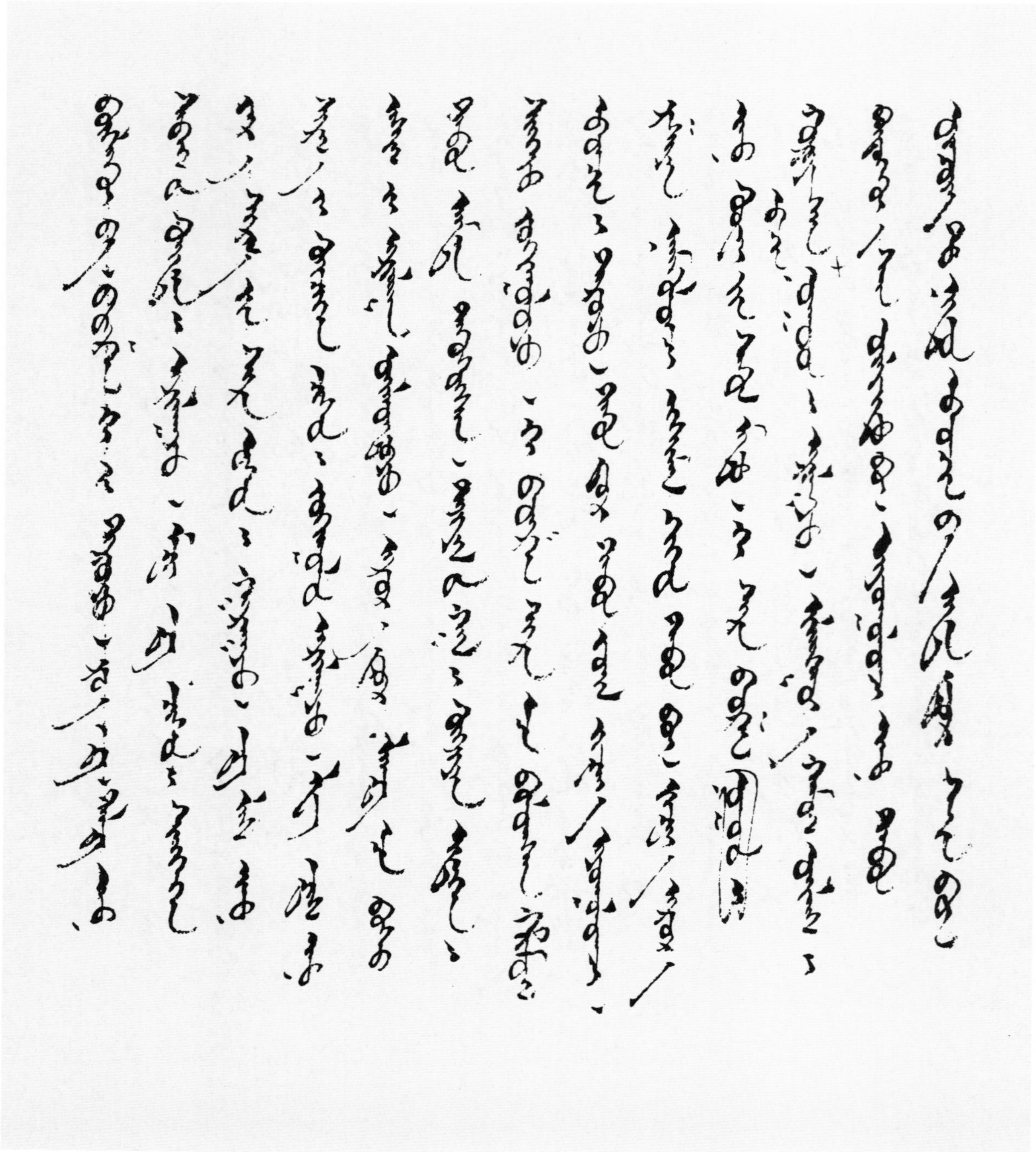

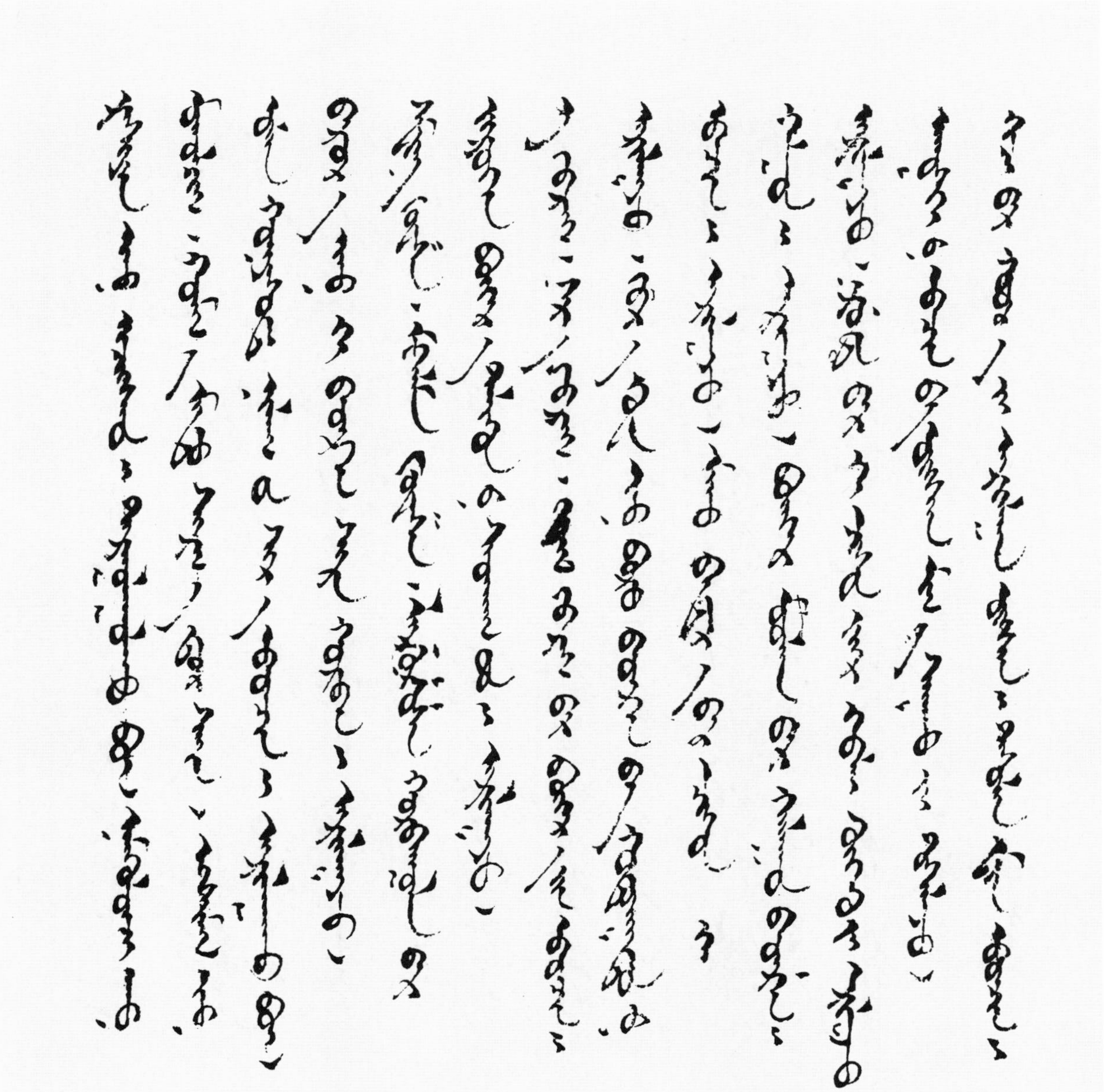

[illegible]

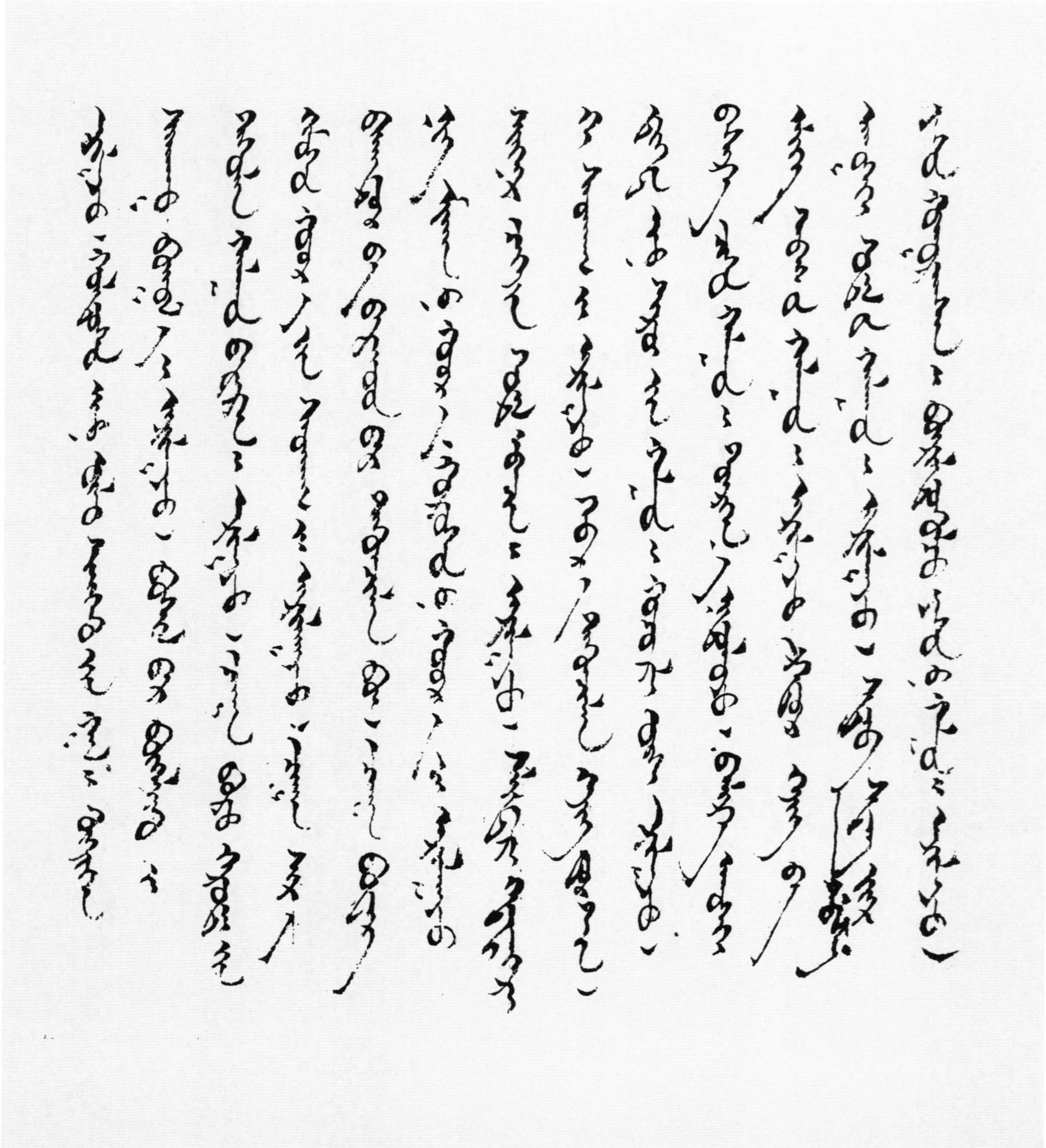

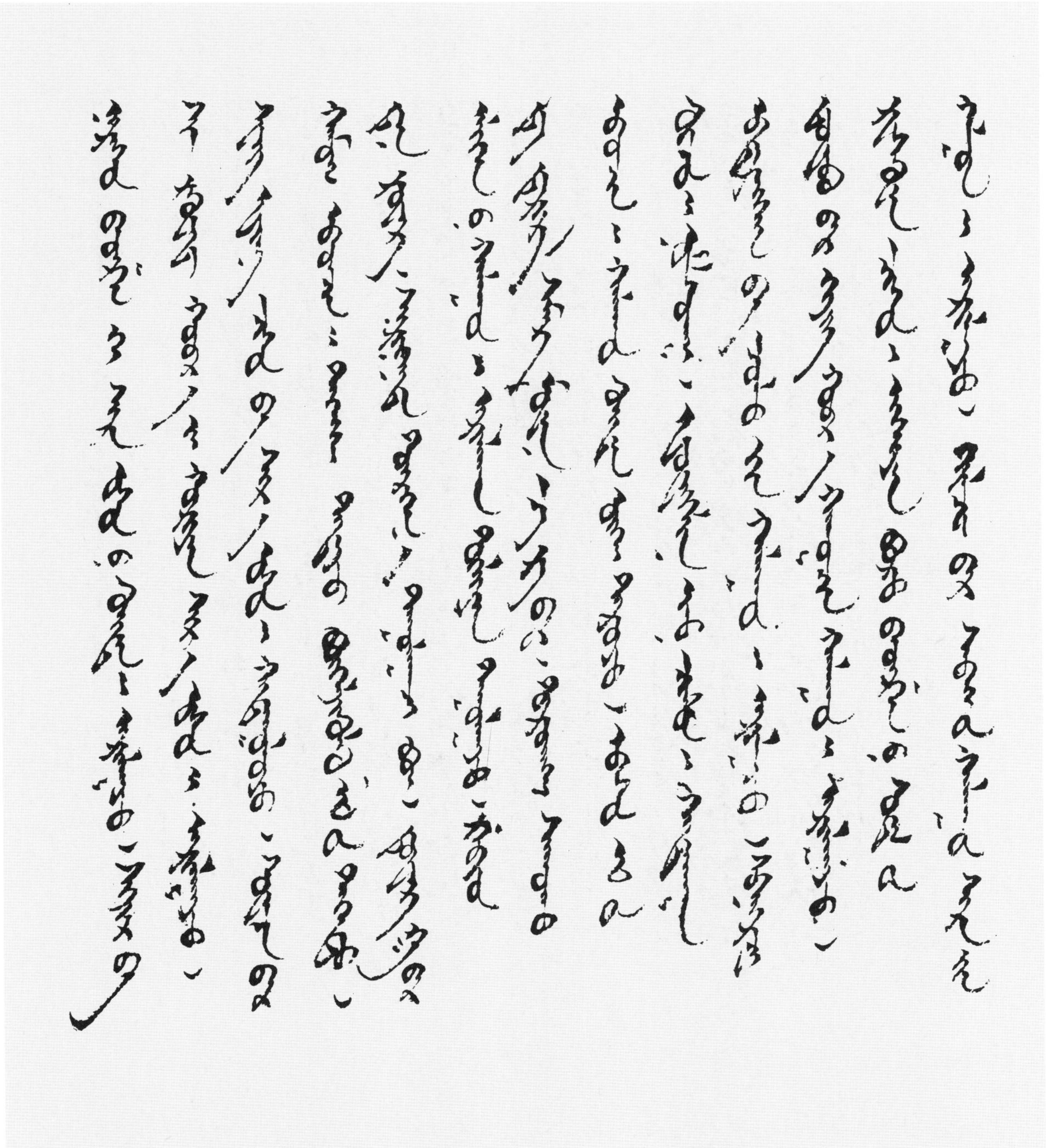

[illegible]
[illegible]
[illegible]
[illegible]
[illegible]
[illegible]
[illegible]
[illegible]
[illegible]
[illegible]
[illegible]
[illegible]

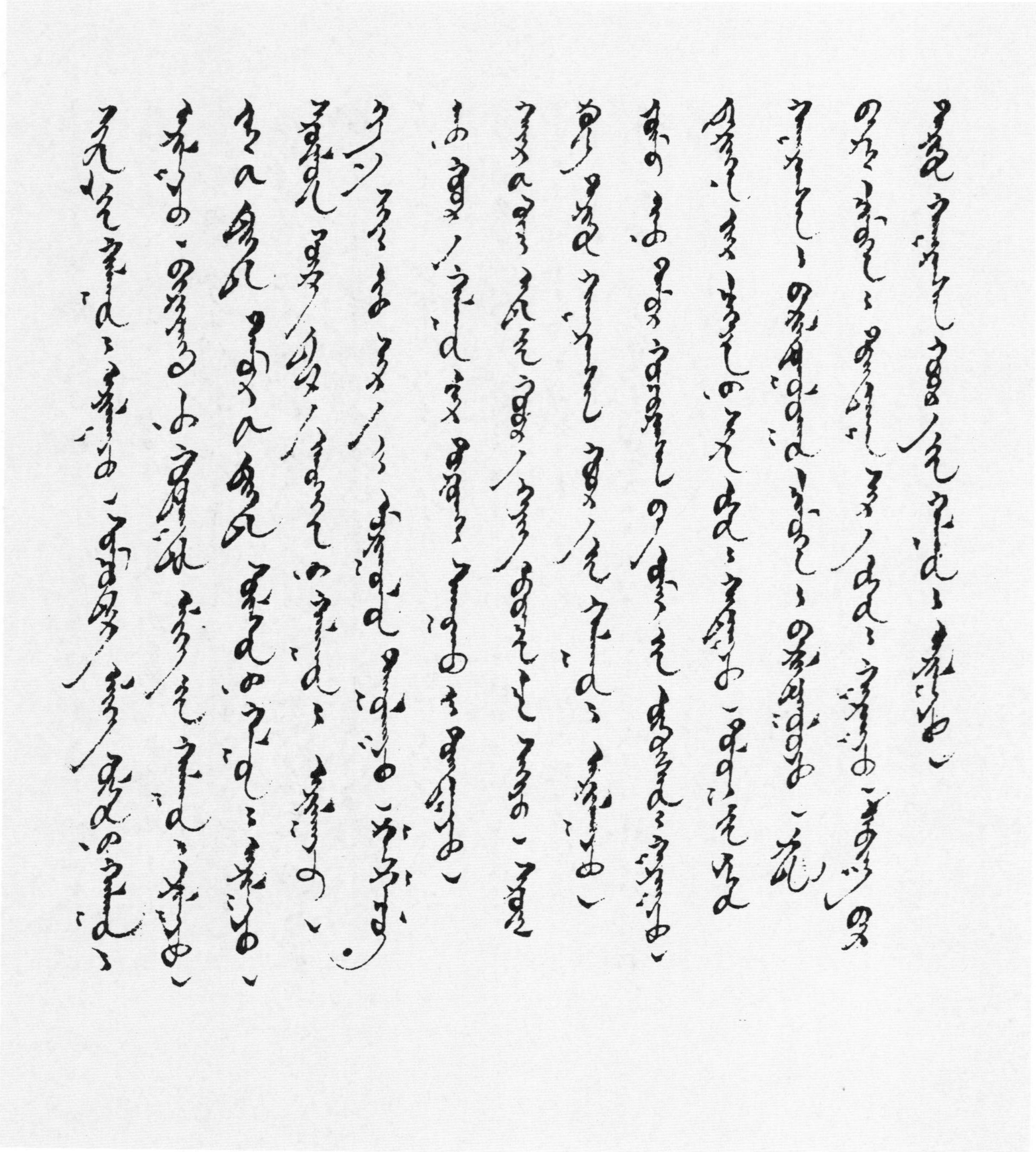

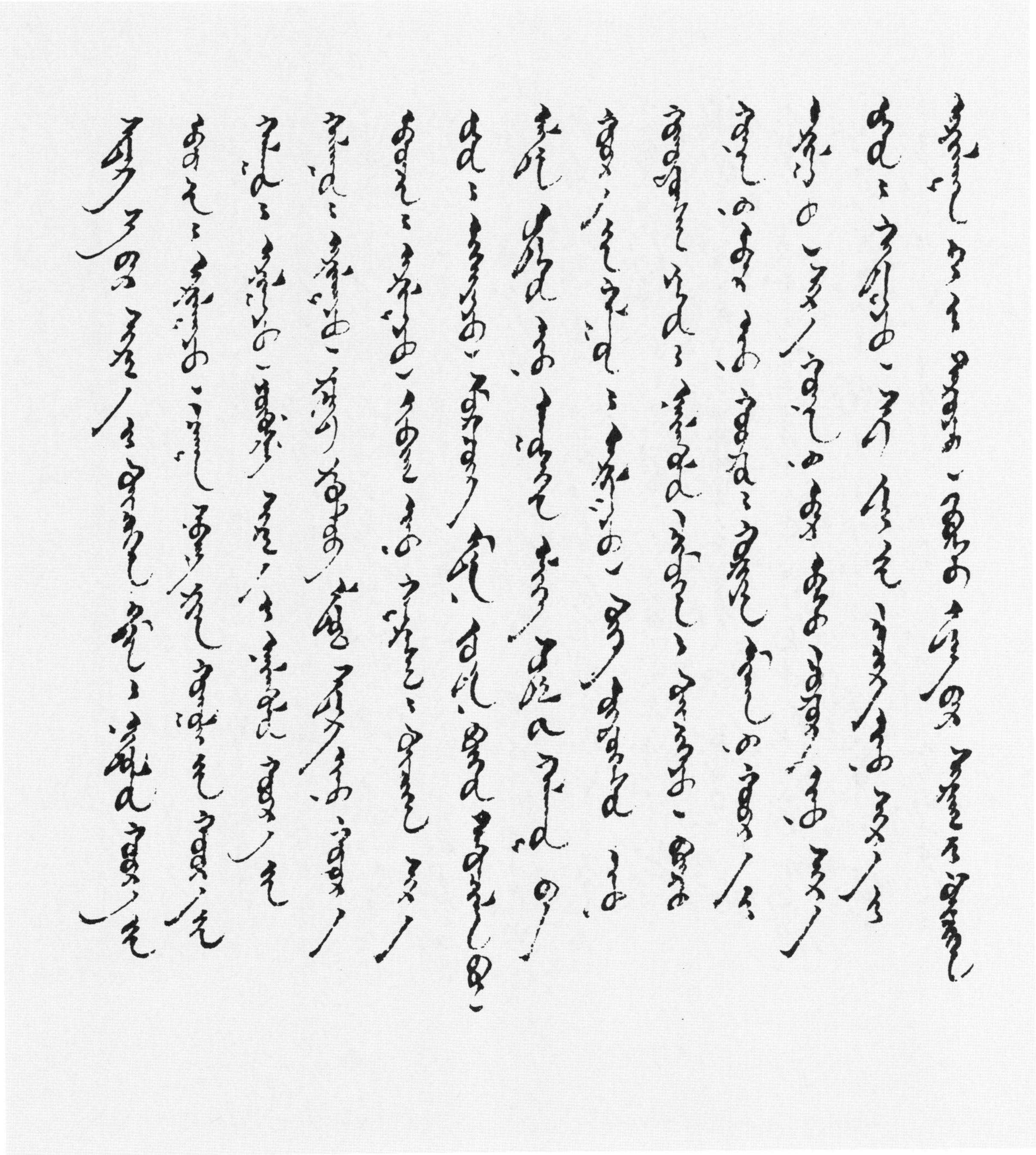

[illegible]
[illegible]
[illegible]
[illegible]
[illegible]
[illegible]
[illegible]
[illegible]
[illegible]
[illegible]
[illegible]
[illegible]
[illegible]
[illegible]

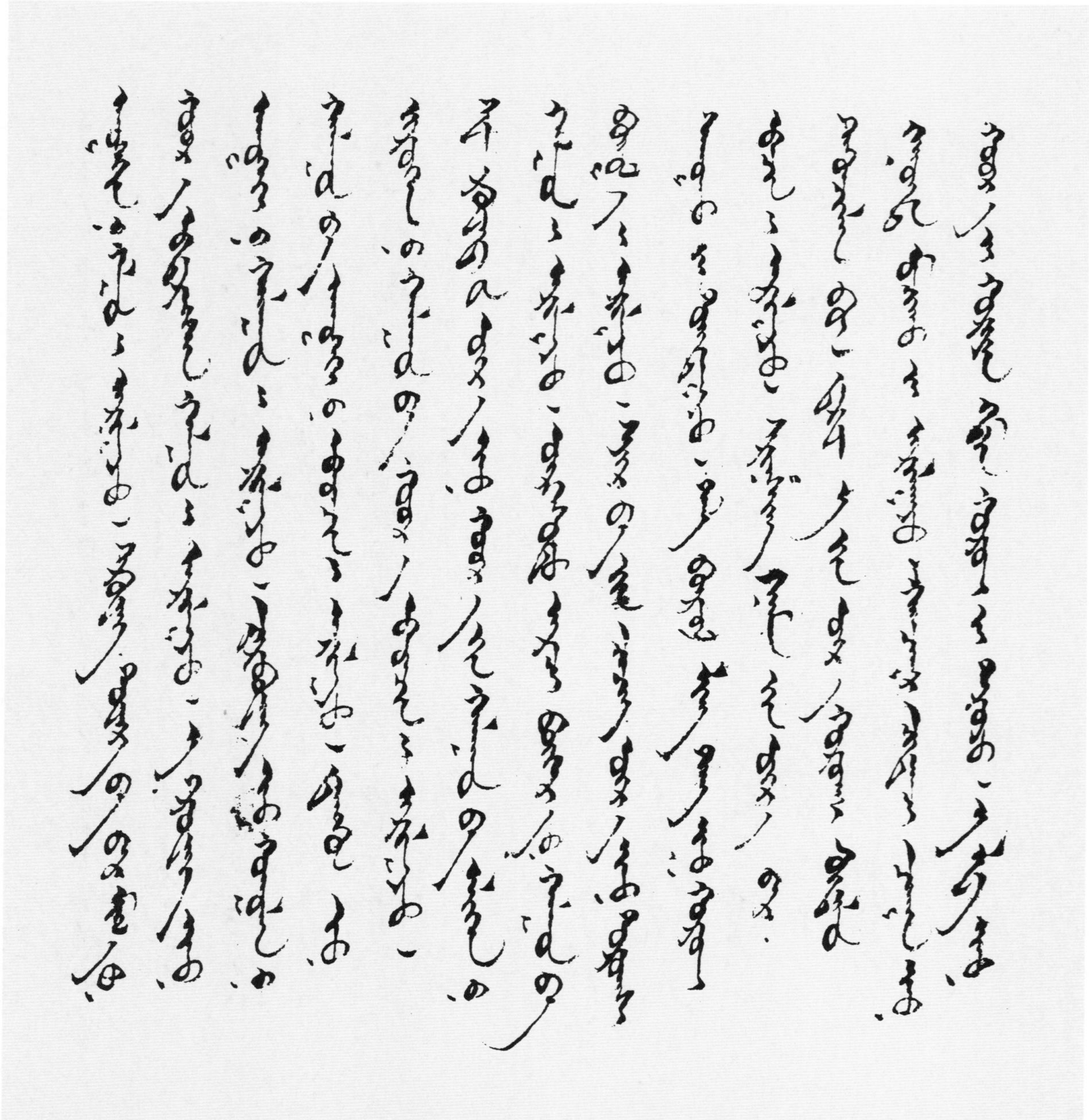

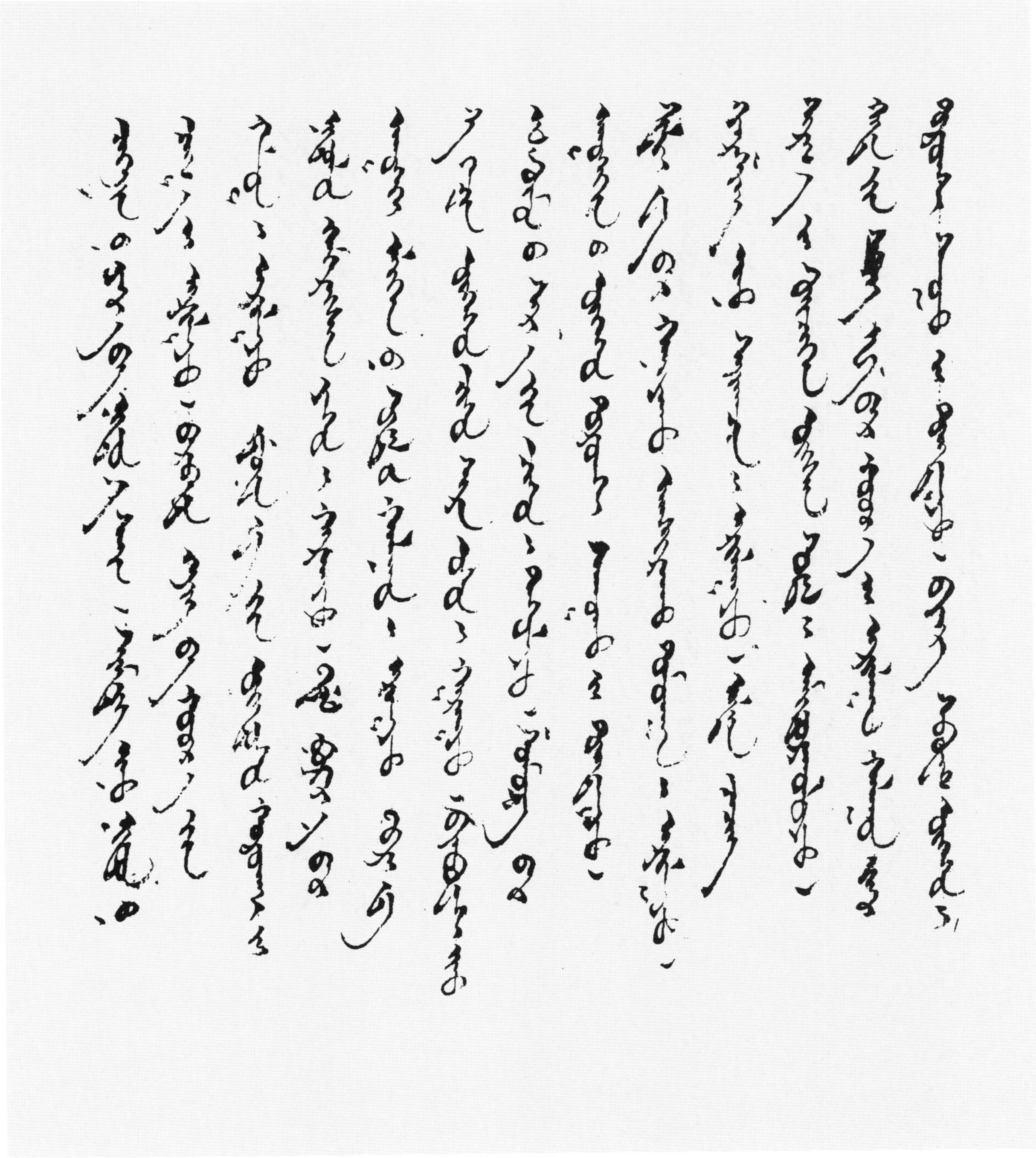

[illegible]

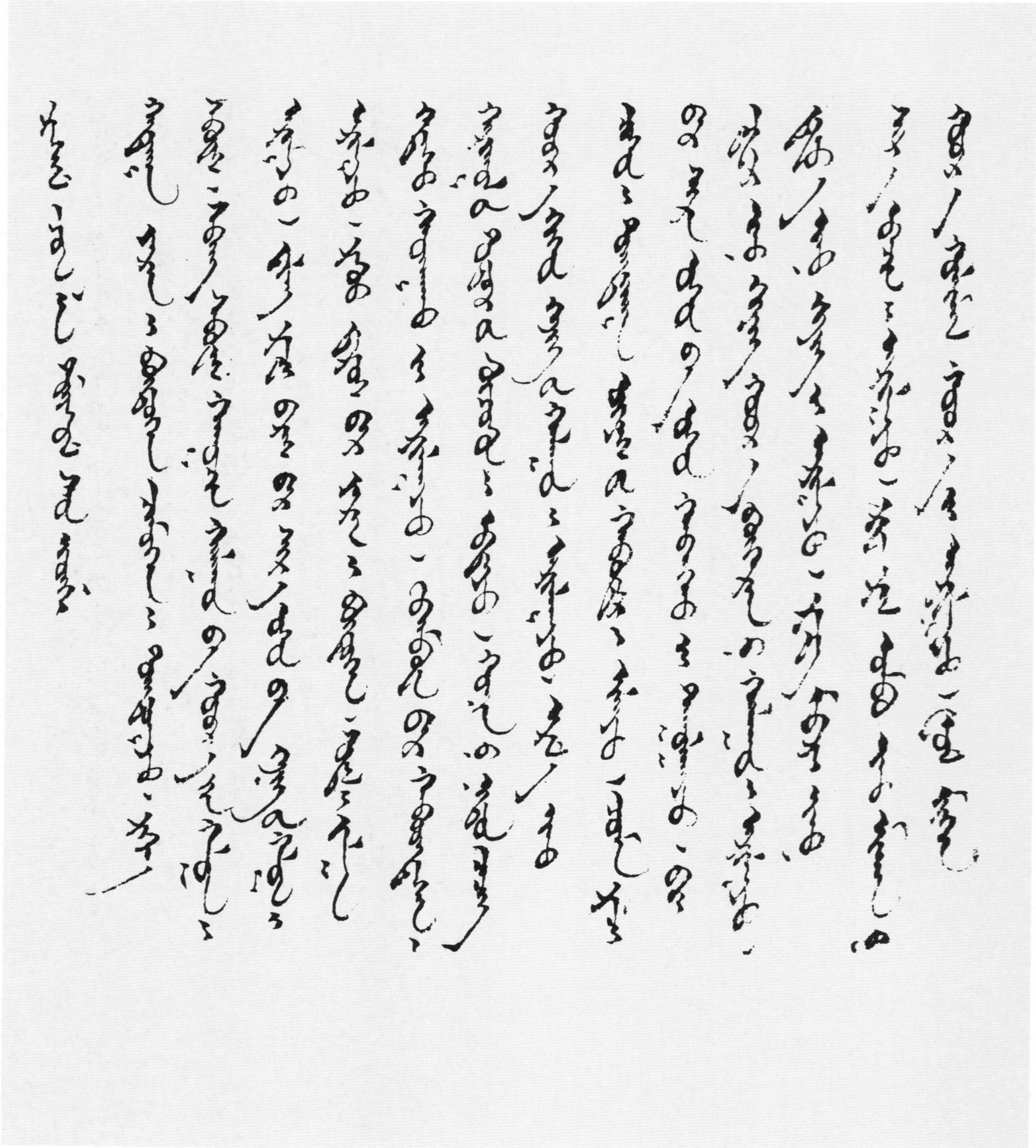

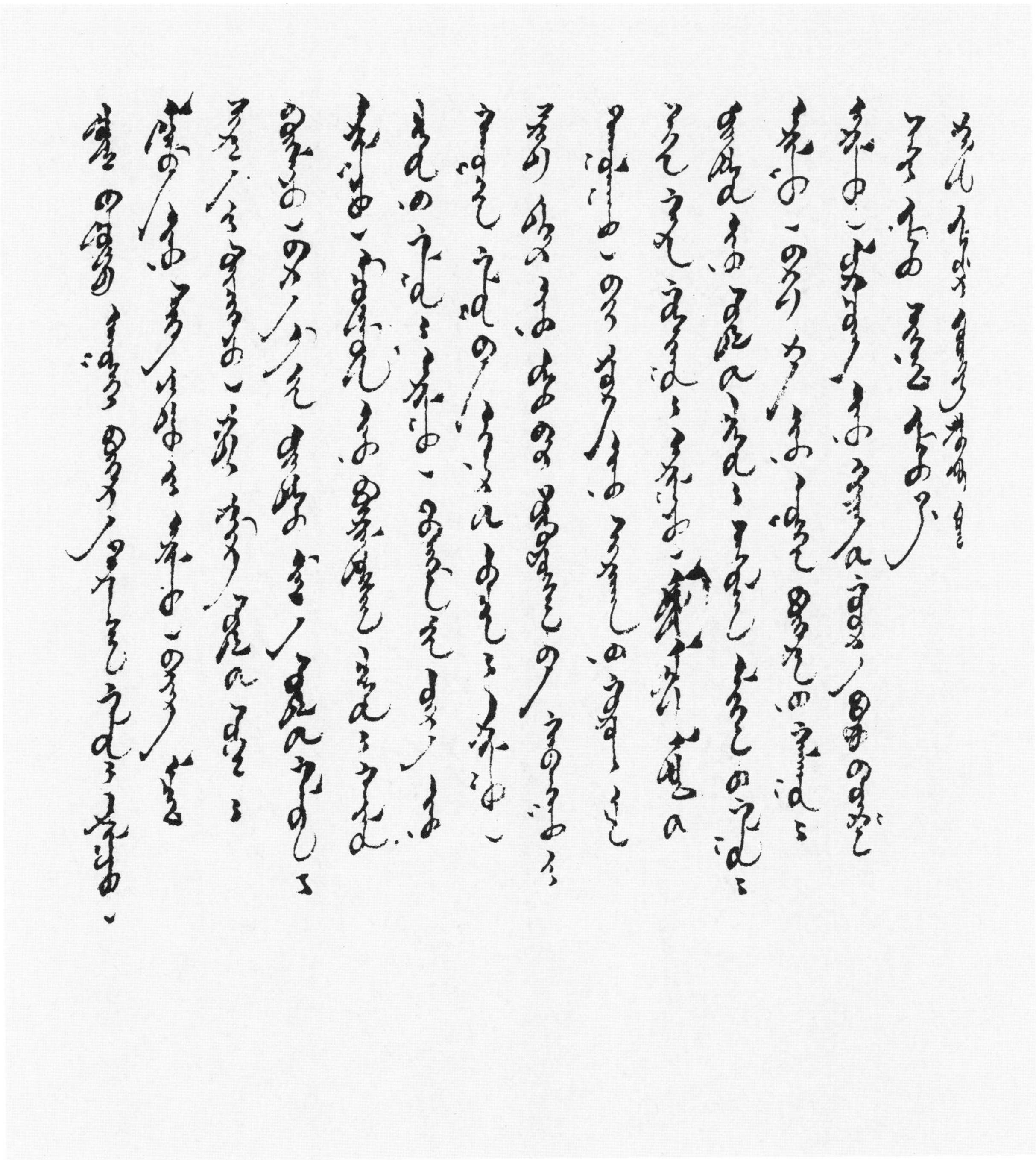

[illegible]

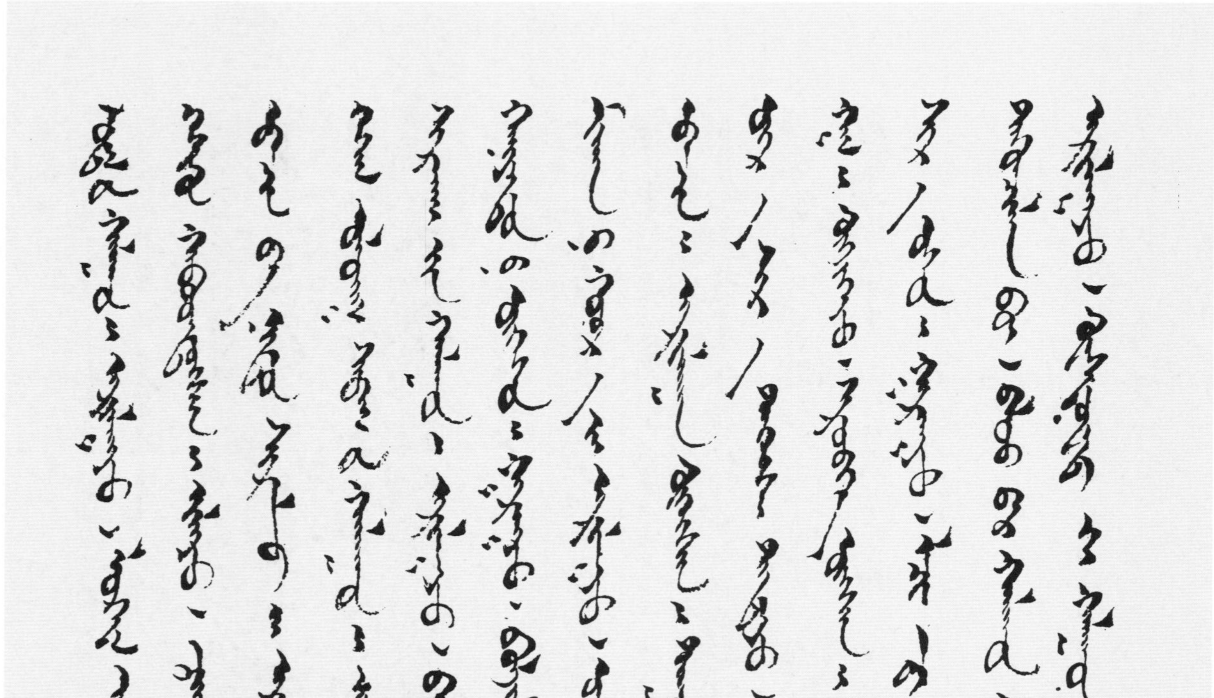

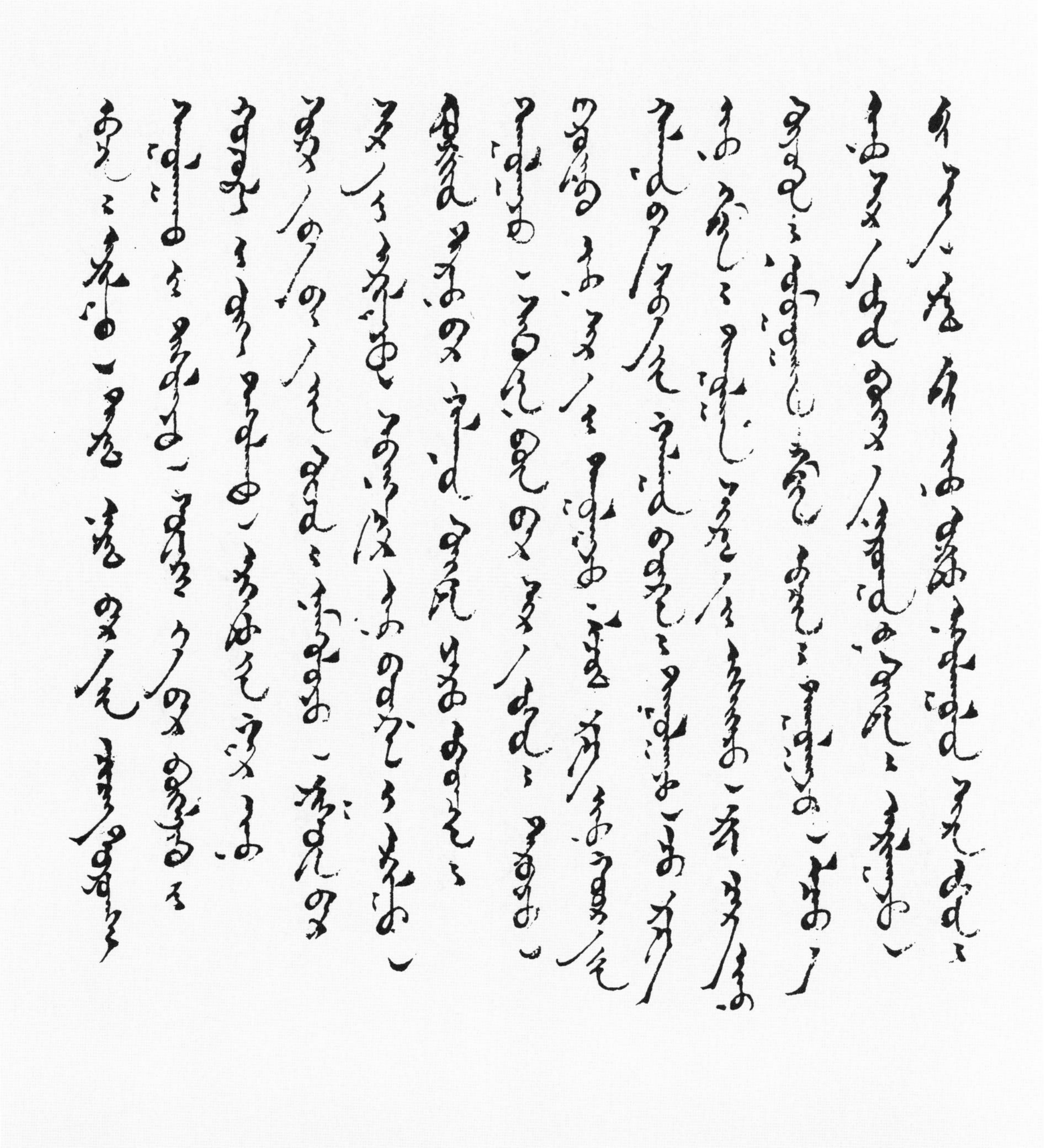

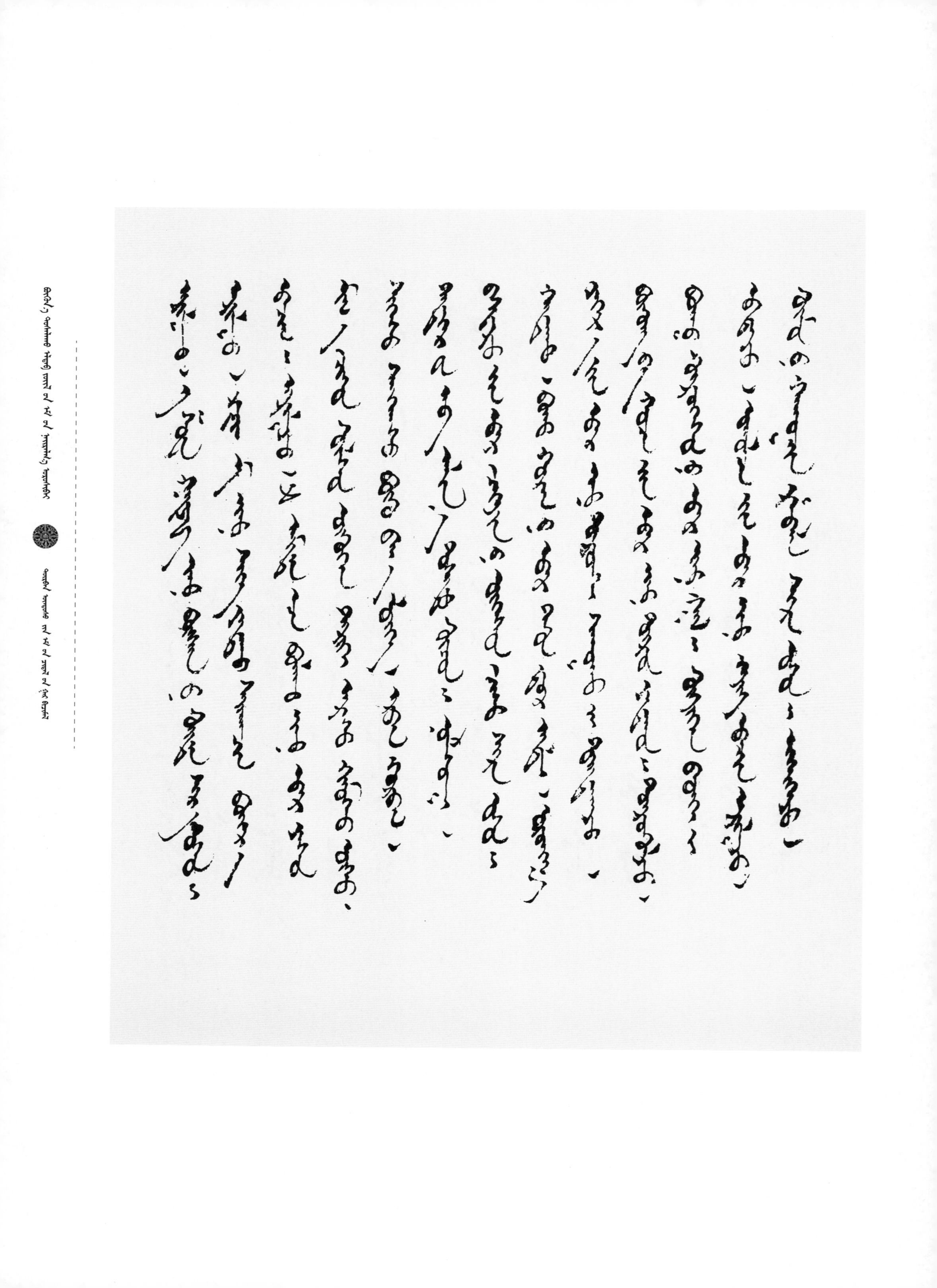

[illegible]
[illegible]
[illegible]
[illegible]
[illegible]
[illegible]
[illegible]
[illegible]
[illegible]
[illegible]
[illegible]
[illegible]

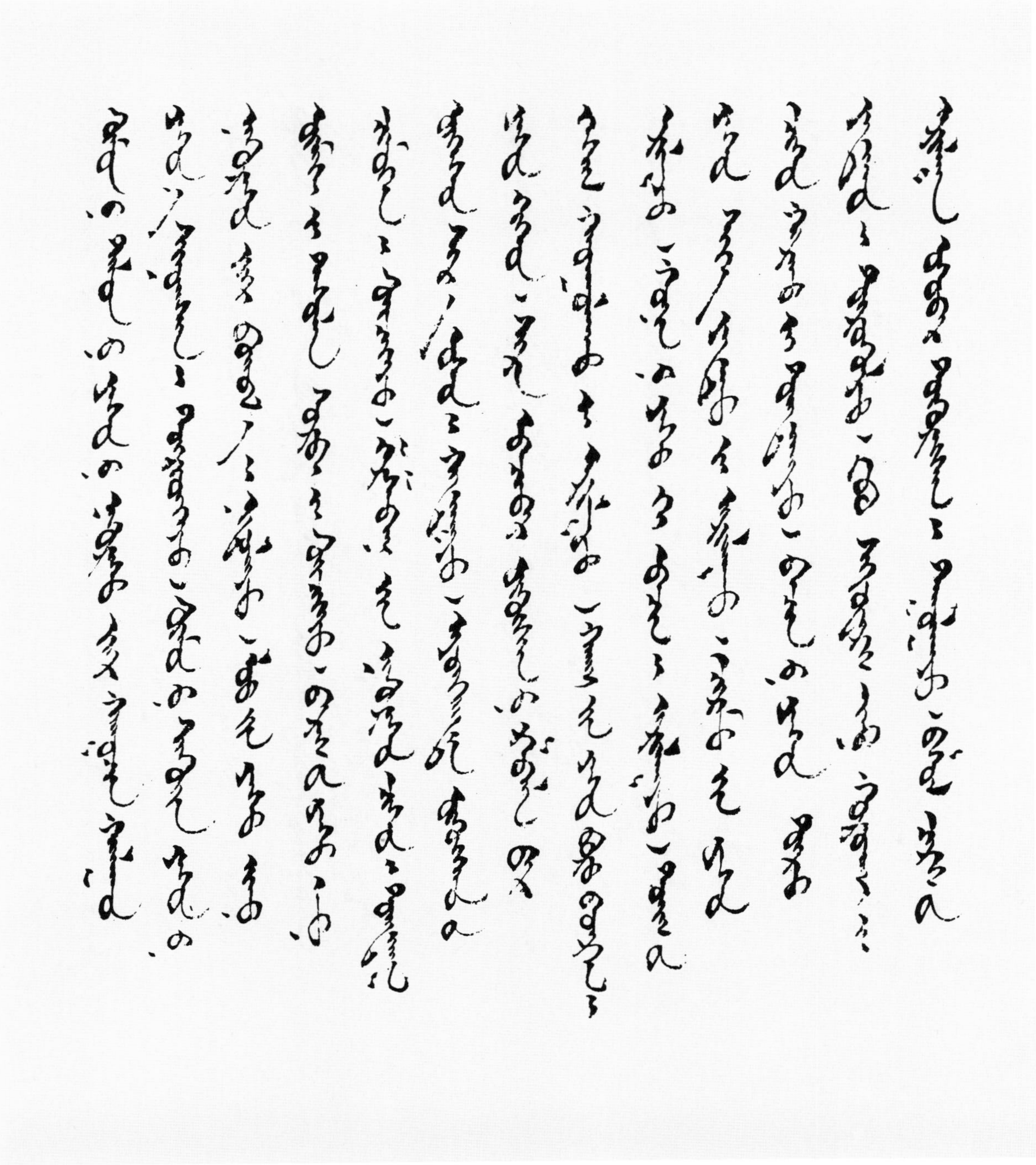

[illegible]
[illegible]
[illegible]
[illegible]
[illegible]
[illegible]
[illegible]
[illegible]
[illegible]
[illegible]
[illegible]
[illegible]
[illegible]

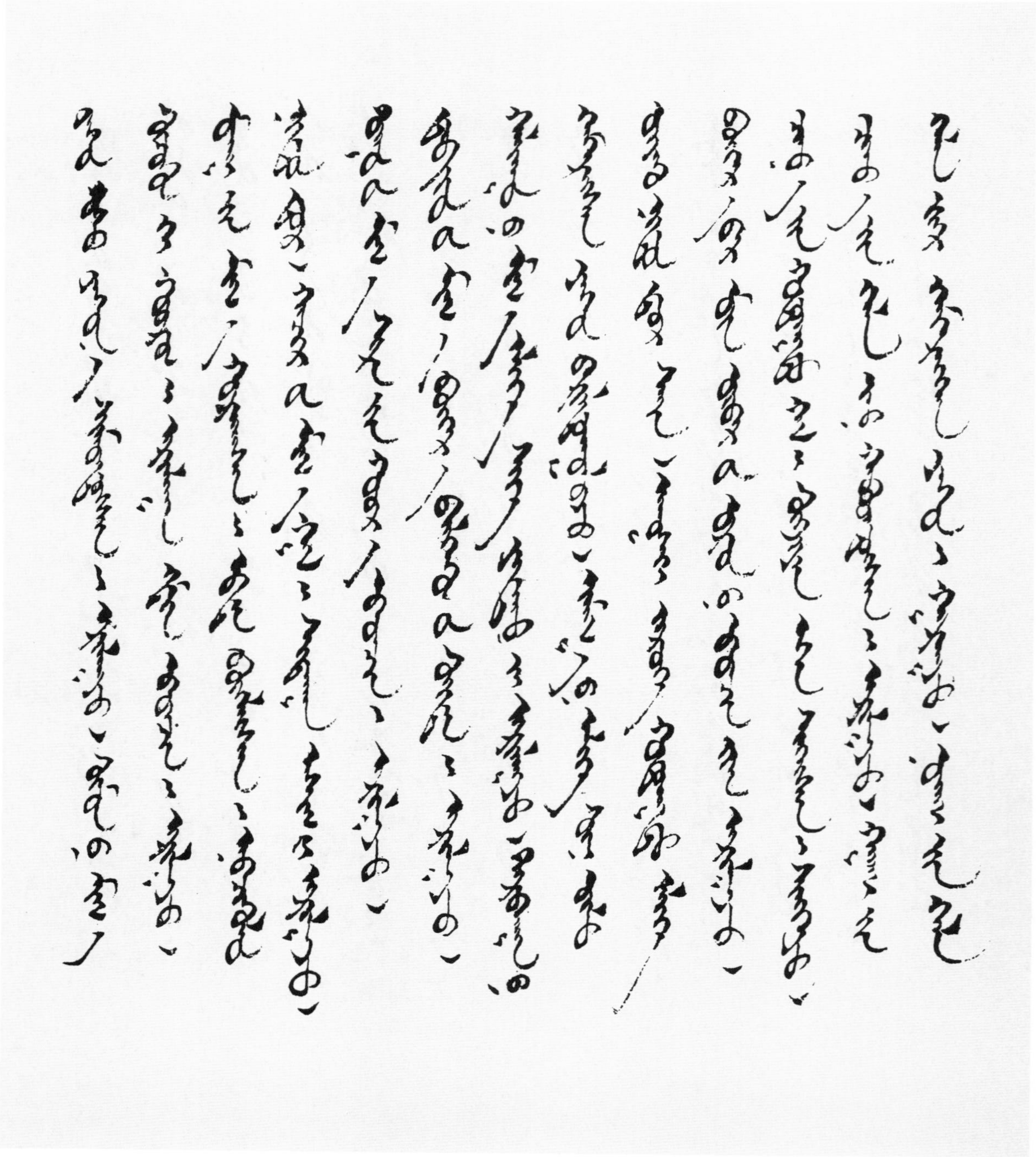

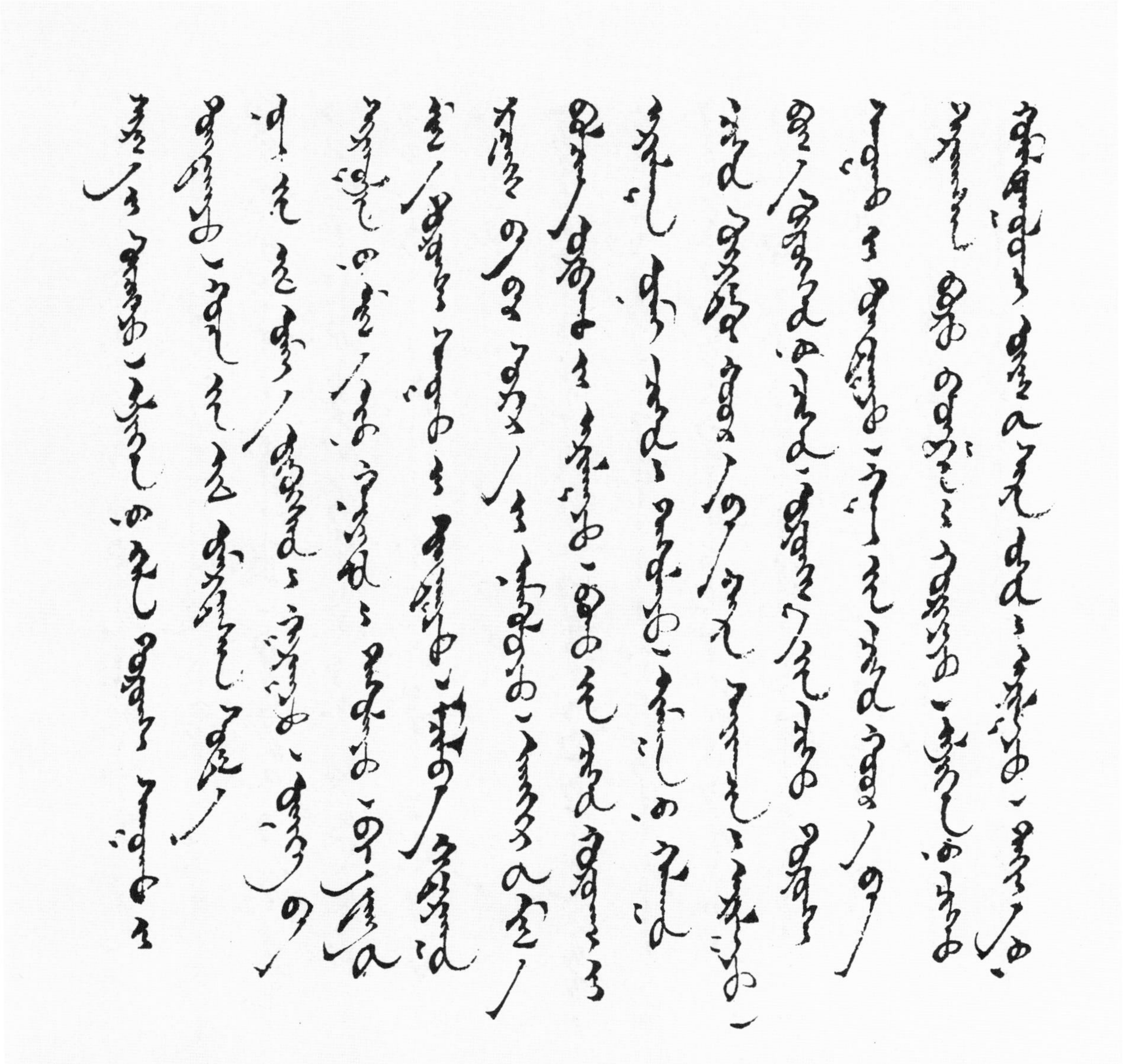

[illegible]

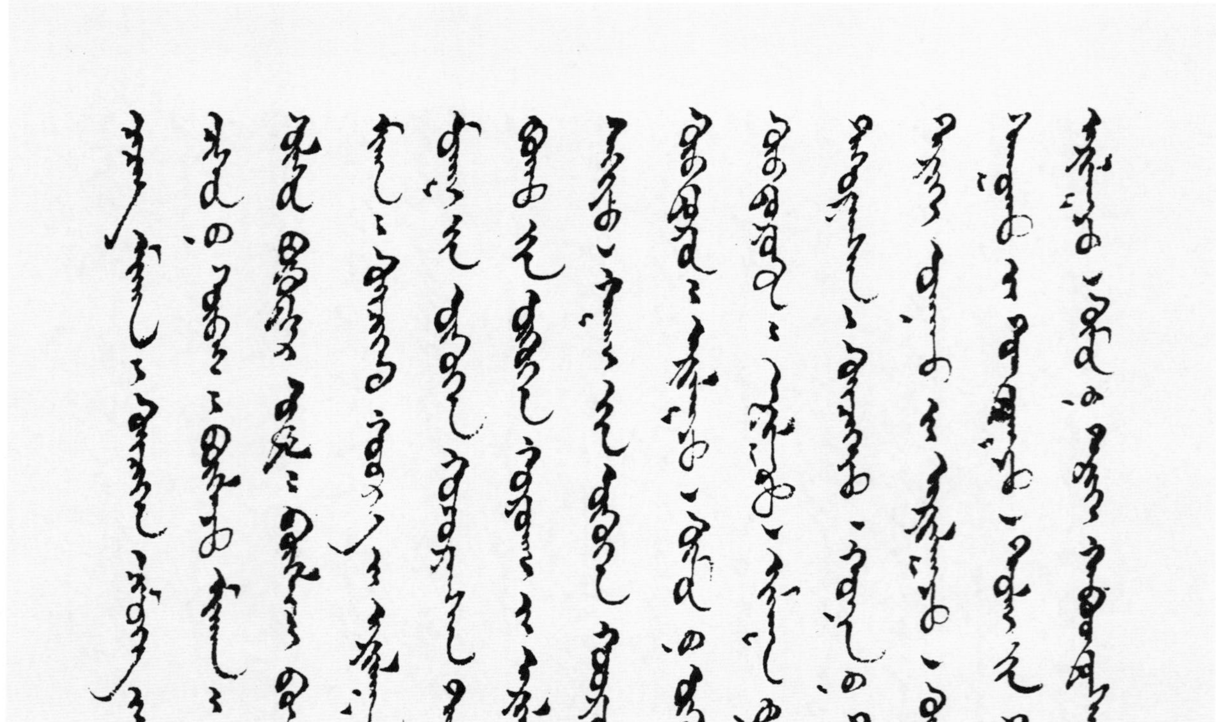

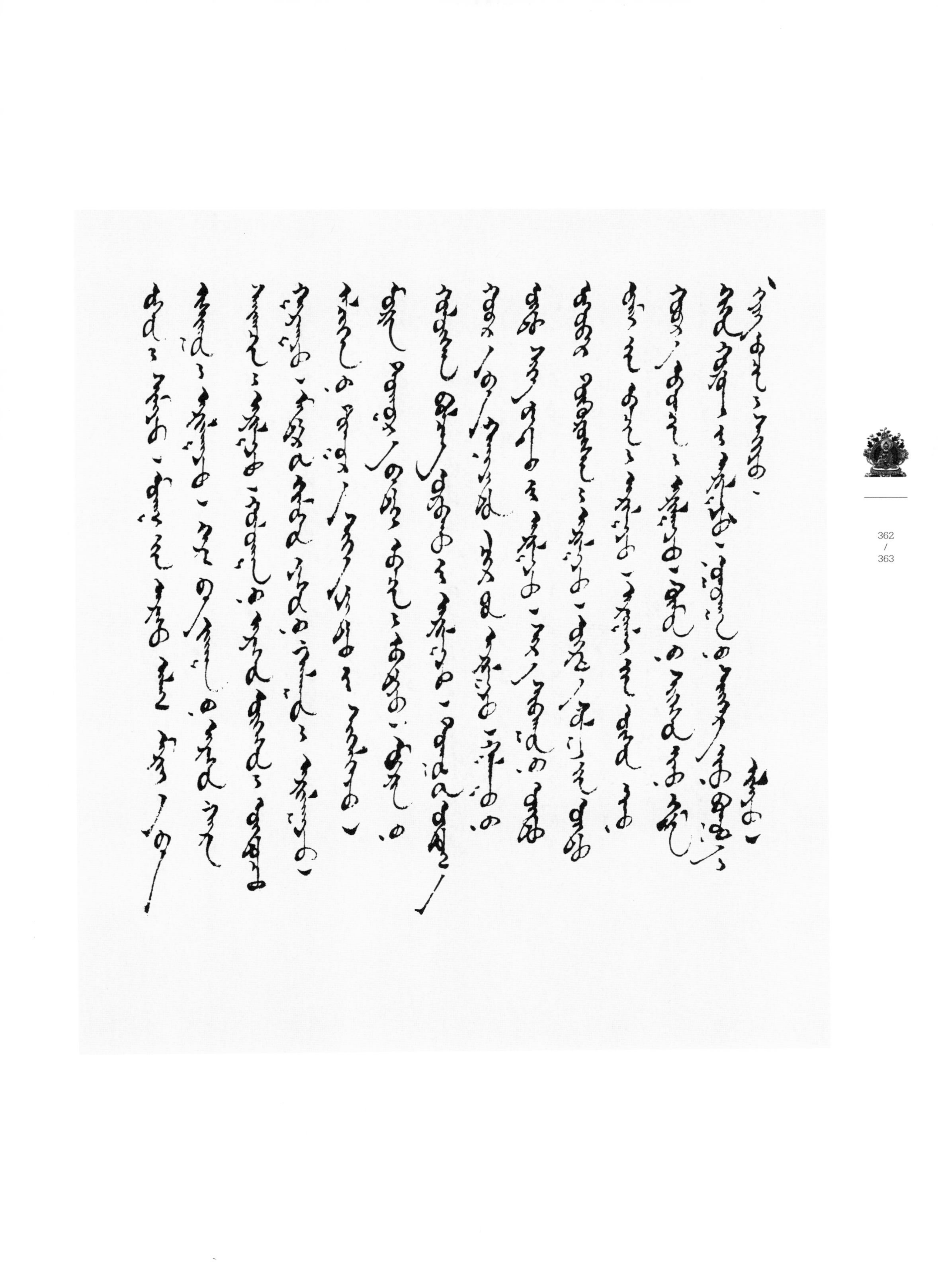

[illegible]

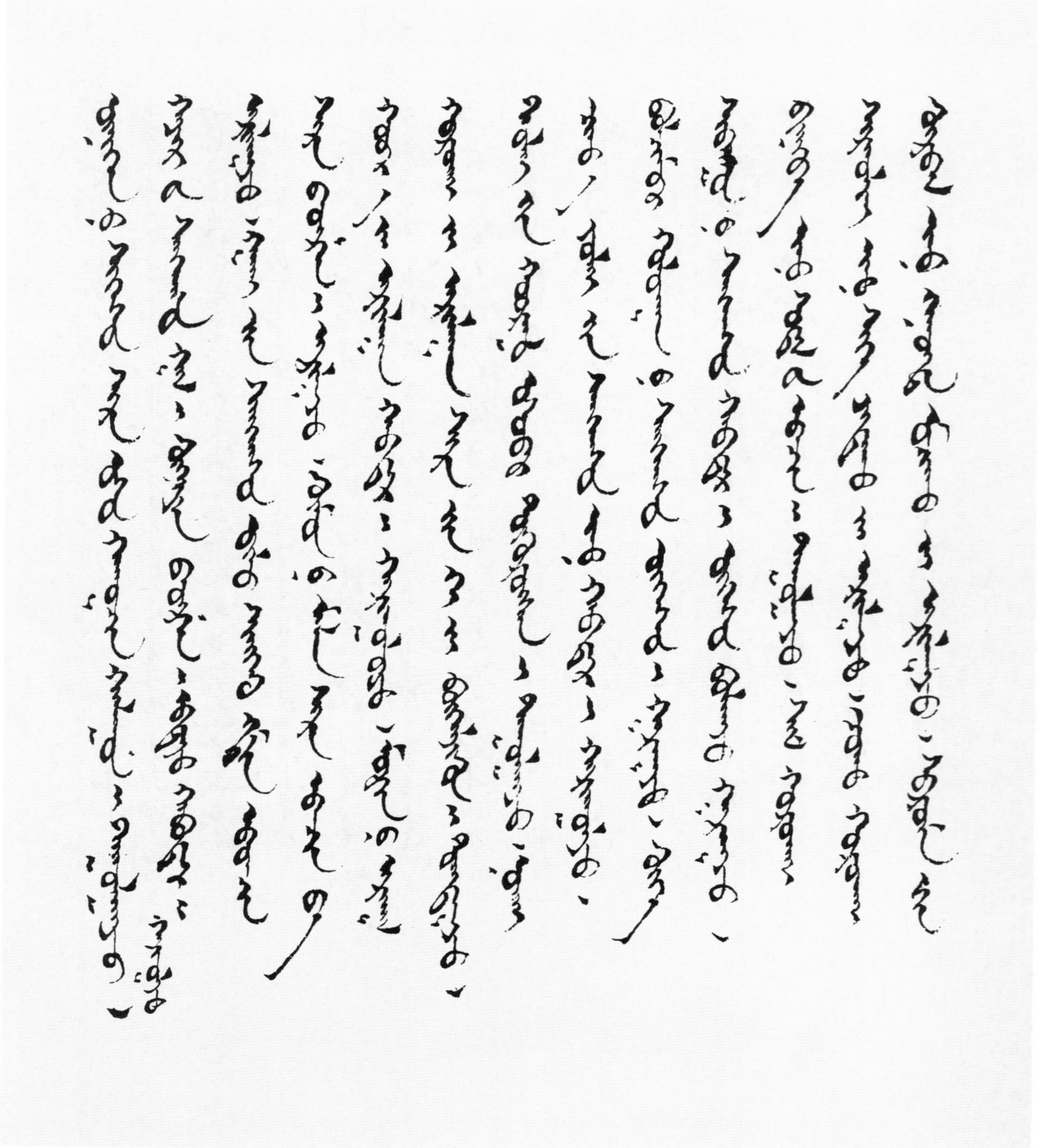

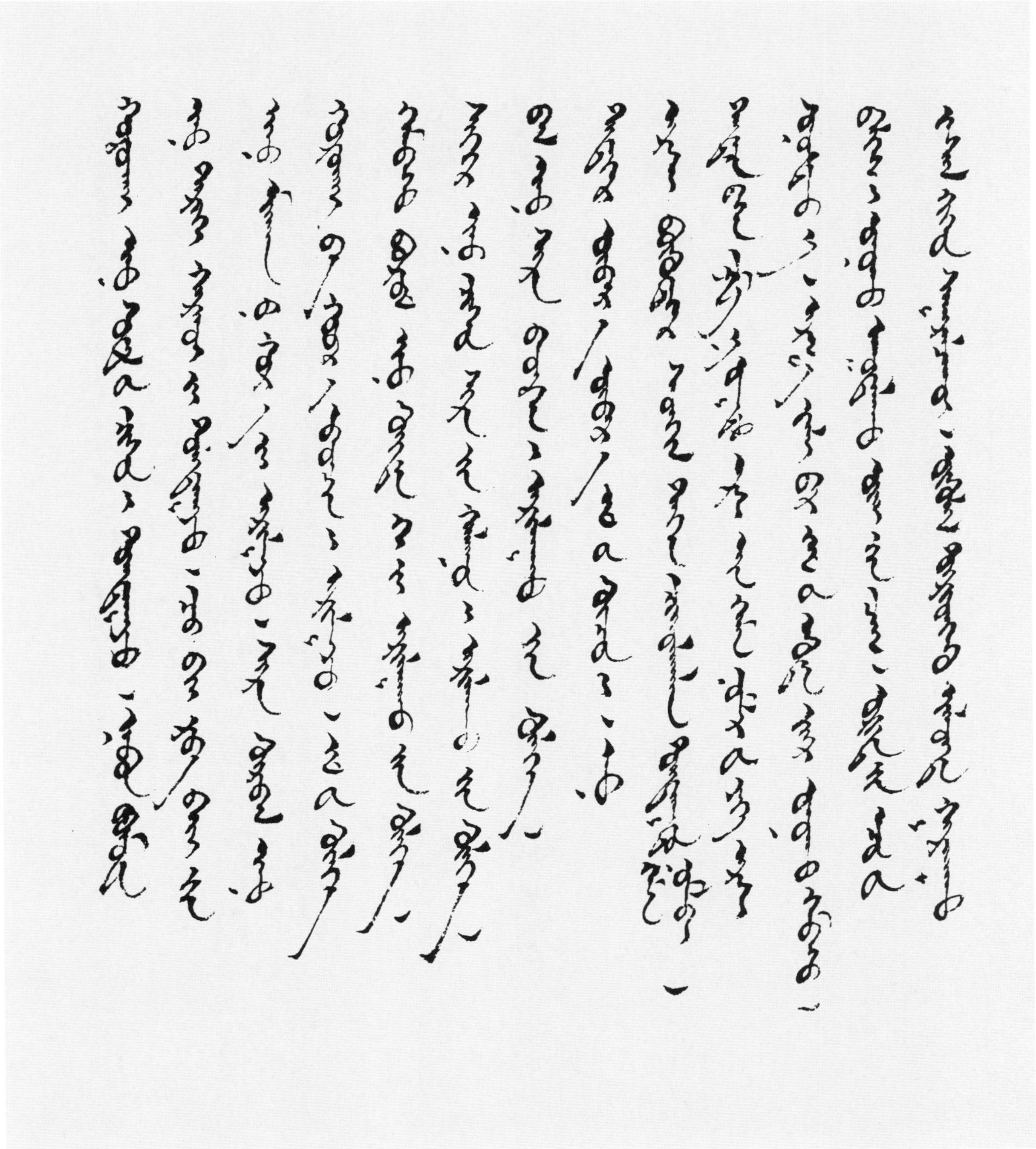

[illegible]

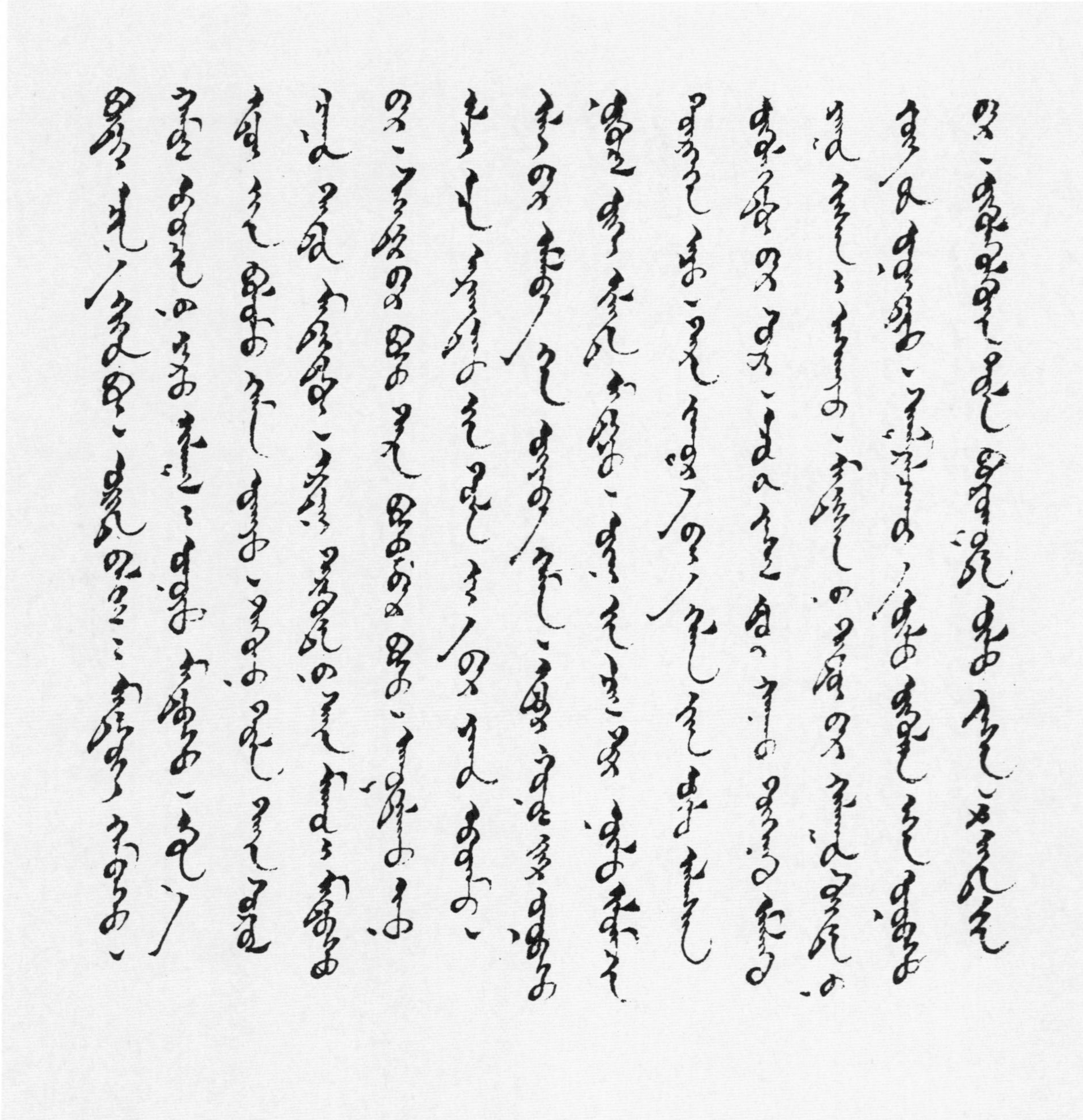

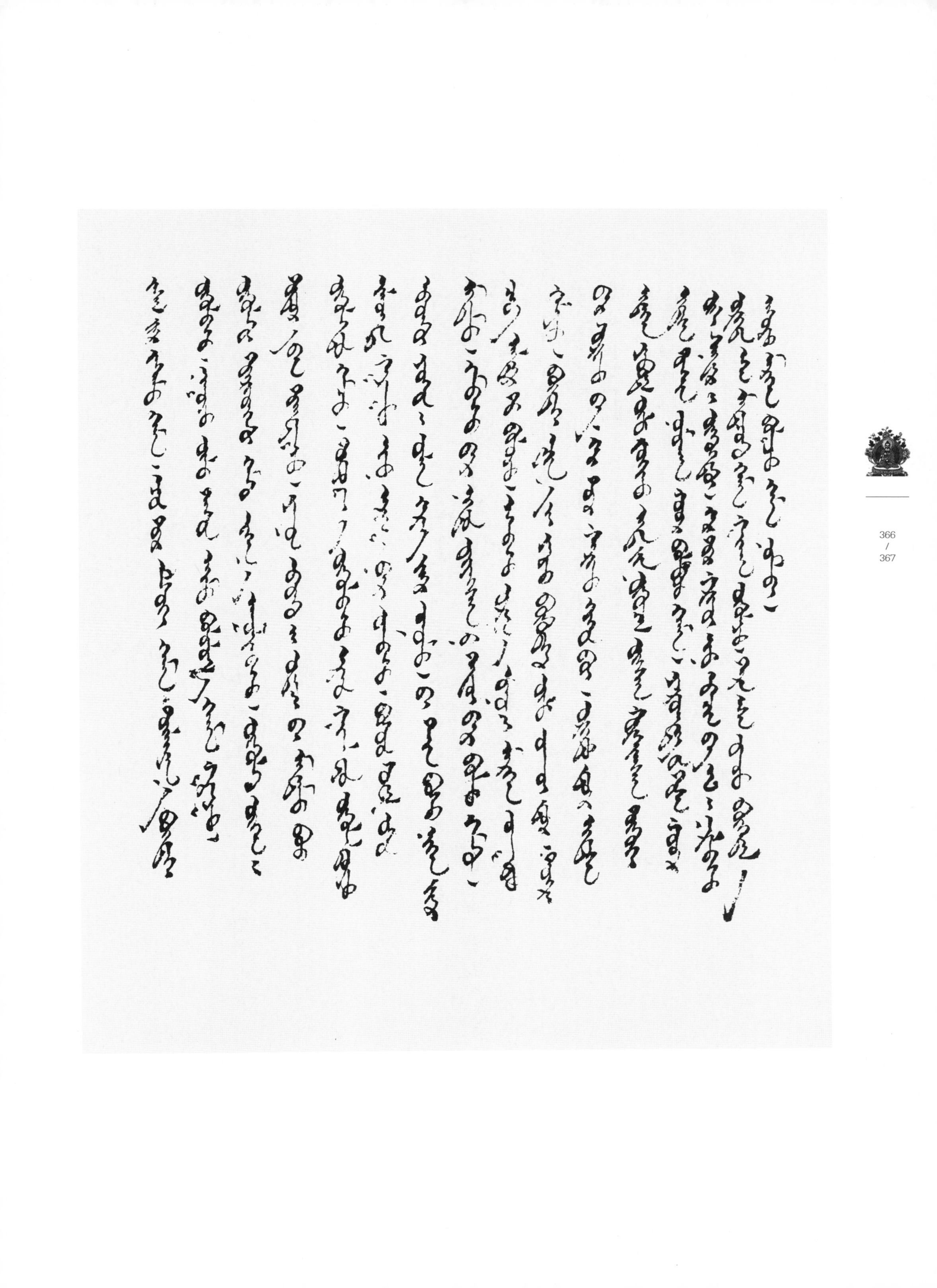

ᠳᠠᠭᠤ ᠳᠠᠭᠤᠯᠠᠬᠤ᠂ ᠪᠢᠴᠢᠭ ᠬᠡᠯᠡ ᠳᠠᠭᠤ᠂ ᠪᠢᠴᠢ ᠪᠠᠢ ᠪᠢᠴᠢ ᠳᠡᠭᠡᠷ᠎ᠡ ᠠᠯ᠎ᠠ ᠳᠠᠭᠤᠤ 37 ᠳᠠᠭᠤᠤ ᠶᠢ ᠪᠠᠭᠲᠠᠭᠠᠭᠰᠠᠨ ᠪᠡᠷ ᠪᠠᠭᠲᠠᠭᠠᠵᠤ ᠤᠷᠤᠭᠤᠯᠪᠠ ᠶᠣᠰᠣ ᠪᠣᠯᠪᠠ᠃ ᠳᠠᠭᠤᠤ ᠶᠢᠨ ᠬᠥᠭᠵᠢᠮᠳᠡ（ᠬᠥᠭᠵᠢᠮ ᠪᠠᠷ）᠂ ᠬᠥᠭᠡᠯ ᠬᠡᠯᠡ ᠬᠥᠭᠵᠢᠭᠦᠯᠦᠭᠰᠡᠨ ᠳᠤ ᠬᠡᠯᠡ ᠬᠡᠯᠡᠬᠦ᠂ ᠬᠥᠭᠡ ᠪᠢᠴᠢ ᠬᠡᠯᠡᠬᠦ᠂ ᠬᠥᠭᠡᠯ ᠳᠤ ᠬᠡᠯᠡᠬᠦ᠂ ᠳᠤ ᠬᠥᠭ ᠬᠡᠯ᠂ ᠳᠠᠭᠤ᠂ ᠬᠥᠭᠡ ᠲᠠᠢ ᠪᠣ ᠪᠢᠴᠢᠭᠡ᠂ ᠪᠢᠴᠢᠭ ᠬᠡ ᠤᠷᠲᠤ ᠳᠠᠭᠤᠤ ᠪᠠ ᠬᠡᠯ ᠪᠢᠴᠢᠭᠡ ᠪᠣ ᠬᠡ ᠳᠤ ᠳᠠᠭᠤᠤ 12 ᠳᠠᠭᠤᠤ ᠶᠢ ᠪᠠᠭᠲᠠᠭᠠ ᠪᠠᠷ᠂ ᠤᠷ ᠬᠣᠭᠣᠯᠠᠢ ᠲᠠᠢ ᠤᠲᠠᠰᠤ ᠳᠠᠭᠤᠤ 9 ᠳᠠᠭᠤᠤ ᠶᠢ ᠬᠠᠮᠲᠤ ᠪᠠᠷ᠂ ᠬᠡ ᠪᠣᠢ ᠬᠣᠭᠣᠯ ᠳᠠᠭᠤᠤ 8 ᠳᠠᠭᠤᠤᠯᠠᠭᠰᠠᠨ ᠬᠡ ᠤᠷᠤᠭᠤᠯᠵᠤ ᠪᠠᠭᠤᠯᠭᠠᠭᠰᠠᠨ ᠳᠠᠭᠤᠯᠠᠭᠰᠠᠨ ᠪᠣᠯ ᠳᠤ ᠬᠡ ᠪᠣᠢ ᠤᠷᠤᠭᠤᠯᠵᠤ ᠪᠠᠭᠤᠯᠭᠠ᠃

ᠪᠣᠢ ᠤᠨ ᠬᠡᠮᠵᠢᠶ᠎ᠡ ᠬᠡ : 26cm×26cm ᠪᠤᠶᠤ᠂ ᠬᠠᠭᠤᠳᠠᠰᠤ 22 ᠬᠠᠭᠤᠳᠠᠰᠤ ᠤᠷᠤ᠃

ᠤᠷᠳᠤ ᠤᠷᠲᠤ ᠳᠤ ᠬᠡᠯᠡᠯᠴᠡᠭᠡ ᠪᠢᠴᠢᠭ ᠤᠨ ᠬᠥᠭ ᠪᠢᠴᠢᠭᠡᠨ ᠤᠷᠲᠤ ᠪᠣᠯᠤᠭᠰᠠᠨ᠃

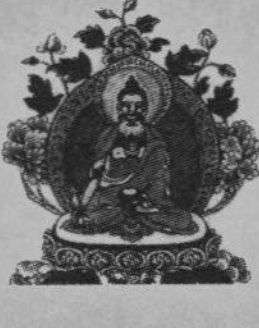

Powerful Effects of Pill, Powder, Cream and Dan

神效丸散膏丹

7

[illegible]

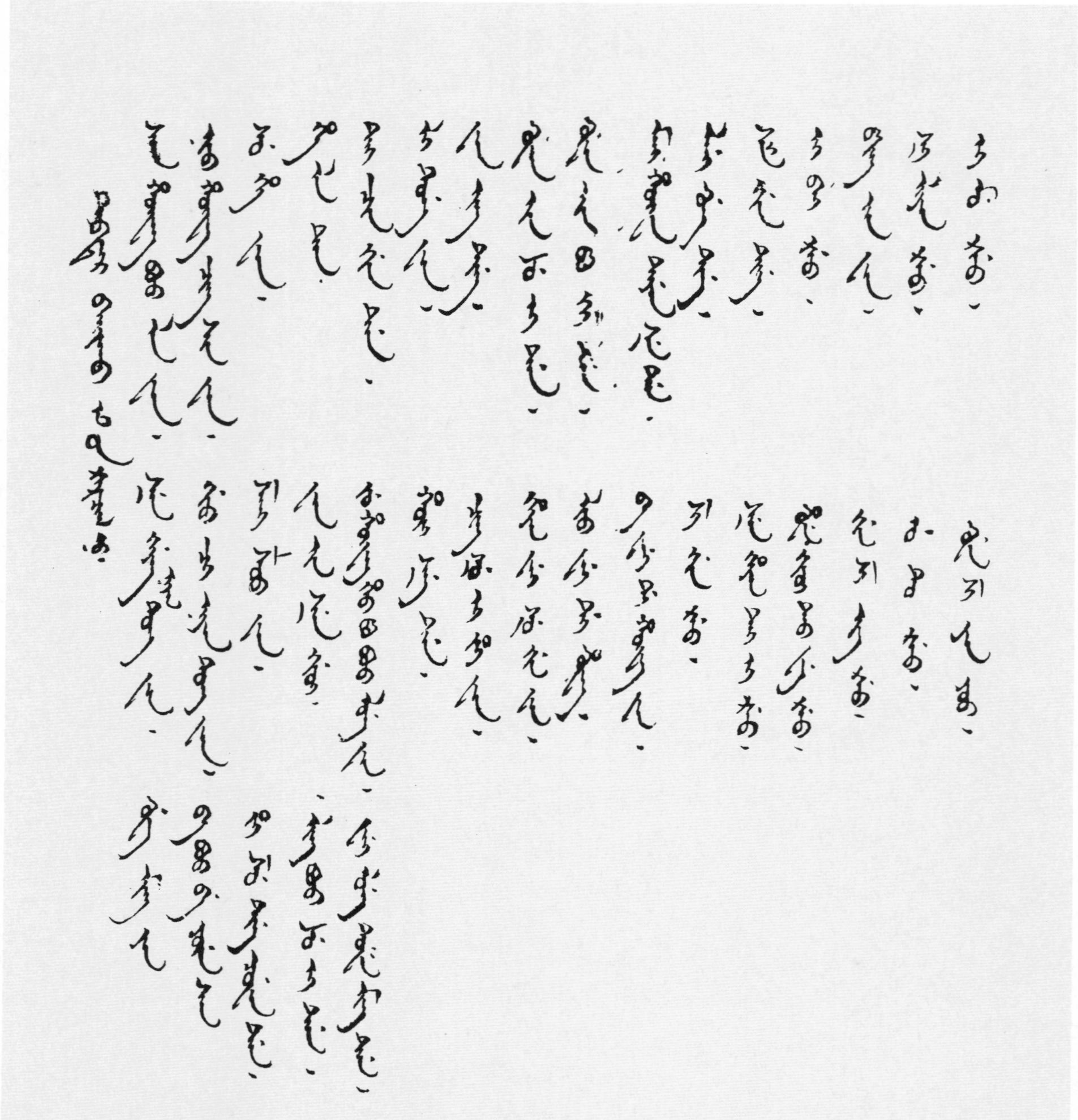

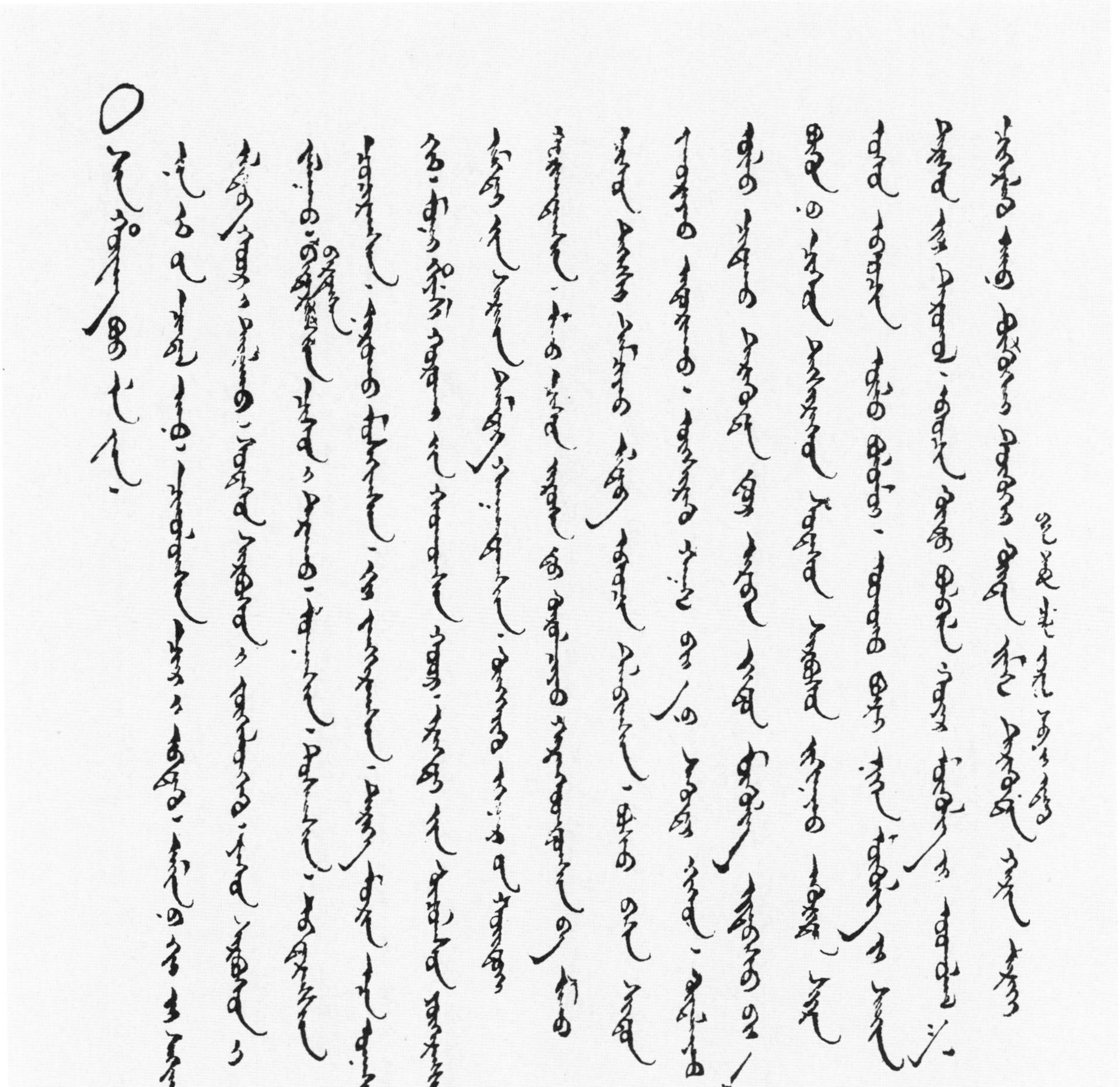

[illegible]
[illegible]
[illegible]
[illegible]
[illegible]
[illegible]
[illegible]
[illegible]
[illegible]
[illegible]
[illegible]
[illegible]
[illegible]
[illegible]
[illegible]
[illegible]

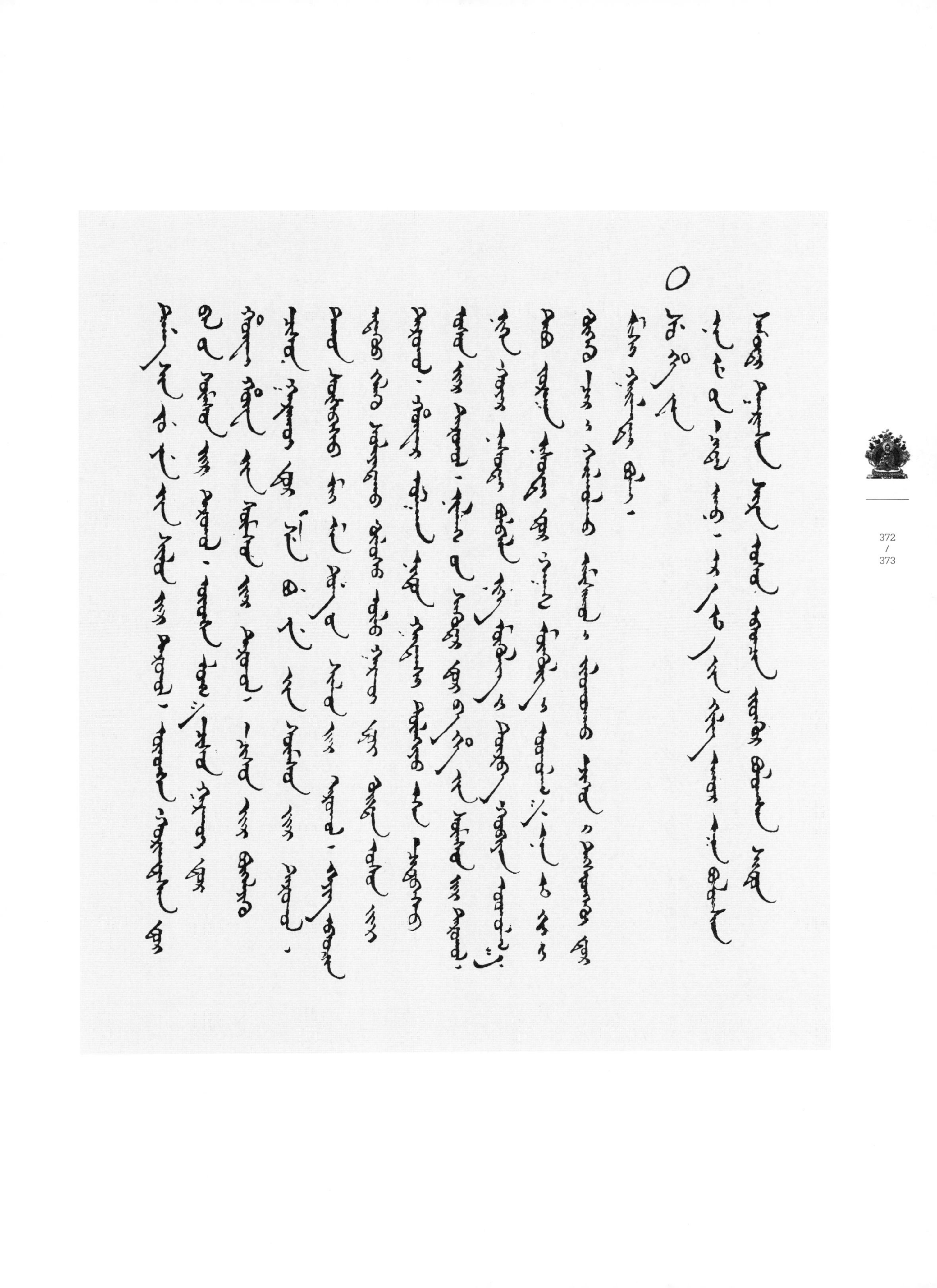

[illegible]

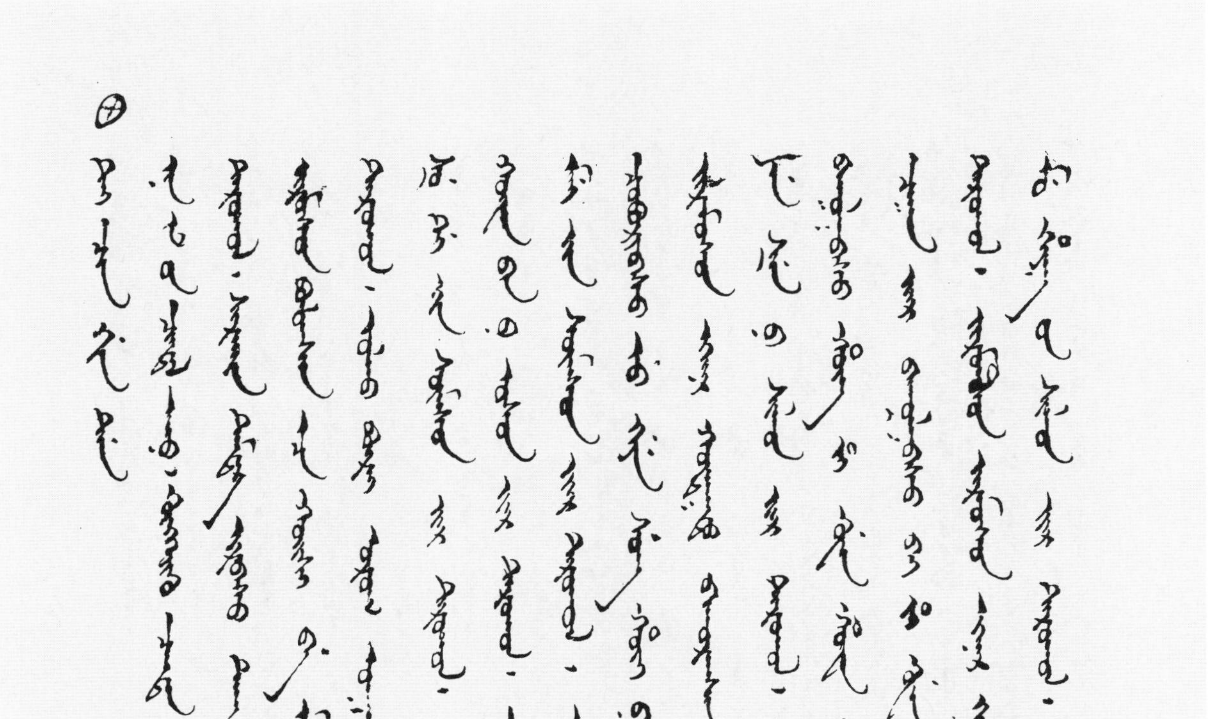

[illegible]
[illegible]
[illegible]
[illegible]
[illegible]
[illegible]
[illegible]
[illegible]
[illegible]
[illegible]
[illegible]
[illegible]
[illegible]
[illegible]
[illegible]
[illegible]
[illegible]

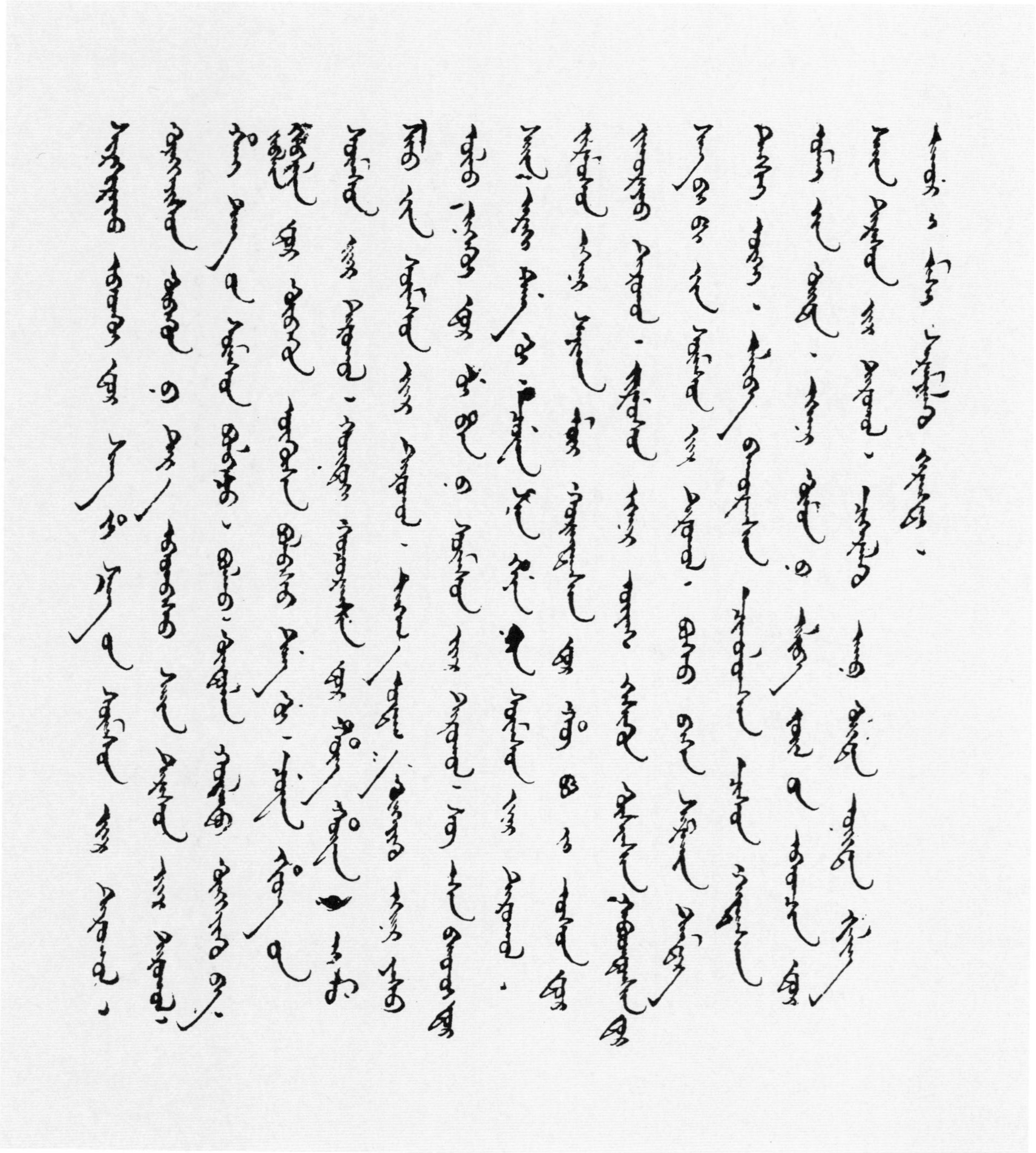

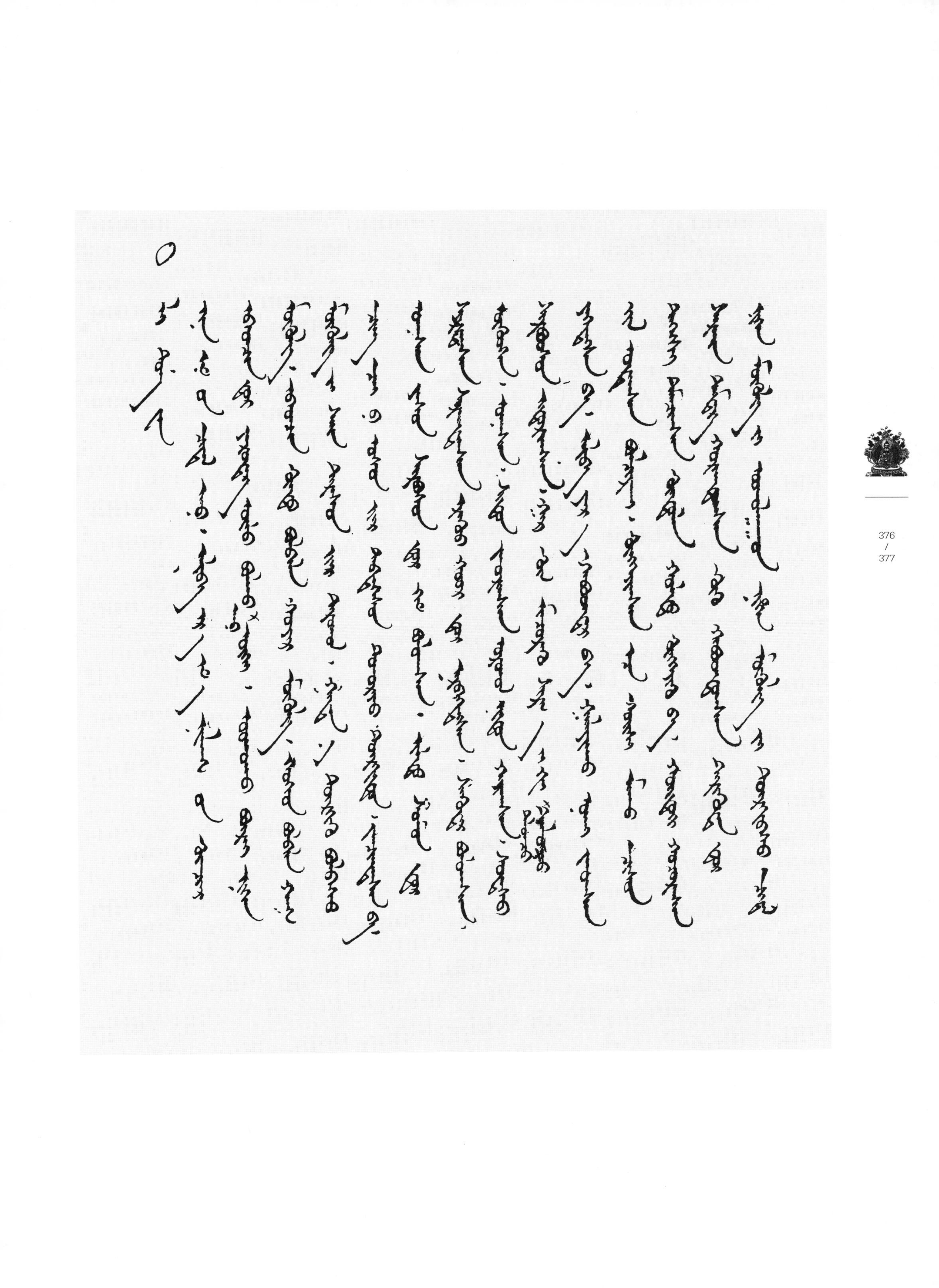

[illegible]

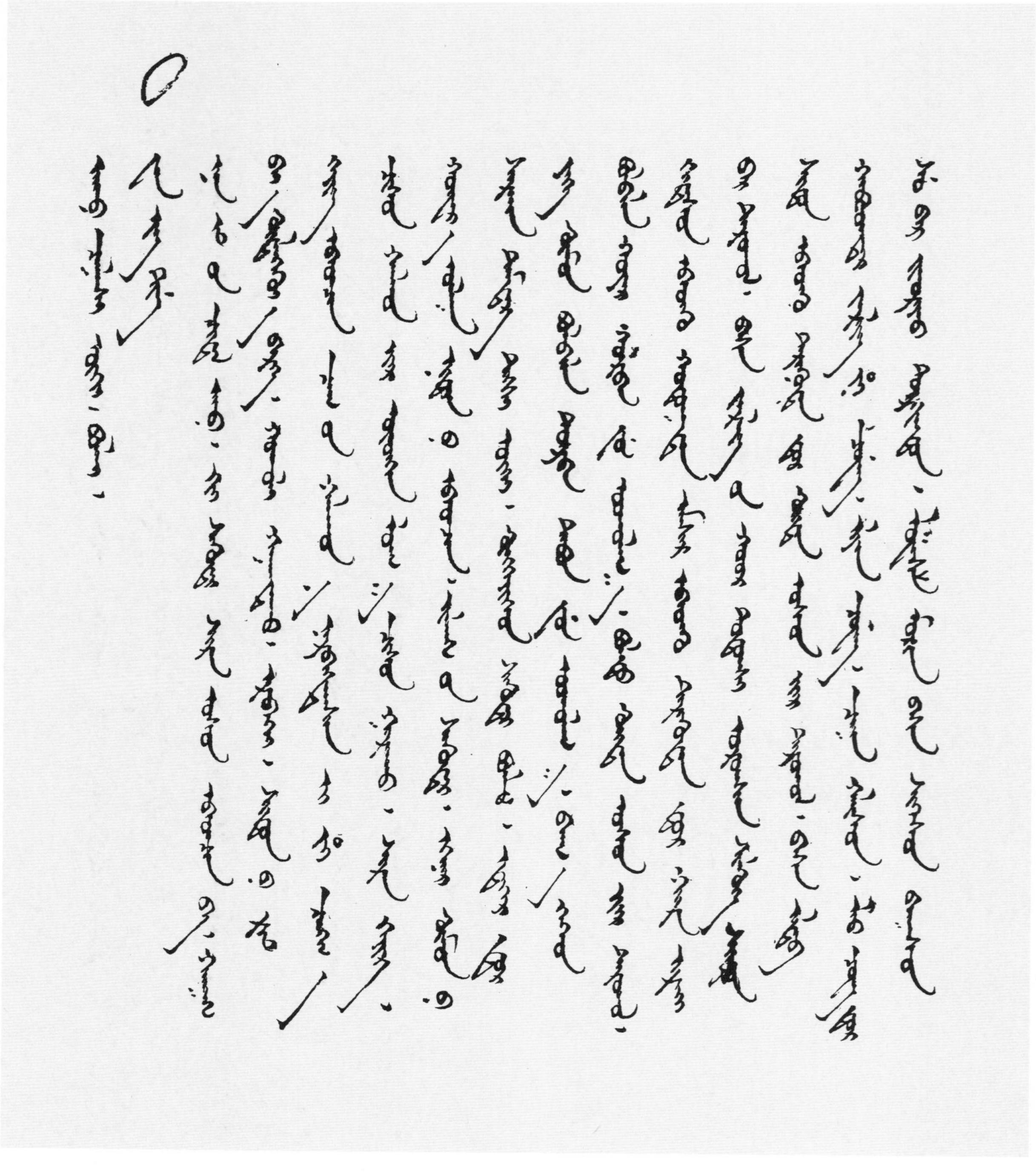

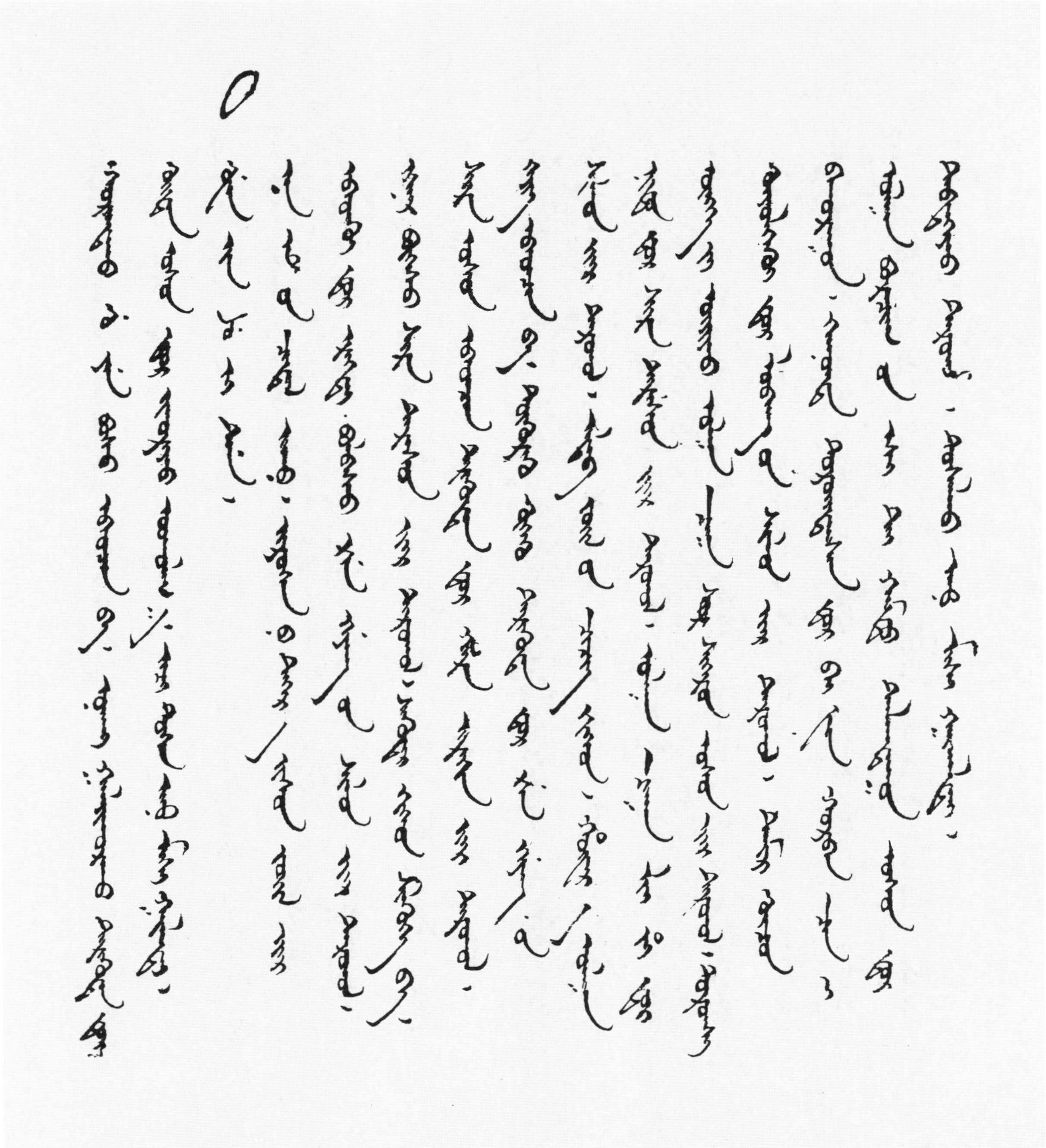

[illegible]

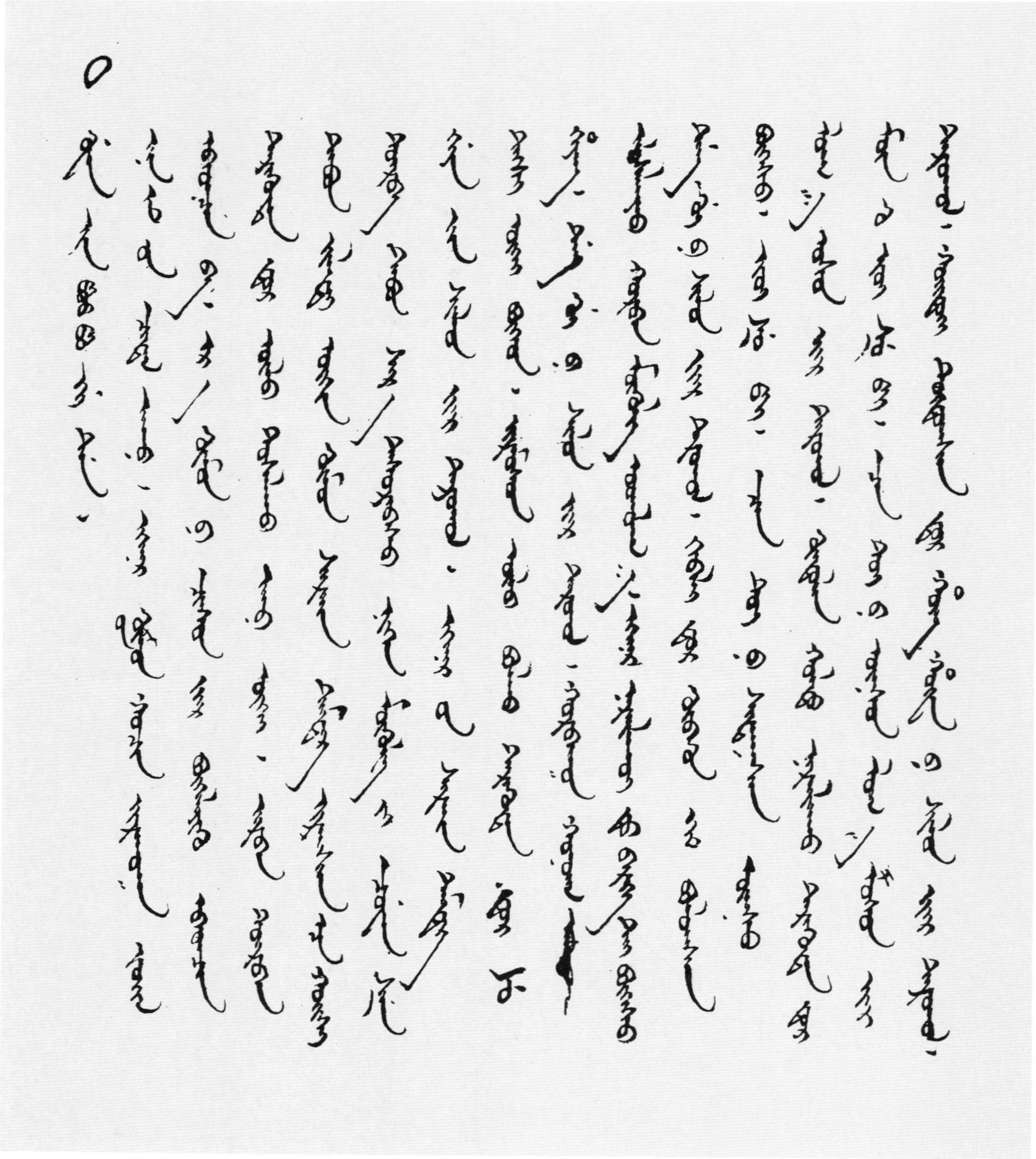

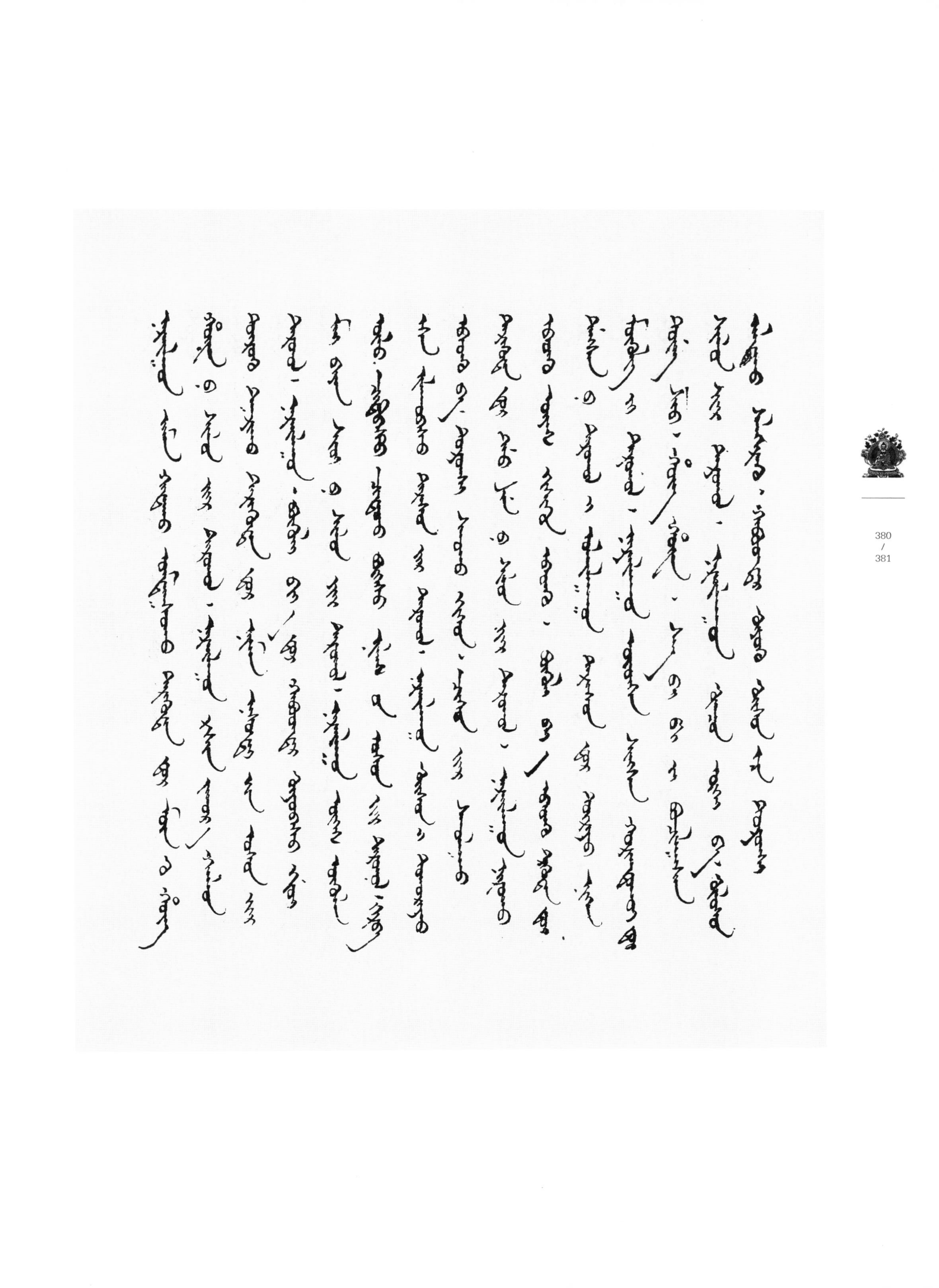

[illegible]

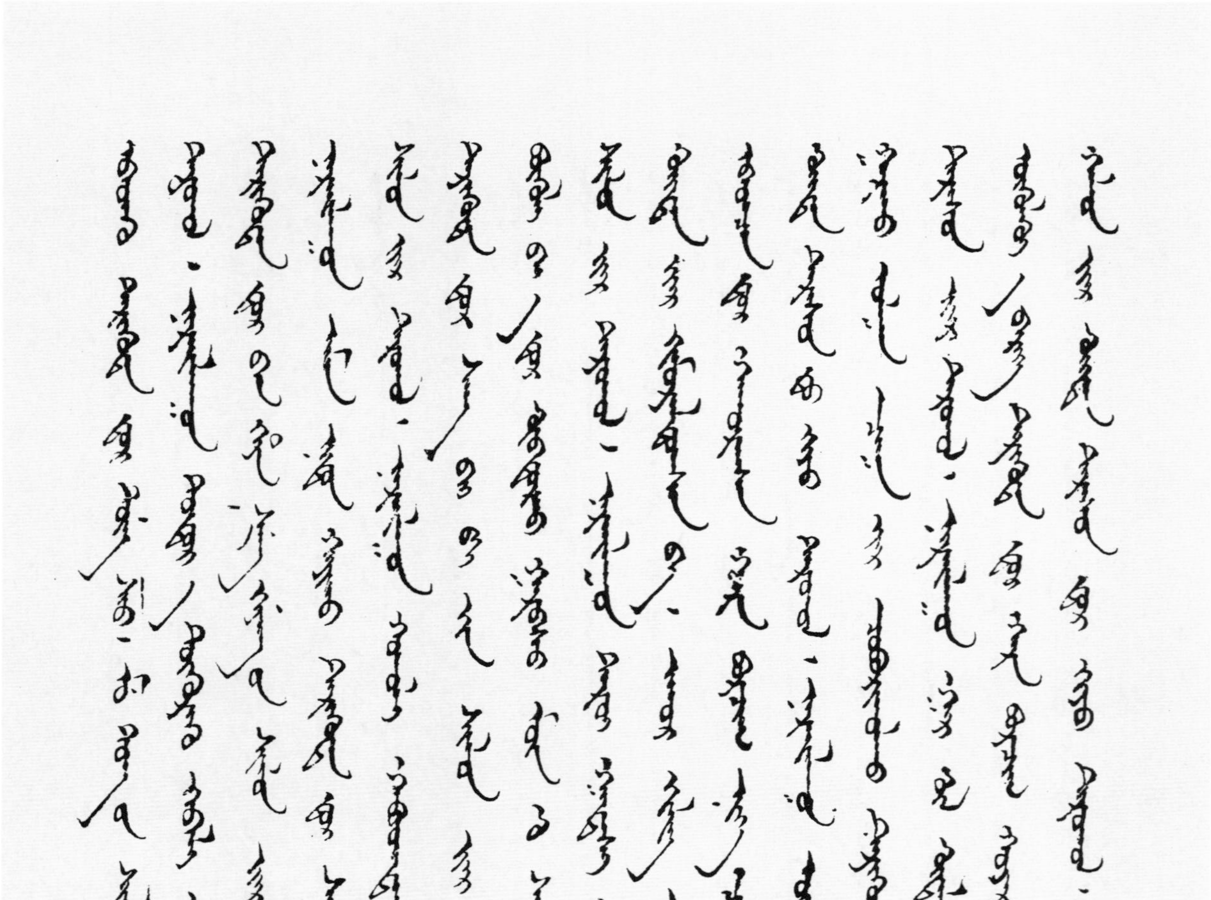

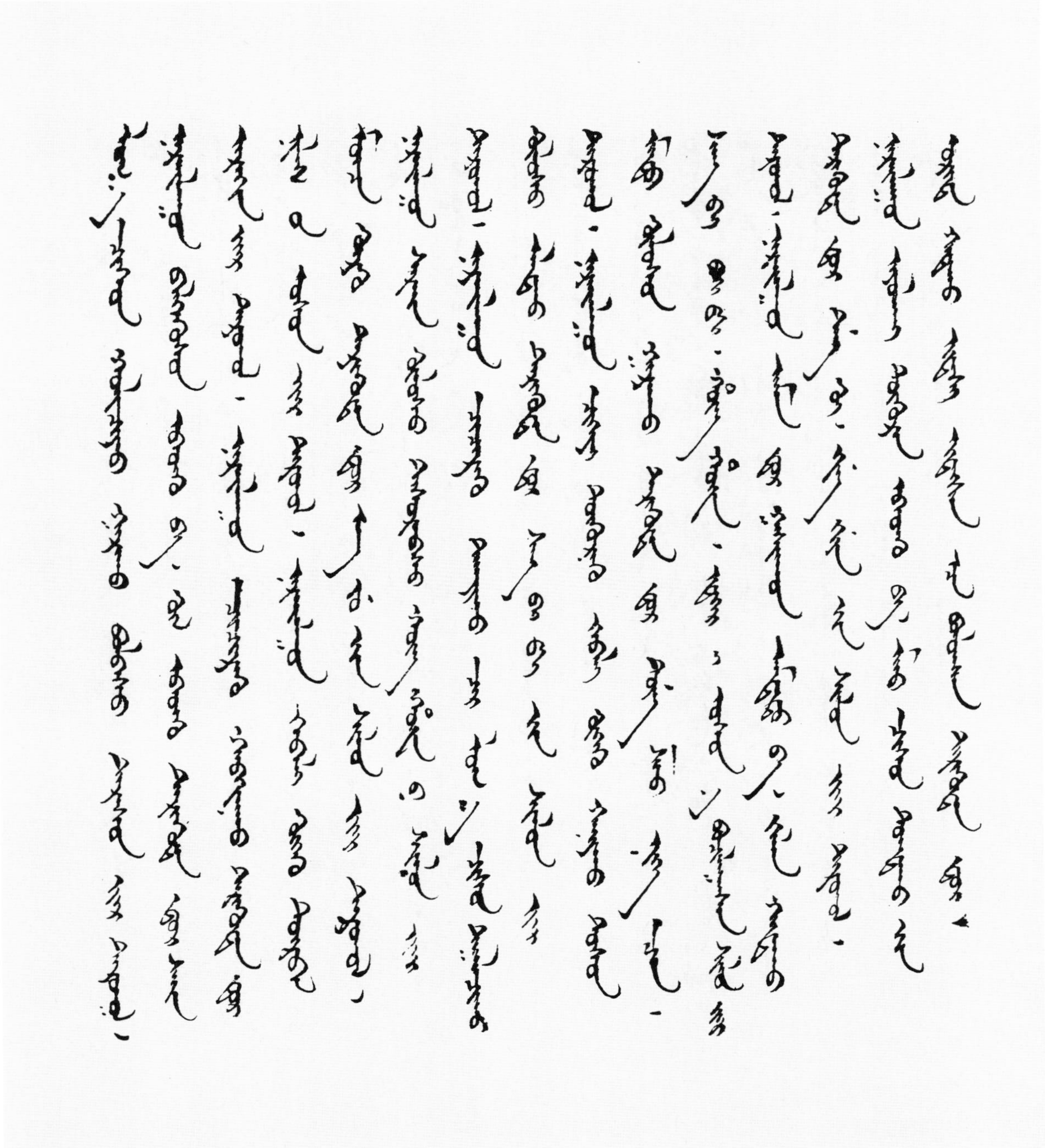

[illegible]

[illegible]

[illegible]

[illegible]

[illegible]

[illegible]

○ [illegible]

[illegible]

[illegible]

[illegible]

[illegible]

[illegible]

[illegible]

[illegible]

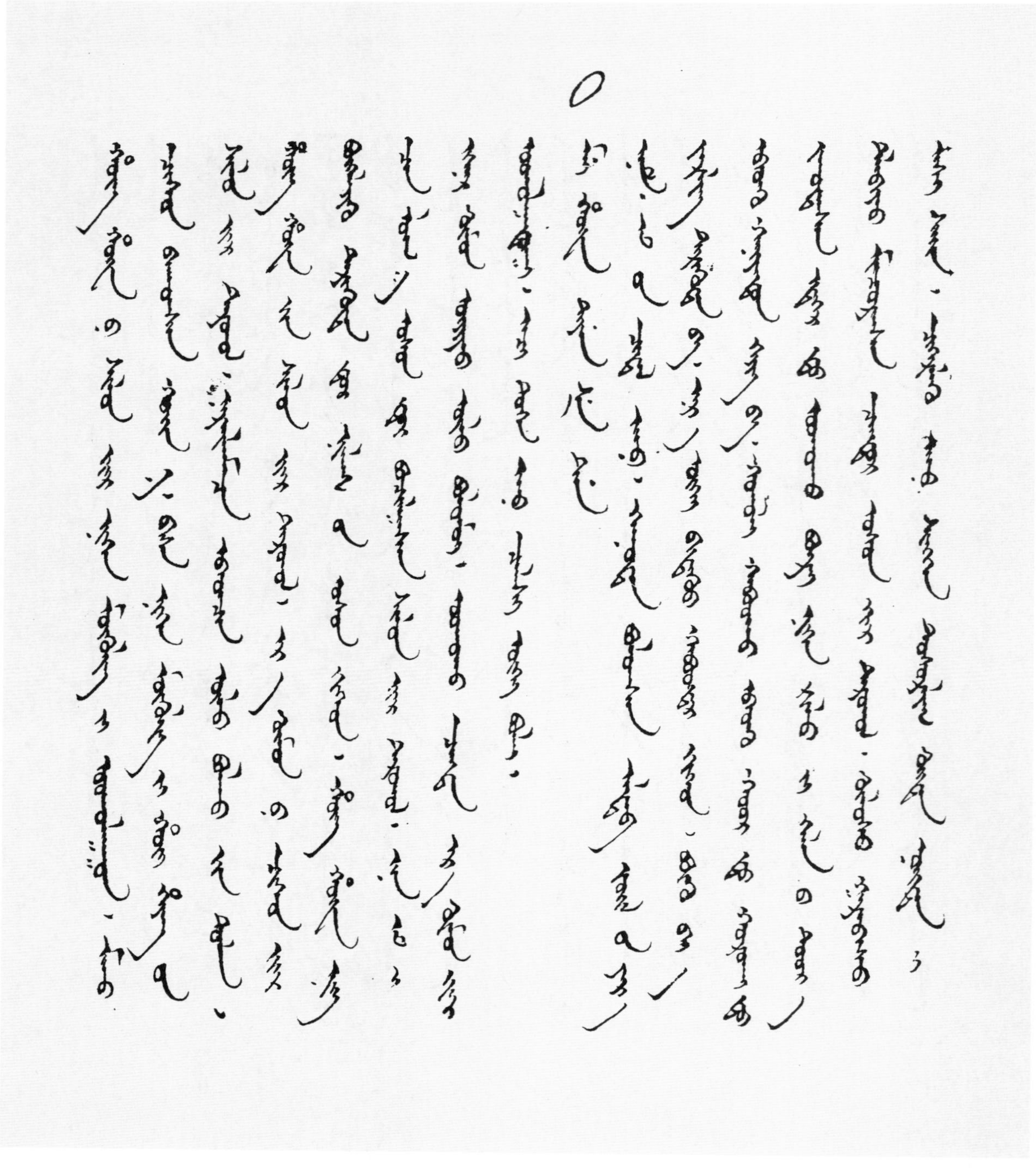

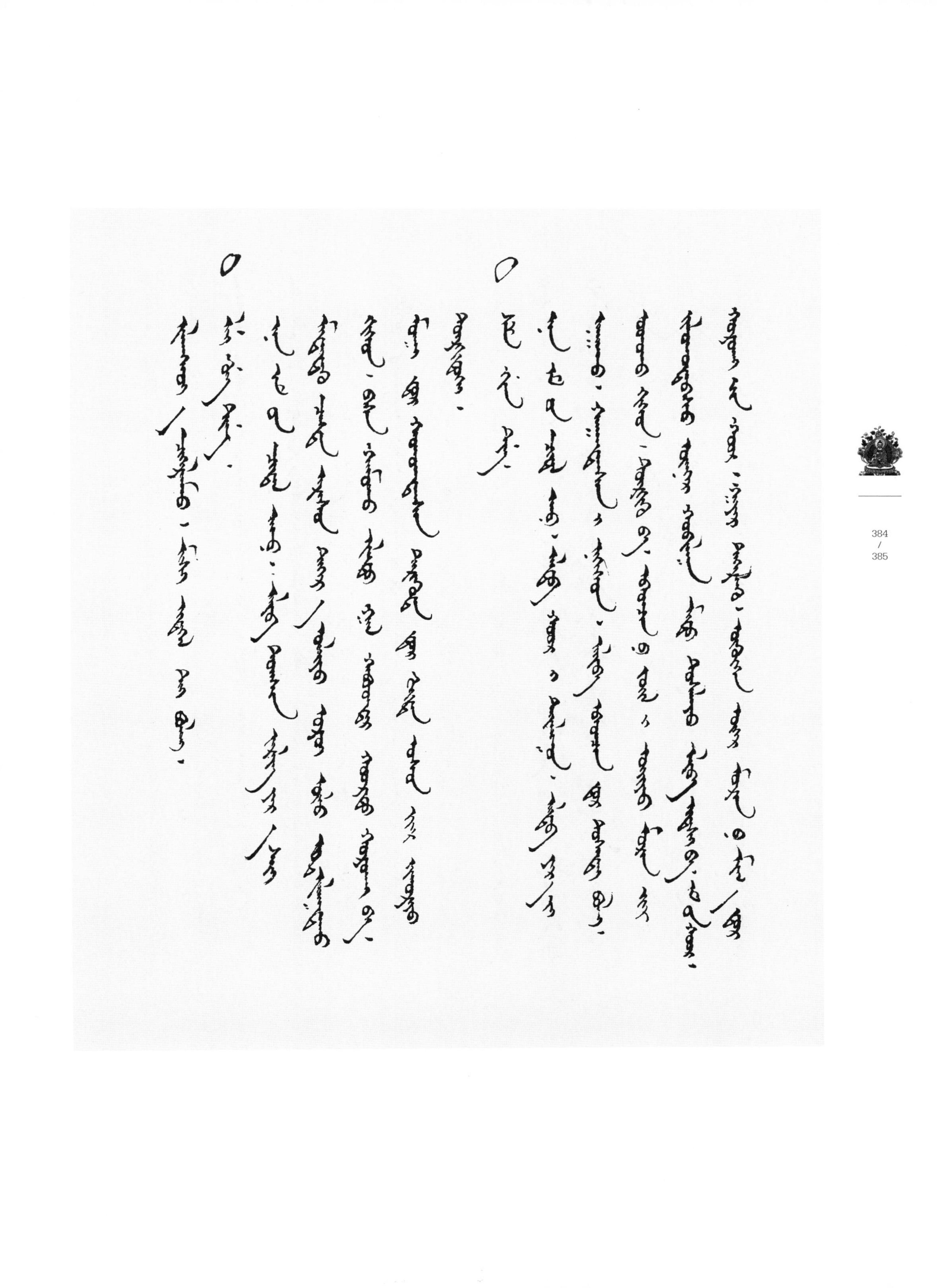

[illegible]
[illegible]
[illegible]
[illegible]
[illegible]
[illegible]
[illegible]
[illegible]
[illegible]
[illegible]
[illegible]
[illegible]
[illegible]

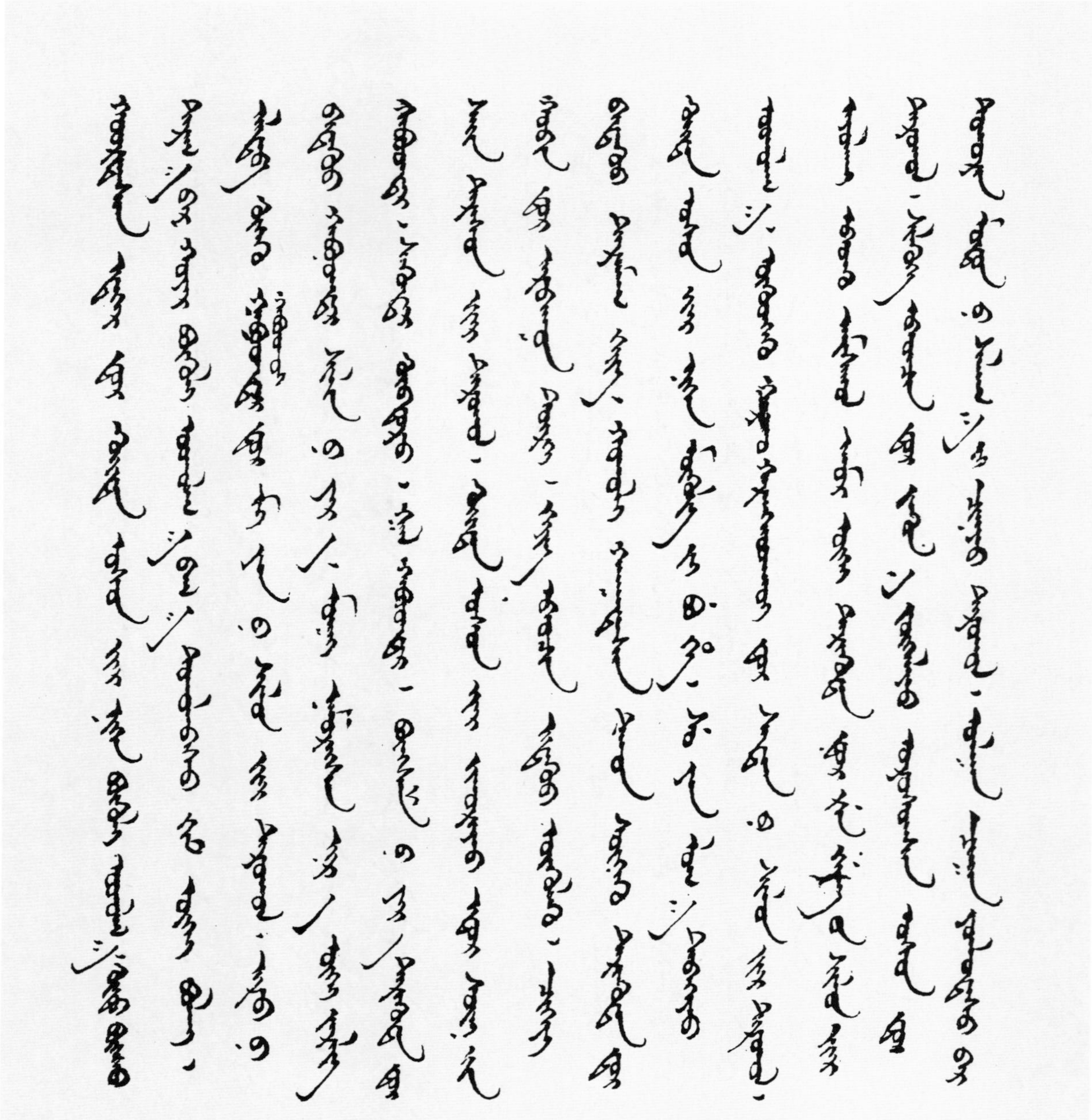

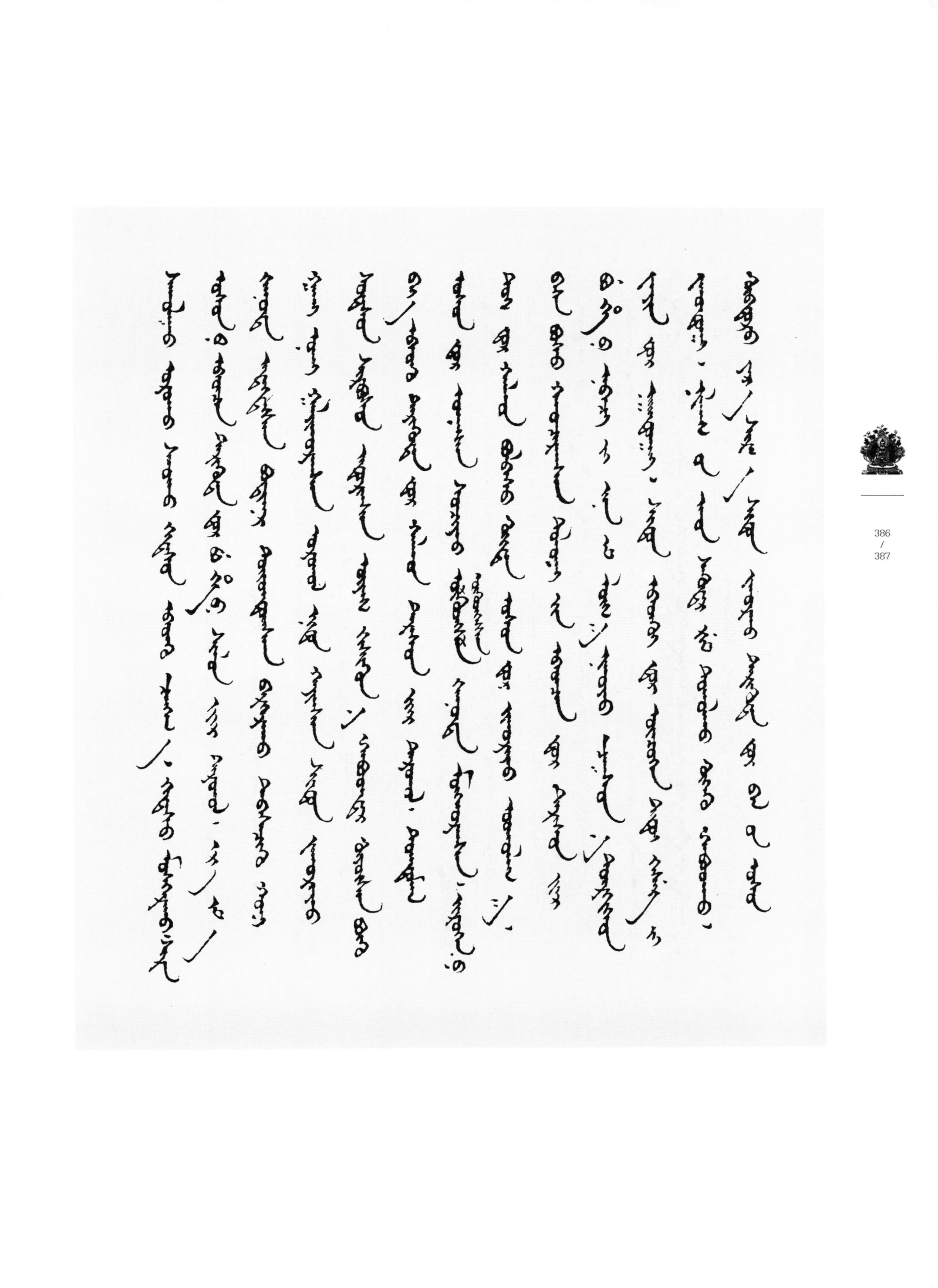

[illegible]

[illegible]

[illegible]

[illegible]

[illegible]

[illegible]

[illegible]

[illegible]

[illegible]

[illegible]

[illegible]

[illegible]

[illegible]

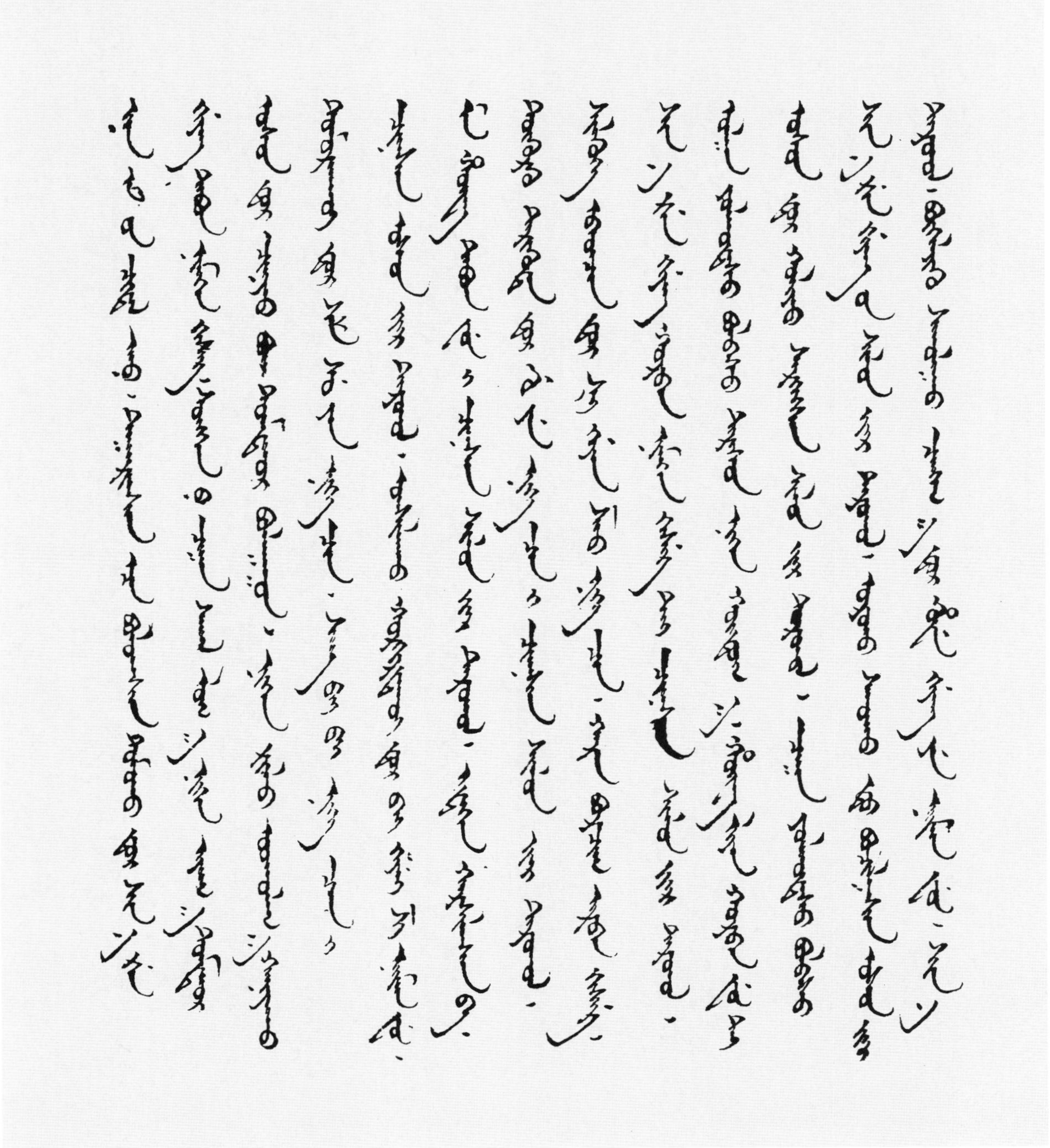

[illegible]

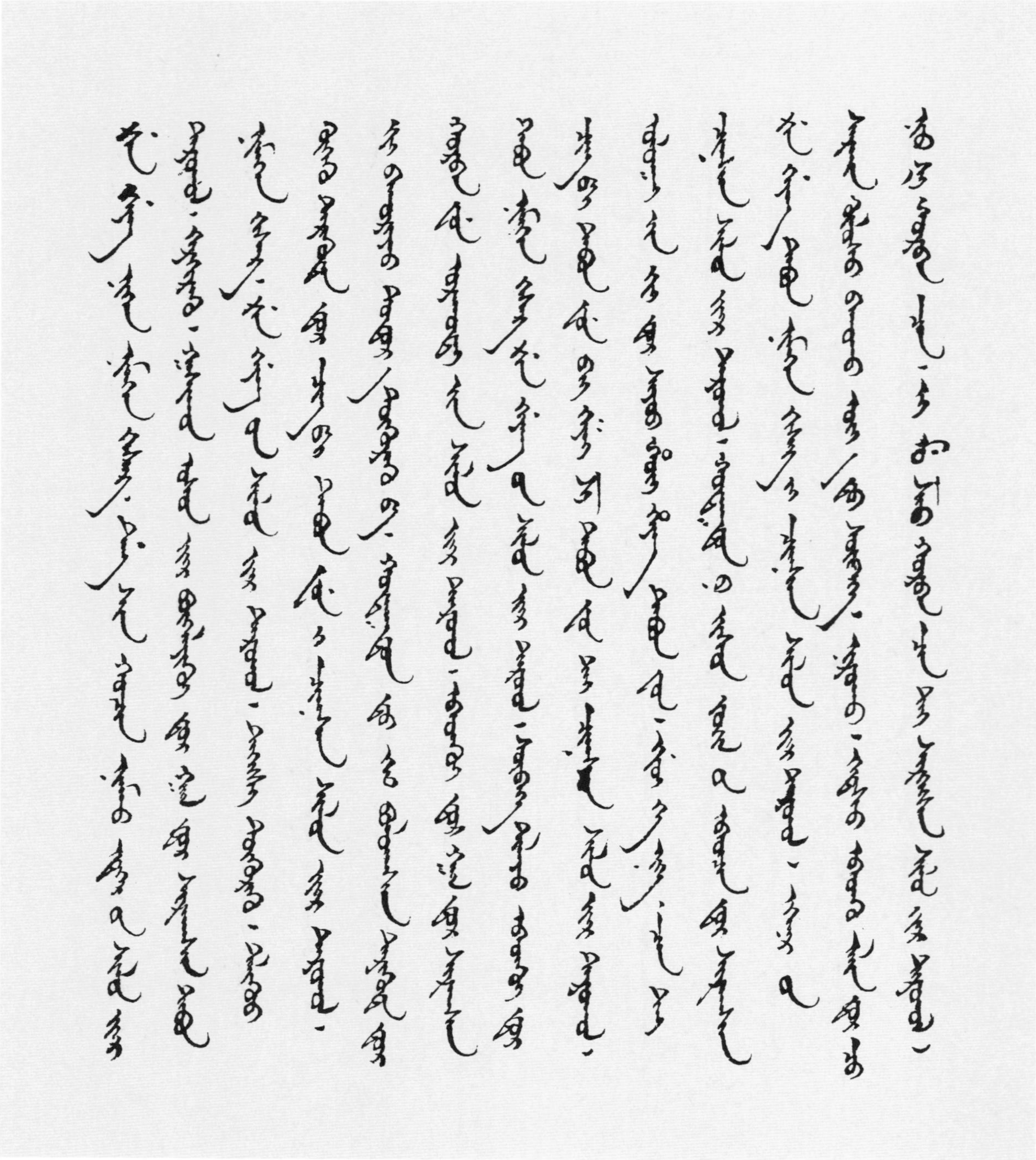

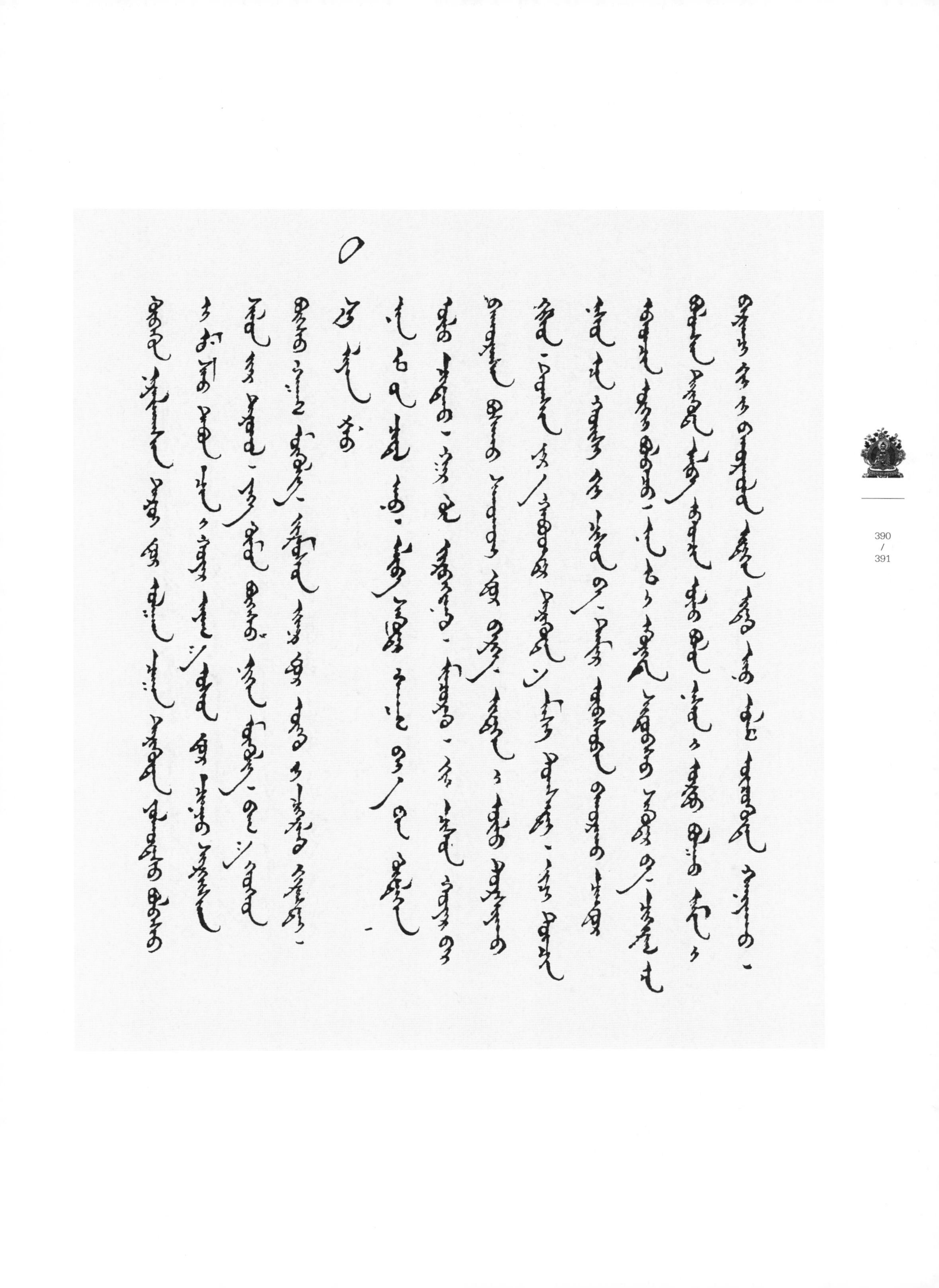

[illegible]

[illegible]

[illegible]

[illegible]

[illegible]

[illegible]

[illegible]

[illegible]

[illegible]

[illegible]

[illegible]

[illegible]

[illegible]

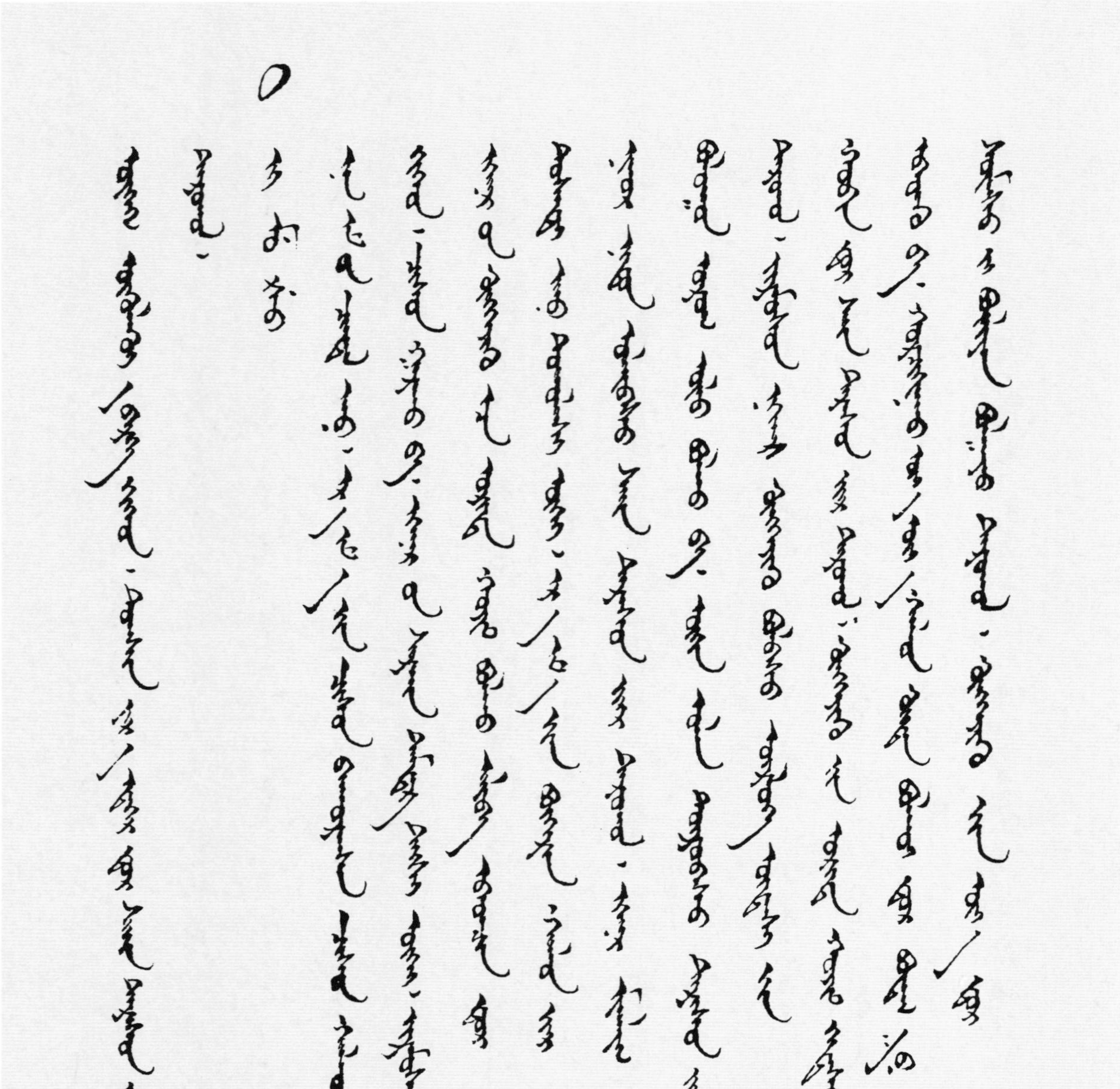

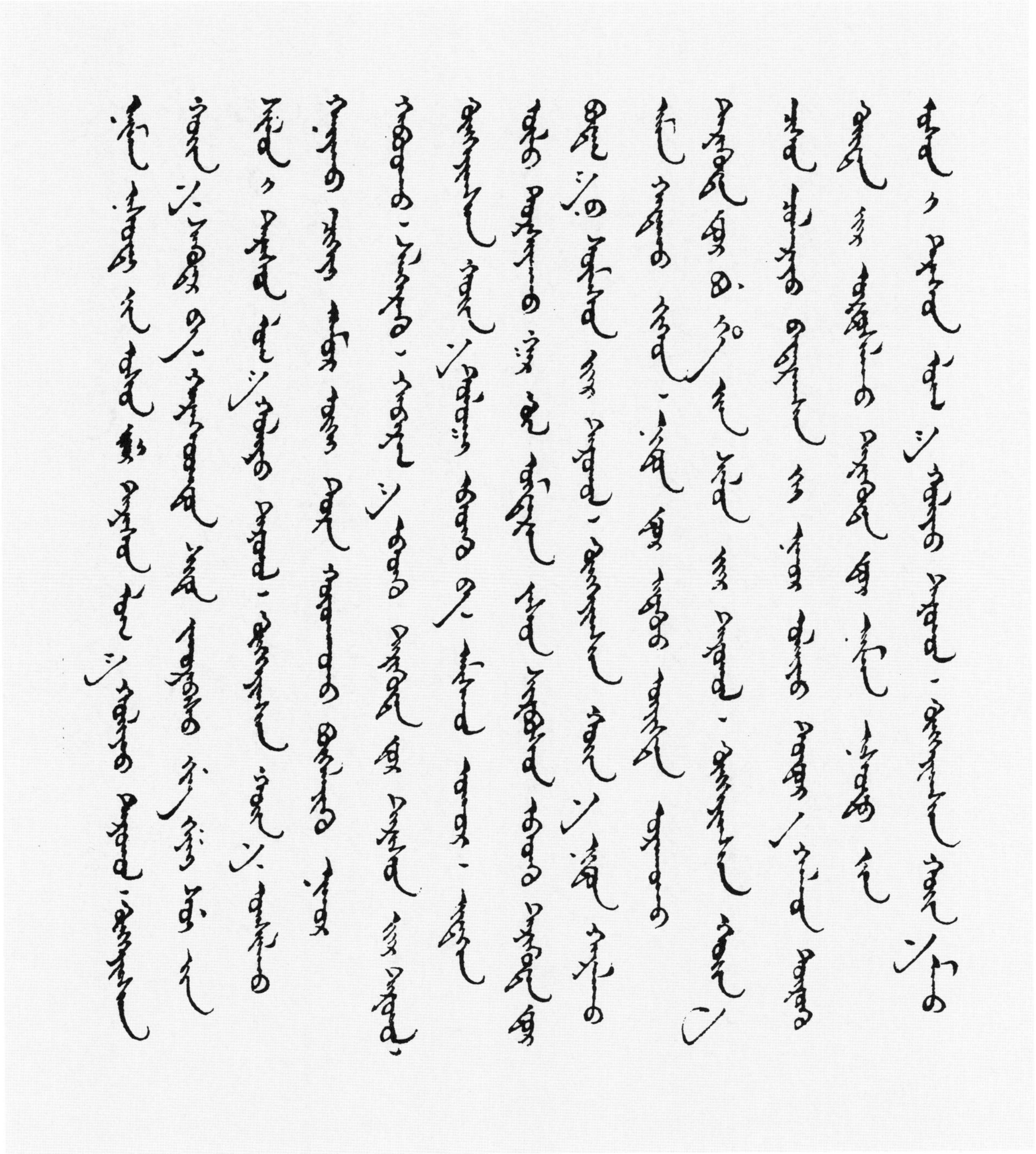

[illegible]

[illegible]

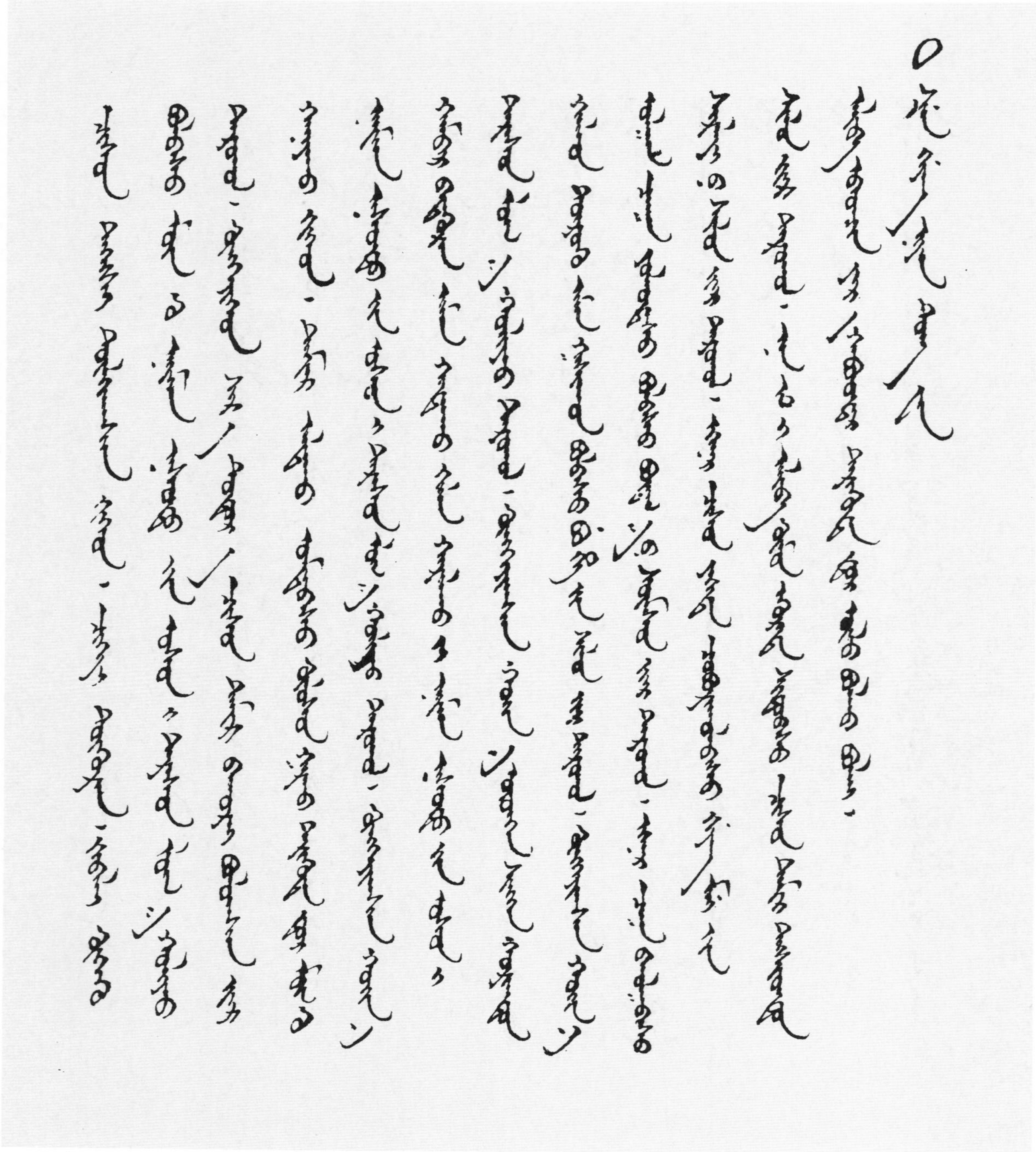

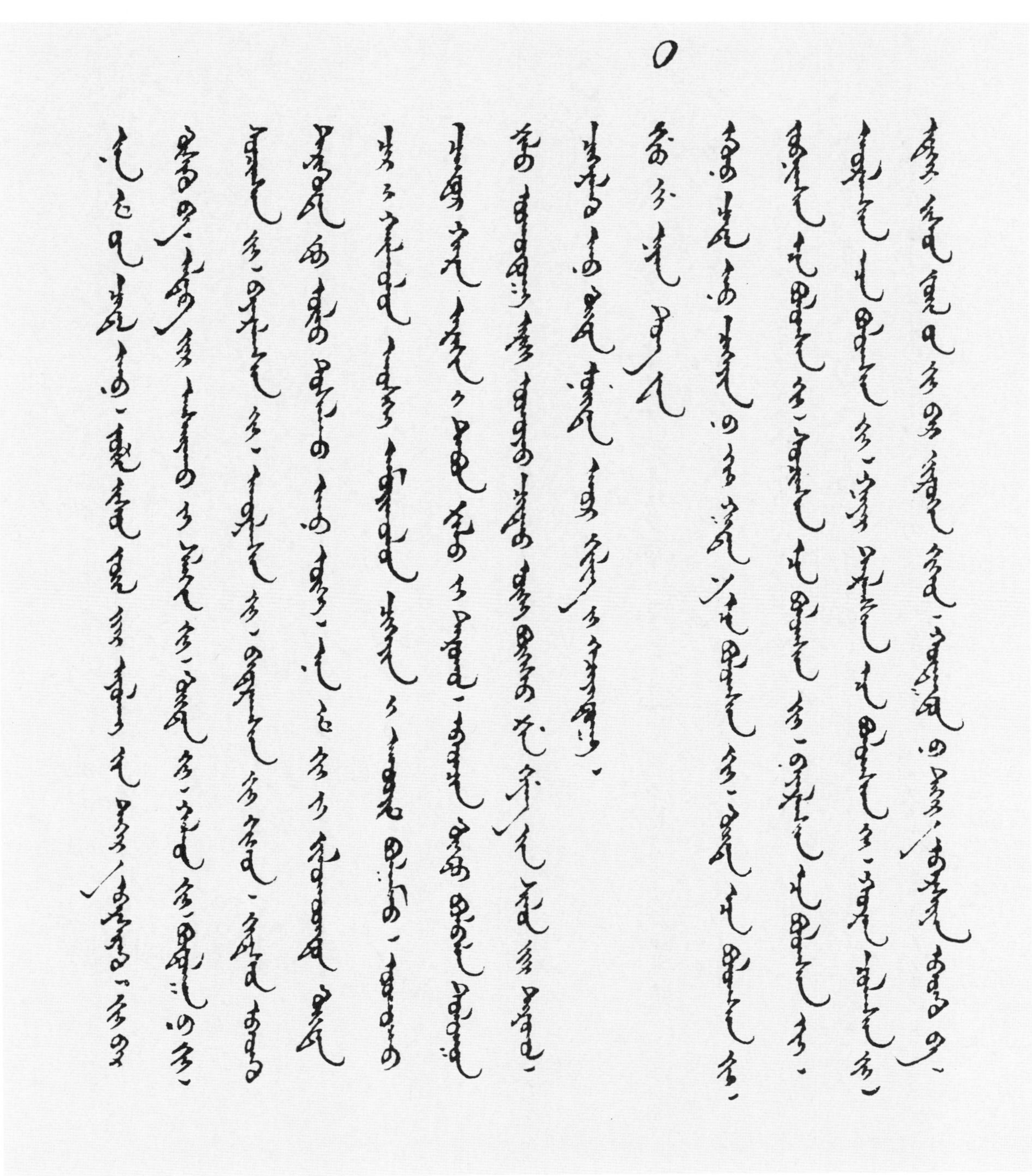

[illegible]
[illegible]
[illegible]
[illegible]
[illegible]
[illegible]
[illegible]

[illegible]
[illegible]
[illegible]
[illegible]
[illegible]
[illegible]

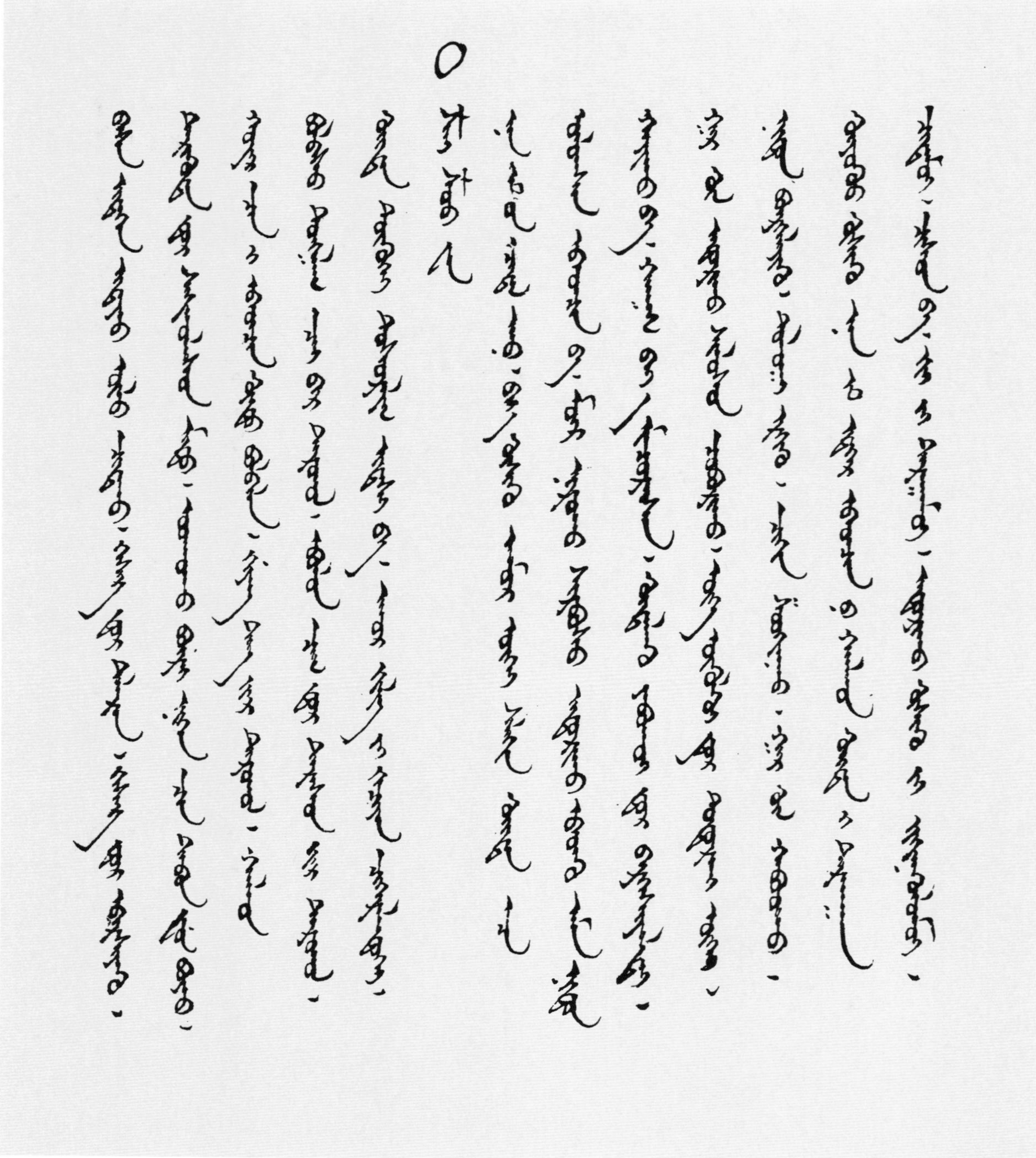

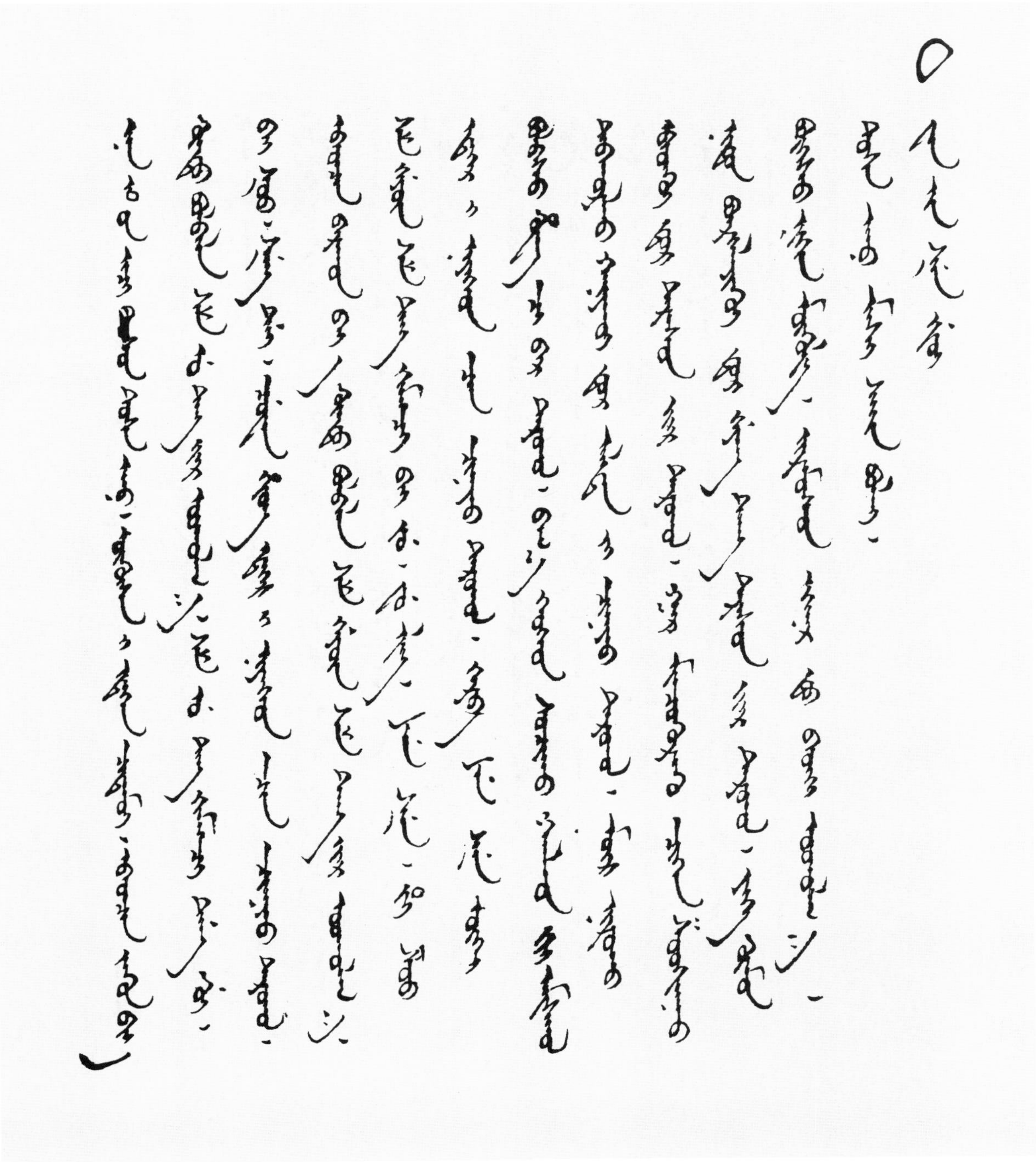

[illegible]
[illegible]
[illegible]
[illegible]
[illegible]
[illegible]
[illegible]
[illegible]
[illegible]
[illegible]
[illegible]
[illegible]

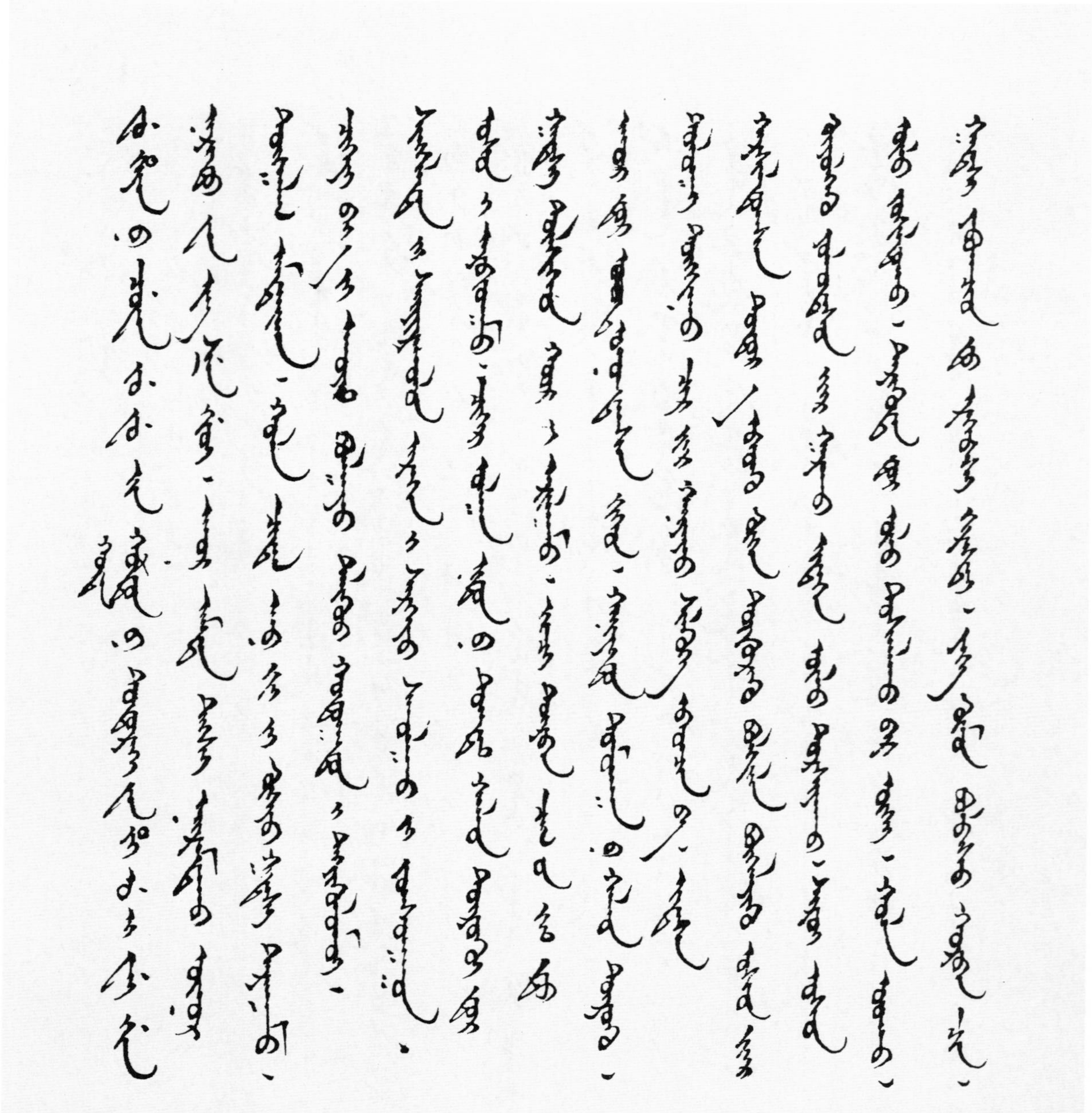

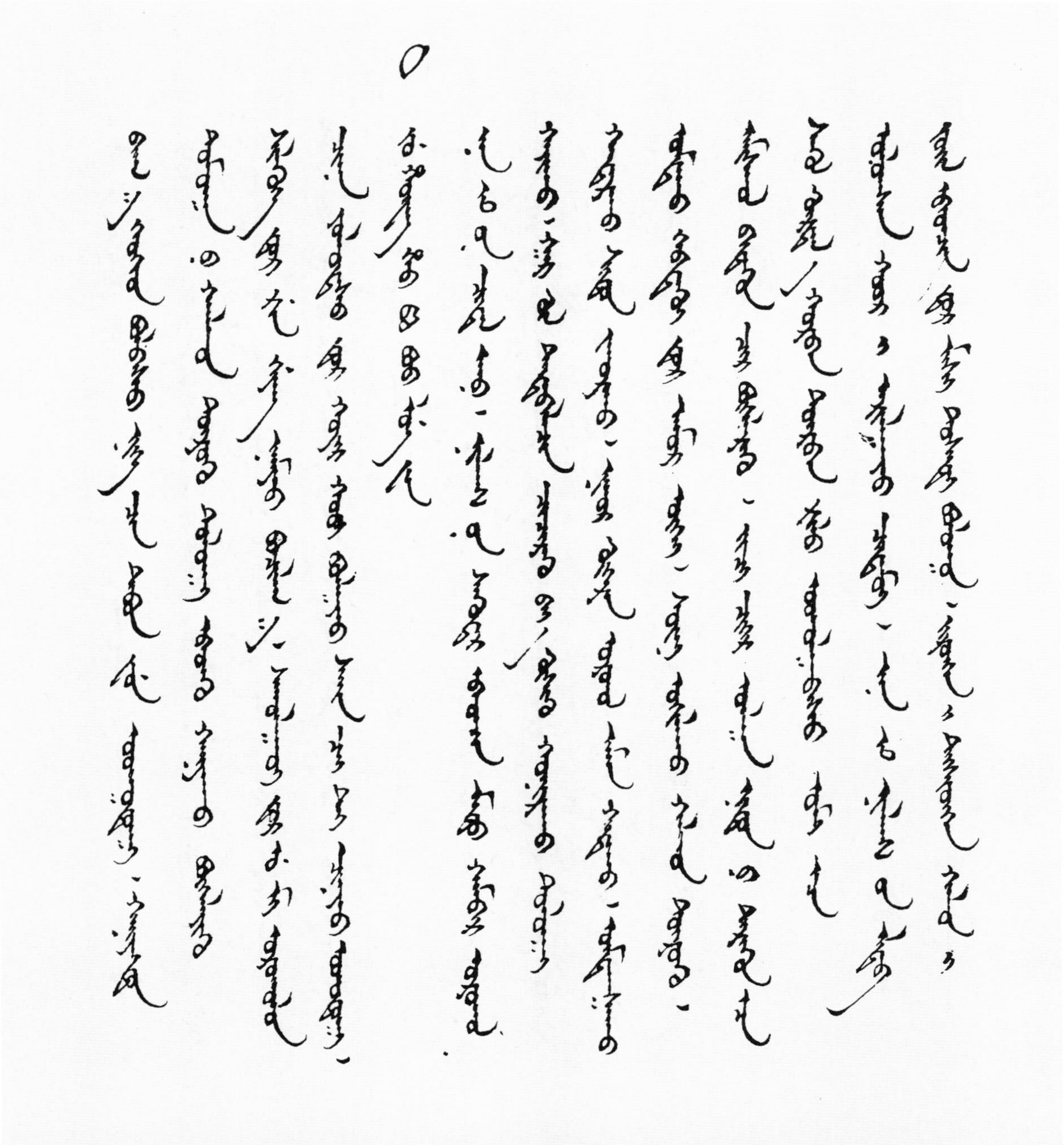

[illegible]
[illegible]
[illegible]
[illegible]
[illegible]
[illegible]
[illegible]
[illegible]
[illegible]

○ [illegible]
[illegible]
[illegible]
[illegible]

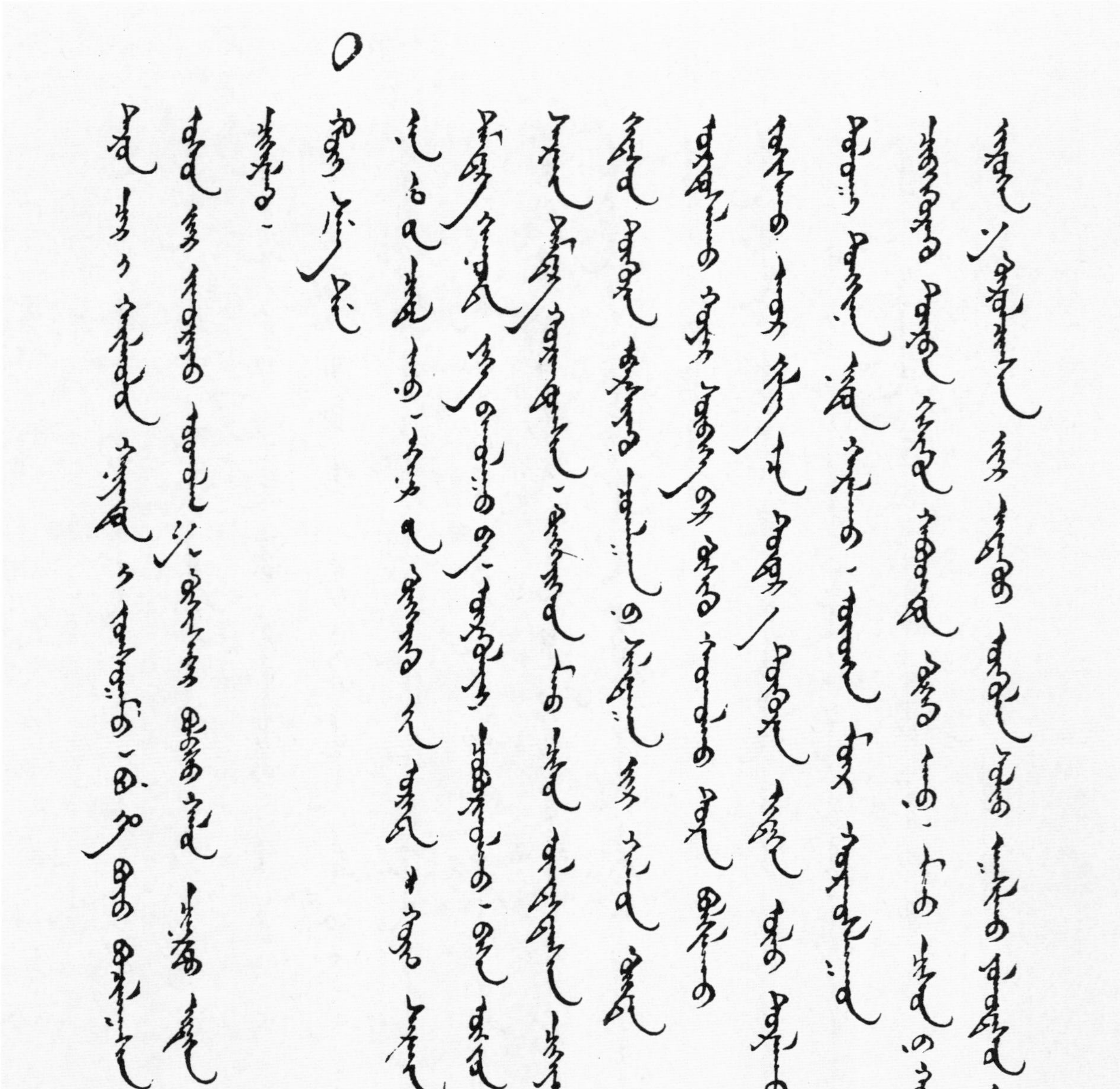

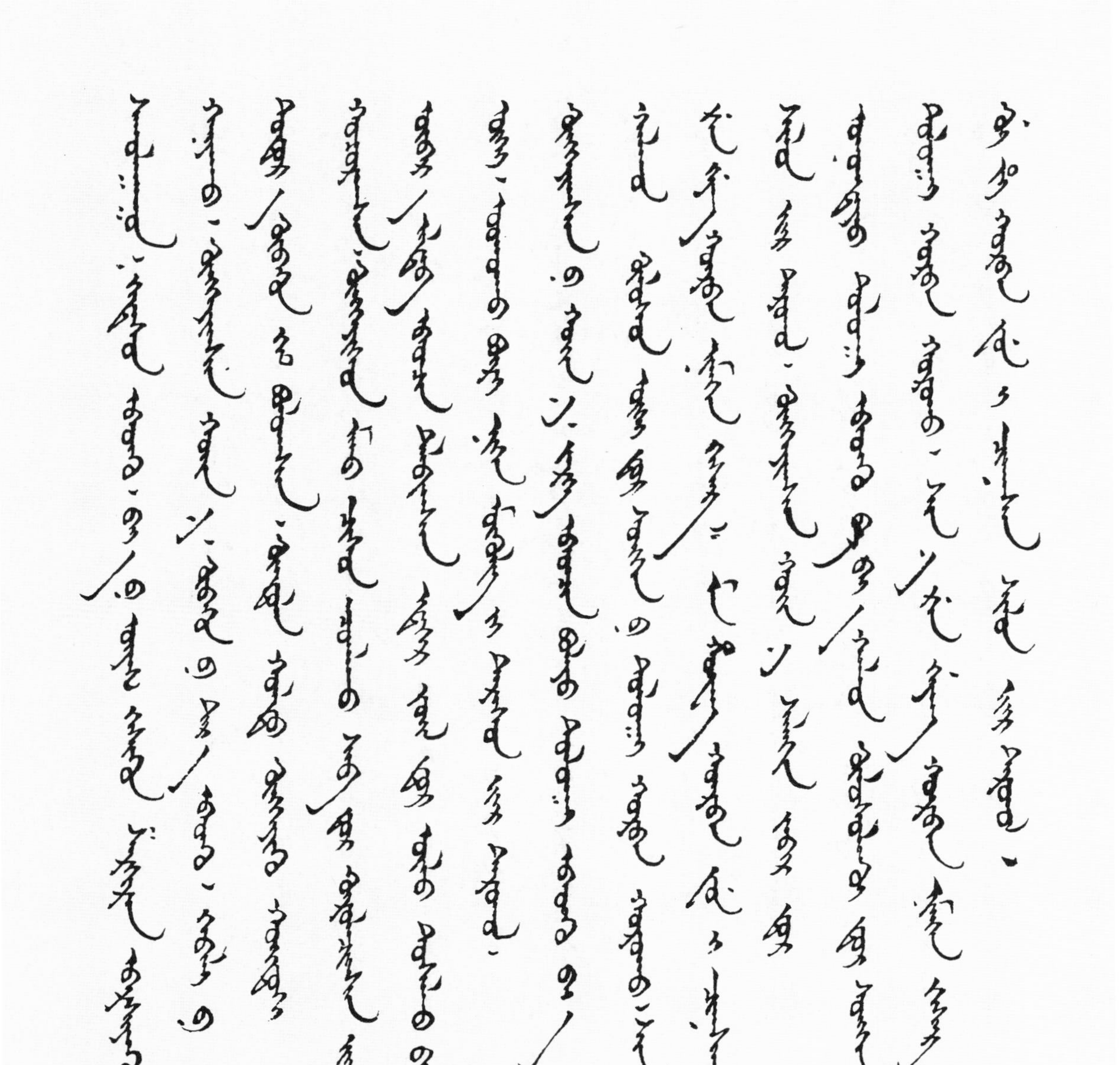

[illegible]

[illegible]

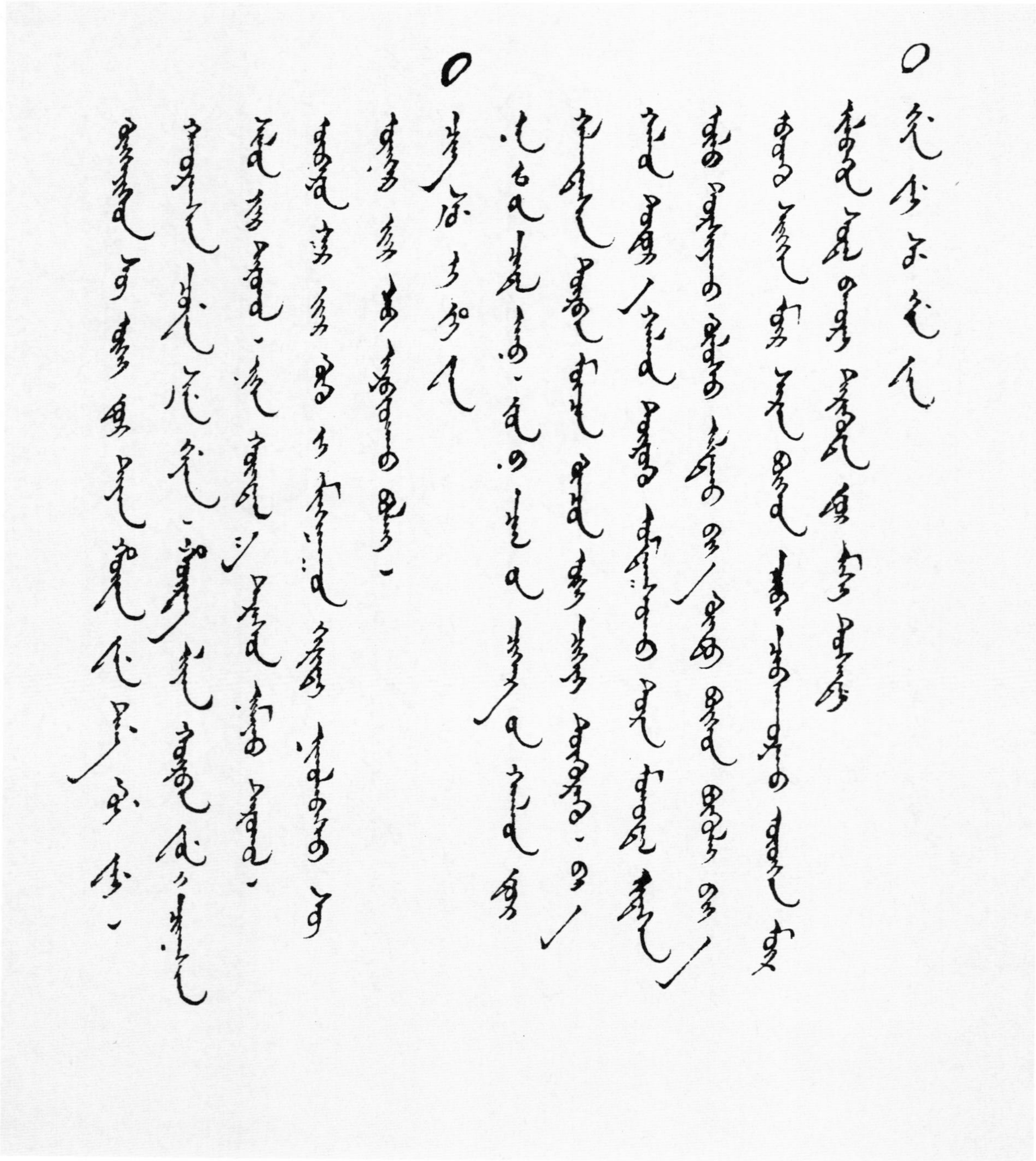

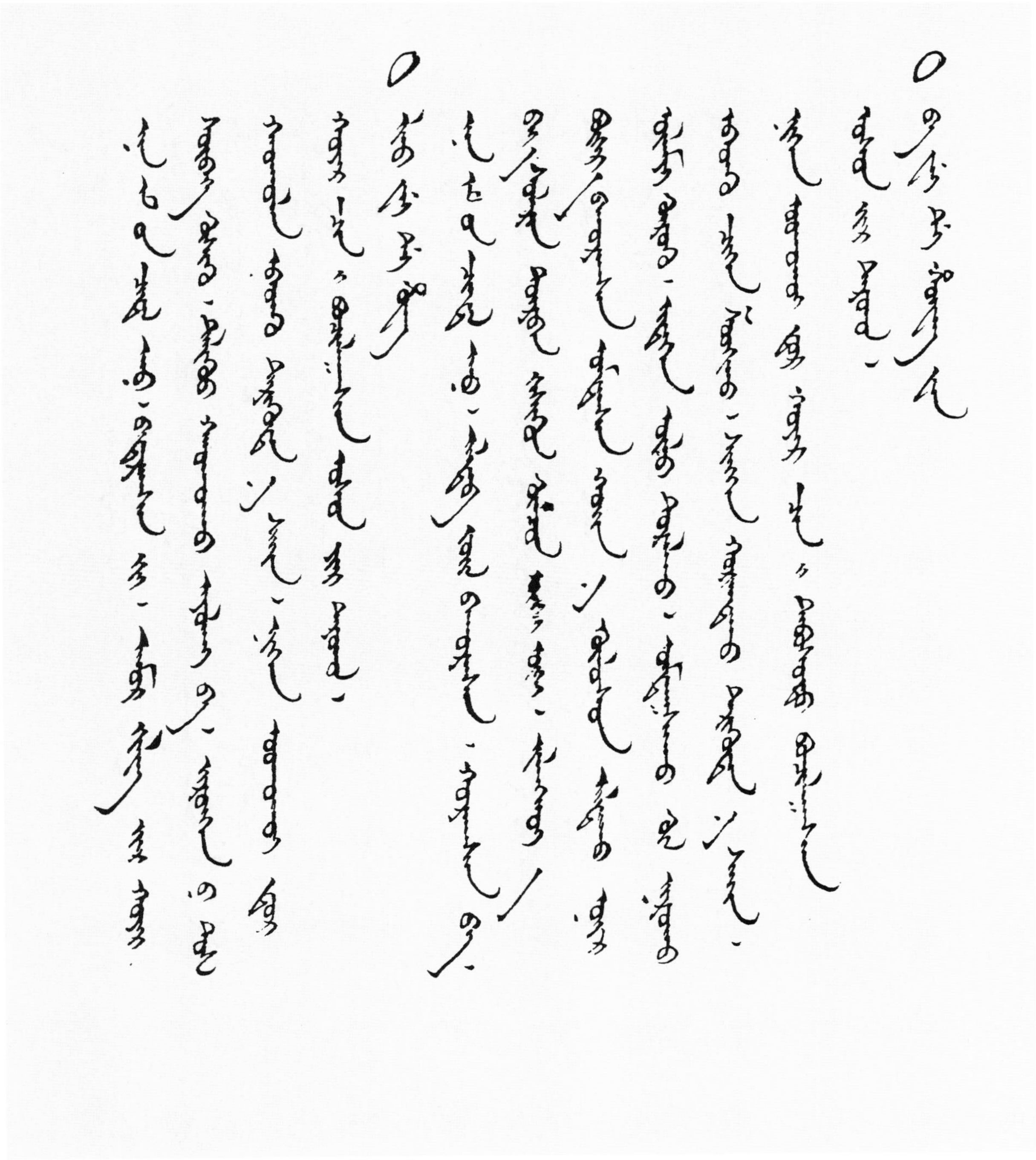

[illegible]
[illegible]
[illegible]
[illegible]
[illegible]
[illegible]
[illegible]
[illegible]

[illegible]
[illegible]
[illegible]
[illegible]

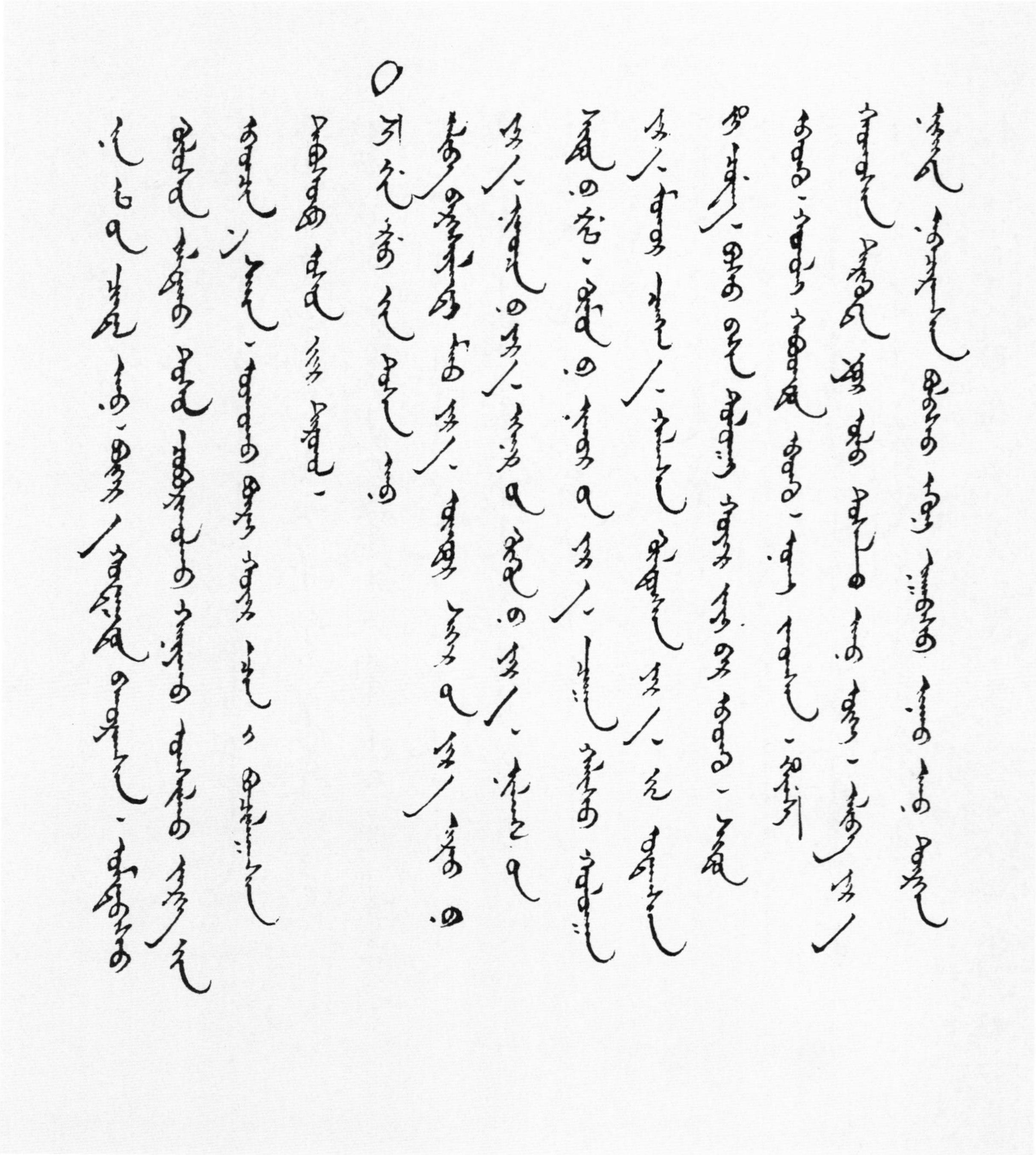

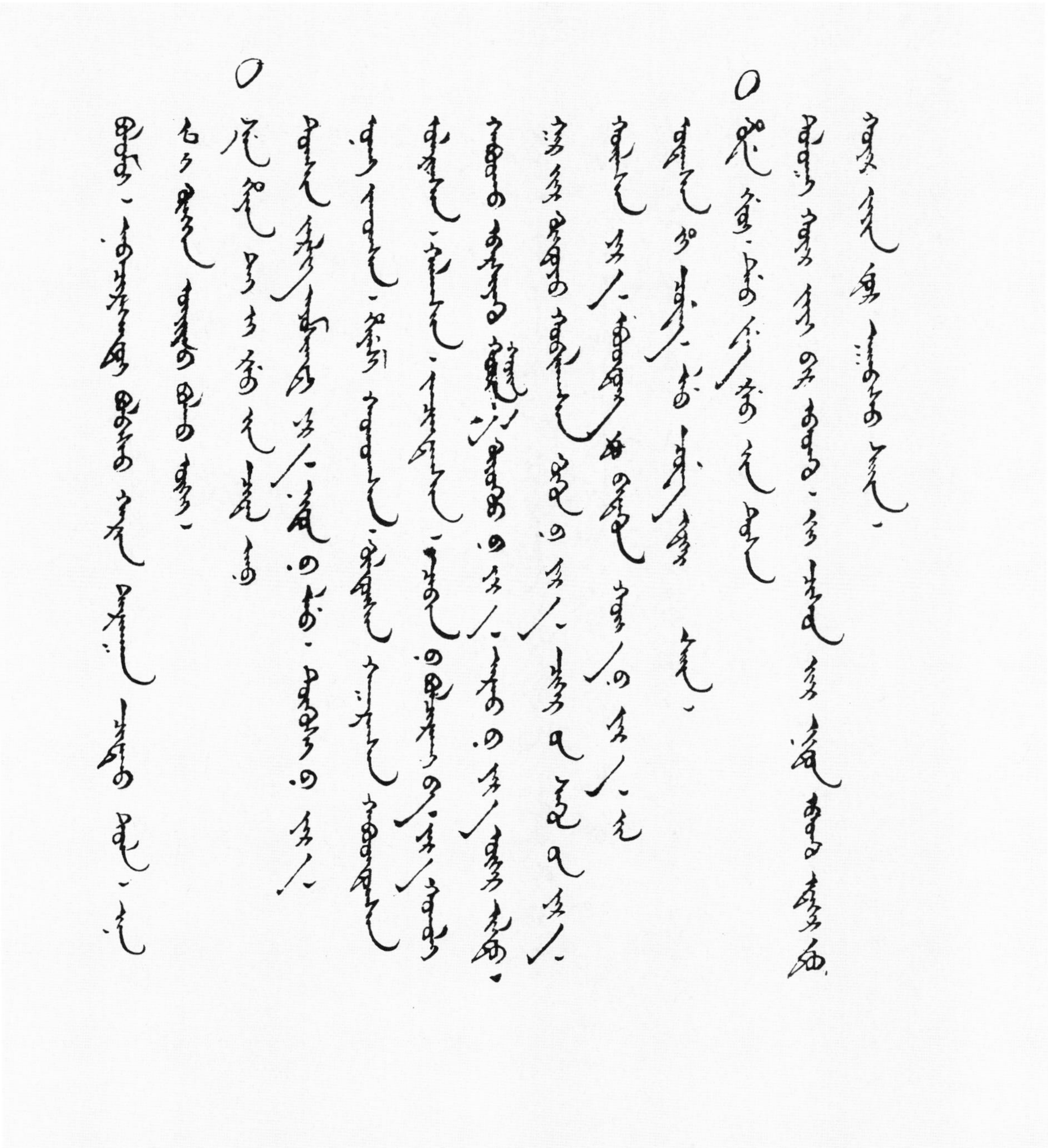

○ [illegible]

○ [illegible]

○ [illegible]

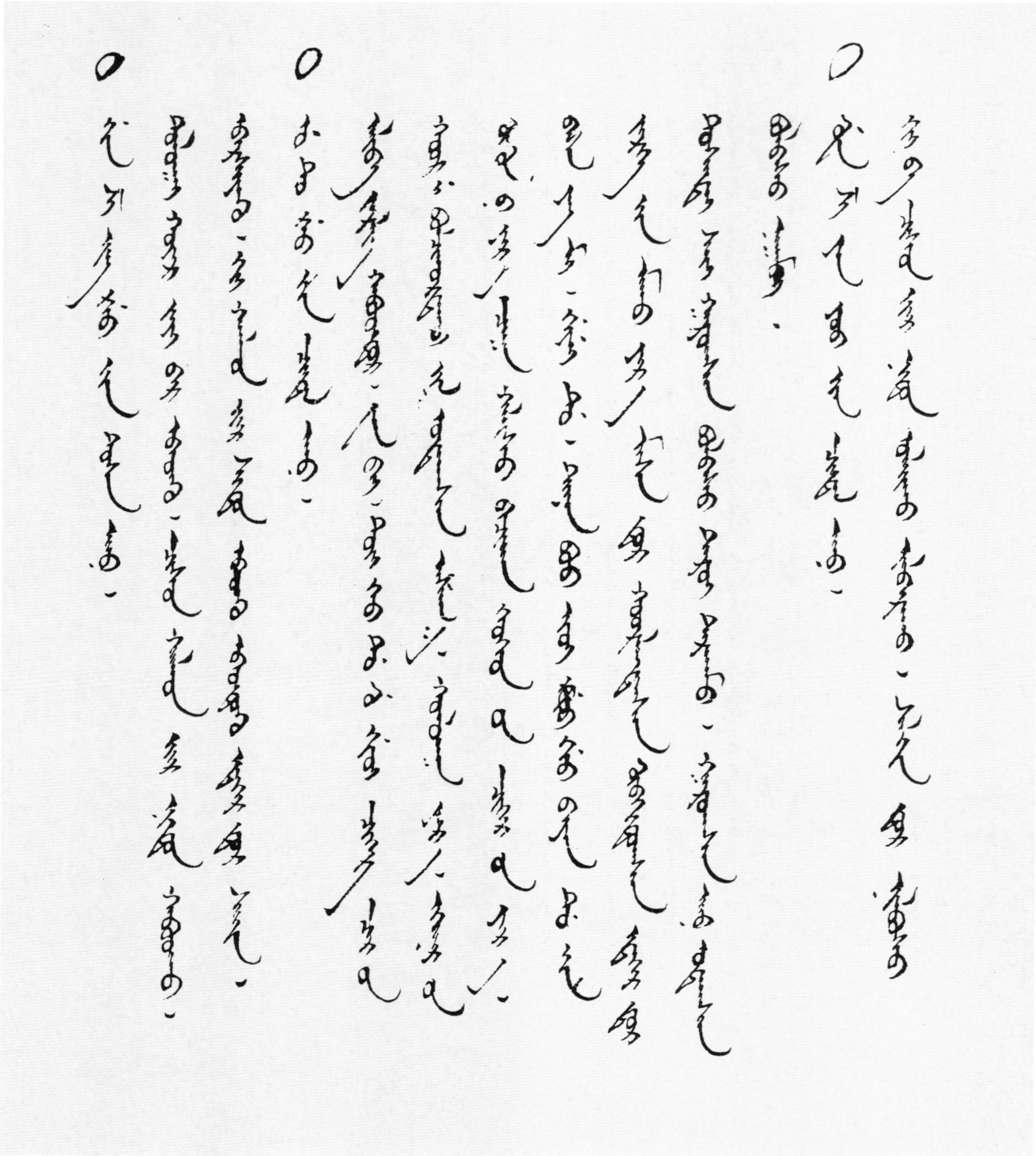

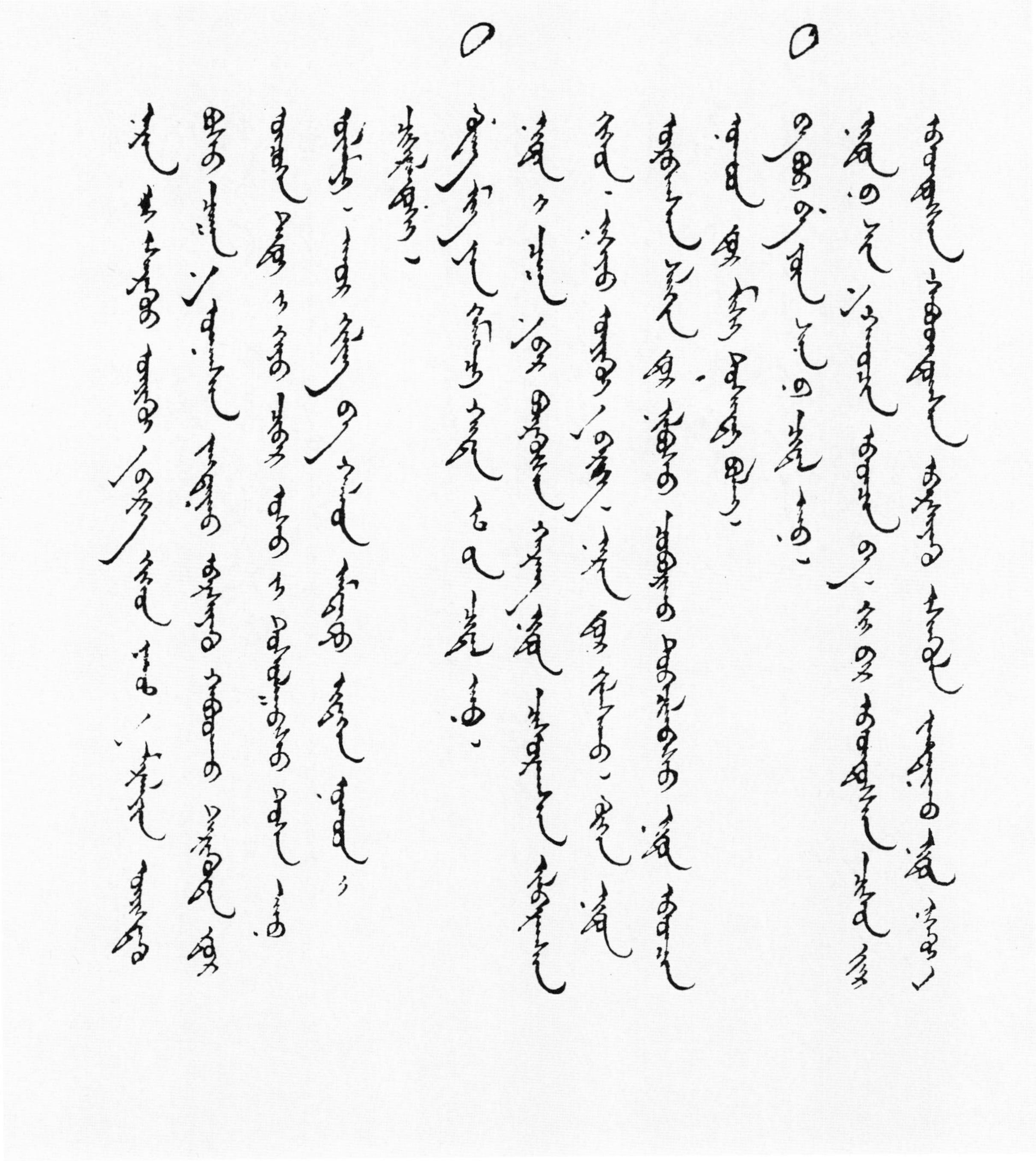

[illegible]

[illegible]

[illegible]

[illegible]

[illegible]

[illegible]

[illegible]

[illegible]

[illegible]

[illegible]

[illegible]

[illegible]

[illegible]

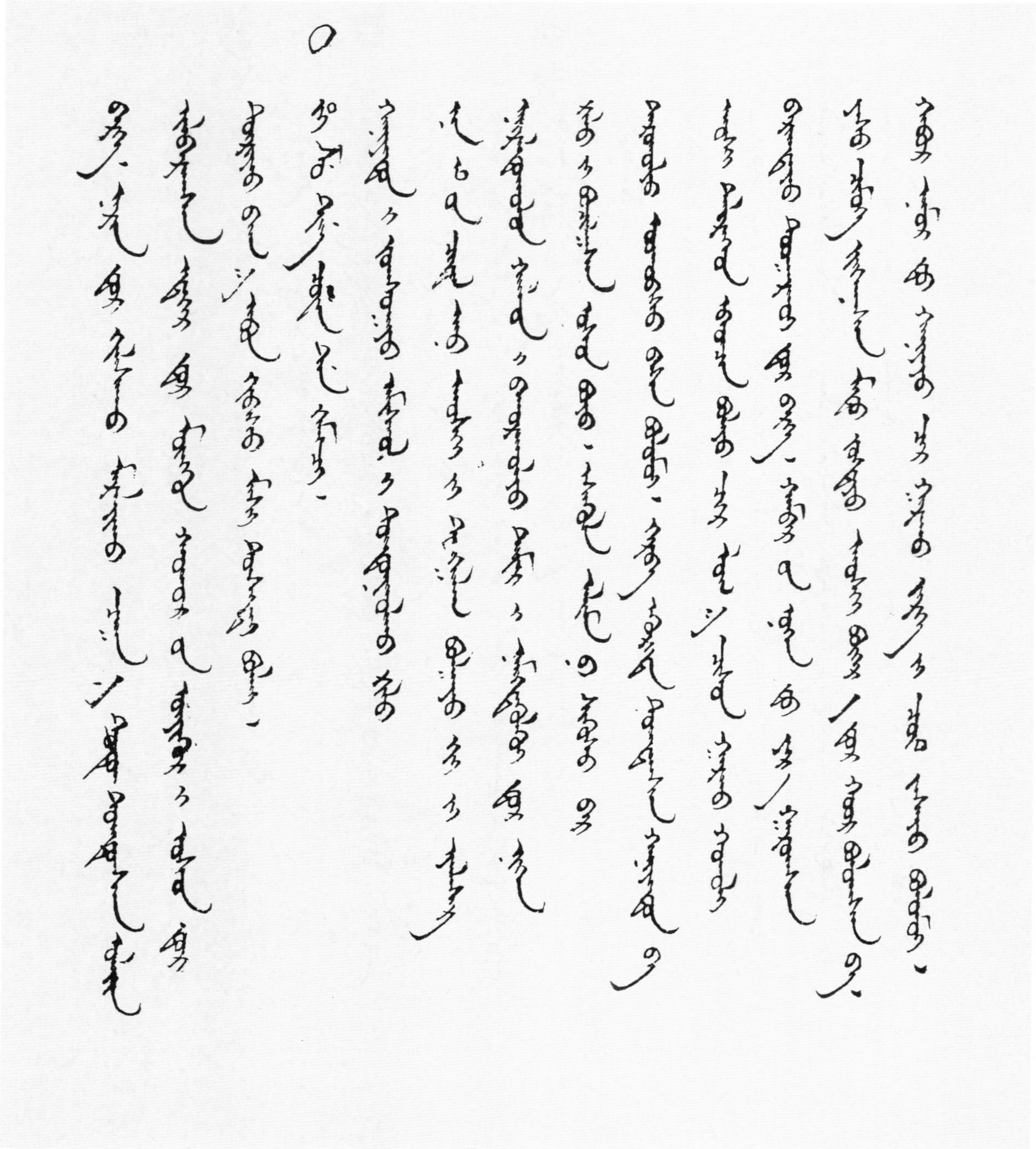

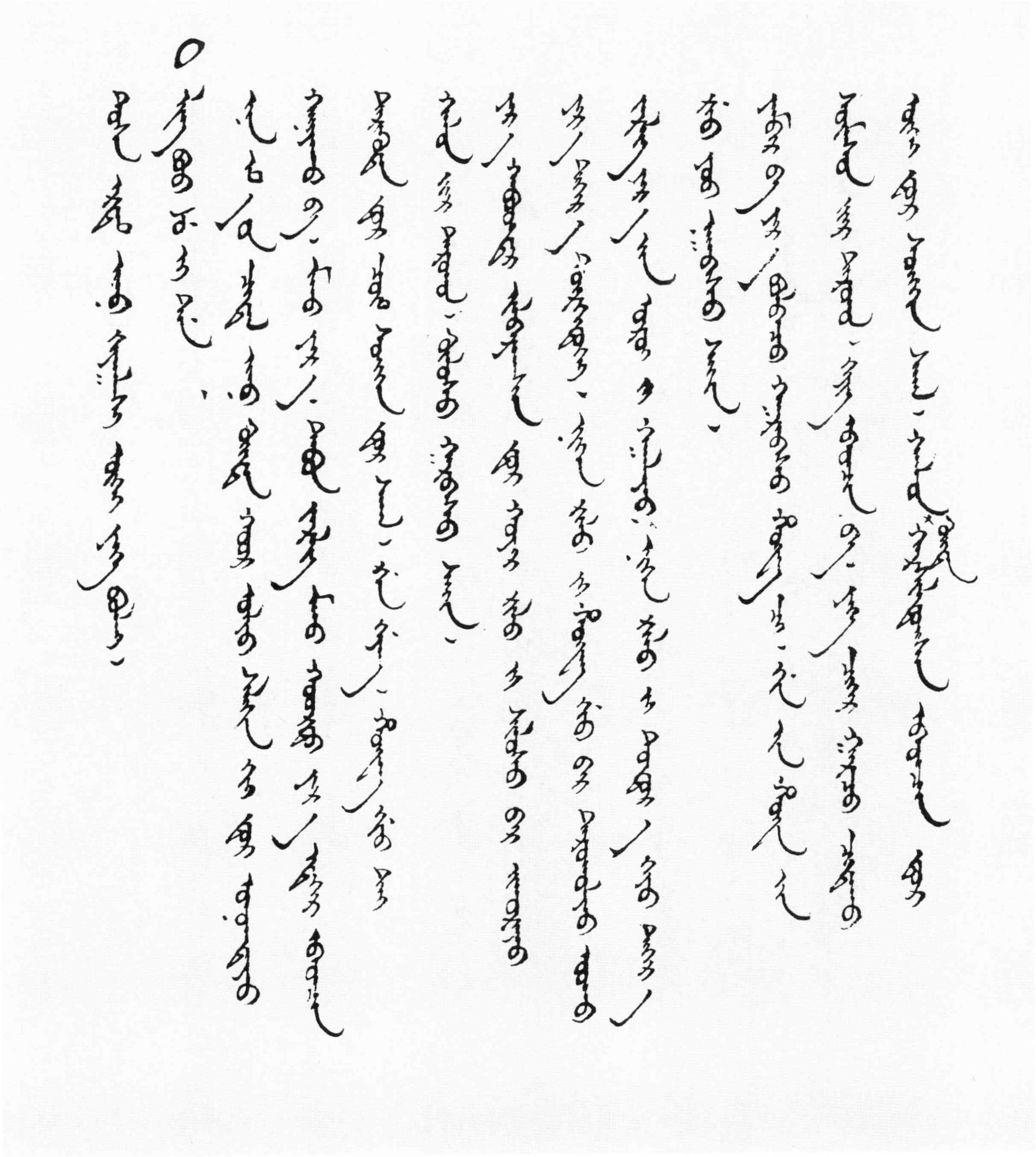

[illegible]
[illegible]
[illegible]
[illegible]
[illegible]
[illegible]
[illegible]
[illegible]
[illegible]
[illegible]
[illegible]

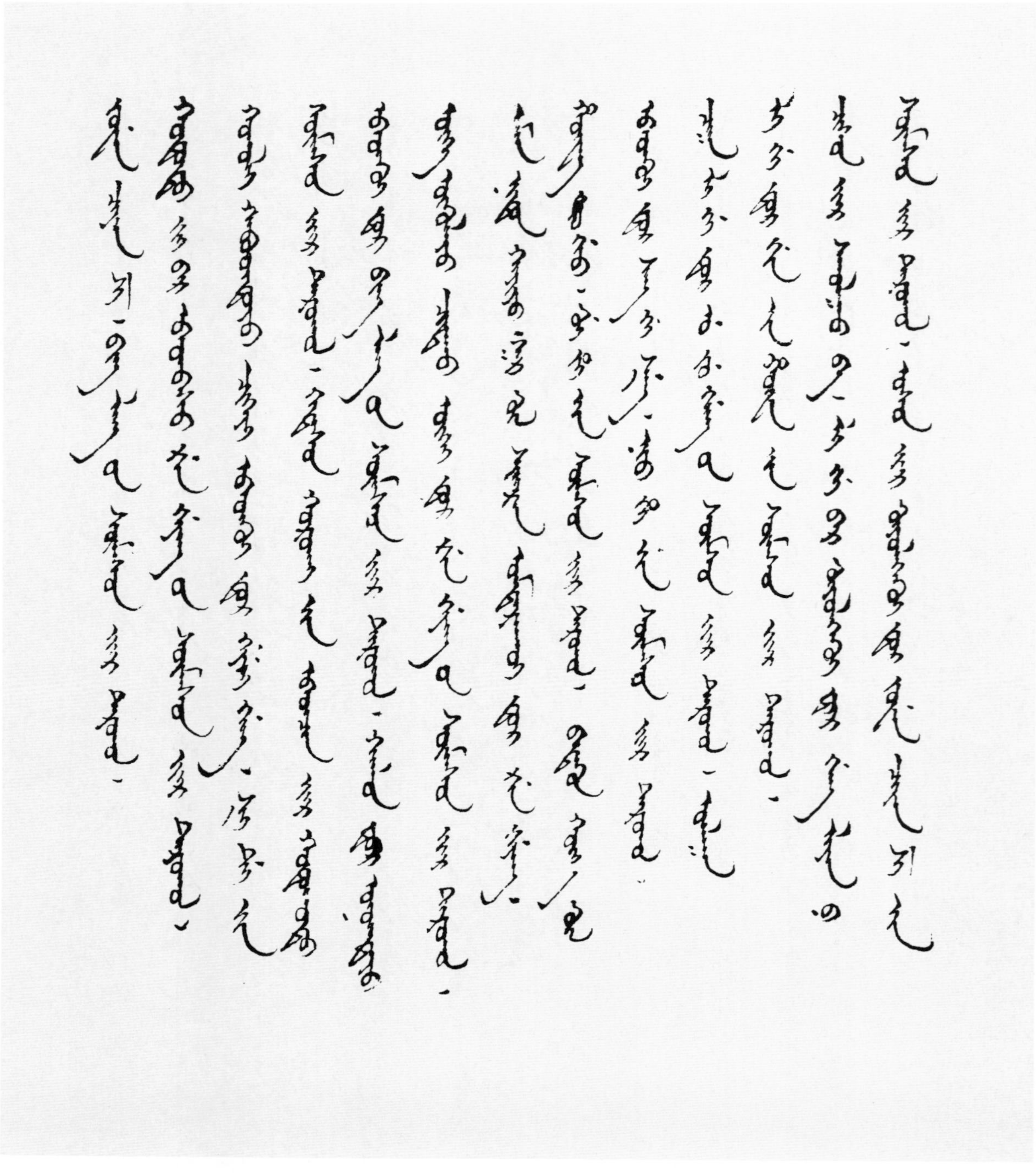

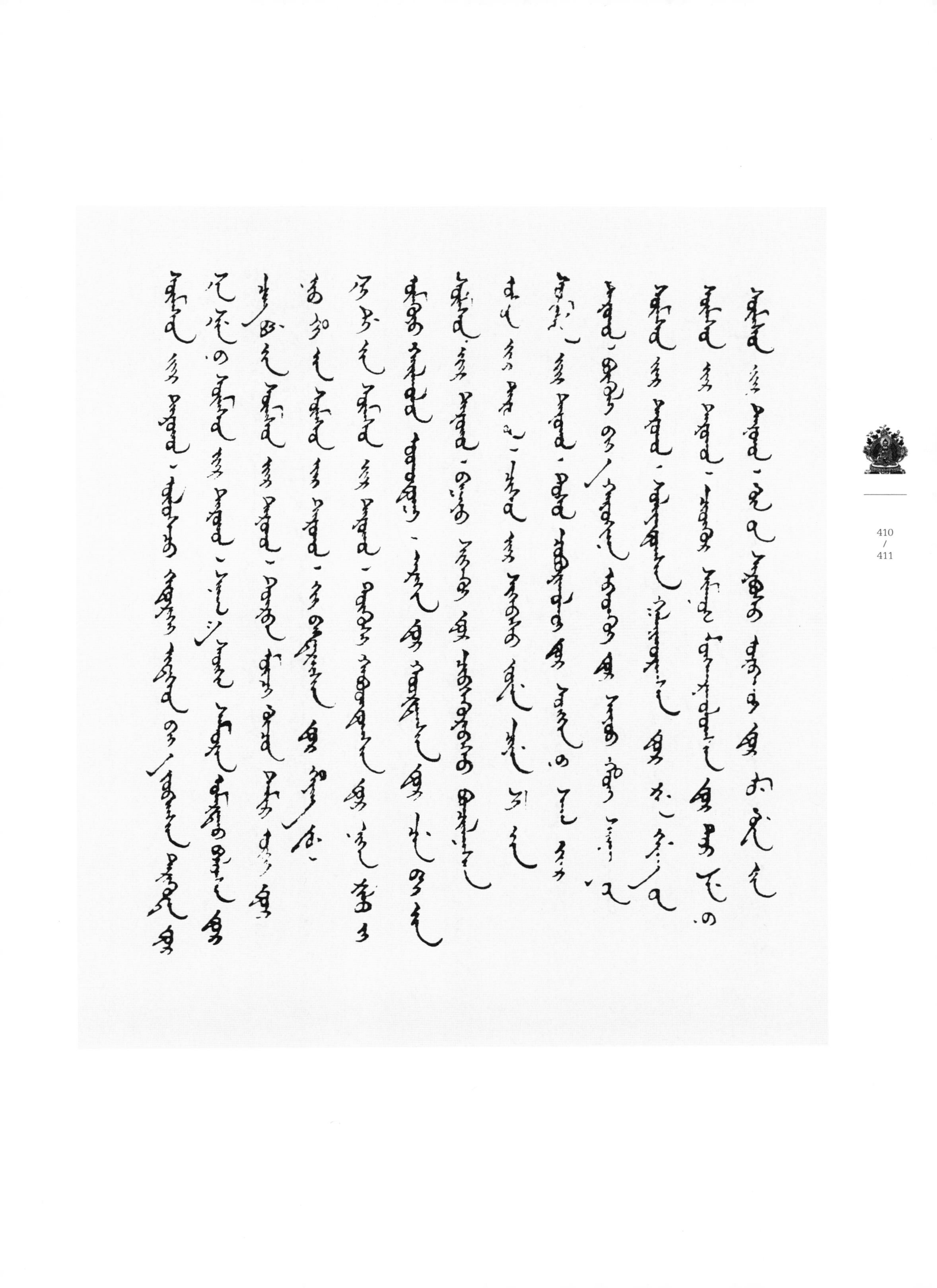

[illegible]

[illegible]

[illegible]

[illegible]

[illegible]

[illegible]

[illegible]

[illegible]

[illegible]

[illegible]

[illegible]

[illegible]

[illegible]

[illegible]

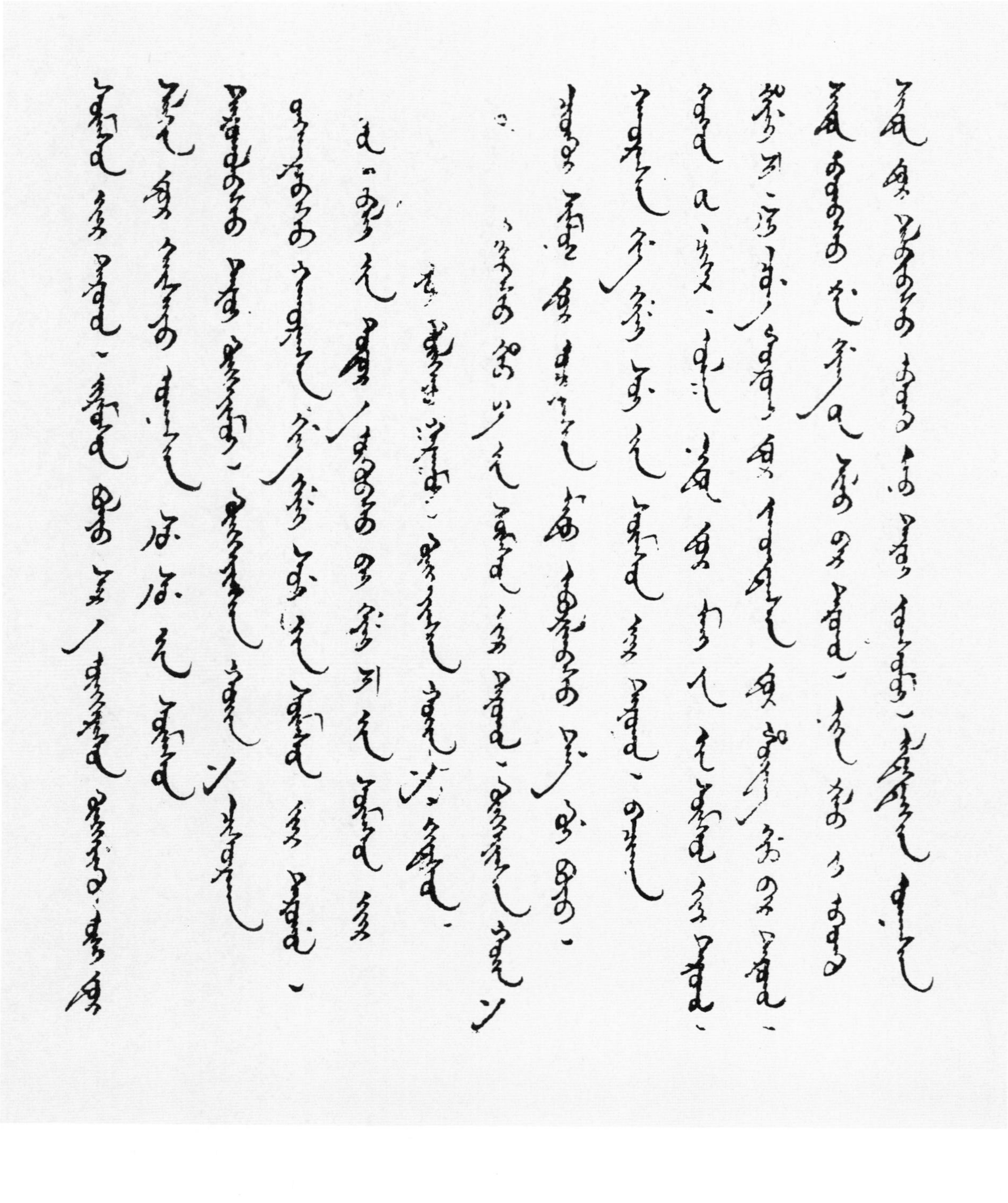

[illegible] ᠪᠠᠢᠨ᠎ᠠ :: [illegible] ::

[illegible] ᠶᠢᠨ 36 [illegible] ᠪᠠᠢᠨ᠎ᠠ :: [illegible] ᠪᠠᠢᠨ᠎ᠠ :: [illegible]

[illegible] ᠨᠢ : 14cm×27.5cm ᠪᠠᠢᠳᠠᠭ᠂ [illegible] 20 ᠨᠢᠭᠤᠷ ᠲᠠᠢ ::

[illegible] ᠪᠠᠢᠨ᠎ᠠ ::

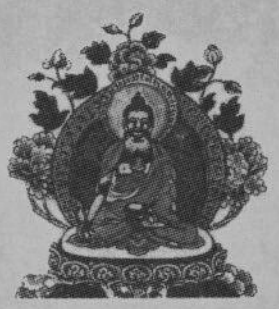

GuanYin Catholicon Medicine Primer

观音普济丹药引书

8

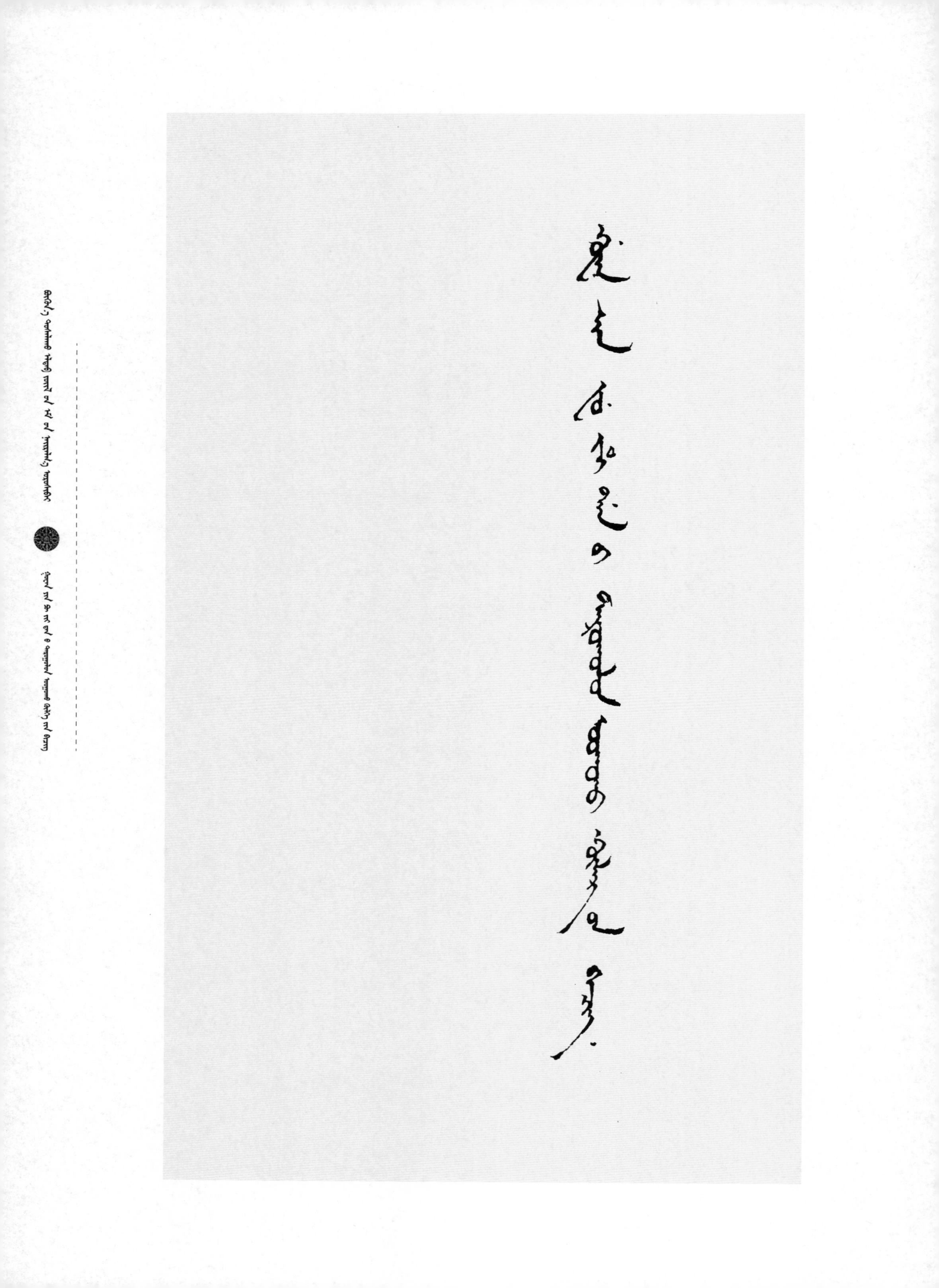

[illegible]

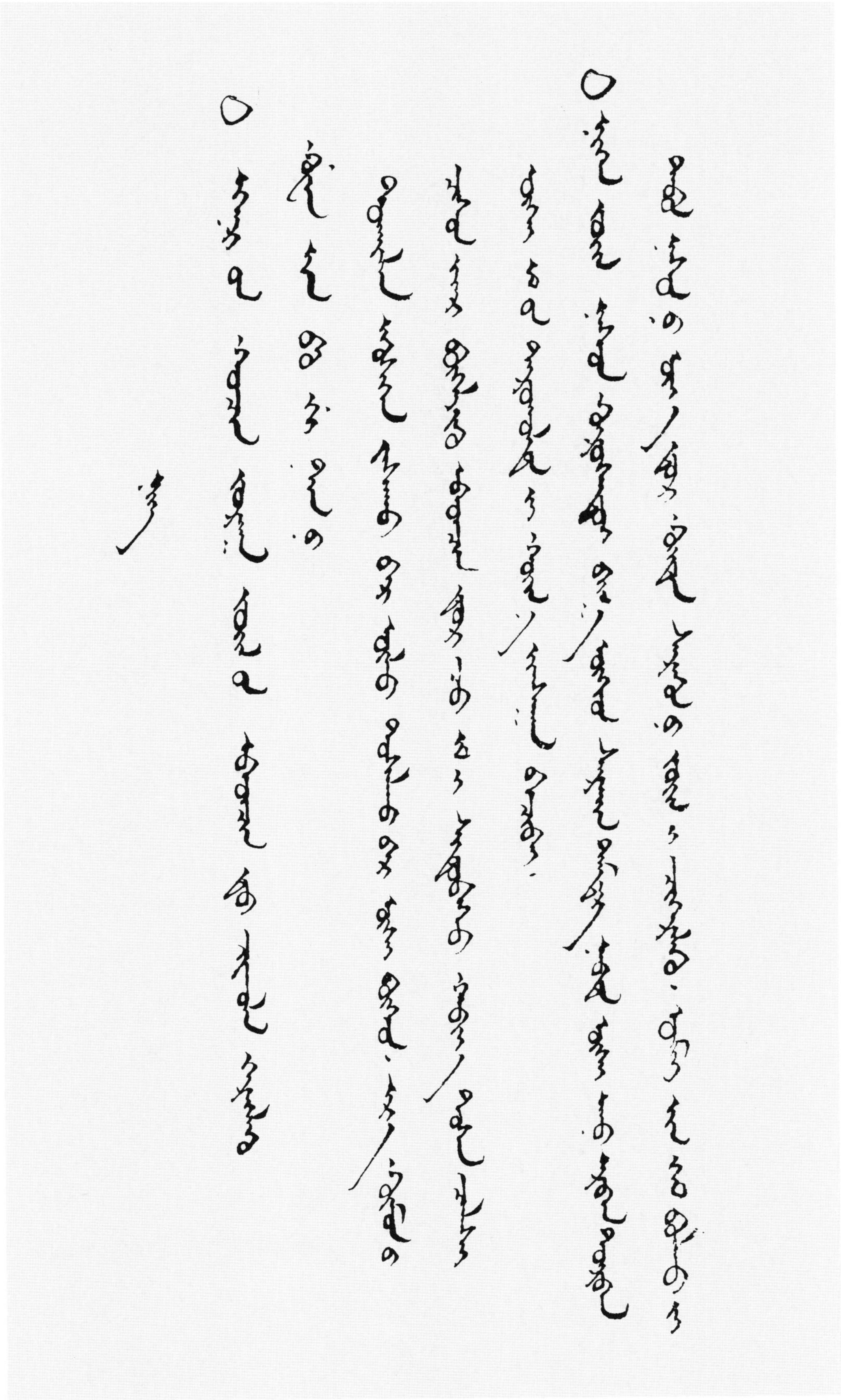

[illegible]

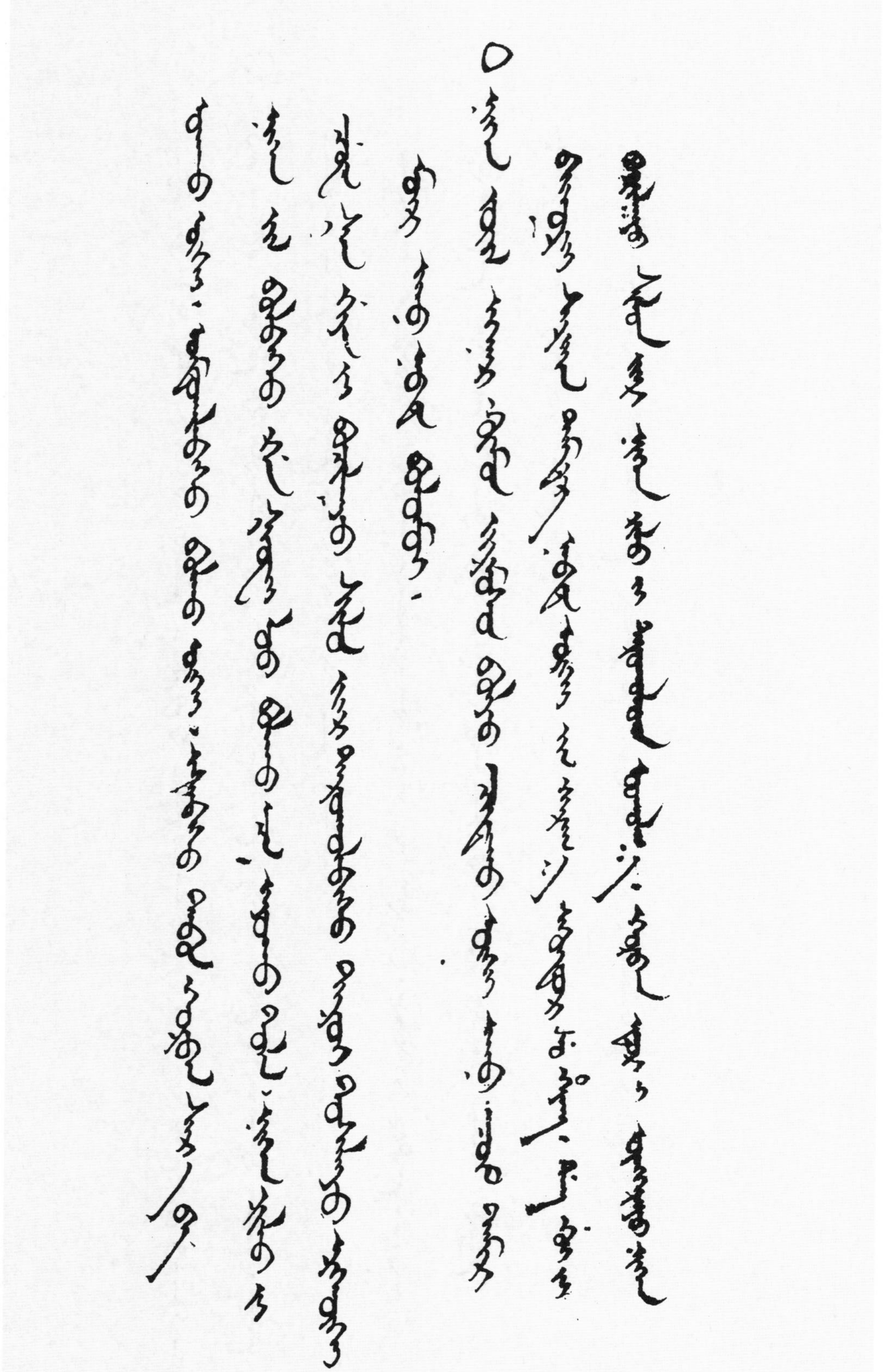

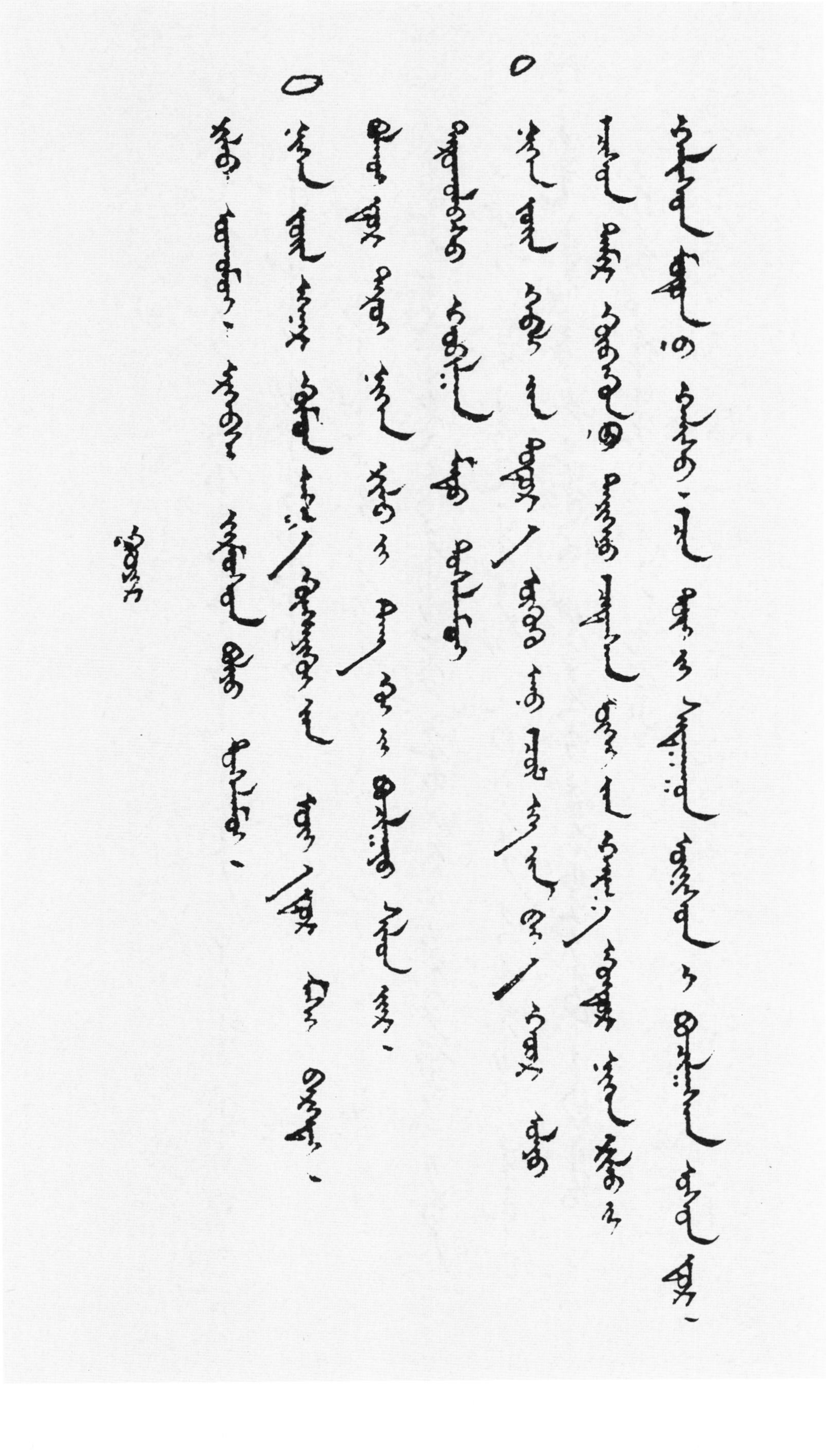

[illegible]

[illegible]

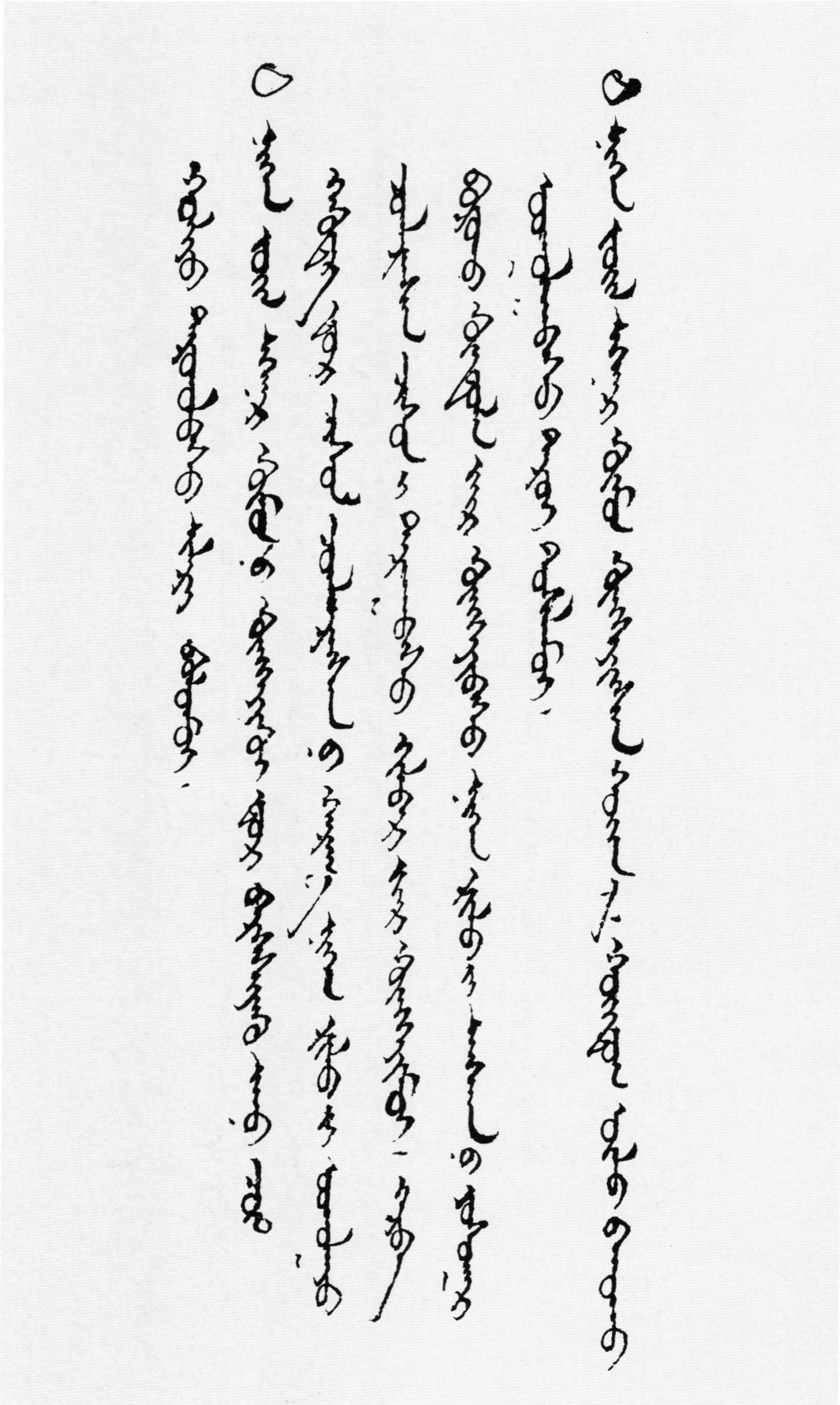

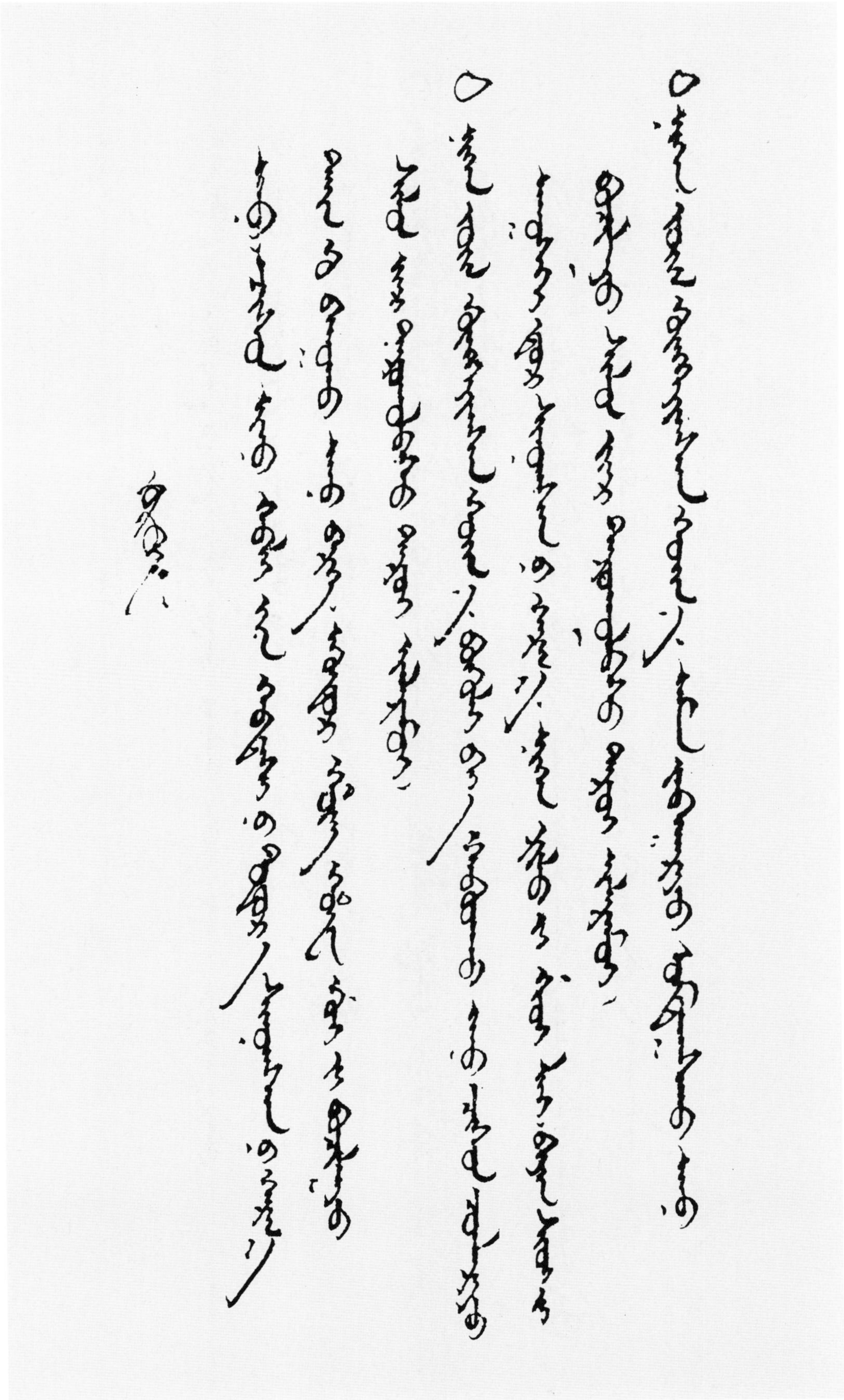

[illegible]

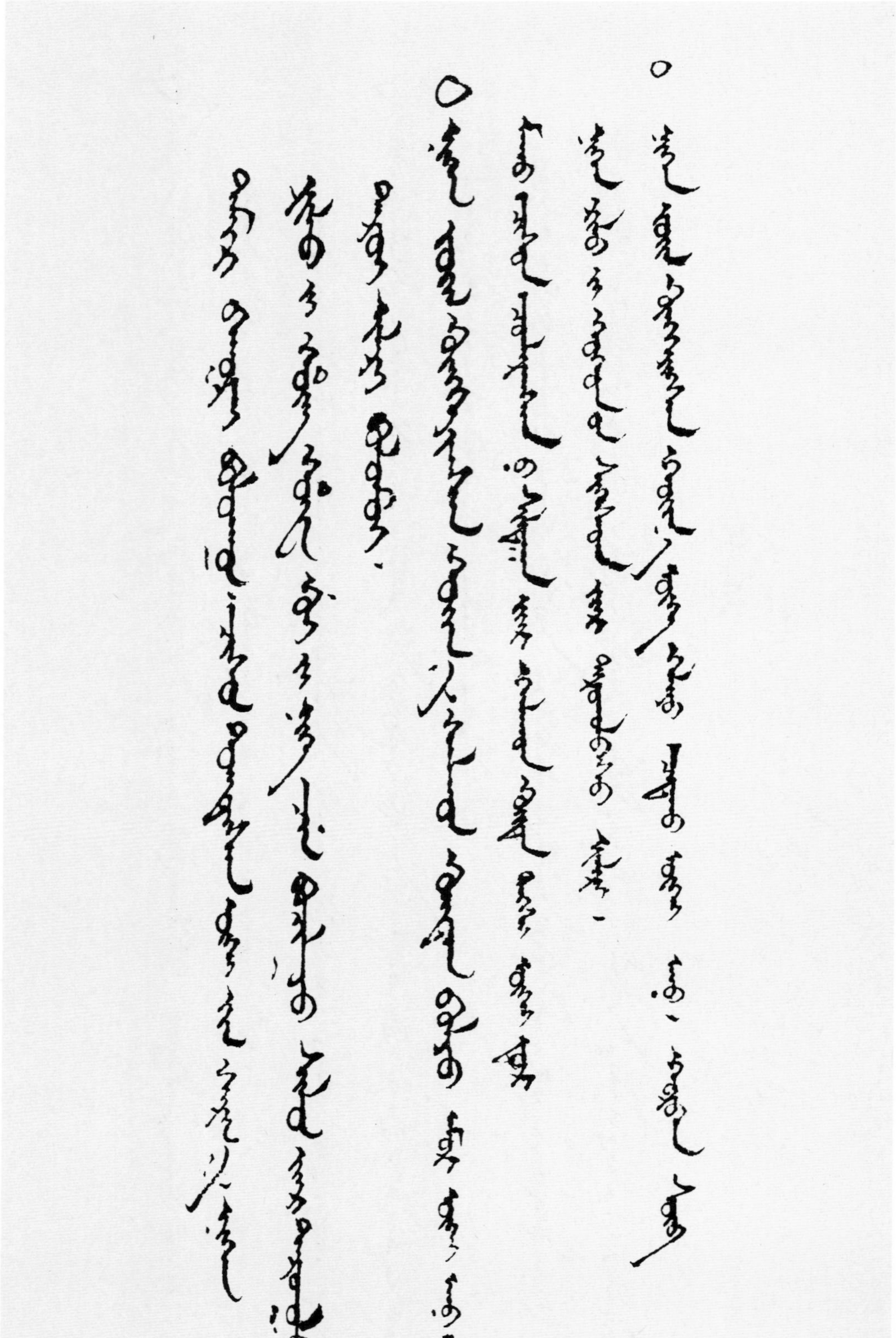

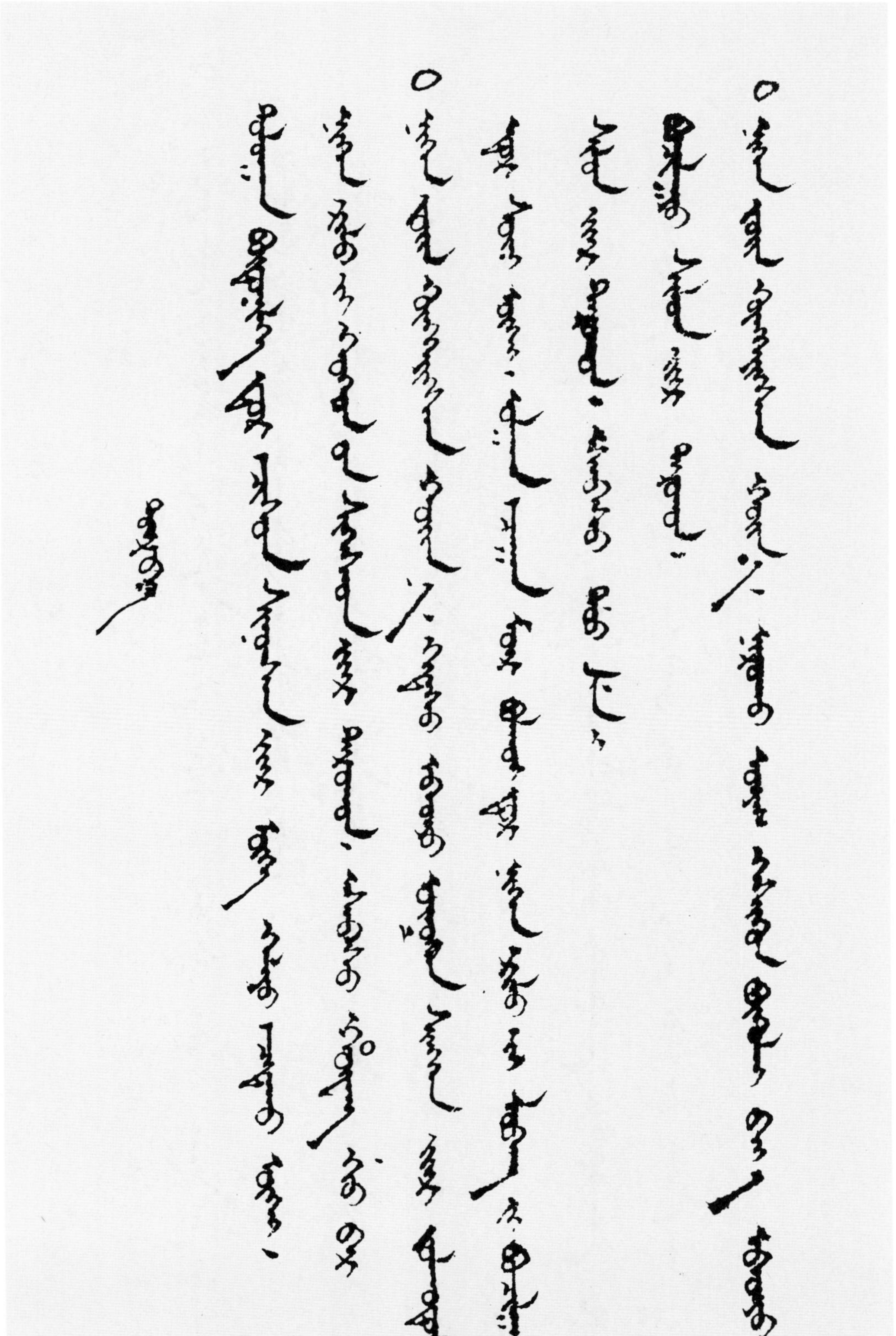

[illegible]

[illegible]

[illegible]

[illegible]

[illegible]

[illegible]

[illegible]

[illegible]

○ [illegible]

[illegible]

[illegible]

○ [illegible]

[illegible]

[illegible]

[illegible]

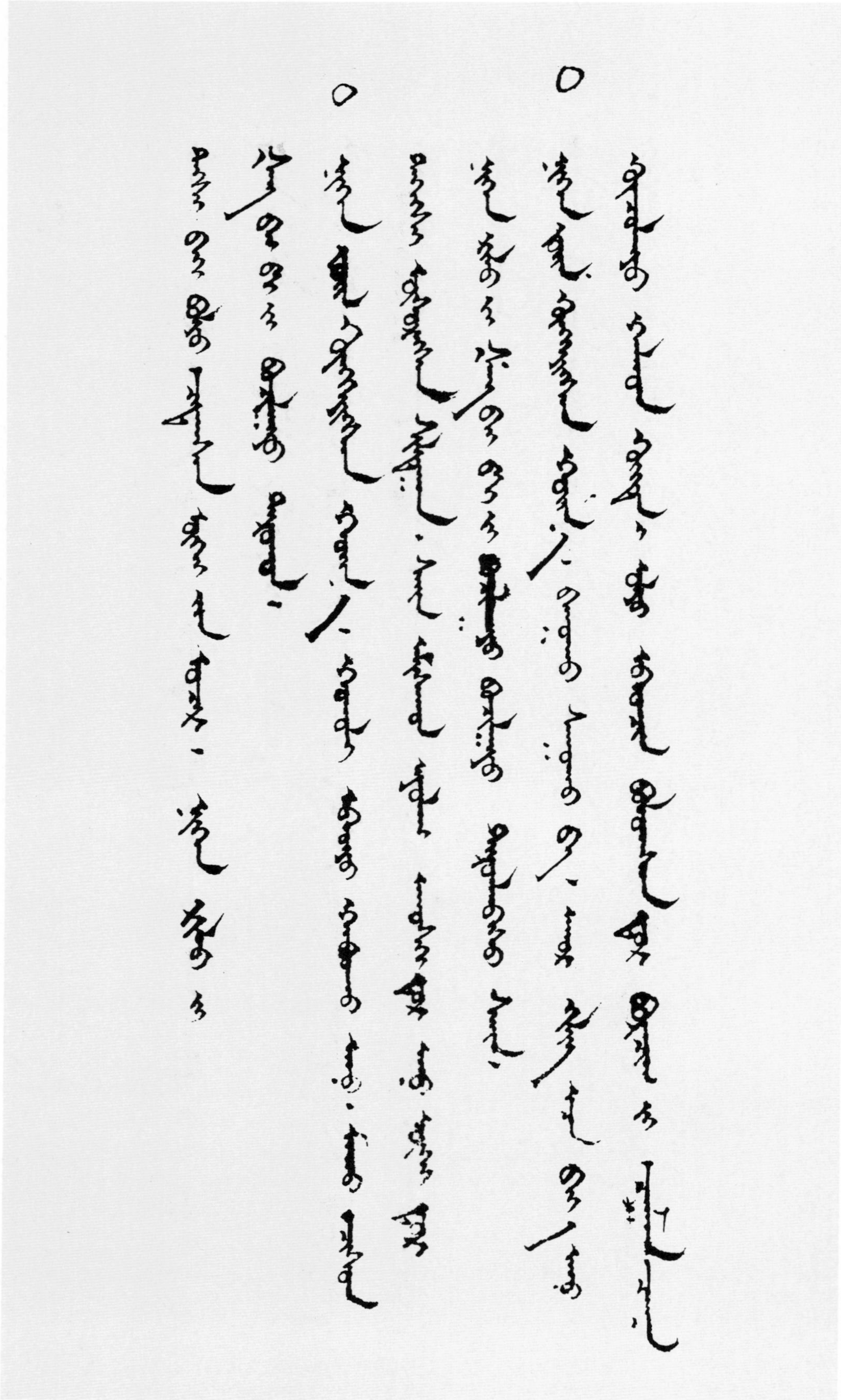

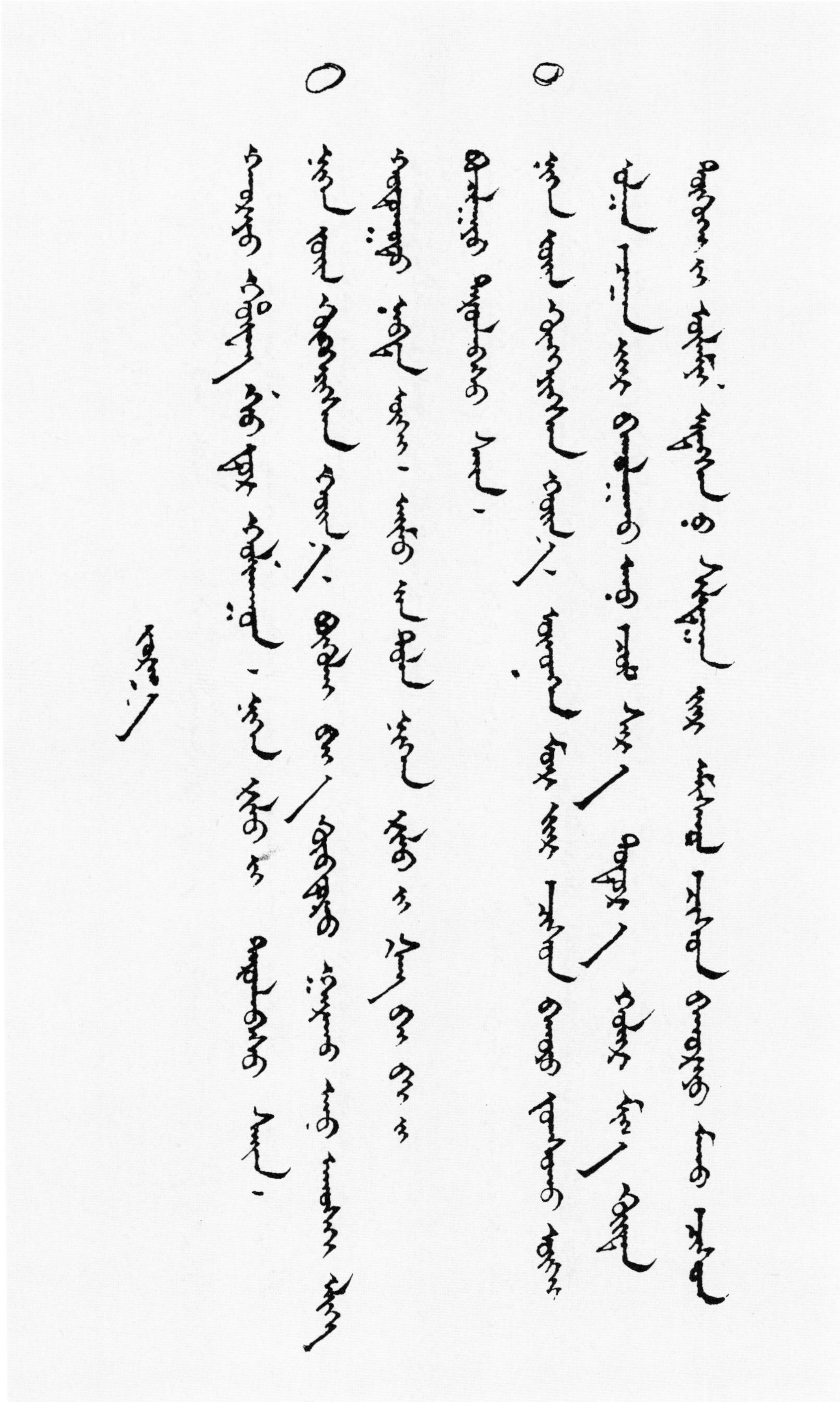

[illegible]

[illegible]

[illegible]

[illegible]

[illegible]

[illegible]

[illegible]

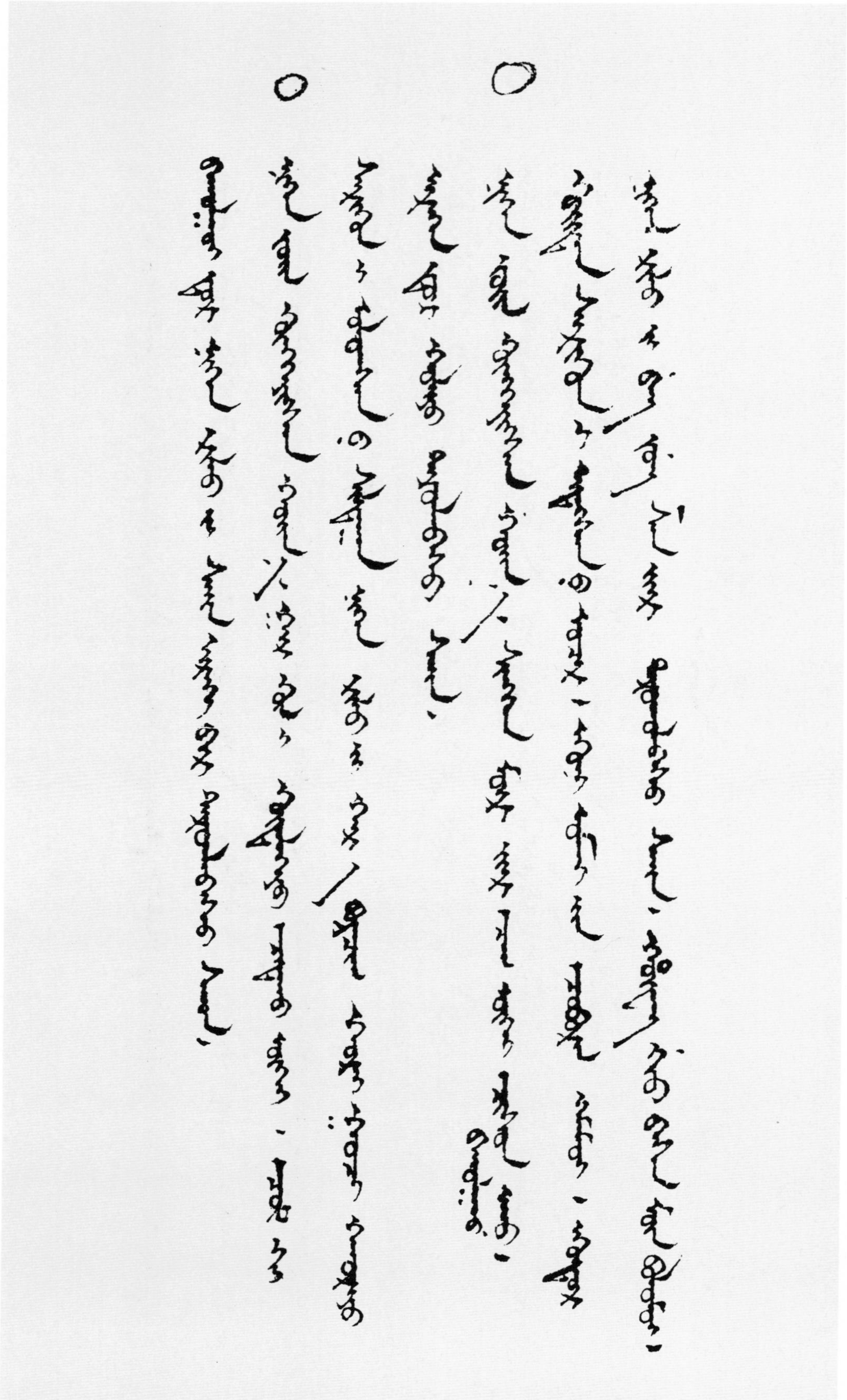

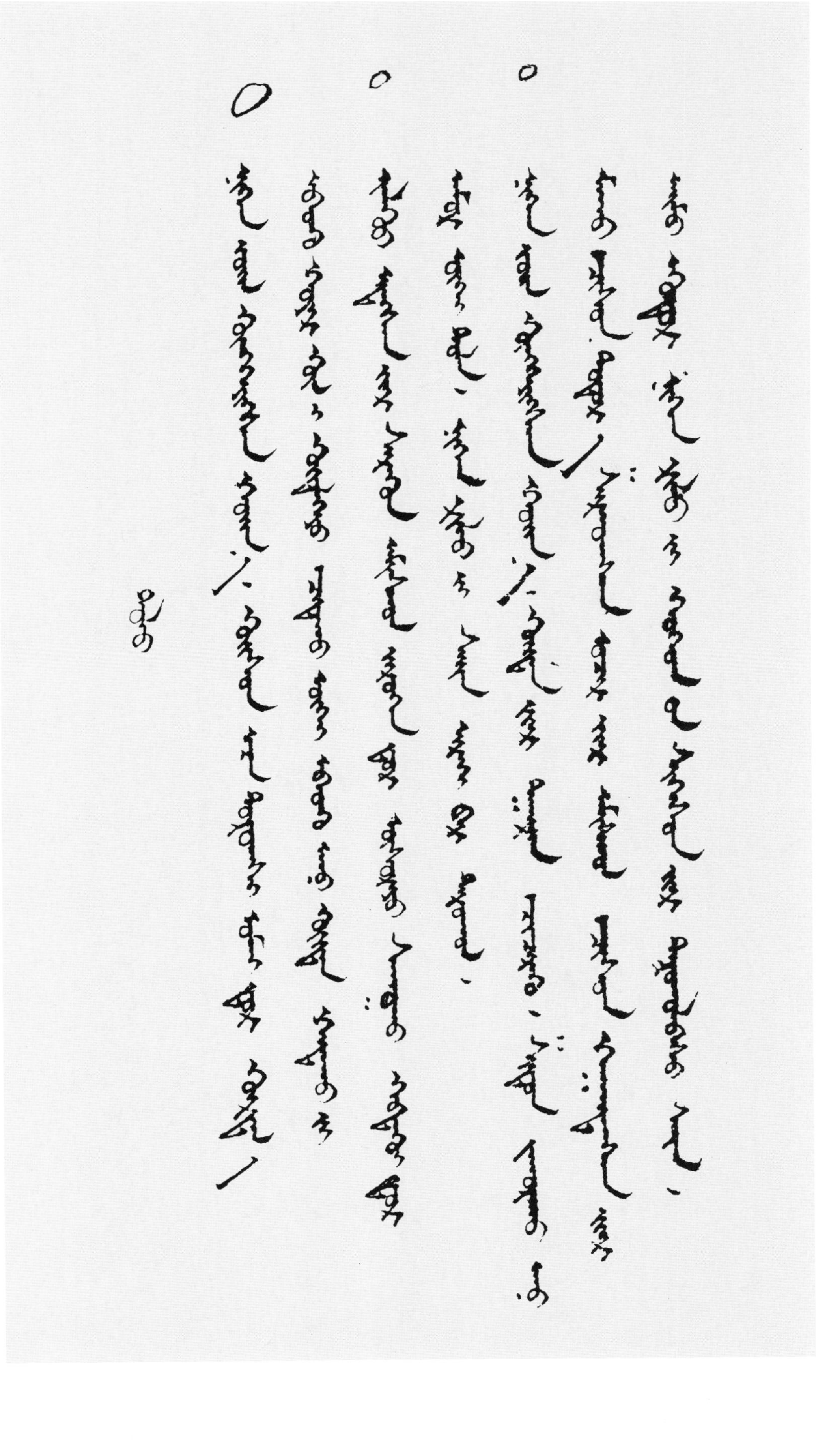

[illegible]

[illegible]

[illegible]

[illegible]

[illegible]

[illegible]

[illegible]

[illegible]

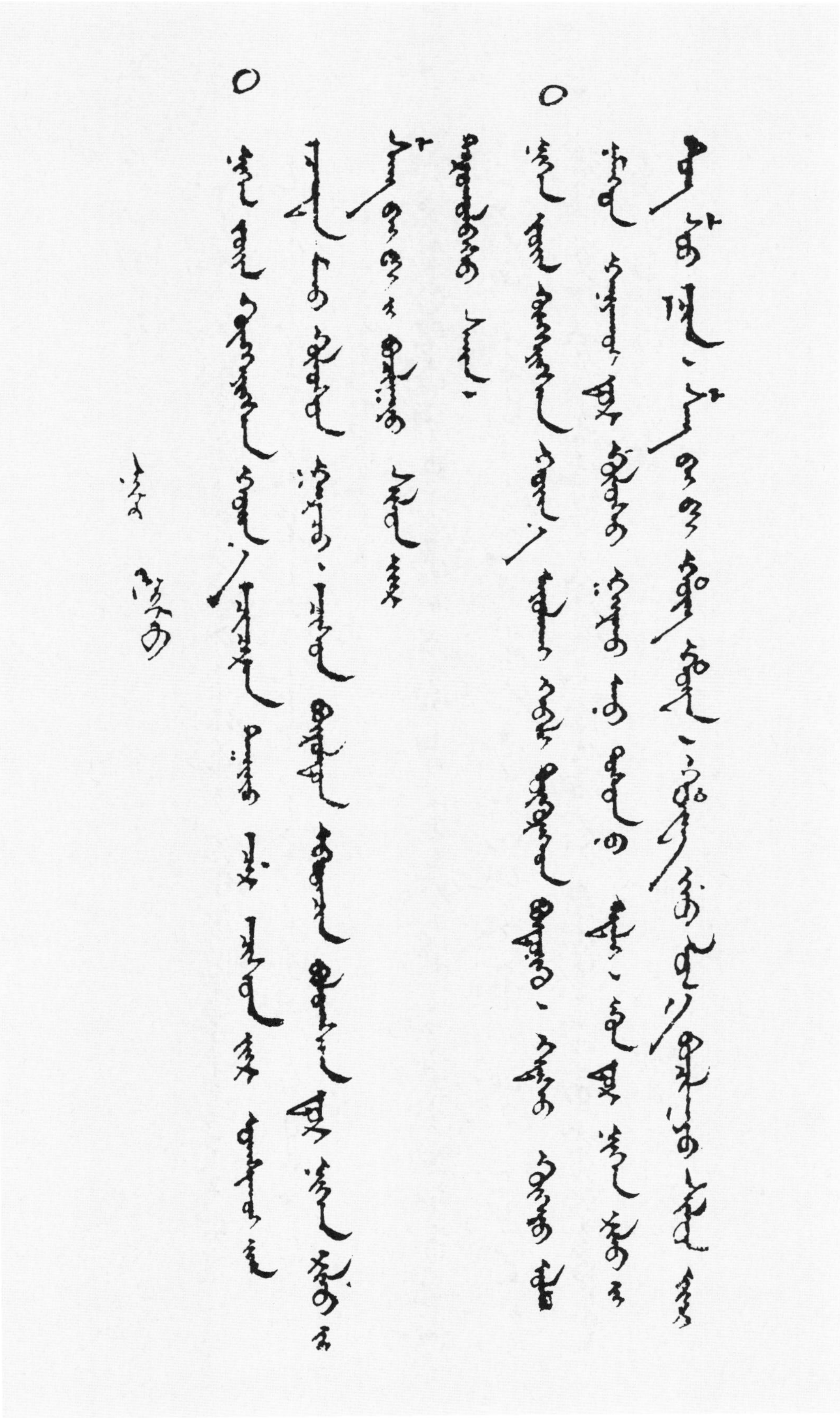

[illegible]

◯ [illegible]

[illegible]

◯ [illegible]

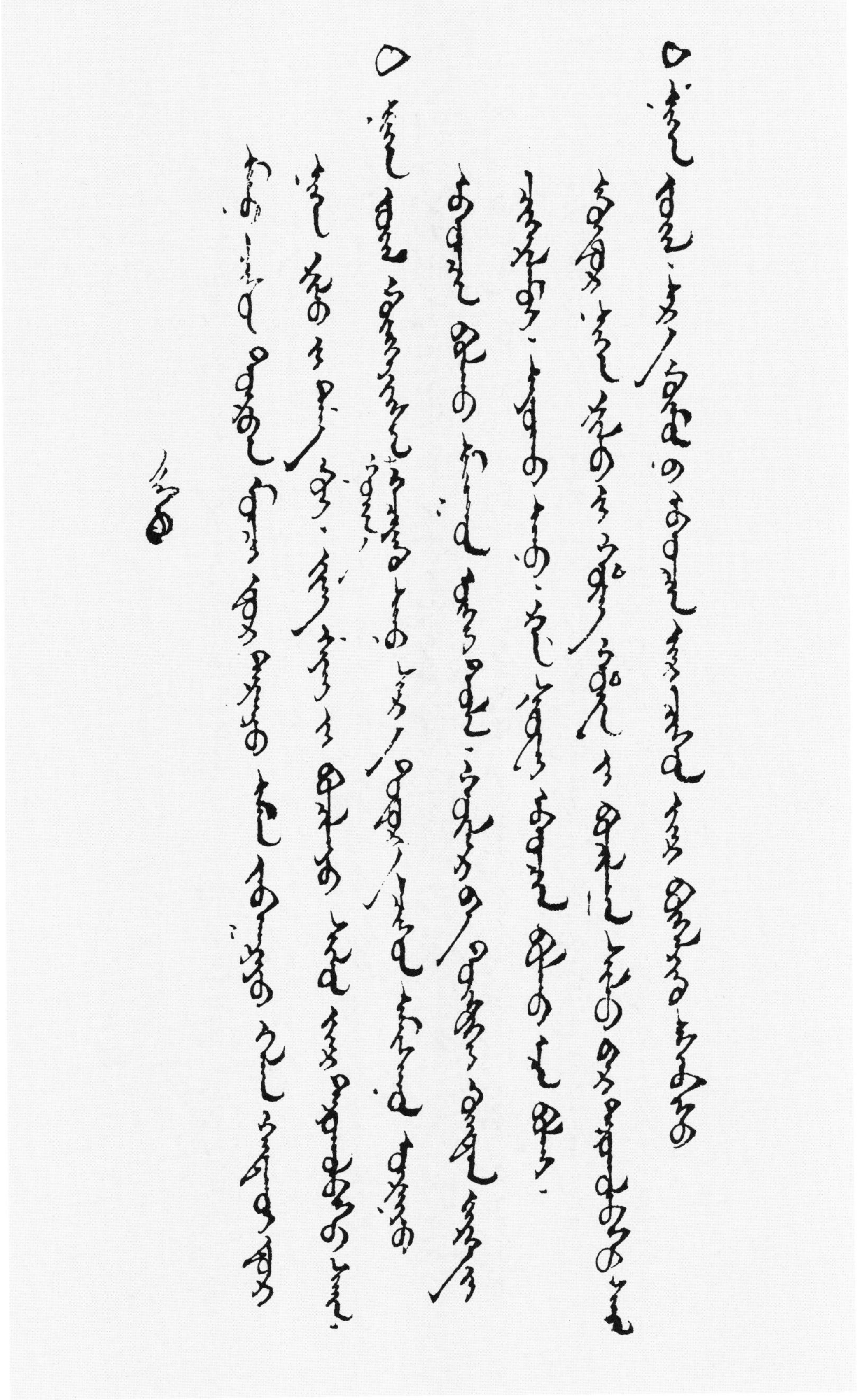

[illegible]
[illegible]
[illegible]
[illegible]
[illegible]
[illegible]
[illegible]

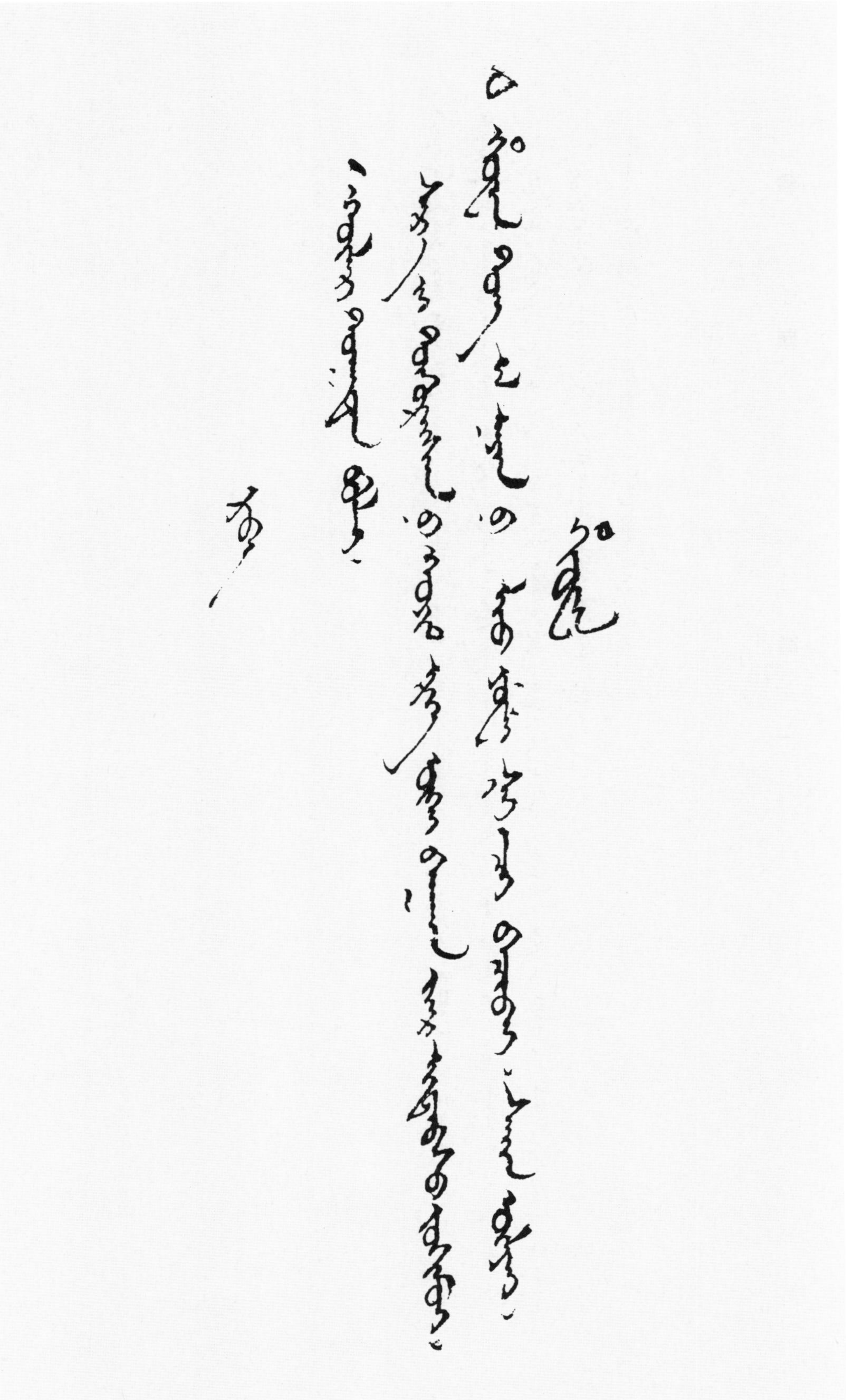

ᠠ ᠰᠢᠨᠵᠢᠯᠡᠯᠲᠡ ᠶᠢᠨ ᠪᠢᠴᠢᠭ ᠮᠣᠩᠭᠣᠯ ᠬᠡᠯᠡ ᠪᠡᠷ ᠪᠢᠴᠢᠭᠳᠡᠭᠰᠡᠨ ᠠ ᠪᠢᠴᠢᠭ ᠲᠠᠢ ᠬᠣᠯᠪᠣᠭᠳᠠᠬᠤ ᠬᠡᠷᠡᠭᠯᠡᠭᠳᠡᠬᠦᠨ ᠦ ᠬᠡᠪᠯᠡᠯ ᠦᠨ ᠳᠤᠷᠠᠰᠬᠠᠯ ᠪᠣᠯᠤᠨ᠎ᠠ ᠃
ᠬᠠᠪᠰᠤᠷᠤᠯᠲᠠ ᠪᠠᠨ ᠃ ᠮᠣᠩᠭᠣᠯ ᠪᠢᠴᠢᠭ ᠲᠤ ᠰᠢᠨᠵᠢᠯᠡᠯᠲᠡ ᠪᠣᠯᠤᠨ᠎ᠠ ᠃ ᠲᠤᠰ ᠨᠣᠮ ᠤᠨ ᠪᠢᠴᠢᠭ ᠮᠣᠩᠭᠣᠯ ᠬᠡᠯᠡ ᠪᠡᠷ ᠵᠢᠷᠤᠭ ᠤᠨ ᠬᠡᠷᠡᠭᠯᠡᠭᠳᠡᠬᠦᠨ ᠦ ᠬᠡᠪᠯᠡᠯ ᠦᠨ ᠳᠤᠷᠠᠰᠬᠠᠯ
ᠬᠠᠳᠠᠭᠠᠯᠠᠭᠳᠠᠵᠤ ᠪᠠᠢᠭ᠎ᠠ ᠶᠢᠨ ᠦᠢᠯᠡ ᠶᠢᠨ ᠲᠣᠪᠴᠢᠶ᠎ᠠ ᠶᠢᠨ ᠰᠤᠷᠭᠠᠭᠤᠯᠢ ᠳᠤ ᠬᠠᠳᠠᠭᠠᠯᠠᠭᠳᠠᠵᠤ ᠪᠠᠢᠨ᠎ᠠ ᠃ ᠲᠤᠰ ᠨᠣᠮ ᠤᠨ ᠪᠢᠴᠢᠭ ᠤᠨ ᠦᠰᠦᠭ ᠦᠨ ᠪᠢᠴᠢᠯᠭᠡ
ᠪᠣᠳᠠ ᠨᠢ ᠬᠡᠮᠵᠢᠶ᠎ᠡ ᠨᠢ : 15cm×18cm ᠪᠣᠯᠤᠨ᠎ᠠ ᠂ ᠨᠡᠢᠲᠡ 82 ᠨᠢᠭᠤᠷ ᠲᠠᠢ ᠃
ᠣᠳᠣ ᠥᠪᠥᠷ ᠮᠣᠩᠭᠣᠯ ᠤᠨ ᠨᠣᠮ ᠤᠨ ᠰᠠᠩ ᠳᠤ ᠬᠠᠳᠠᠭᠠᠯᠠᠭᠳᠠᠵᠤ ᠪᠠᠢᠨ᠎ᠠ ᠃

120 Kinds of Pill Medicine

丸散药方一百二十种

9

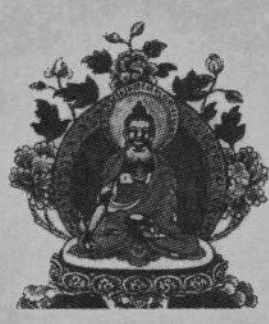

[illegible]

[illegible]

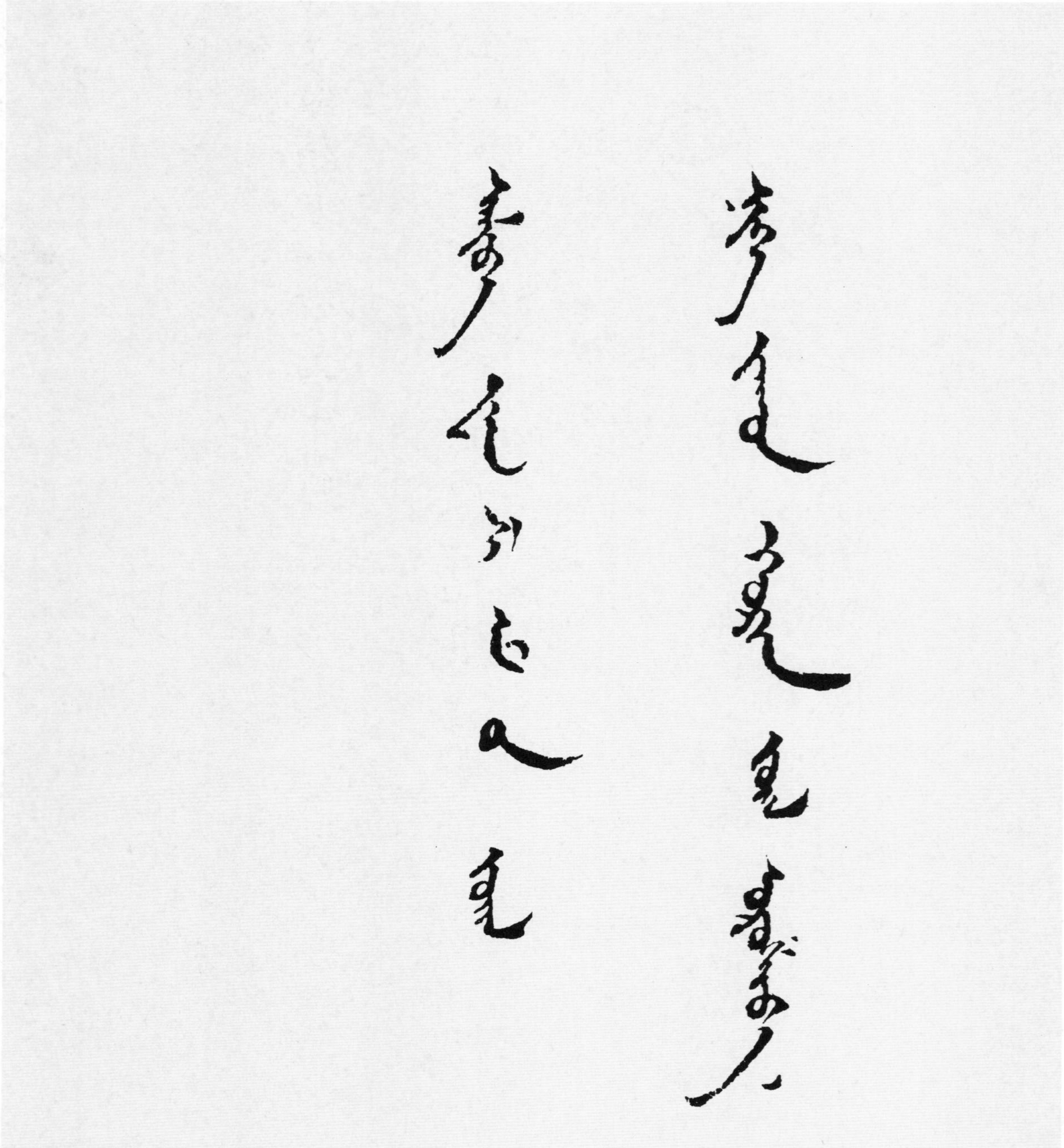

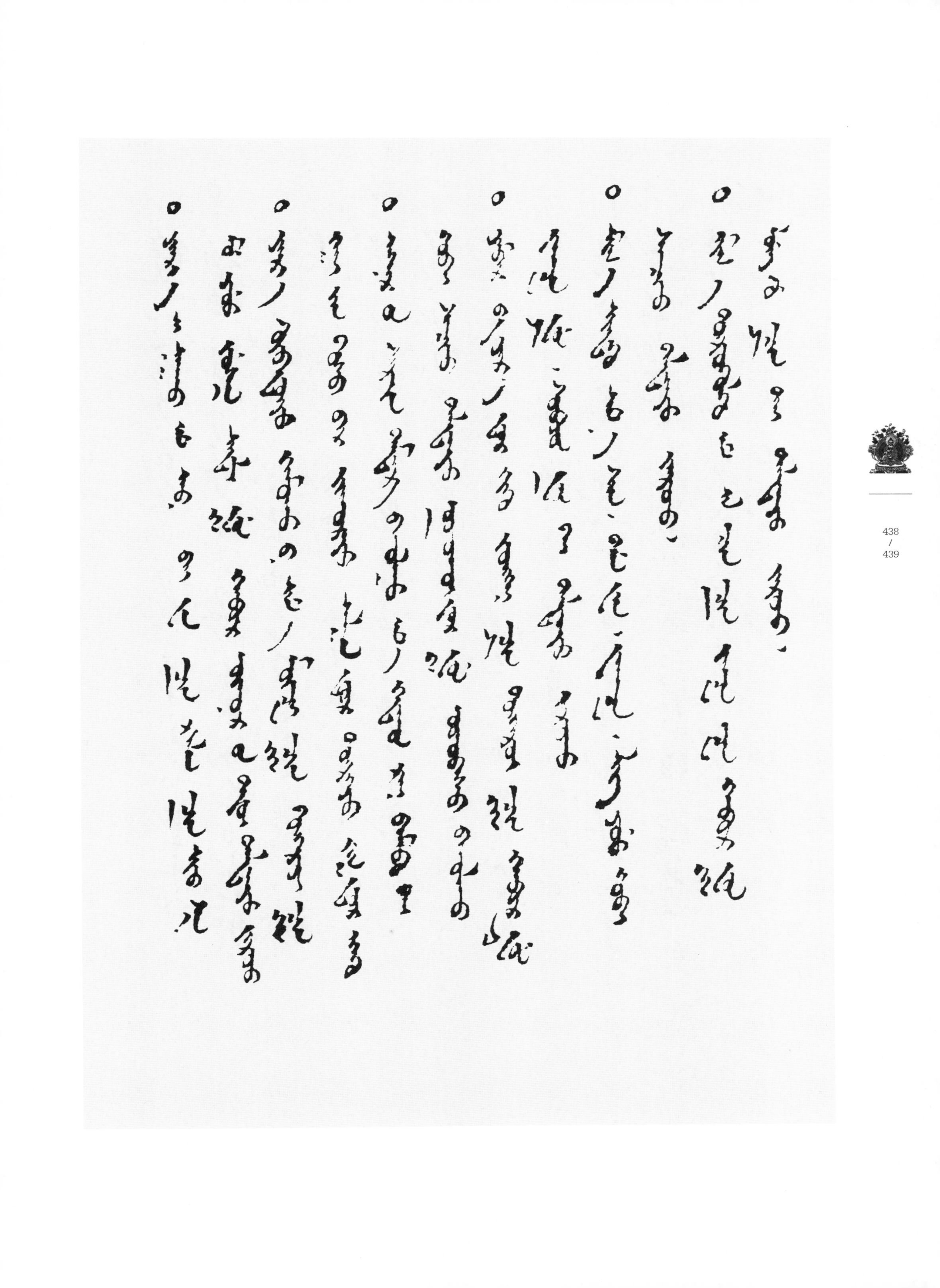

[illegible]

[illegible]

[illegible]

[illegible]

[illegible]

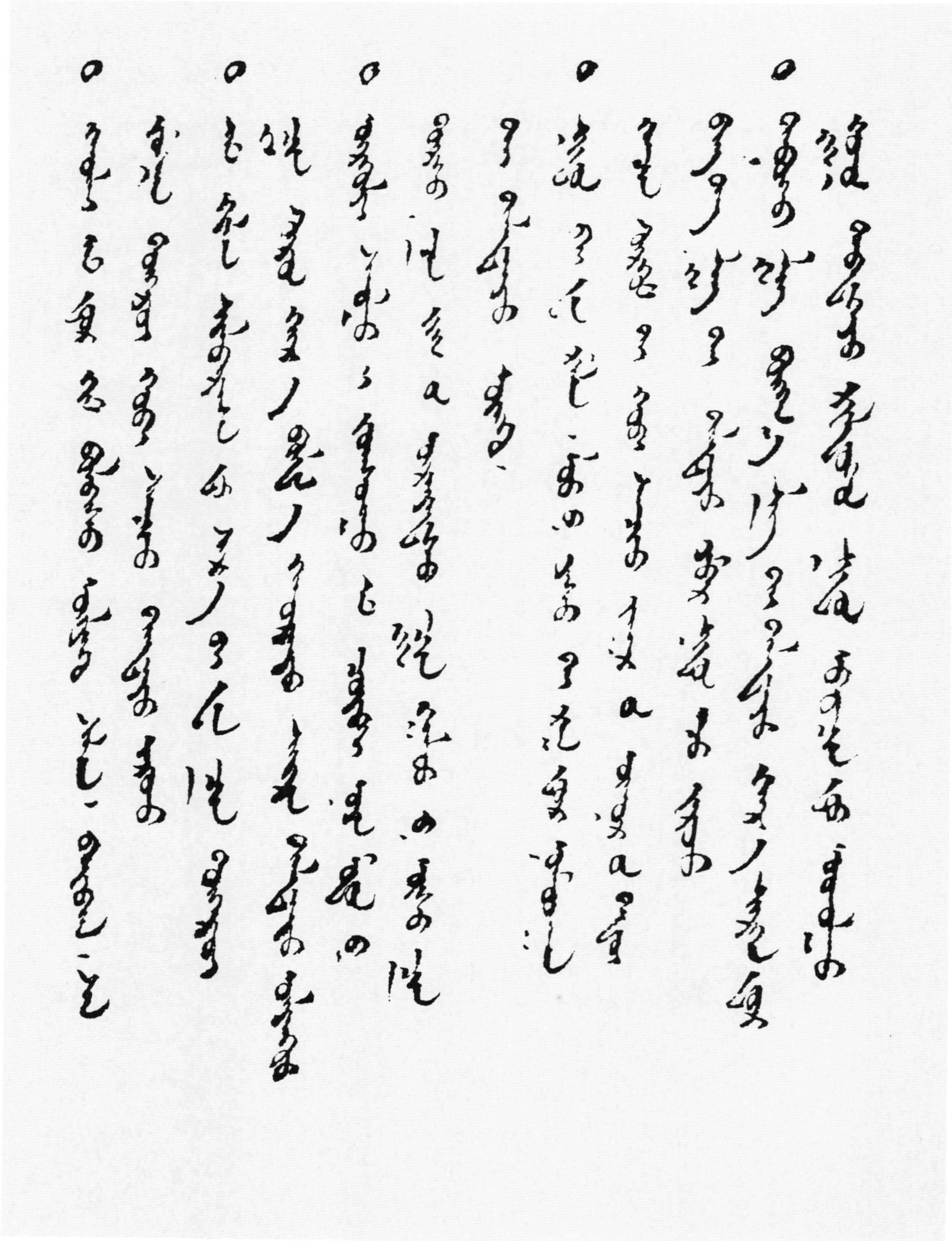

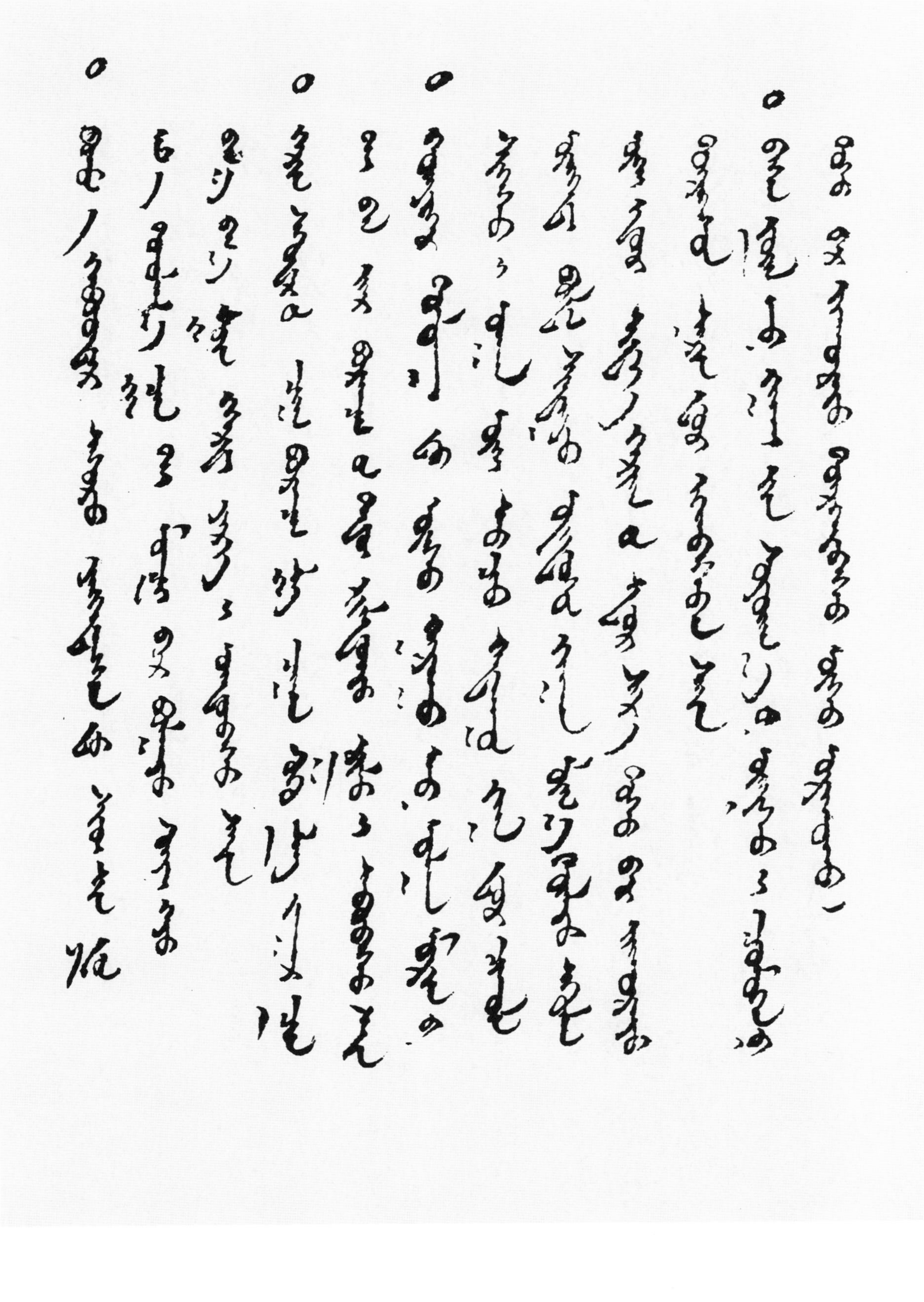

[illegible]

[illegible]

[illegible]

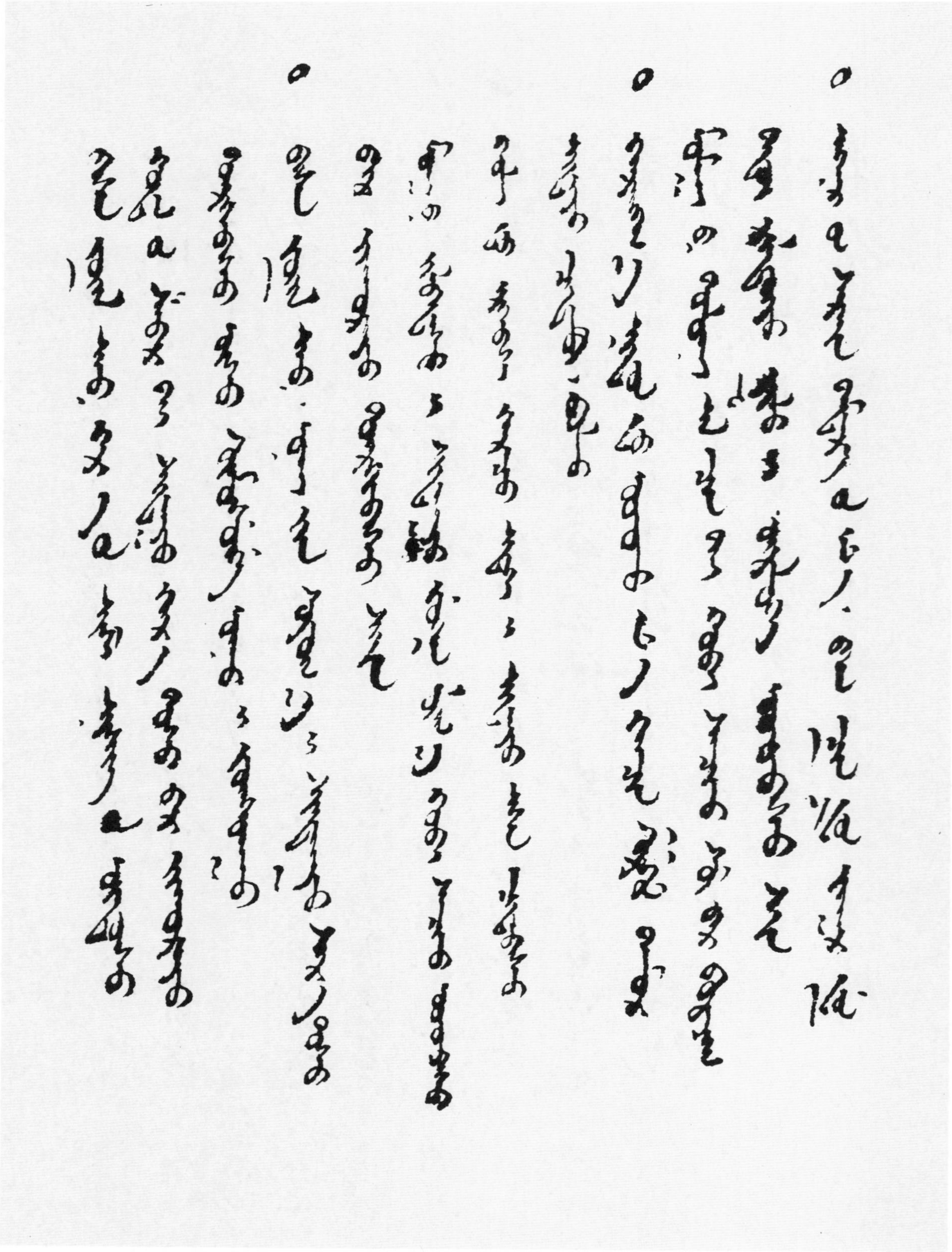

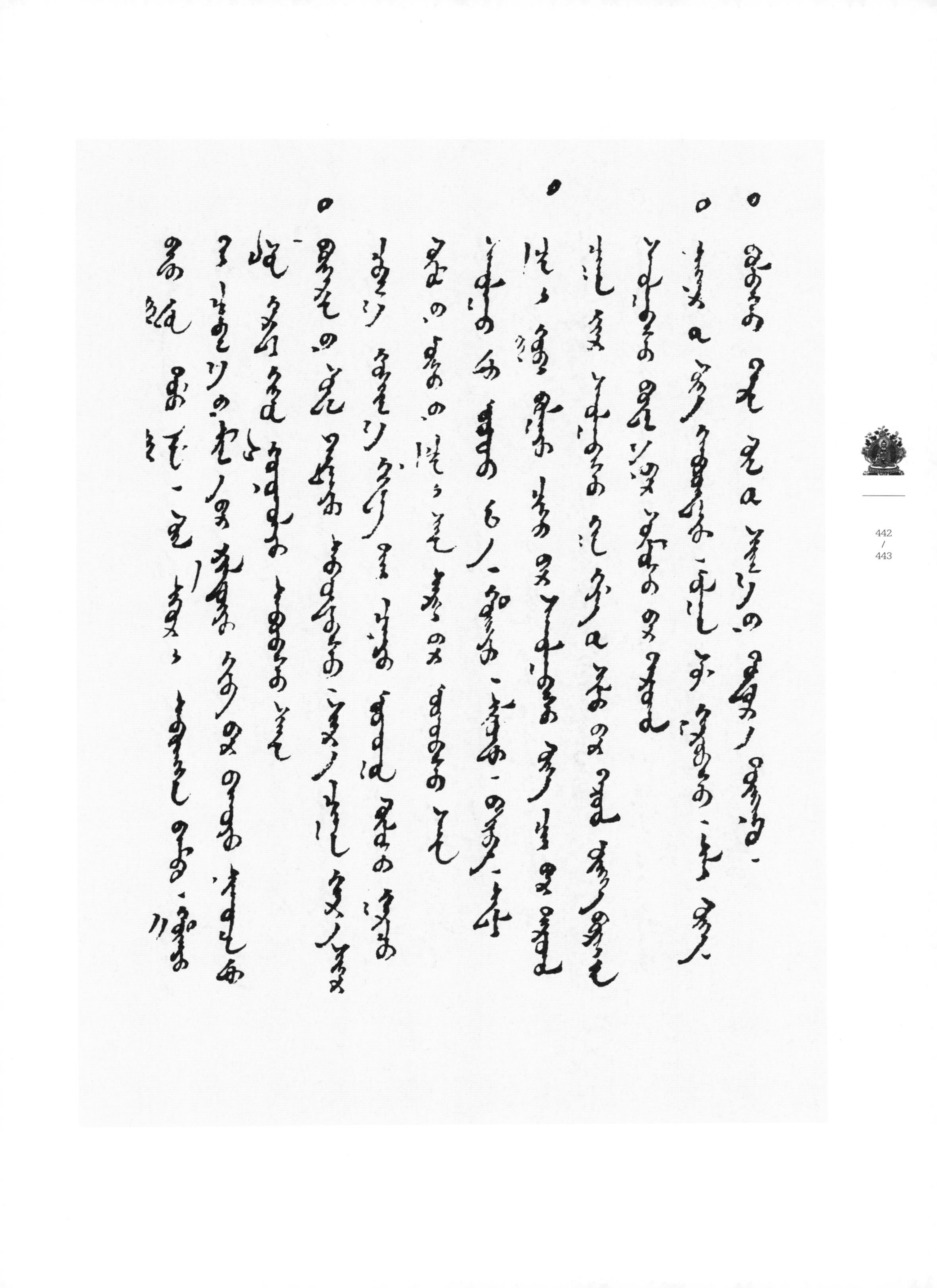

[illegible]

[illegible]

[illegible]

[illegible]

[illegible]

[illegible]

[illegible]

[illegible]

[illegible]

[illegible]

[illegible]

[illegible]

[illegible]

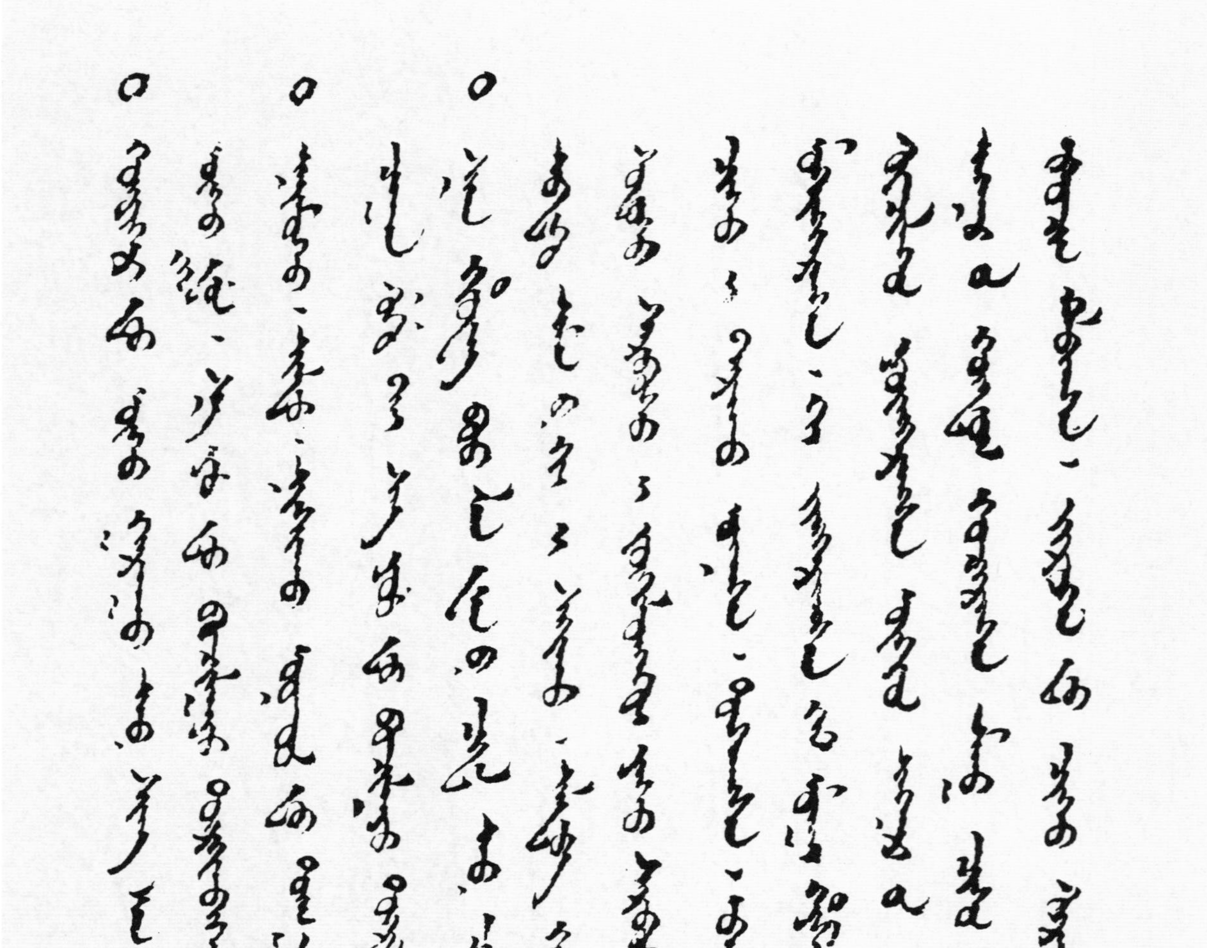

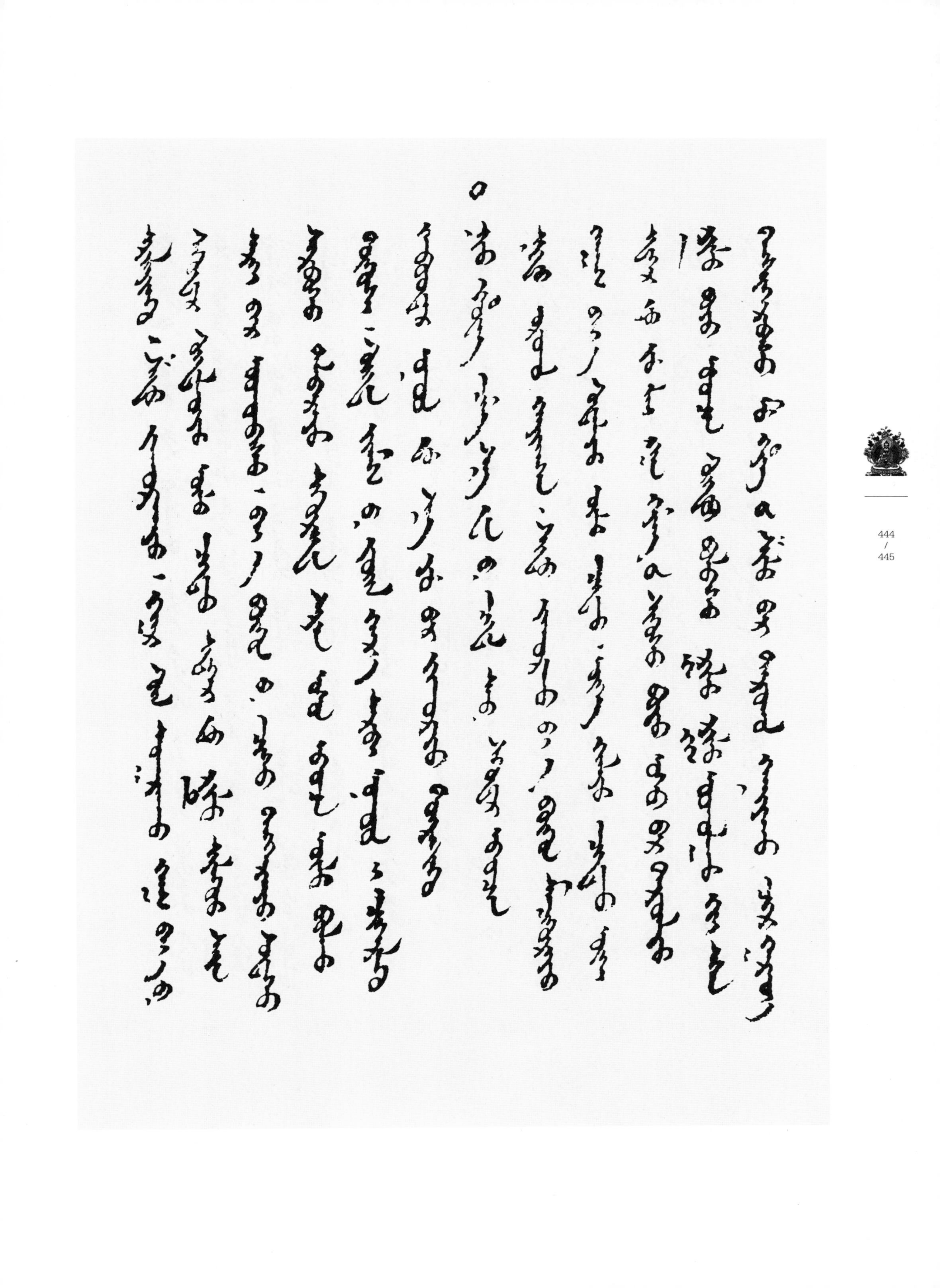

[illegible]

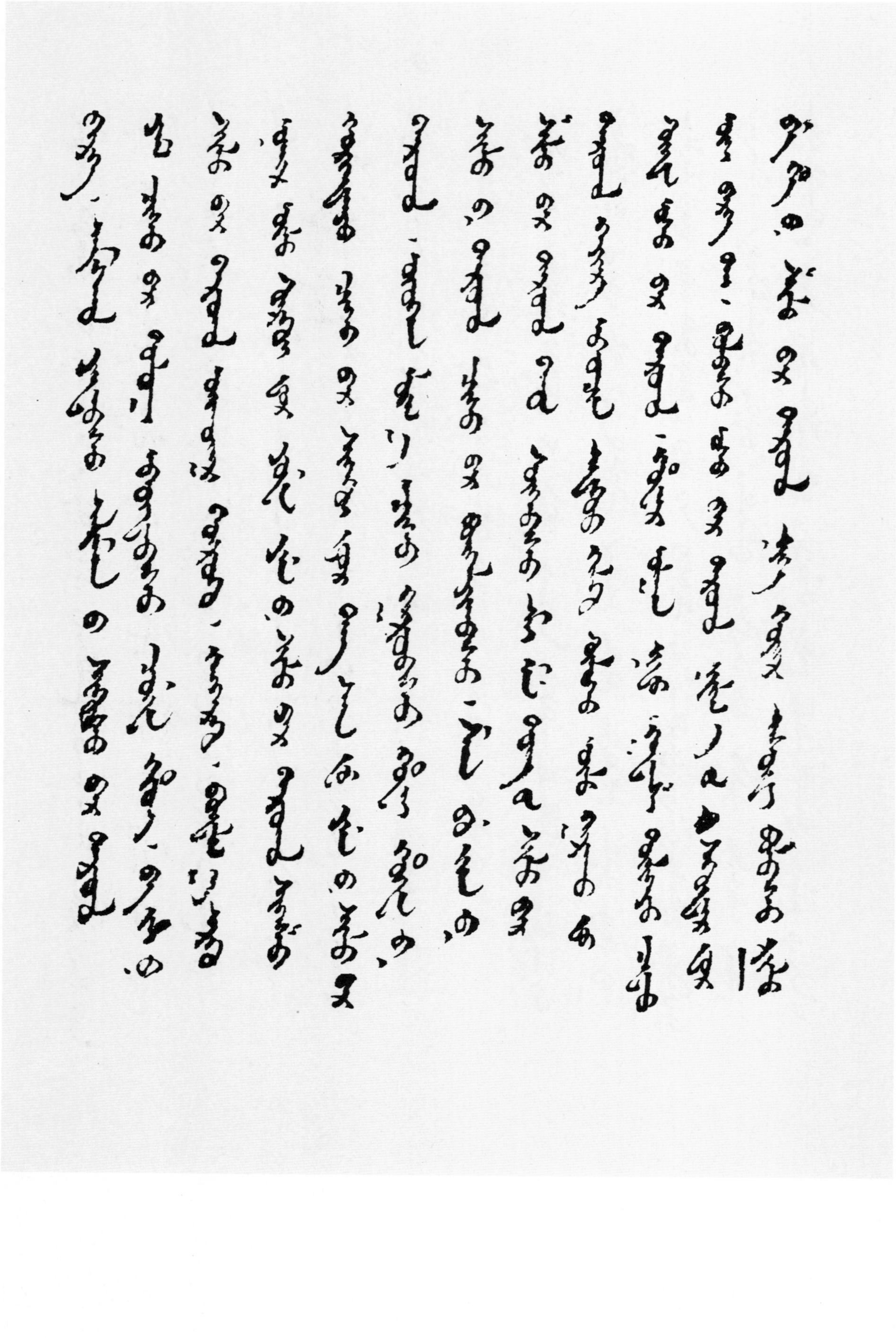

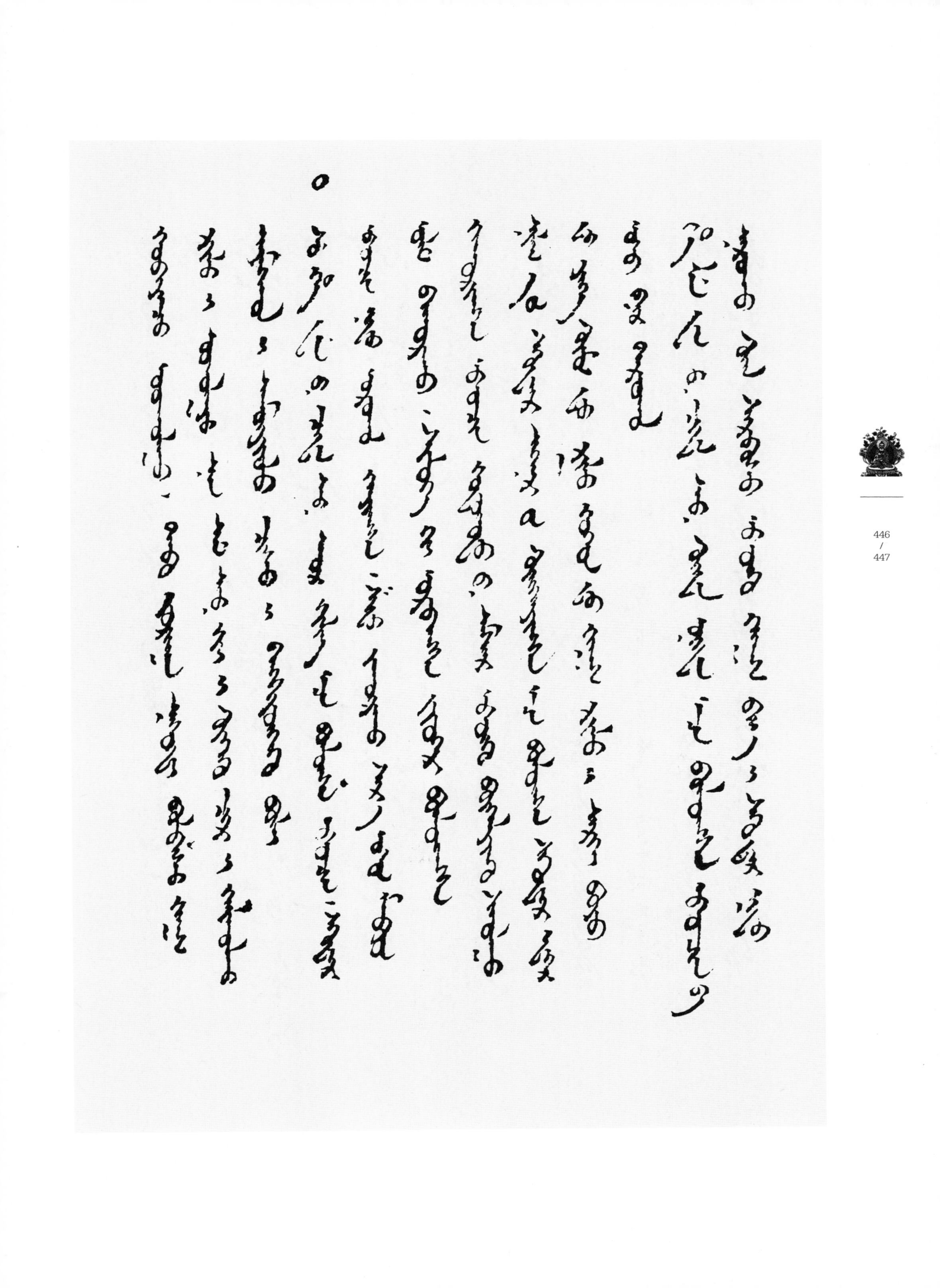

[illegible]

[illegible]

[illegible]

[illegible]

[illegible]

[illegible]

[illegible]

[illegible]

[illegible]

[illegible]

[illegible]

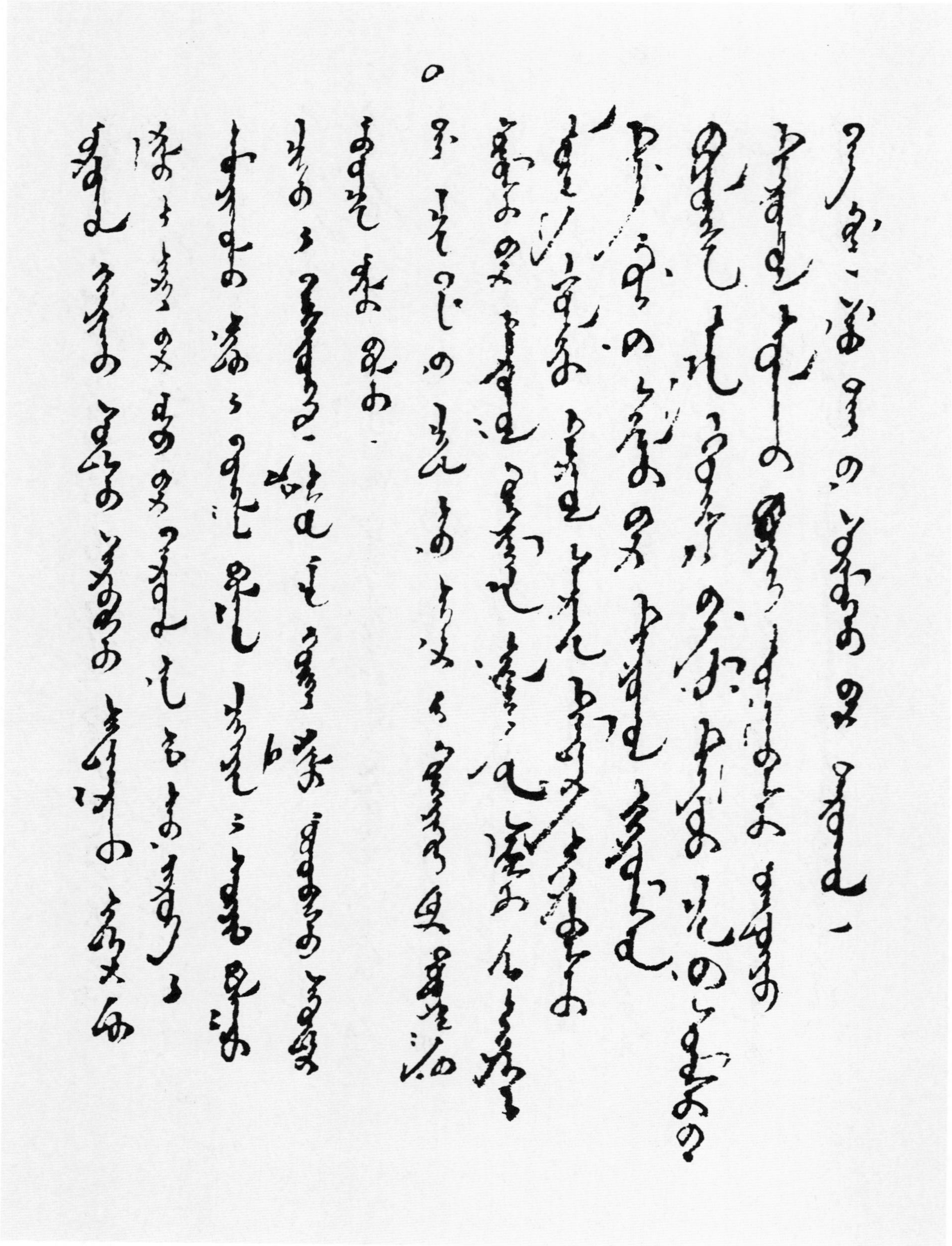

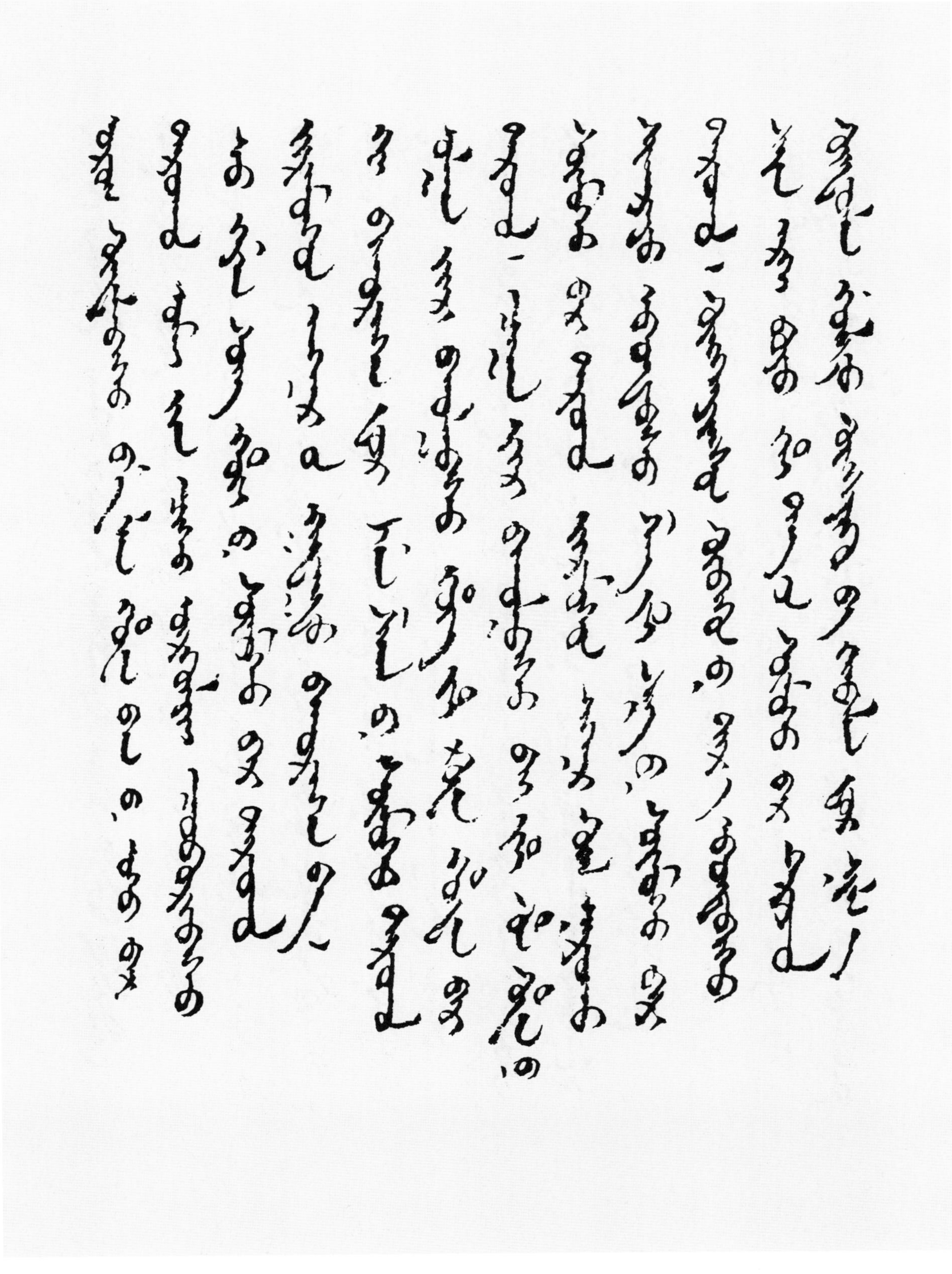

[illegible]
[illegible]
[illegible]
[illegible]
[illegible]
[illegible]
[illegible]
[illegible]
[illegible]
[illegible]
[illegible]
[illegible]

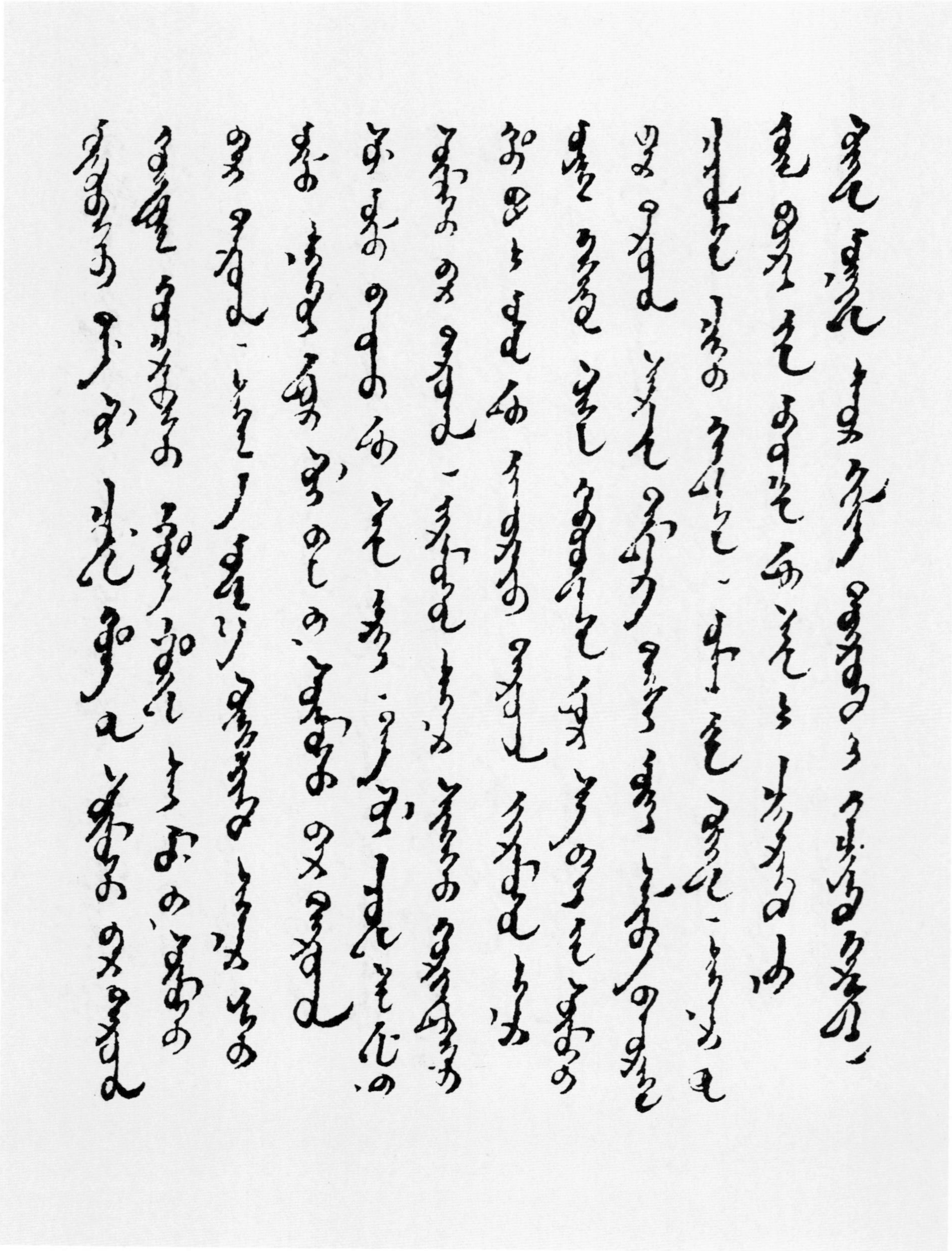

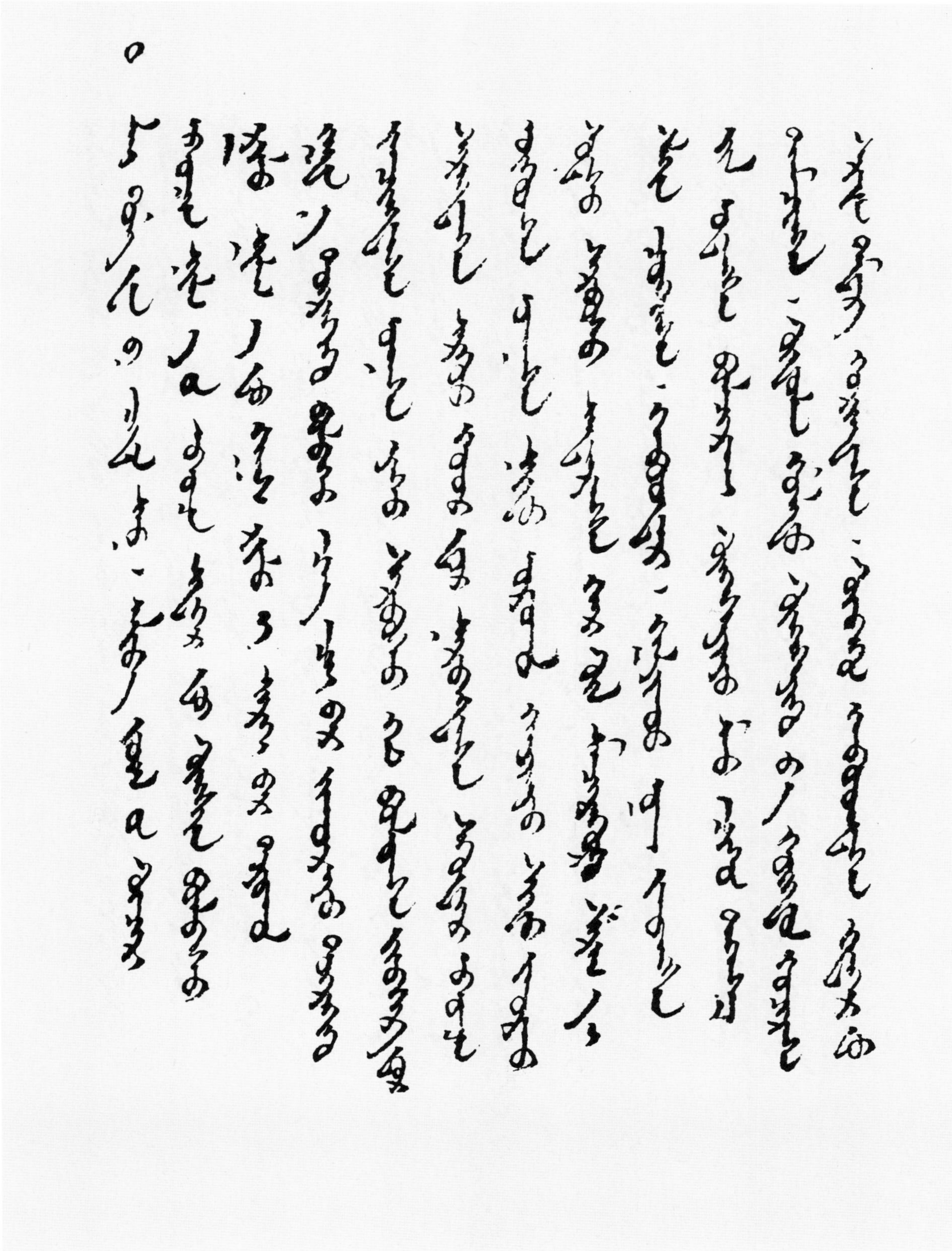

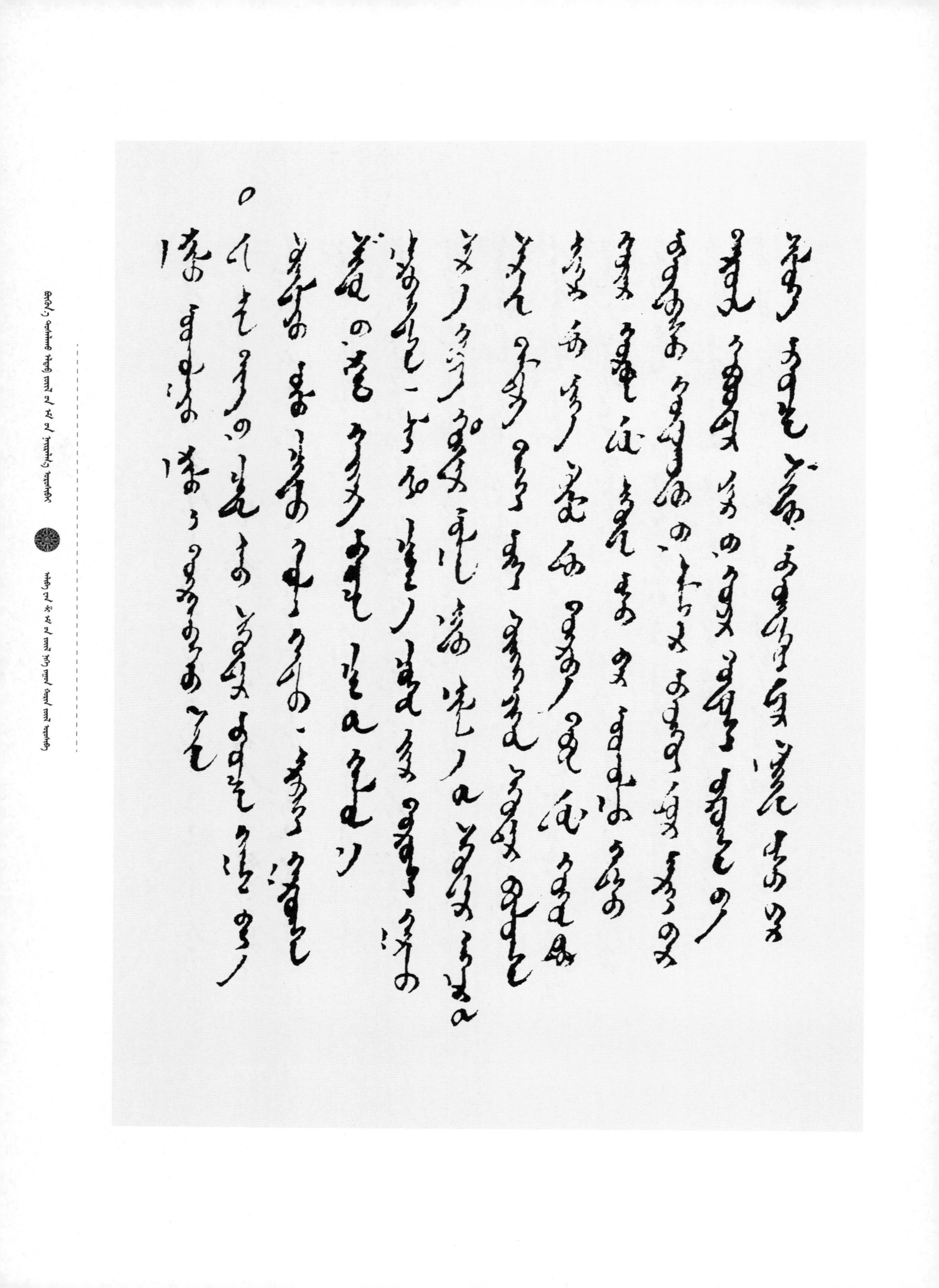

[illegible]

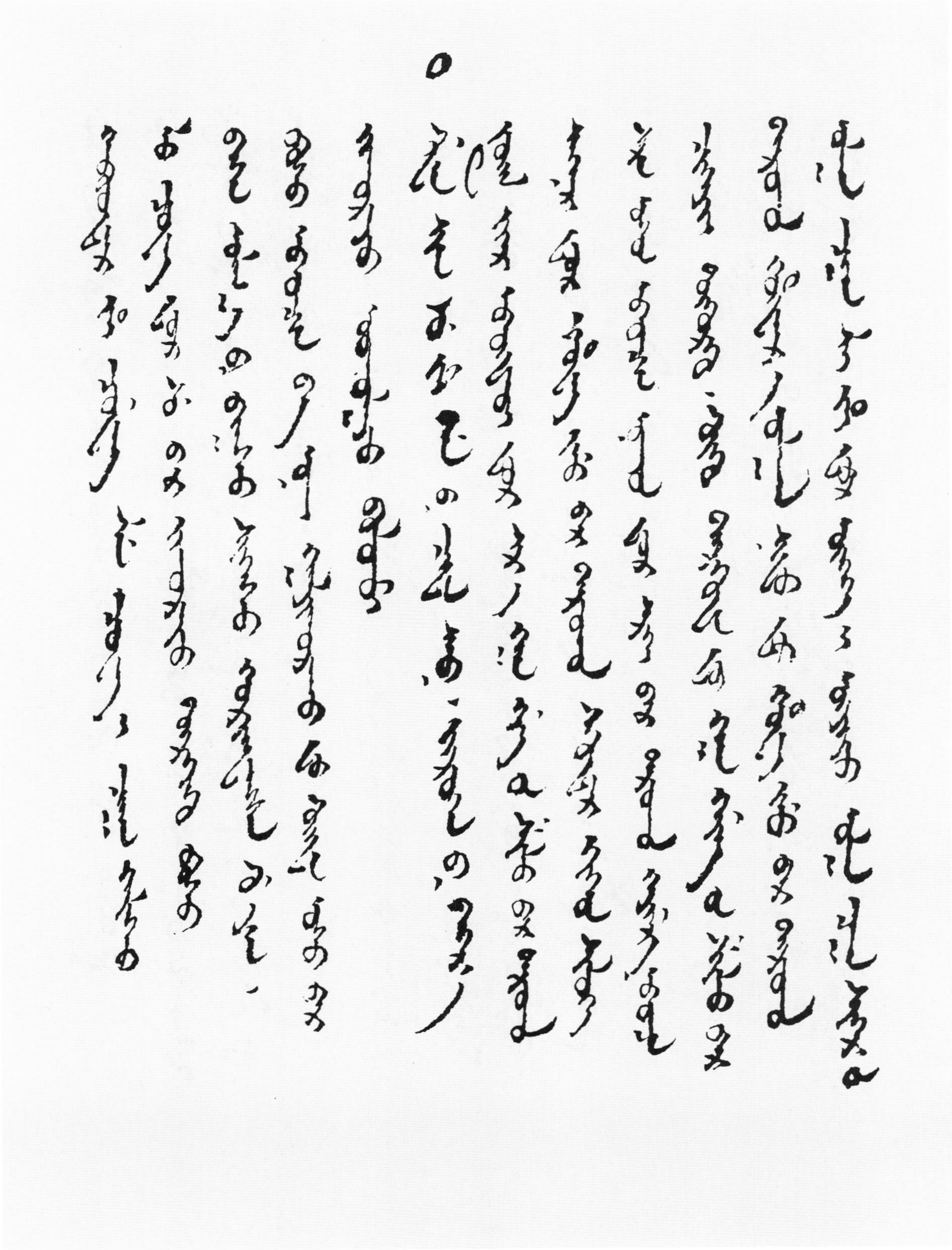

[illegible]
[illegible]
[illegible]
[illegible]
[illegible]
[illegible]
[illegible]
[illegible]
[illegible]
[illegible]
[illegible]
[illegible]

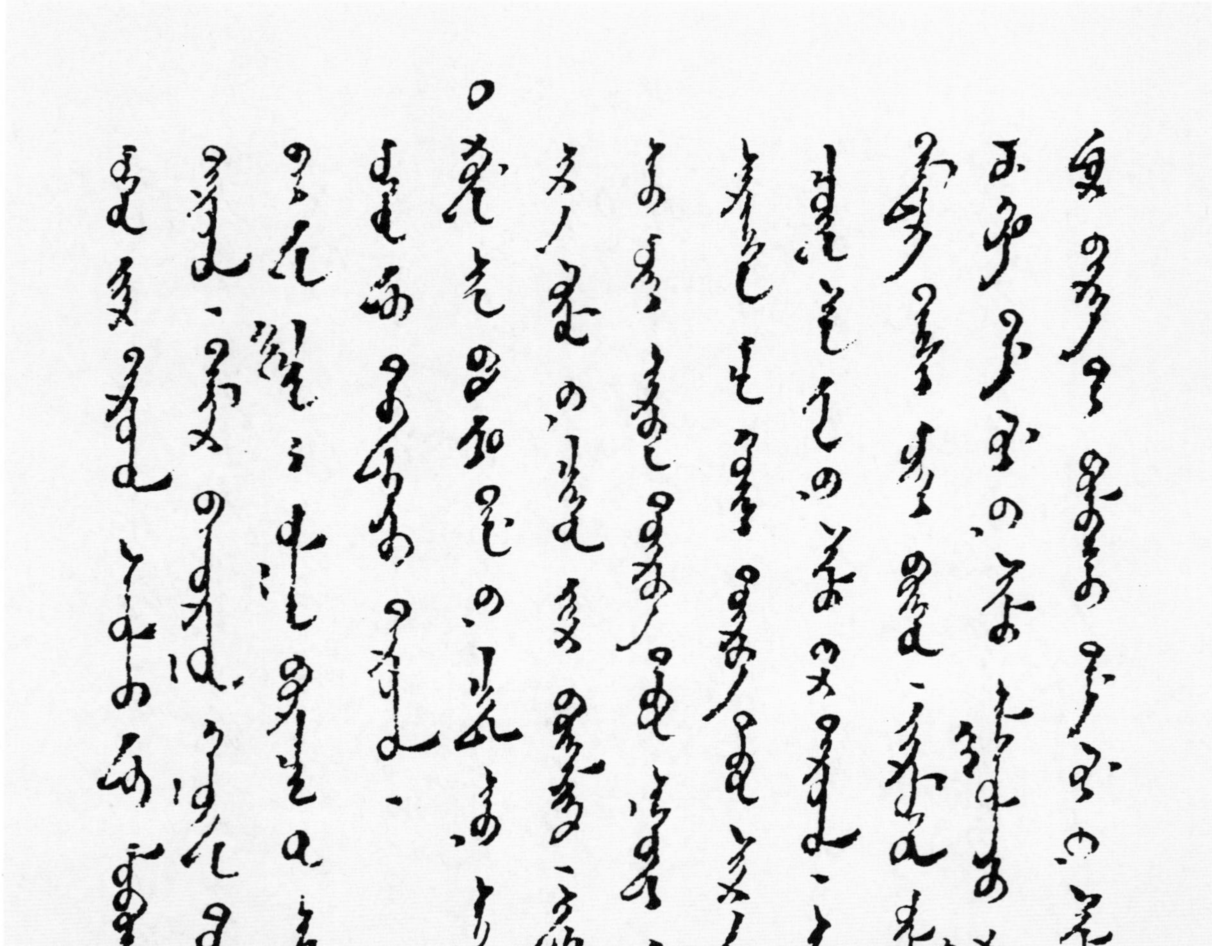

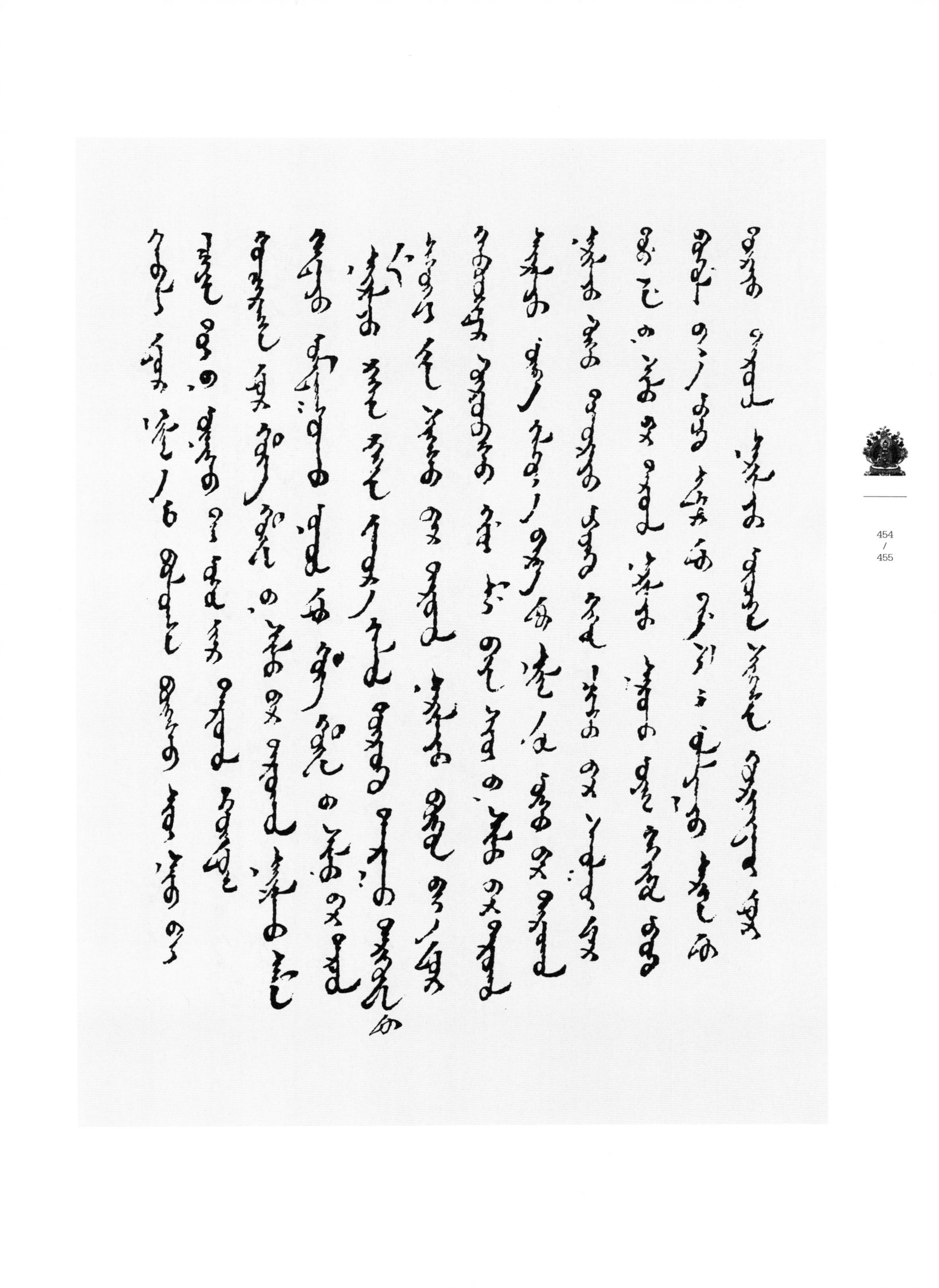

[illegible]
[illegible]
[illegible]
[illegible]
[illegible]
[illegible]
[illegible]
[illegible]
[illegible]
[illegible]
[illegible]
[illegible]
[illegible]
[illegible]

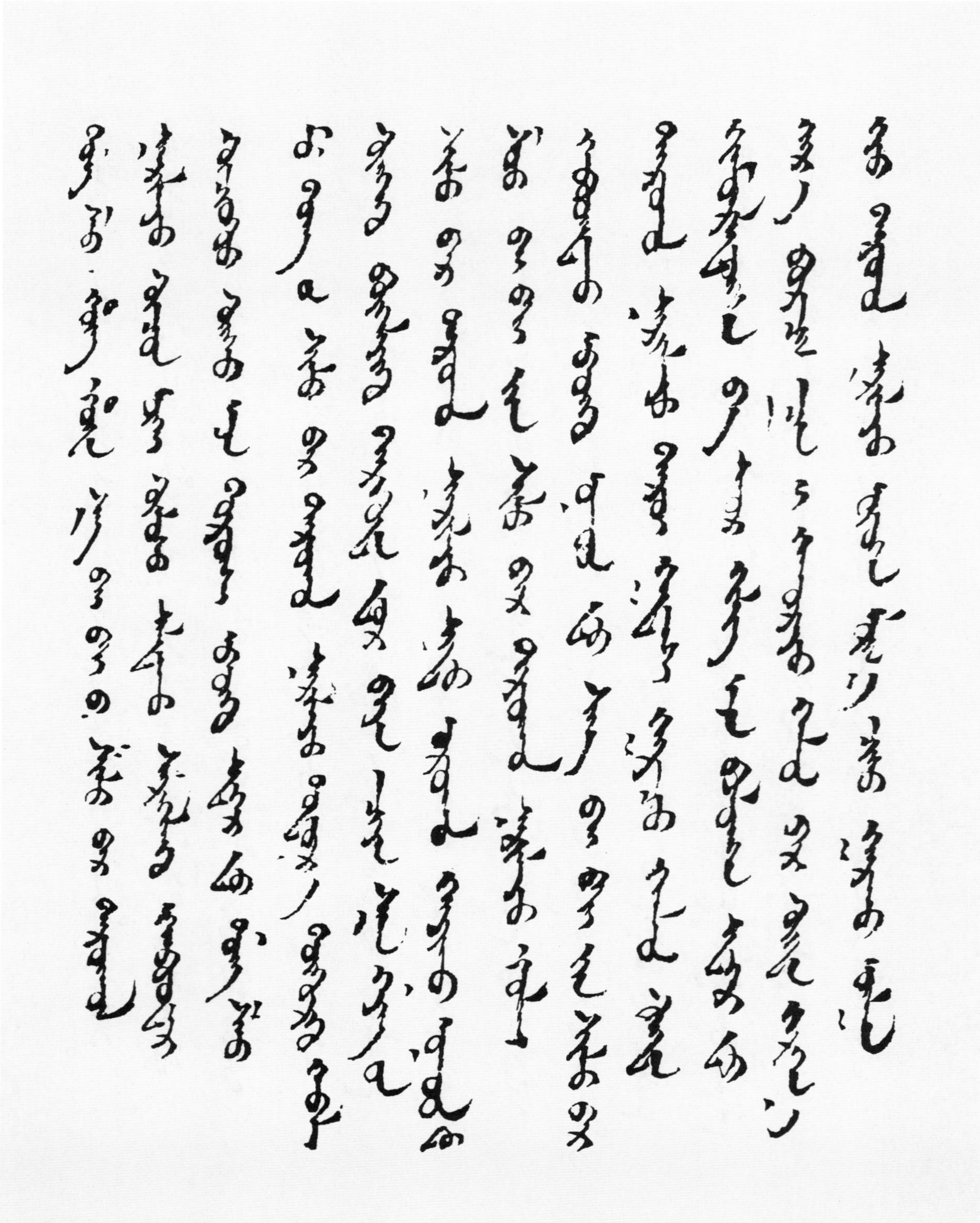

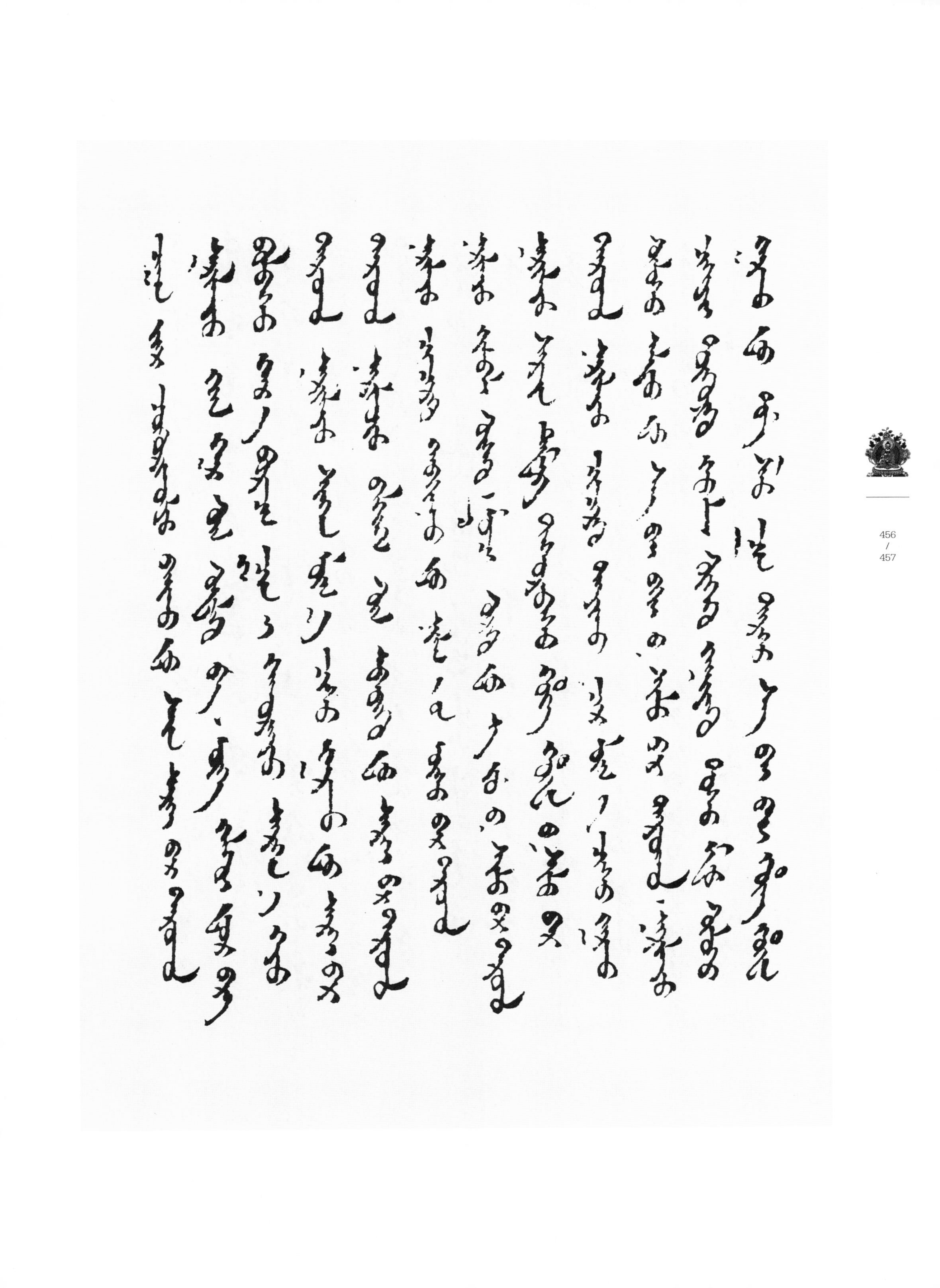

[illegible]

[illegible]

[illegible]

[illegible]

[illegible]

[illegible]

[illegible]

[illegible]

[illegible]

[illegible]

[illegible]

[illegible]

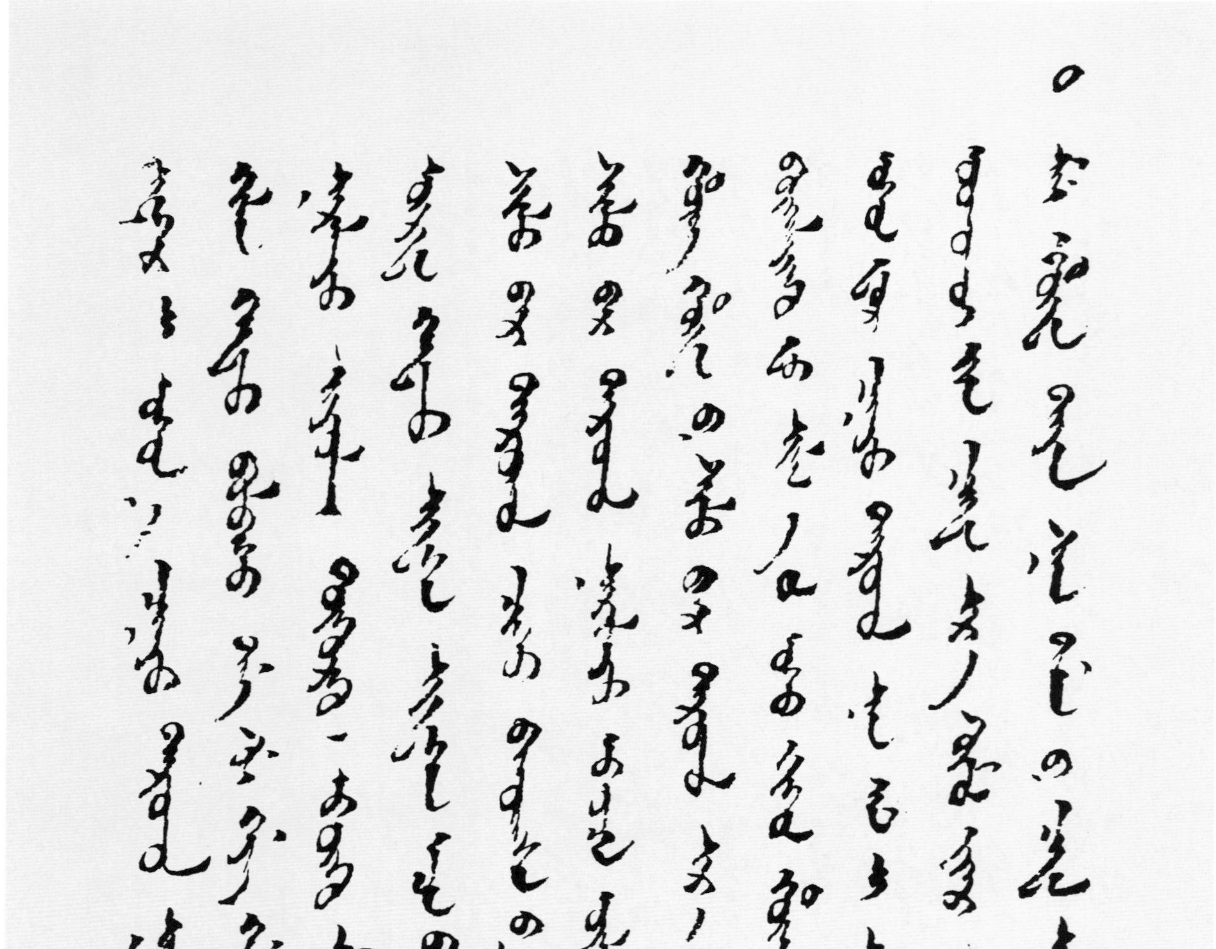

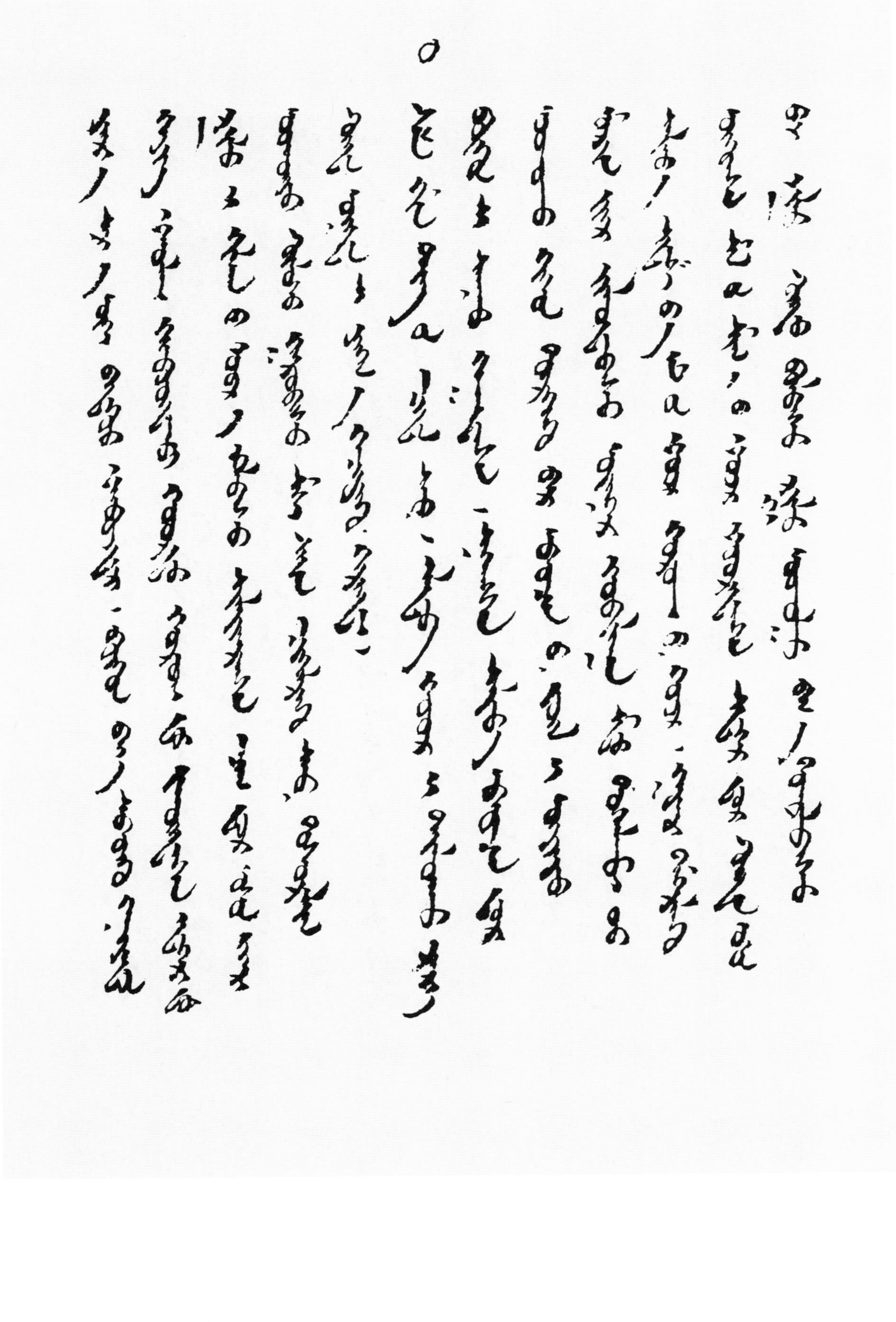

[illegible]
[illegible]
[illegible]
[illegible]
[illegible]
[illegible]
[illegible]
[illegible]
[illegible]
[illegible]
[illegible]
[illegible]
[illegible]
[illegible]

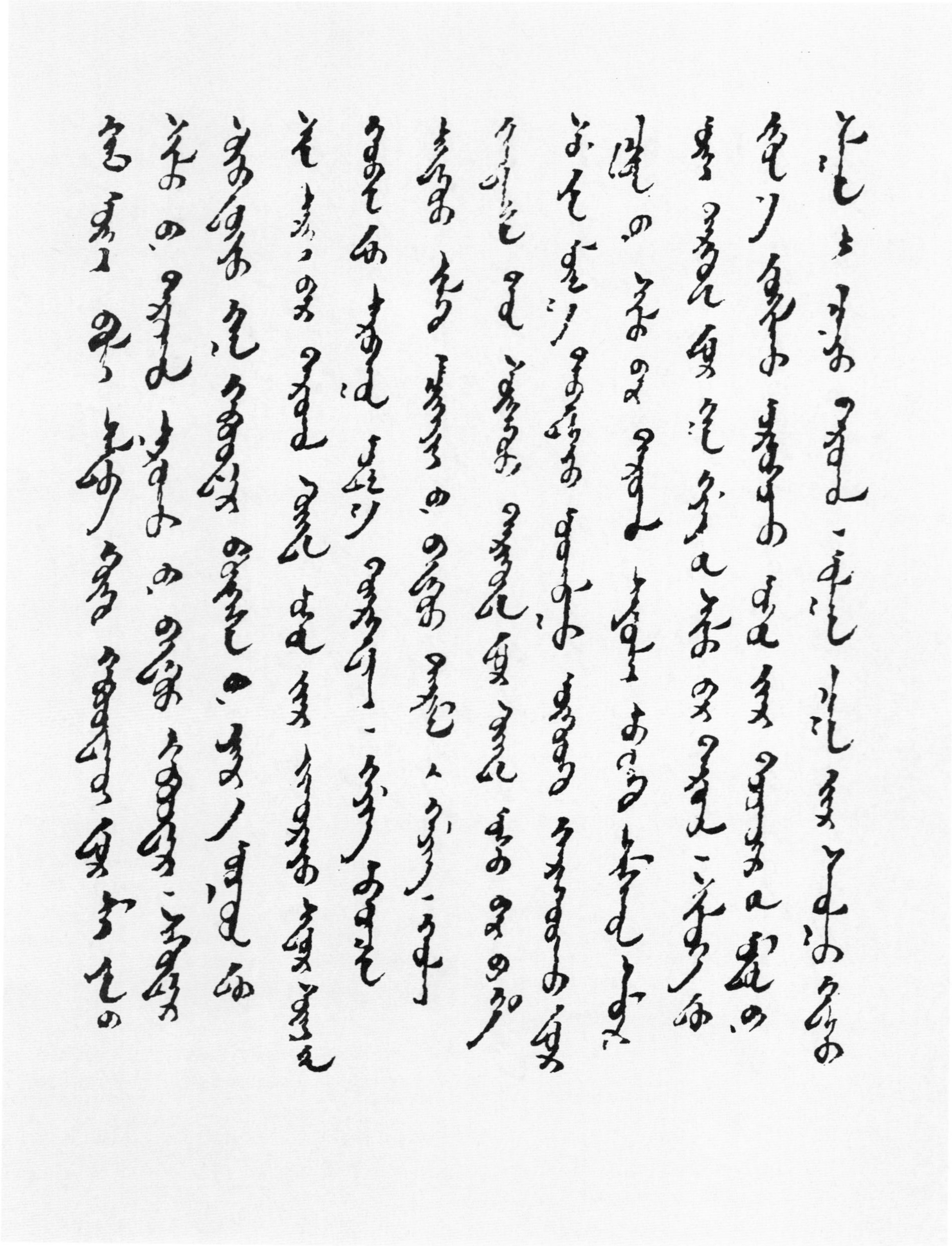

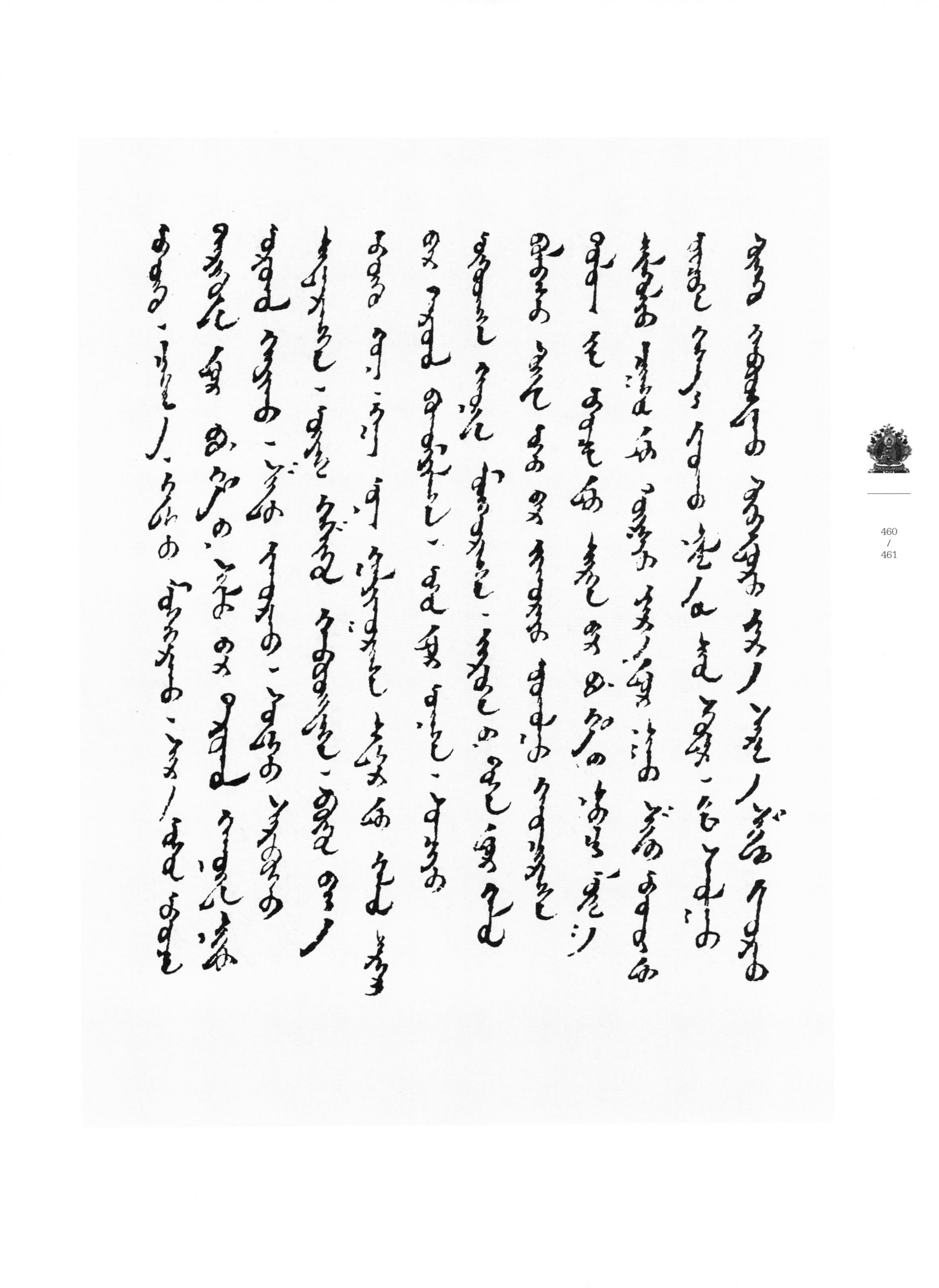

[illegible]

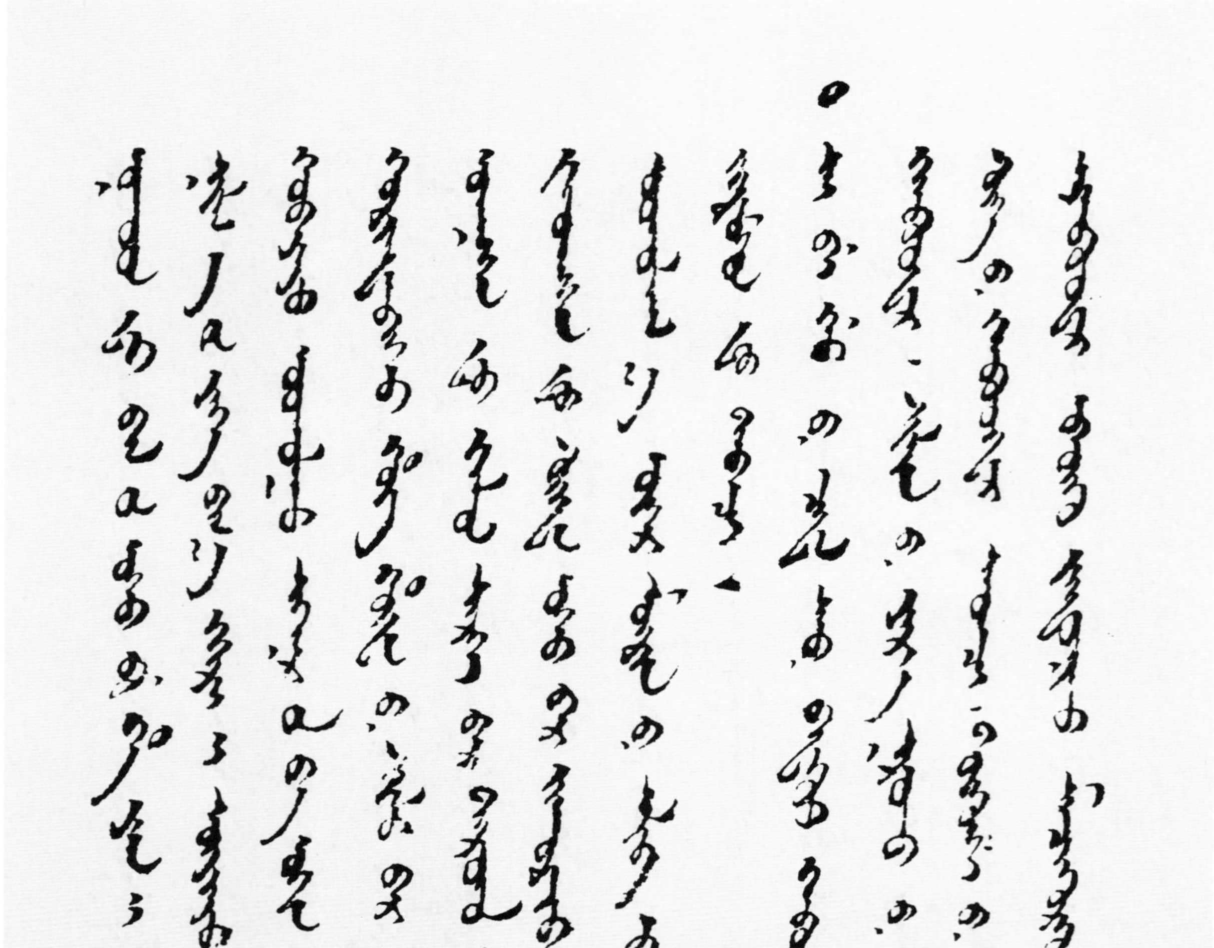

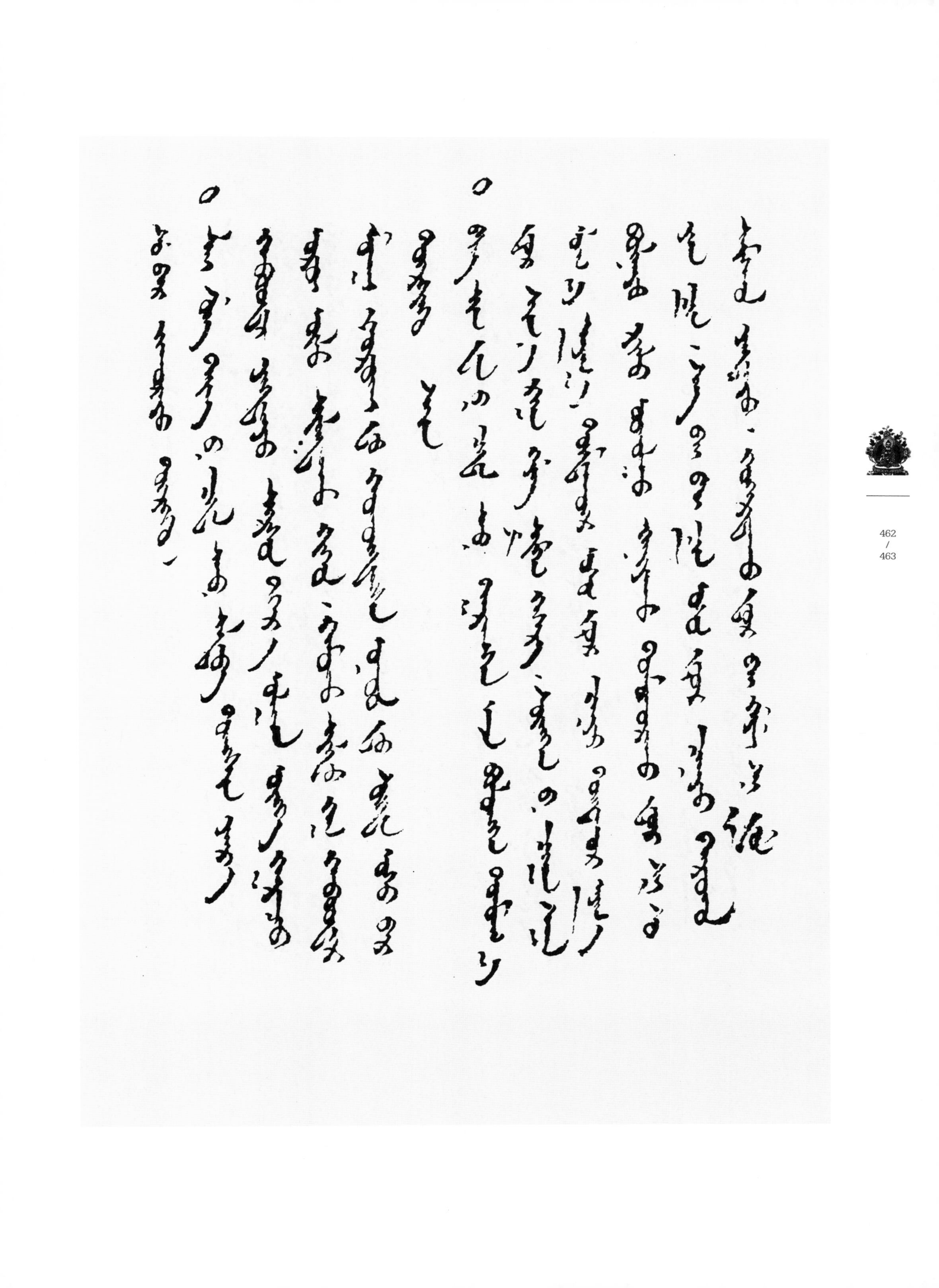

[illegible]
[illegible]
[illegible]
[illegible]
[illegible]
[illegible]
[illegible]
[illegible]
[illegible]
[illegible]
[illegible]
[illegible]

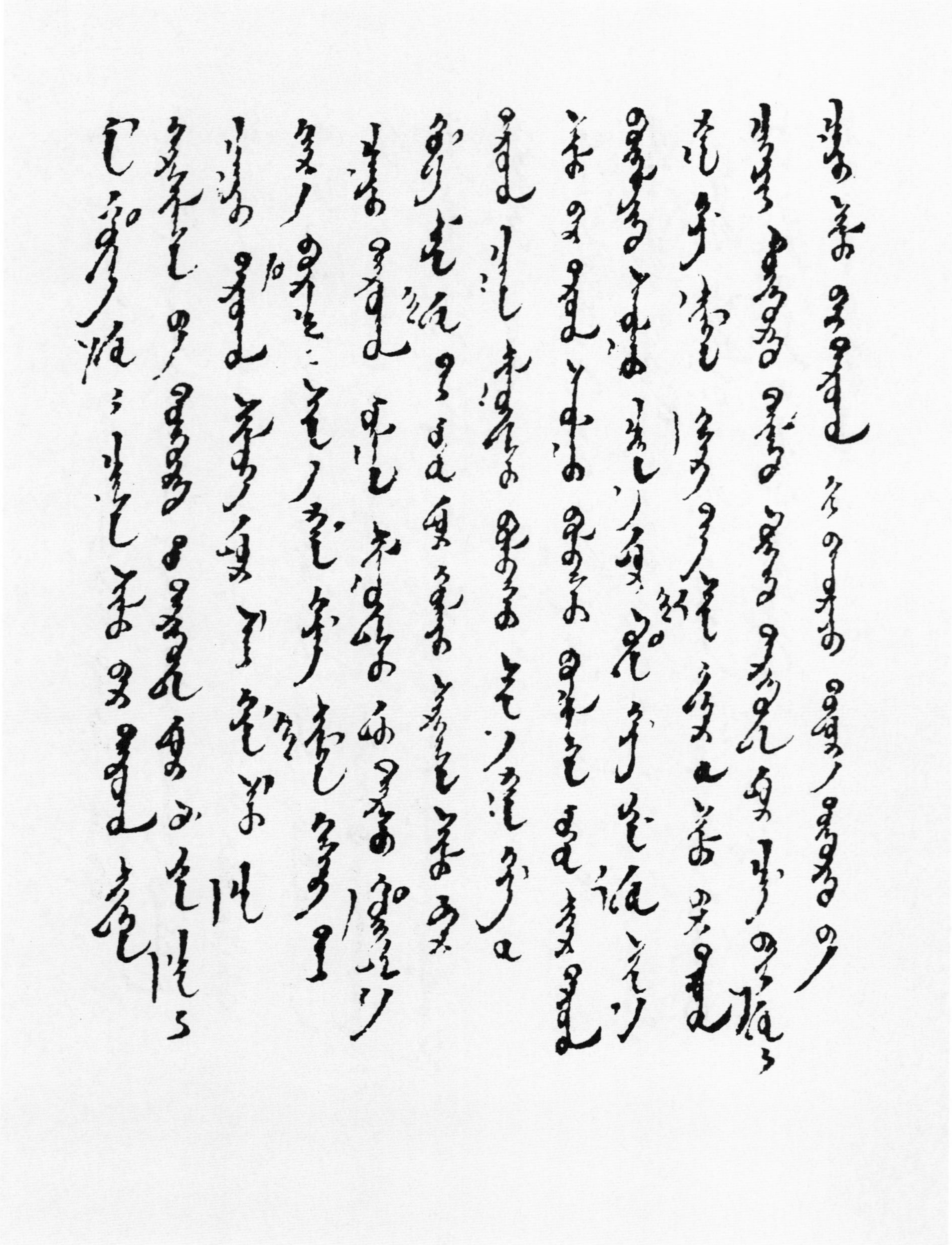

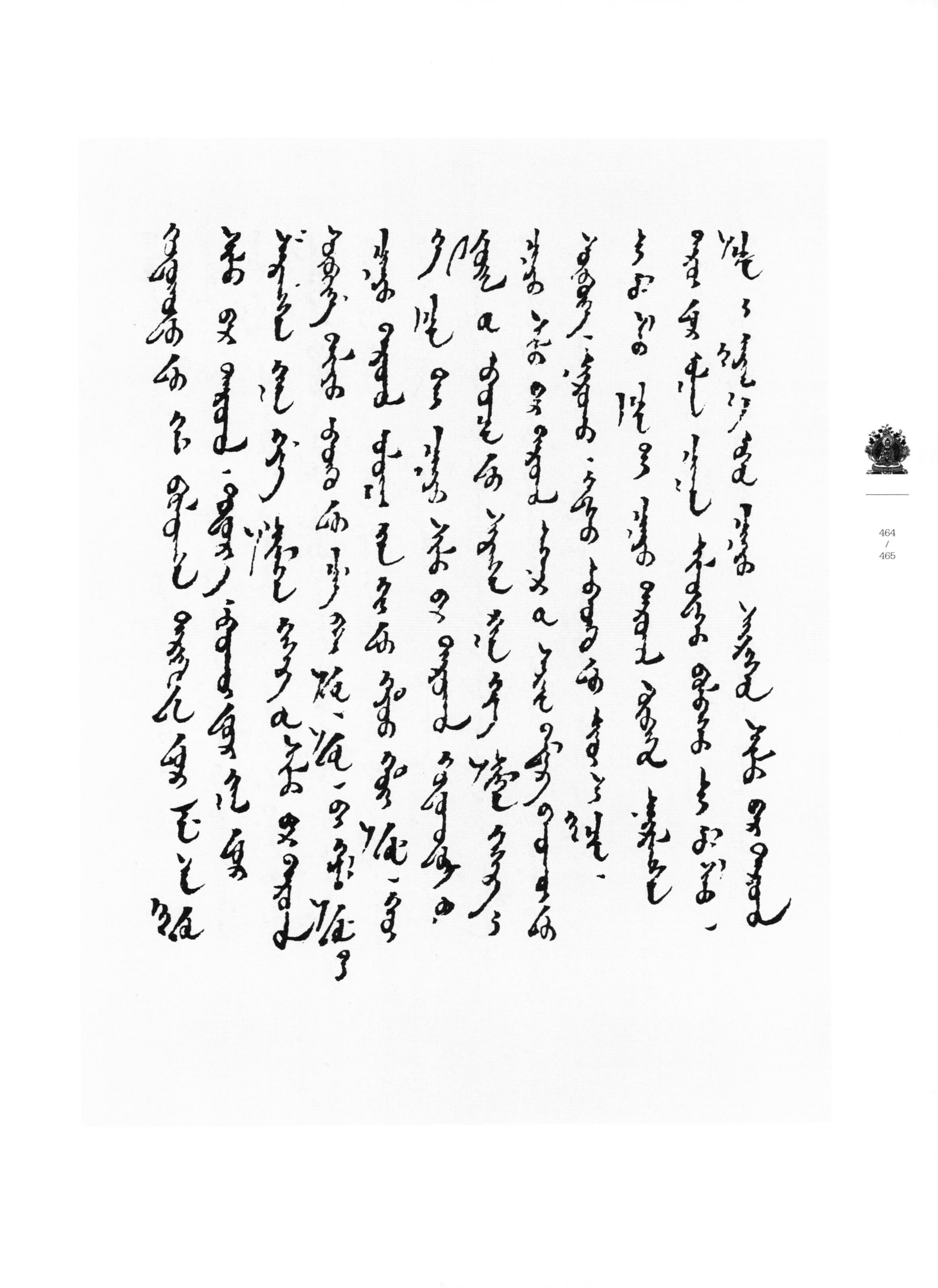

[illegible]

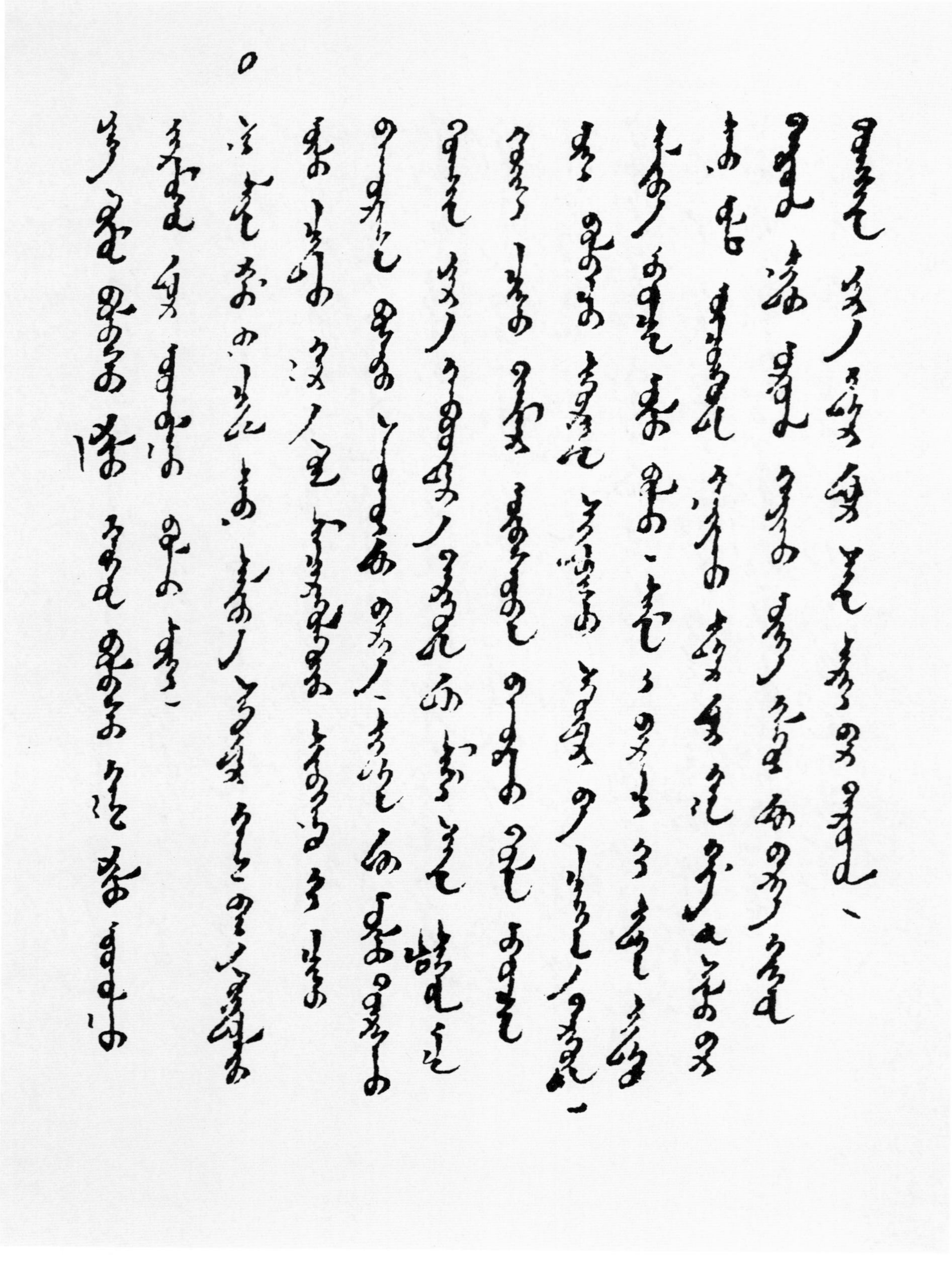

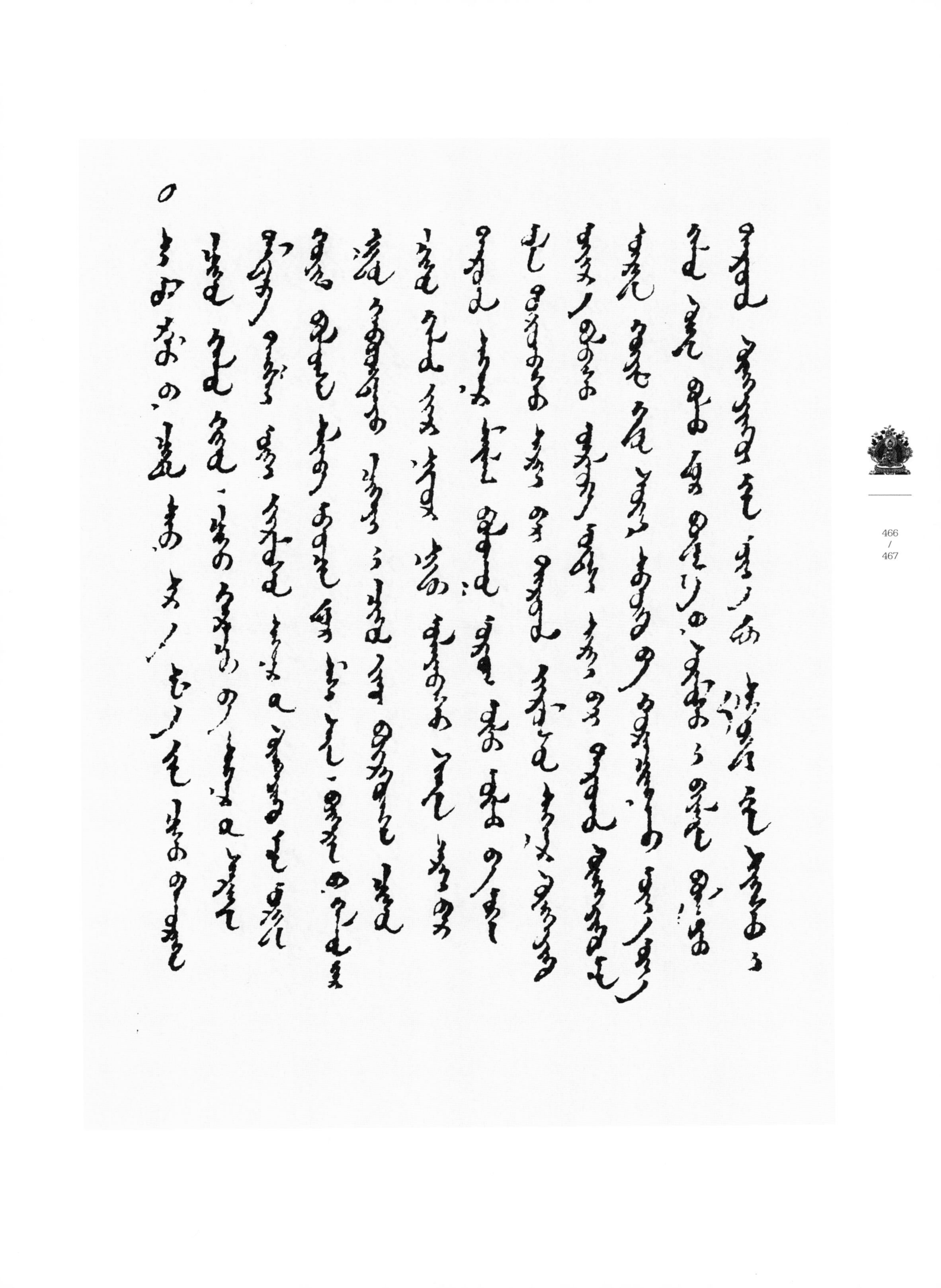

[illegible]
[illegible]
[illegible]
[illegible]
[illegible]
[illegible]
[illegible]
[illegible]
[illegible]
[illegible]
[illegible]
[illegible]

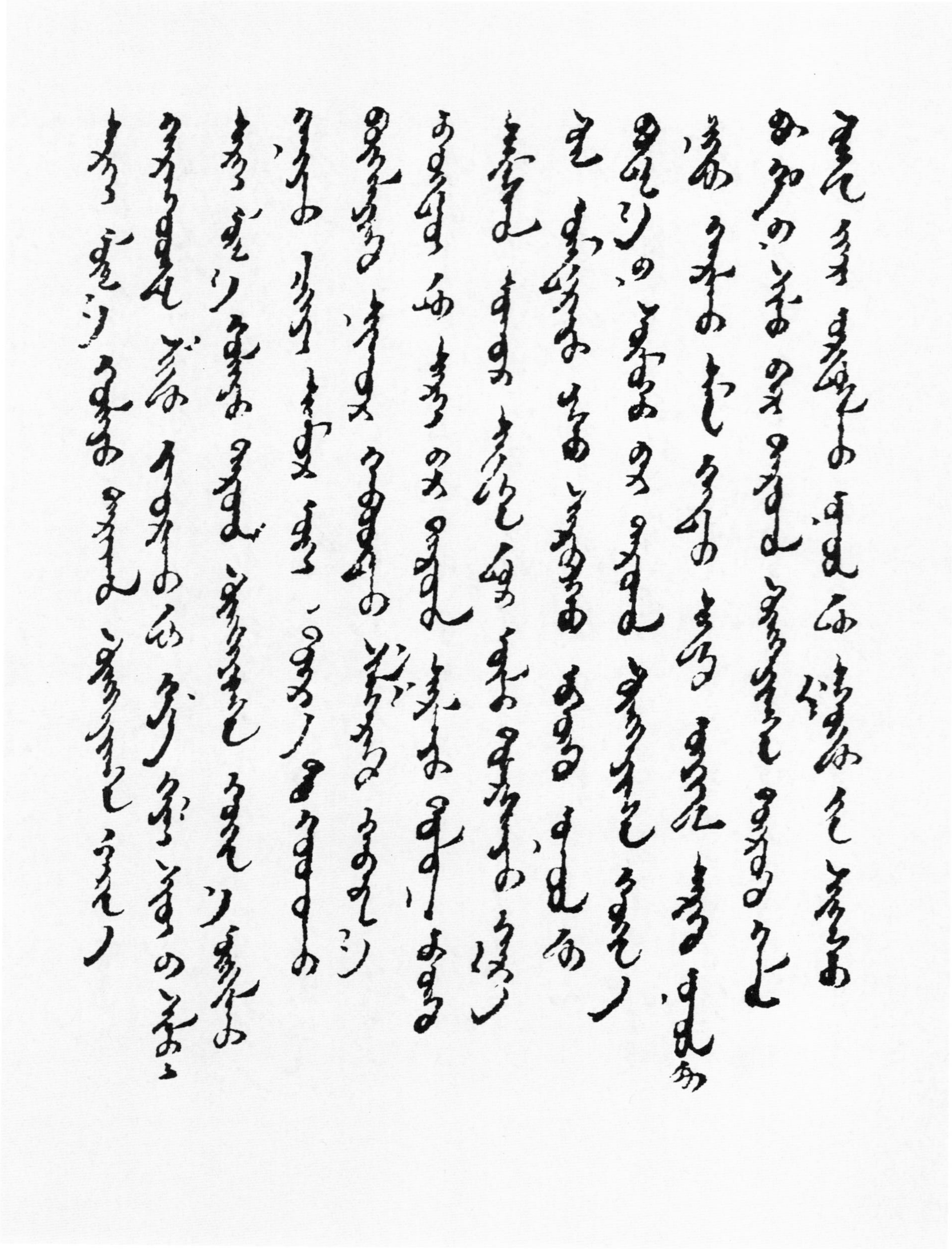

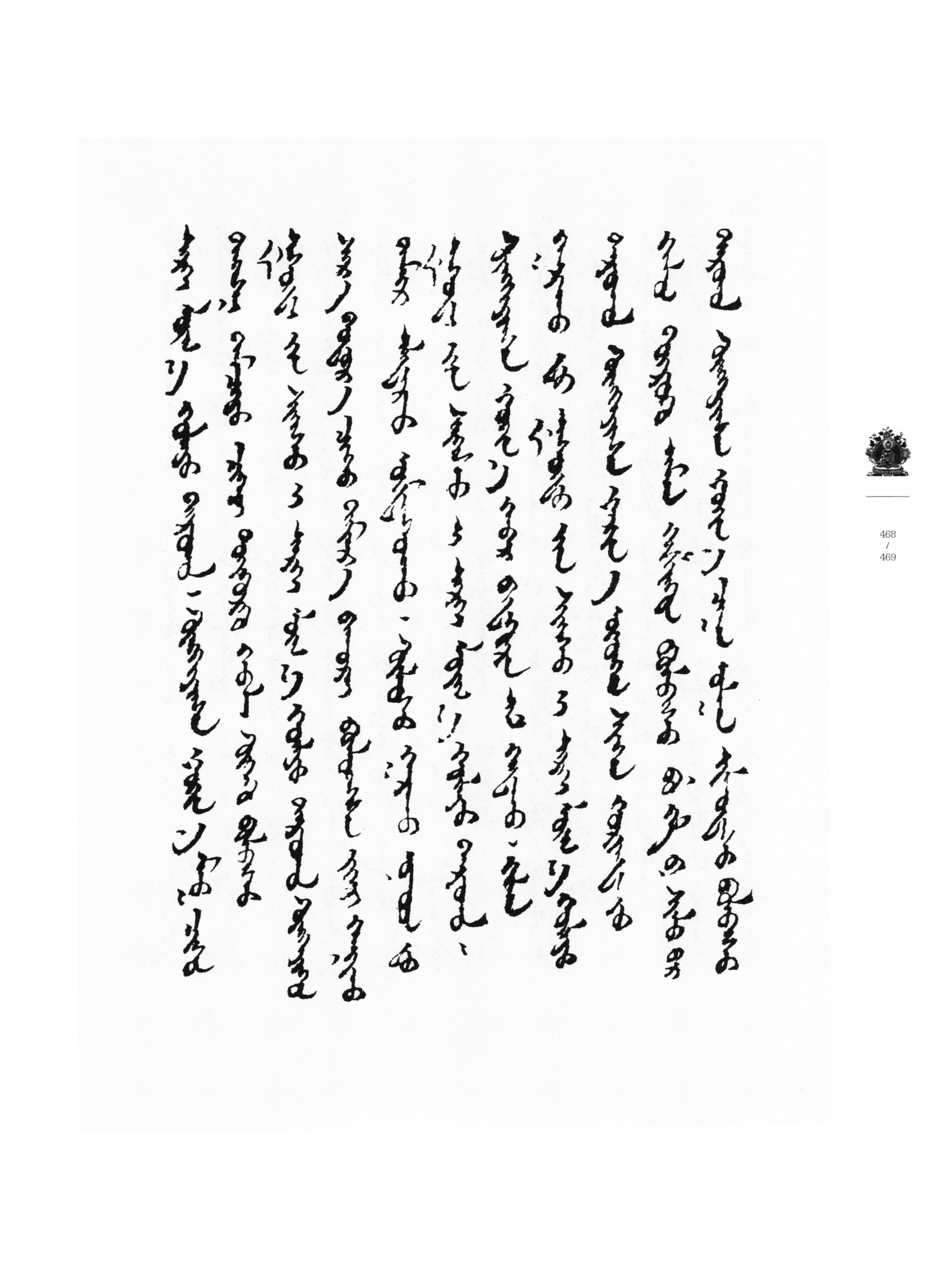

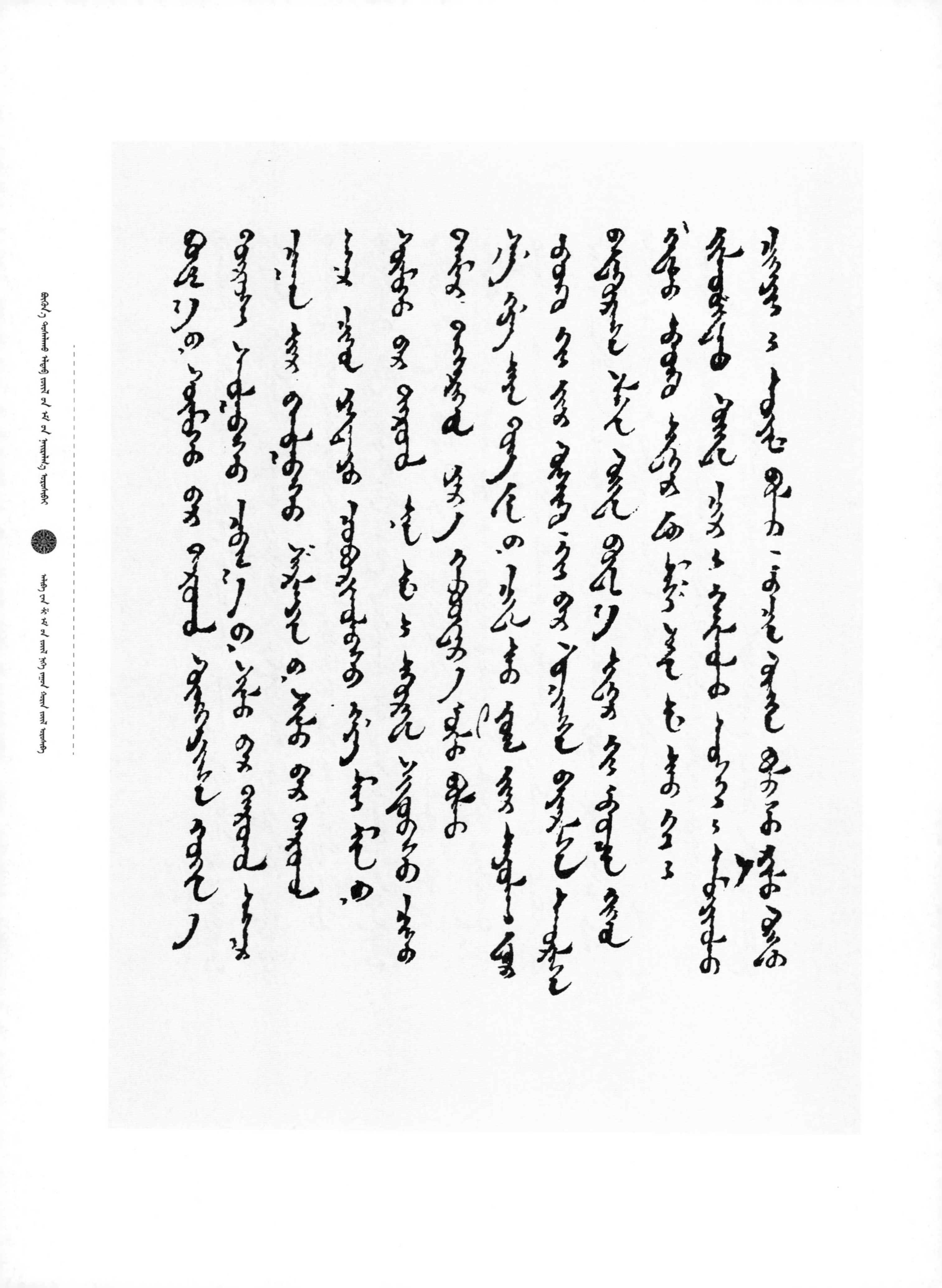

[illegible]
[illegible]
[illegible]
[illegible]
[illegible]
[illegible]
[illegible]
[illegible]
[illegible]
[illegible]
[illegible]
[illegible]
[illegible]

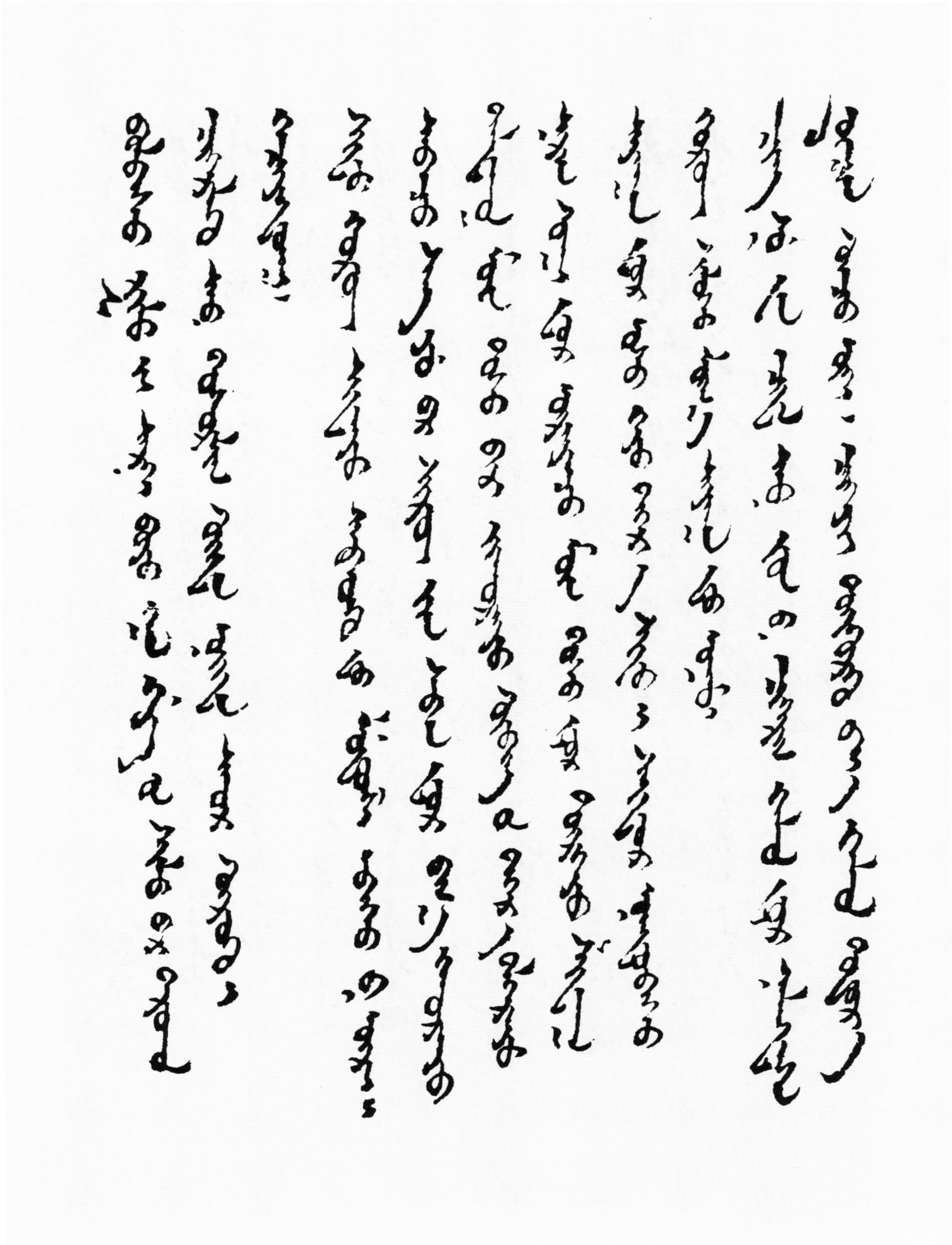

[illegible]
[illegible]
[illegible]
[illegible]
[illegible]
[illegible]
[illegible]
[illegible]
[illegible]
[illegible]
[illegible]
[illegible]
[illegible]

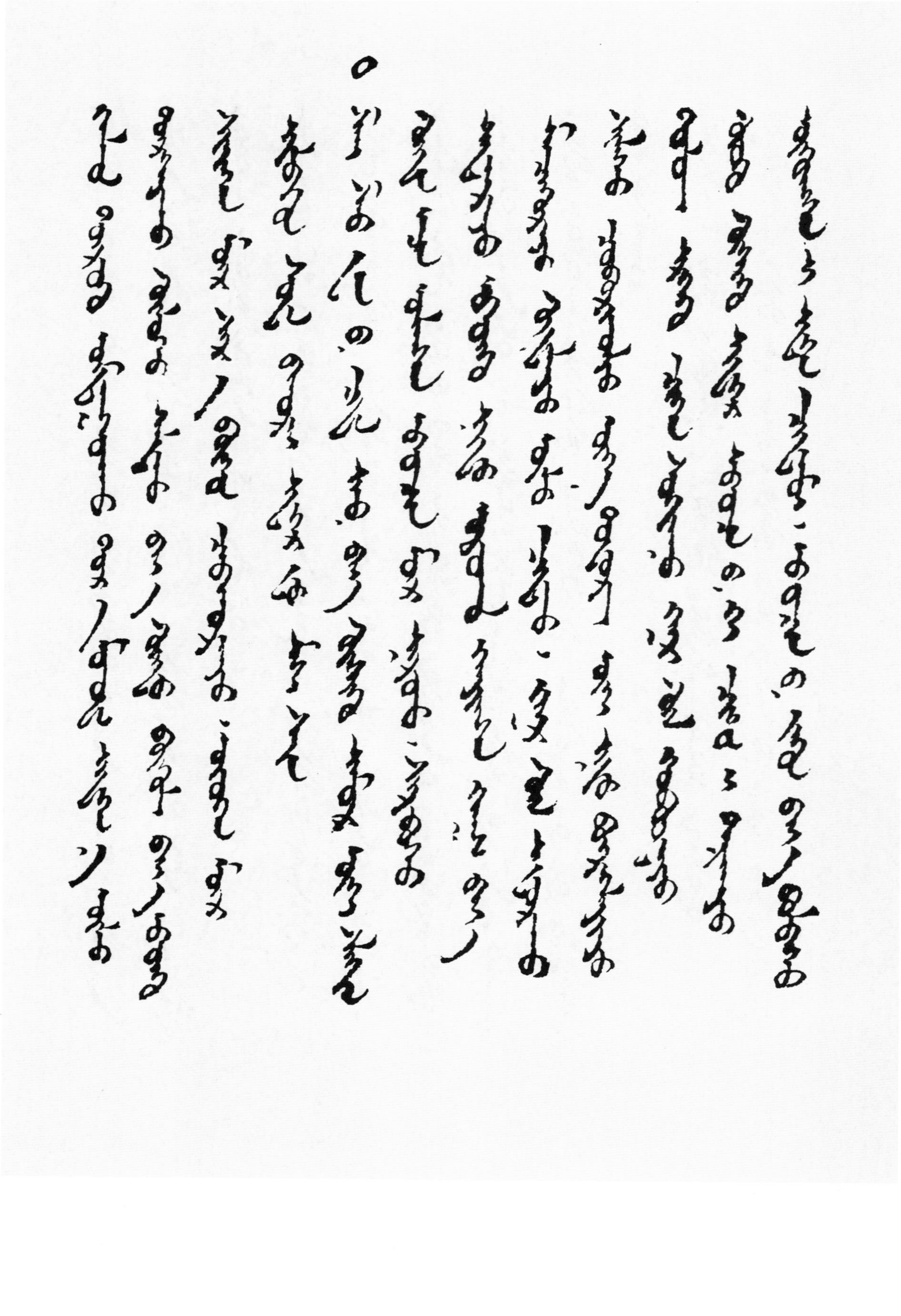

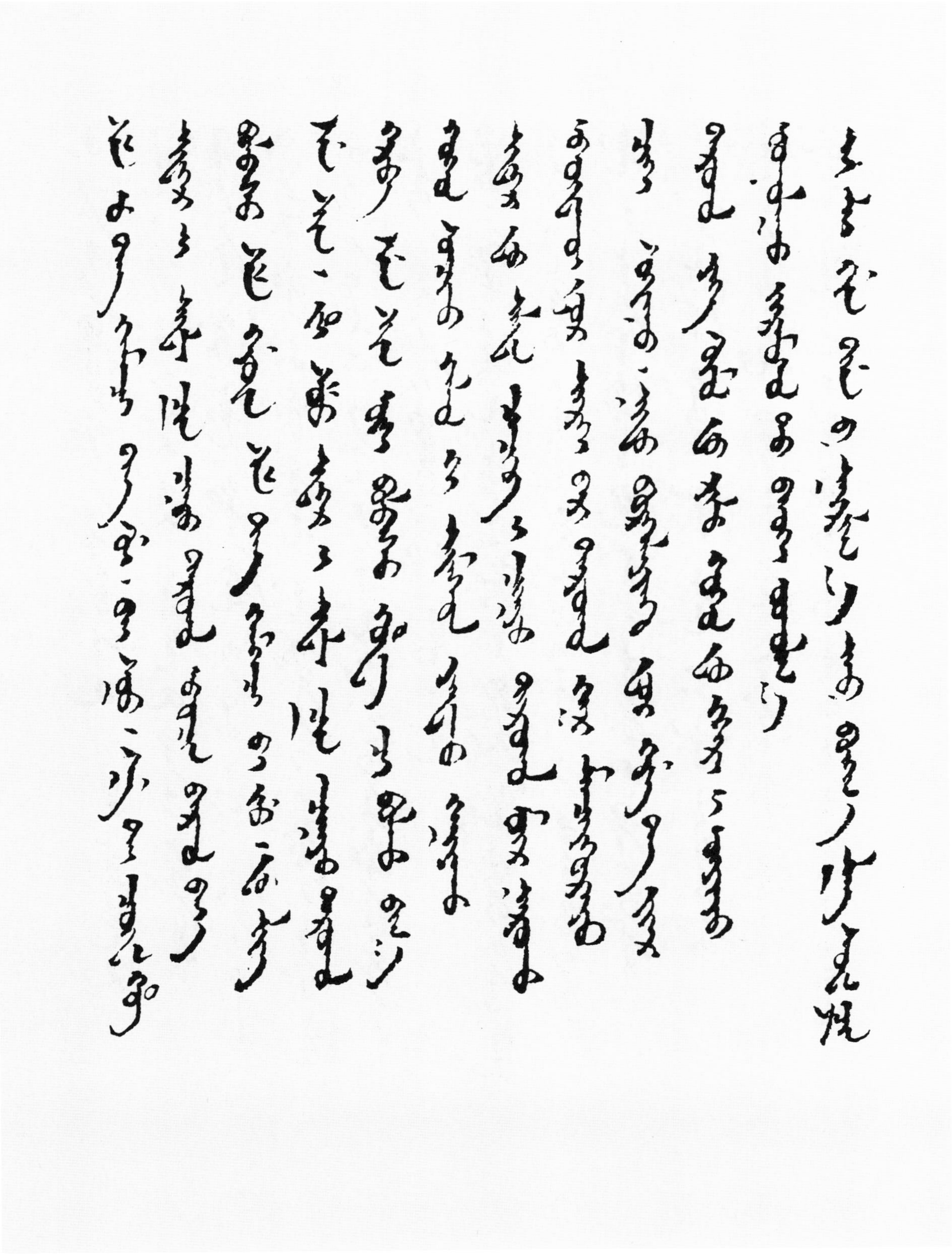

[illegible]

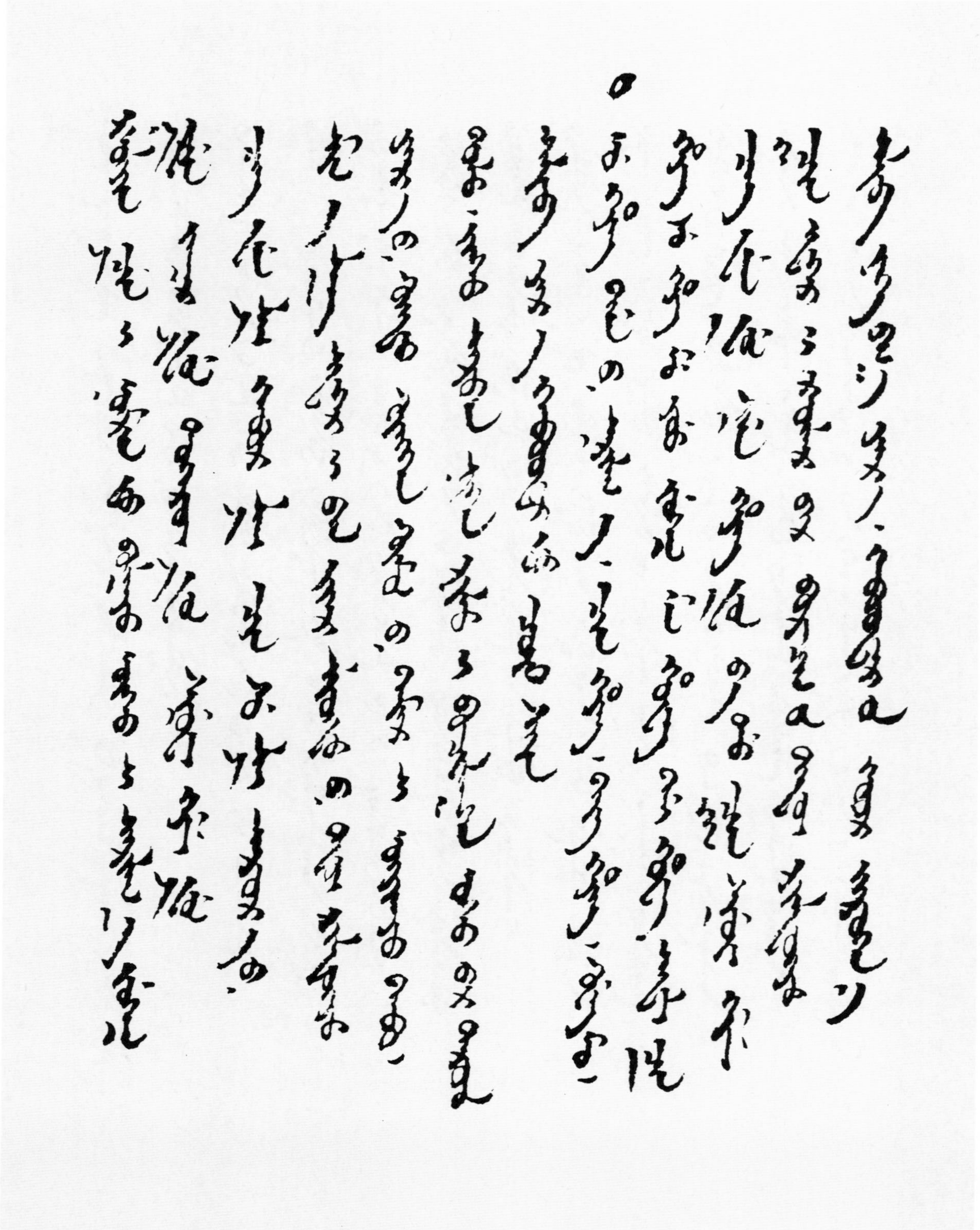

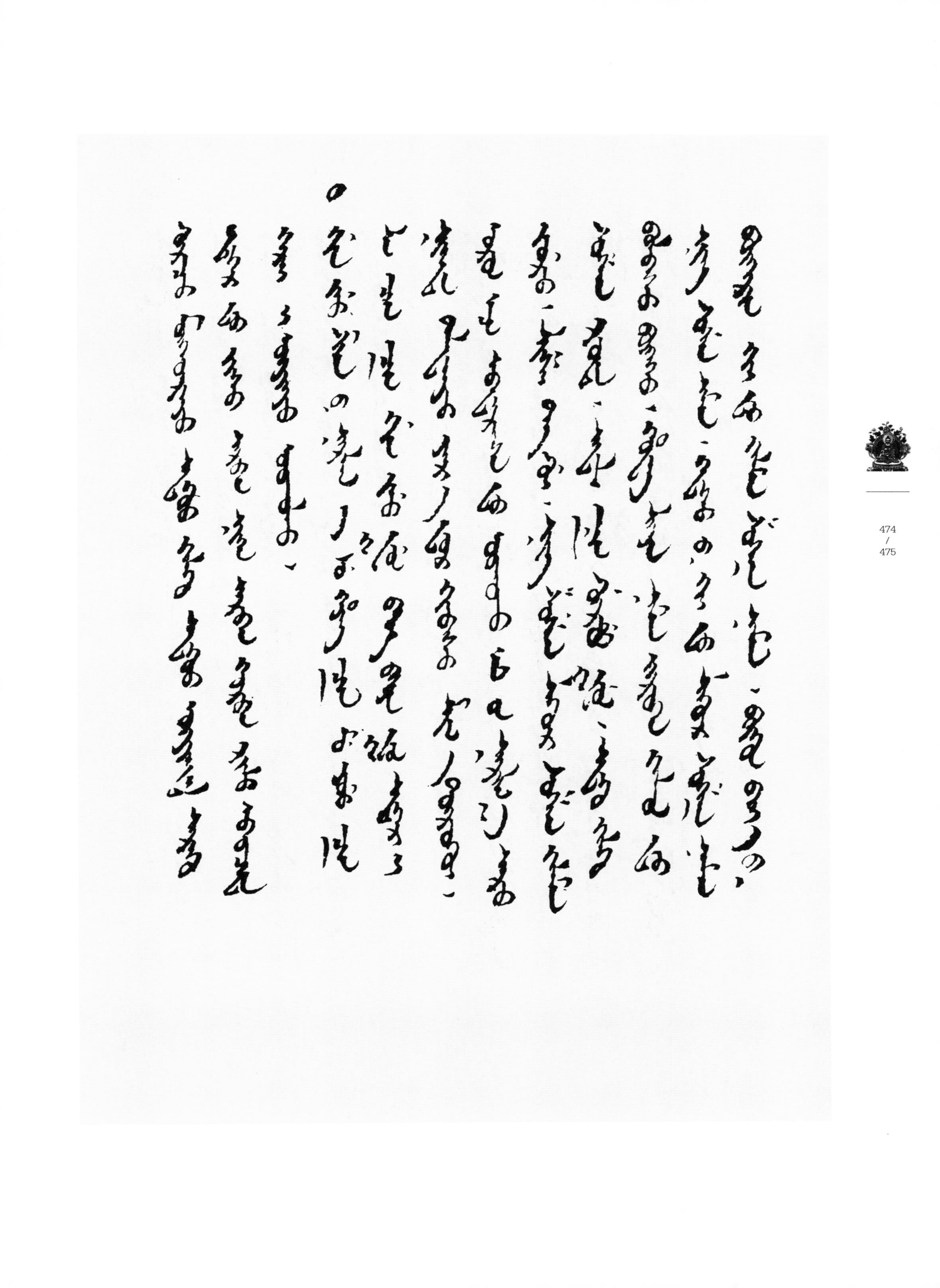

[illegible]

[illegible]

[illegible]

[illegible]

[illegible]

[illegible]

[illegible]

[illegible]

[illegible]

[illegible]

[illegible]

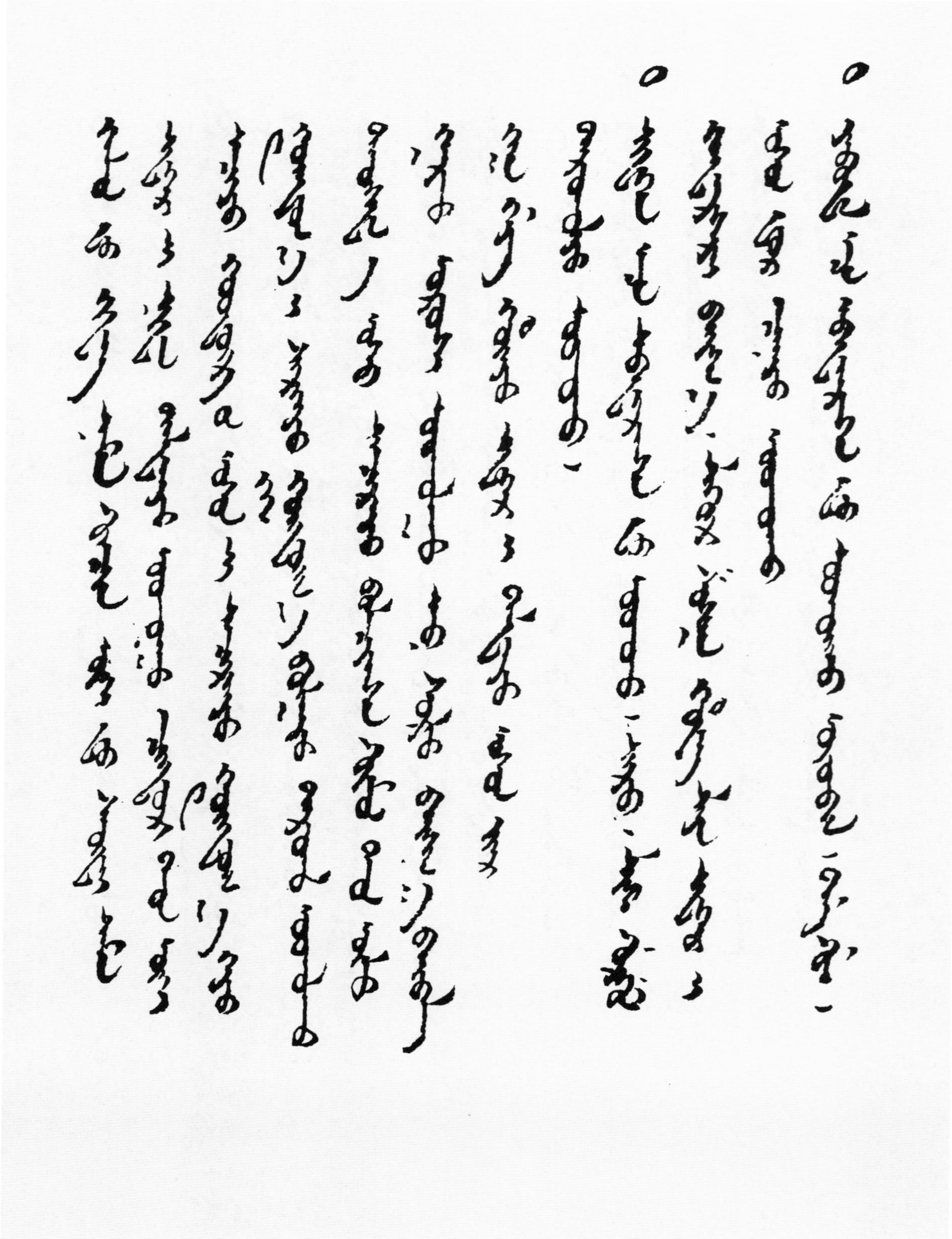

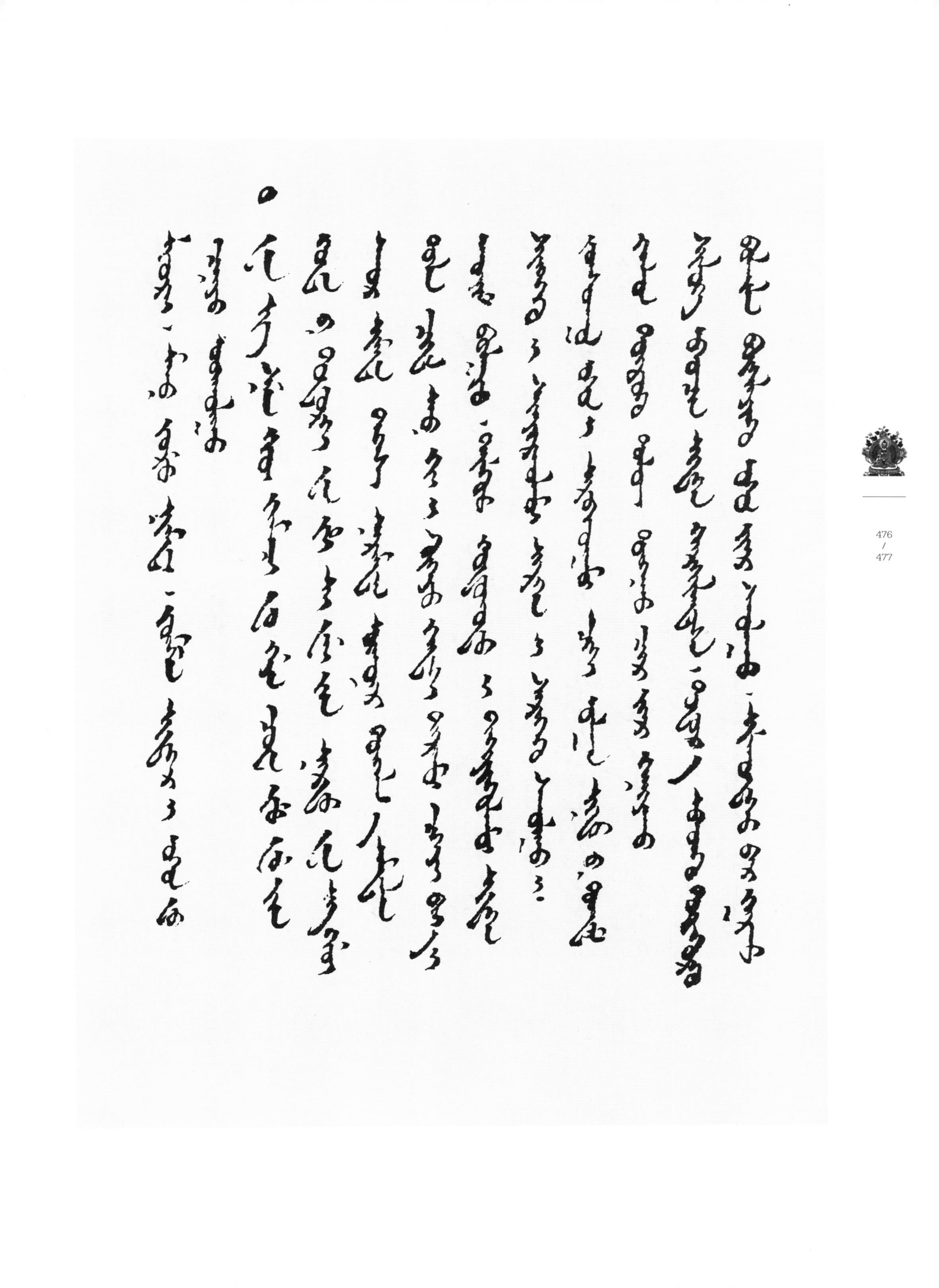

[illegible]
[illegible]
[illegible]
[illegible]
[illegible]
[illegible]
[illegible]
[illegible]
[illegible]
[illegible]
[illegible]
[illegible]

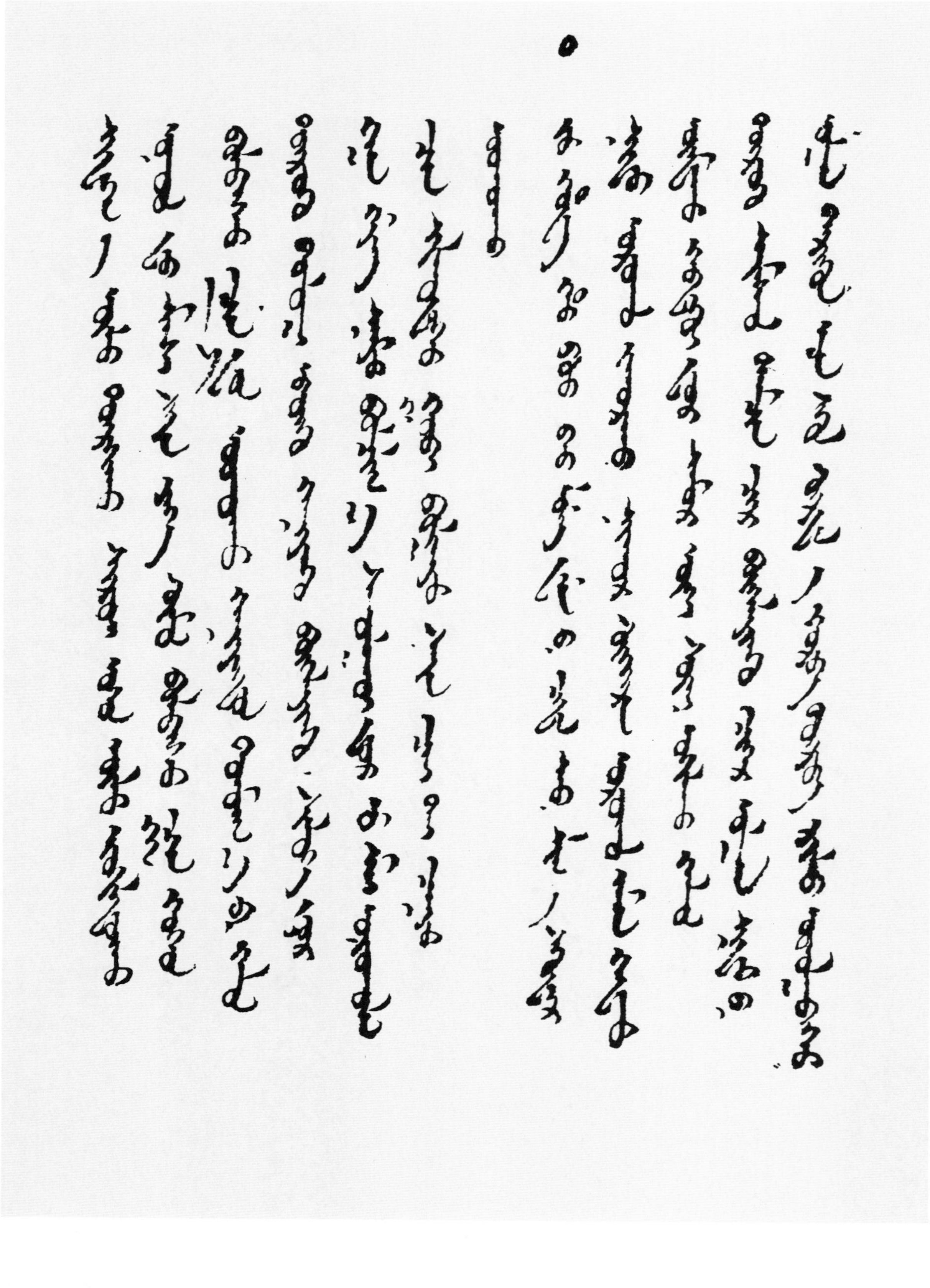

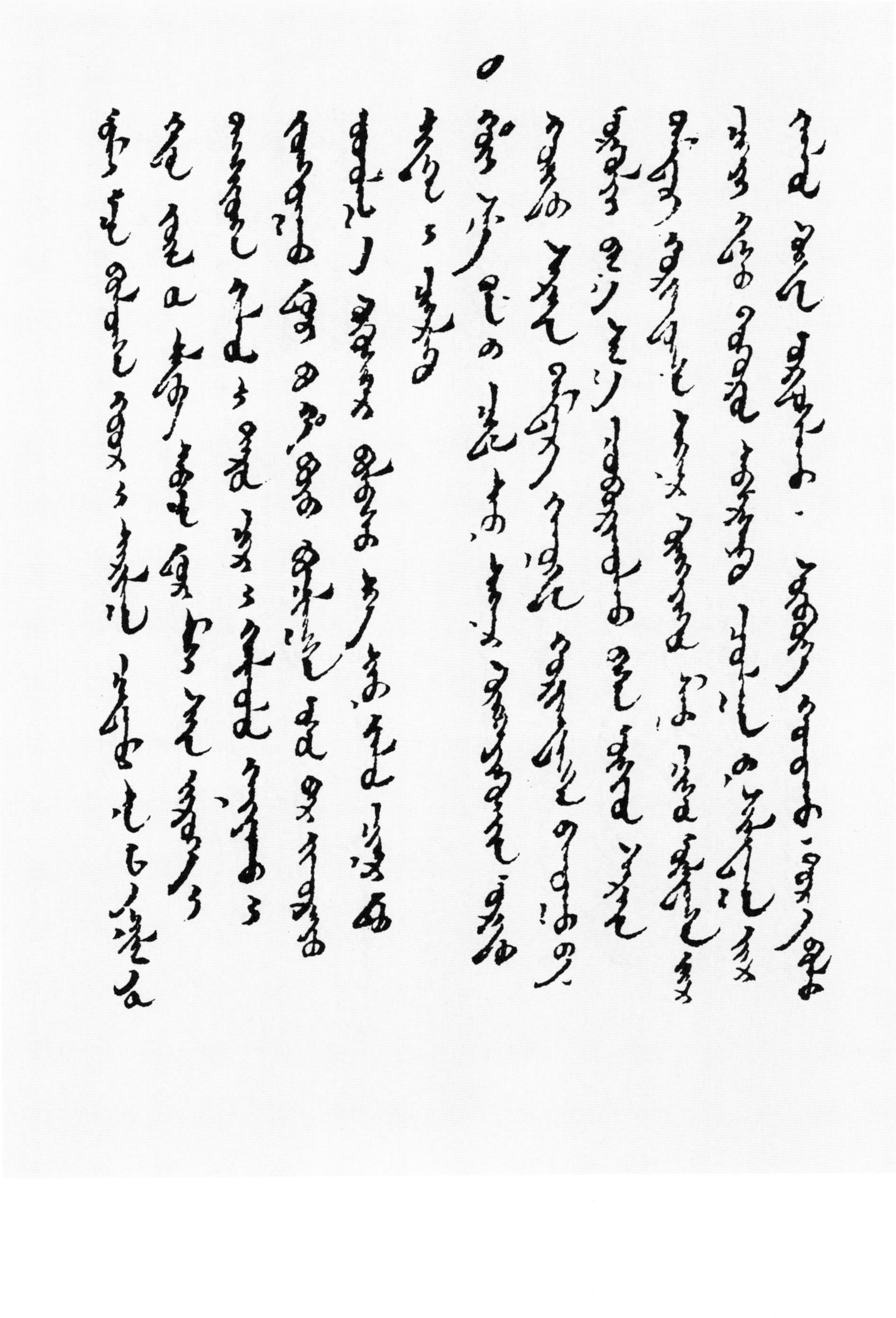

[illegible]
[illegible]
[illegible]
[illegible]
[illegible]
[illegible]
[illegible]
[illegible]
[illegible]
[illegible]
[illegible]
[illegible]
[illegible]

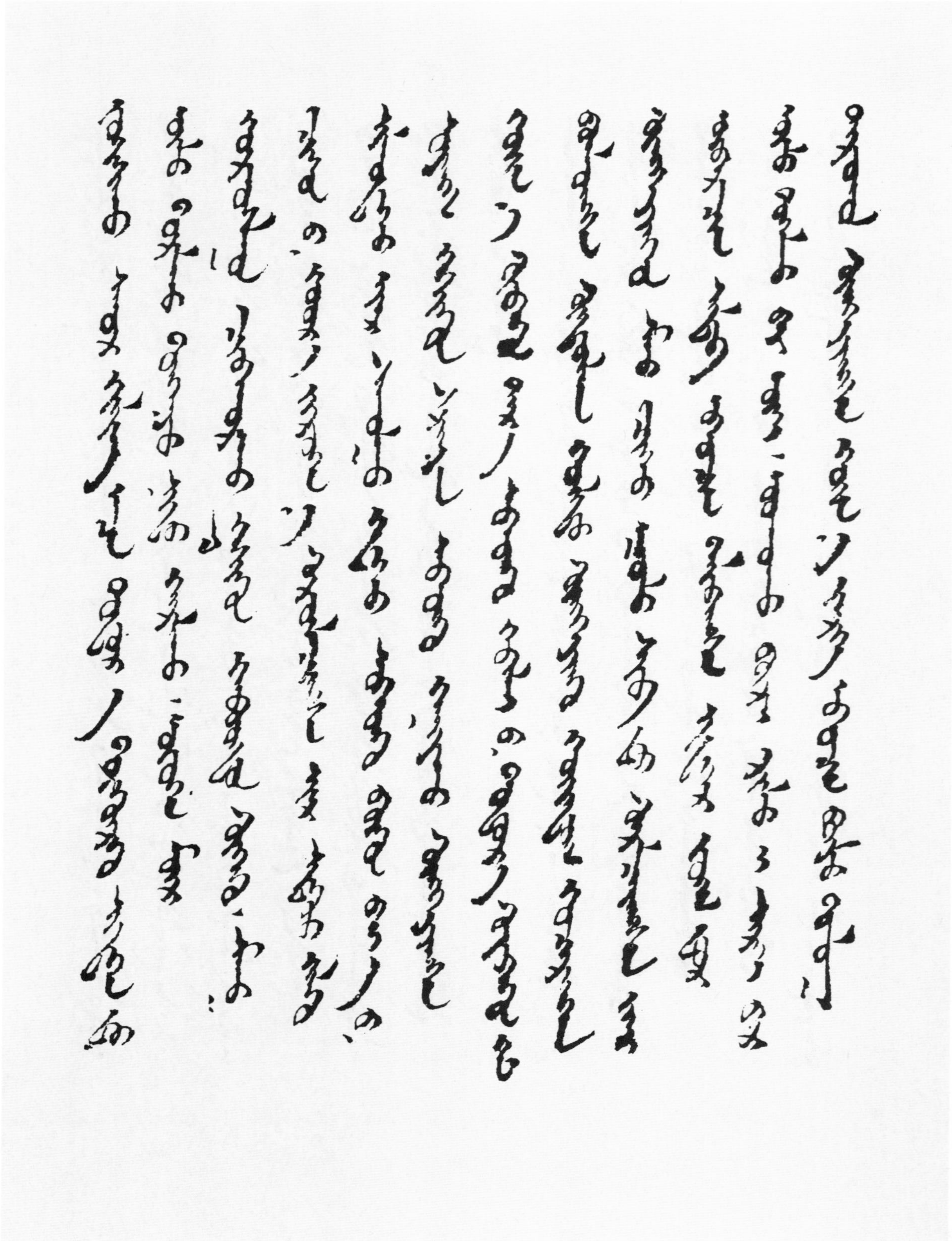

[illegible]

o [illegible]

[illegible]

o [illegible]

[illegible]

o [illegible]

[illegible]

[illegible]

o [illegible]

[illegible]

[illegible]

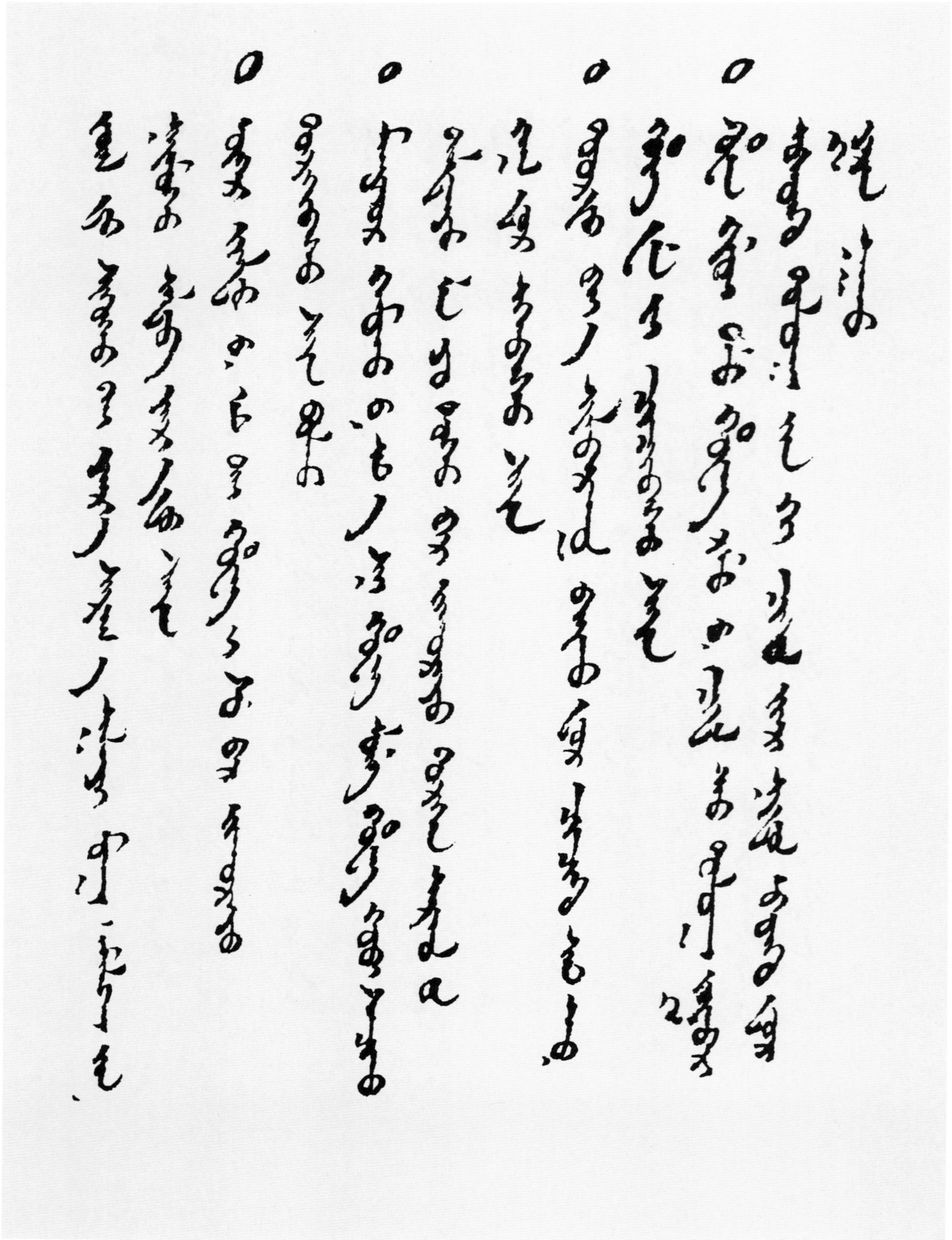

[illegible]

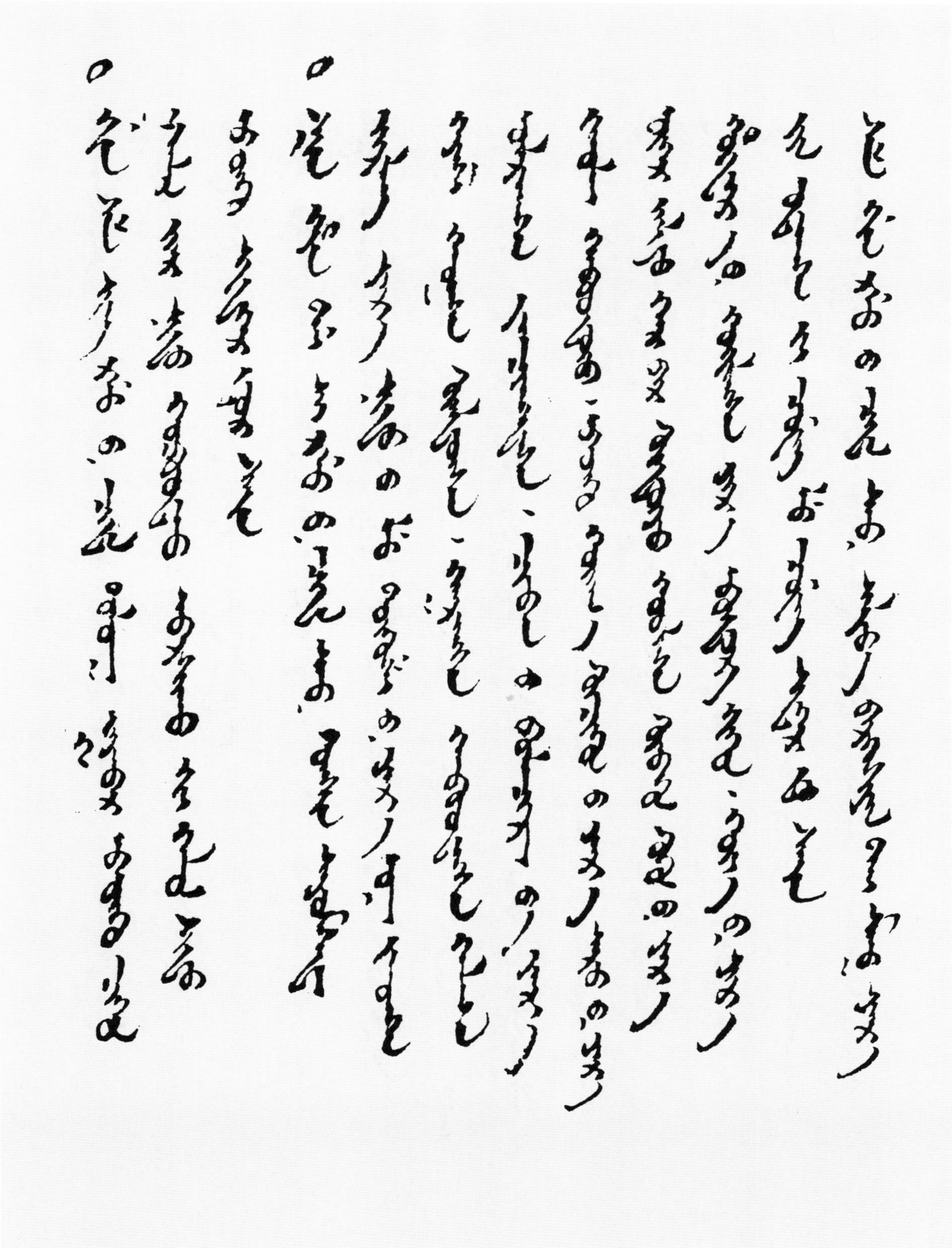

[illegible]

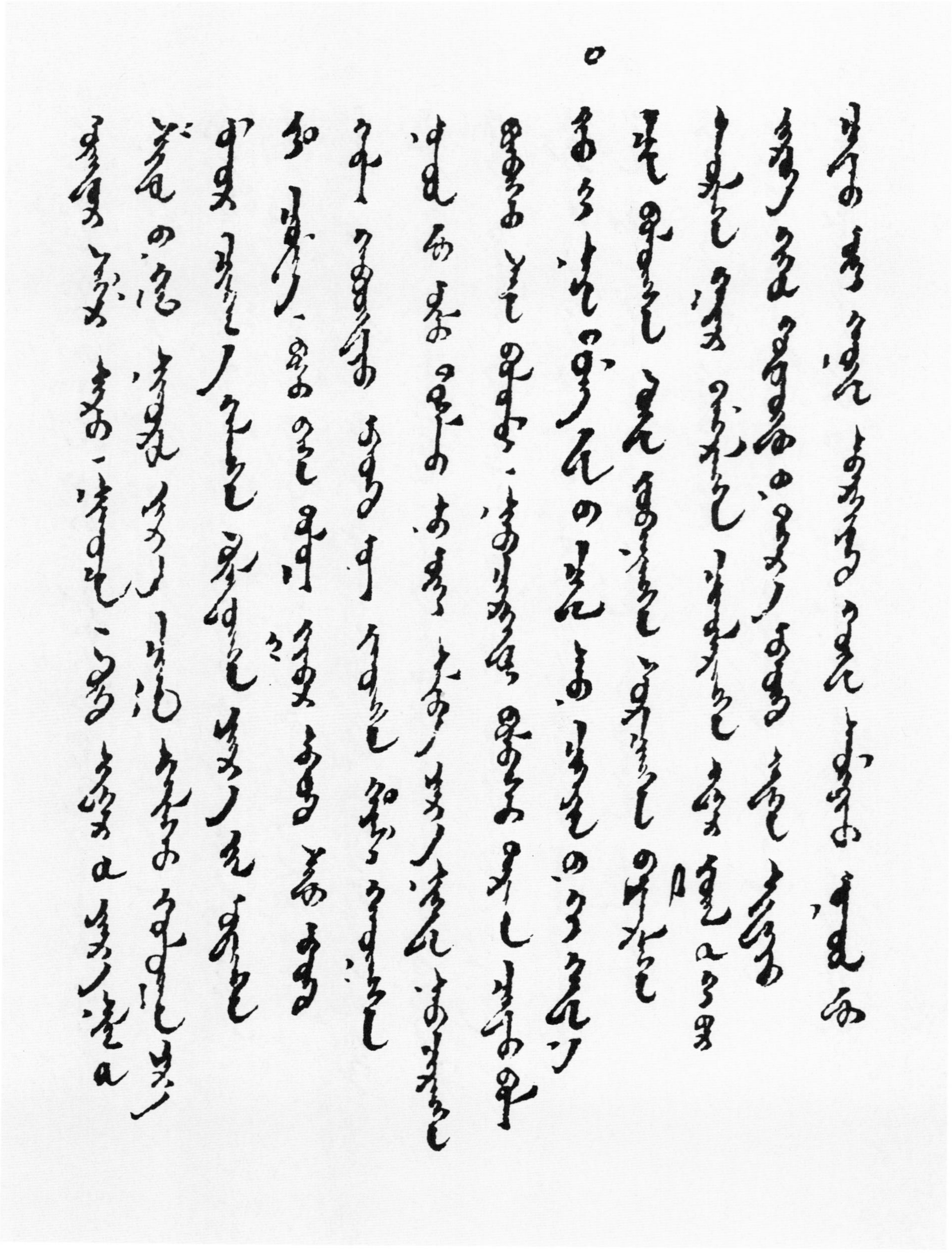

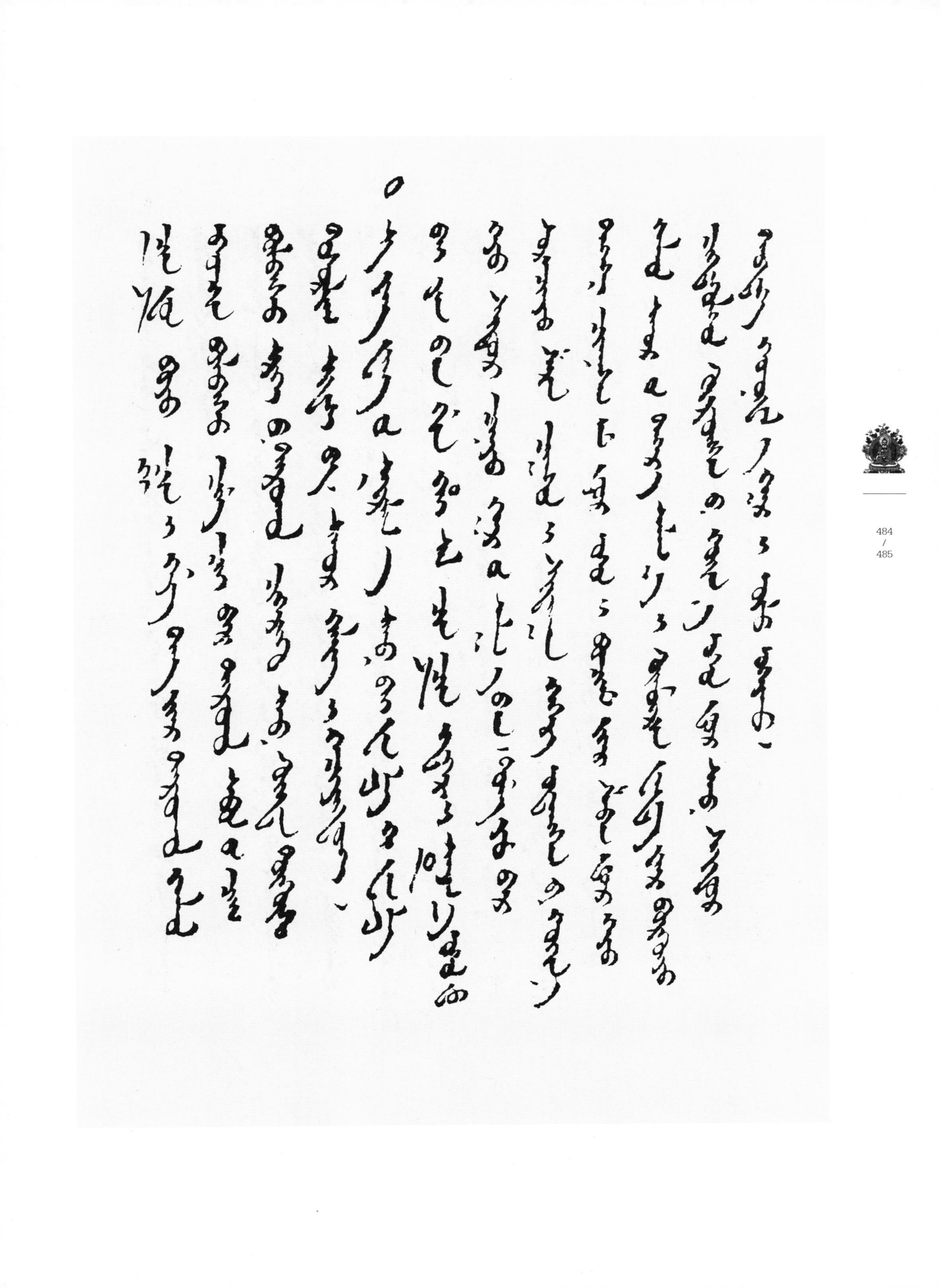

[illegible]

[illegible]

[illegible]

[illegible]

[illegible]

[illegible]

[illegible]

[illegible]

[illegible]

[illegible]

[illegible]

[illegible]

[illegible]

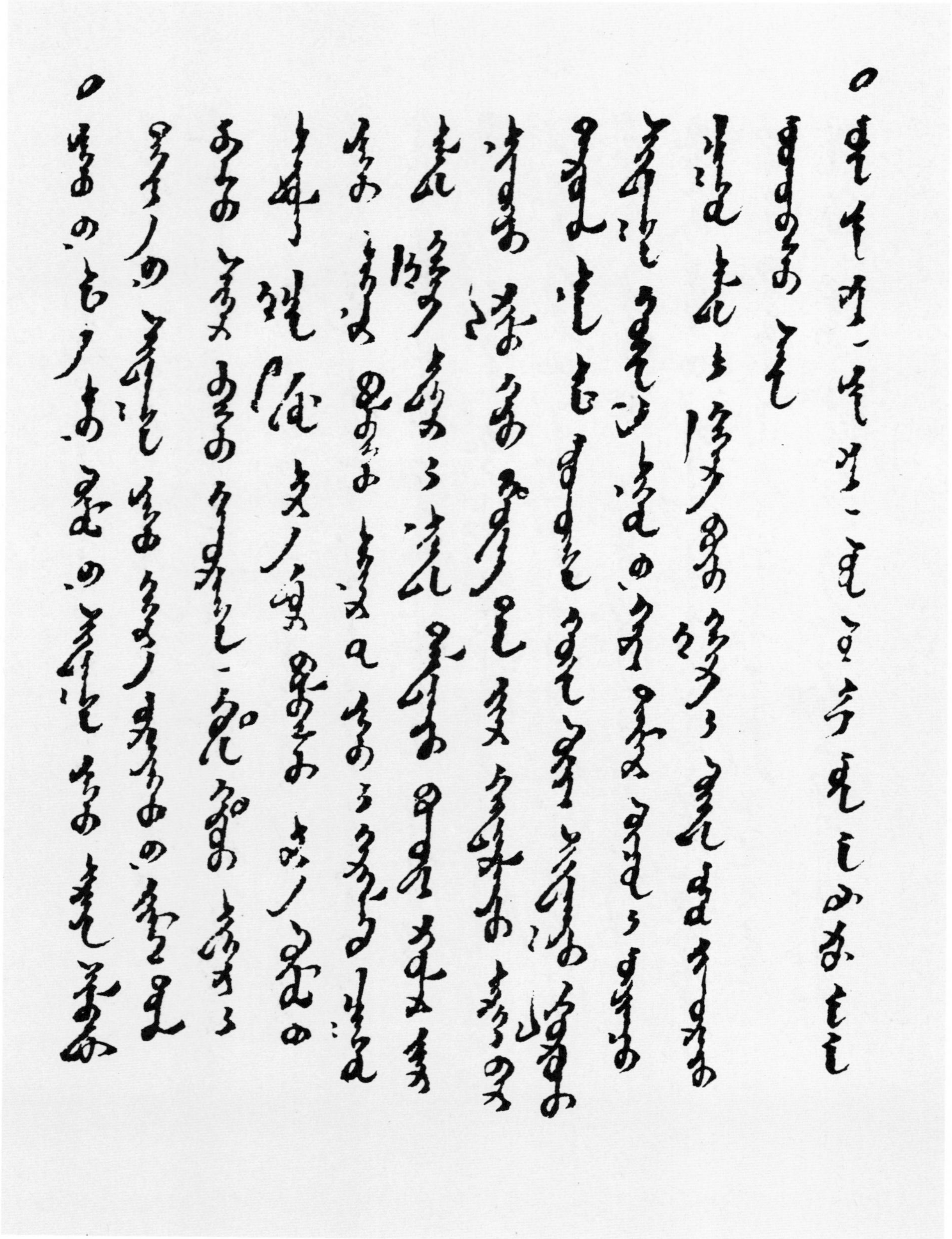

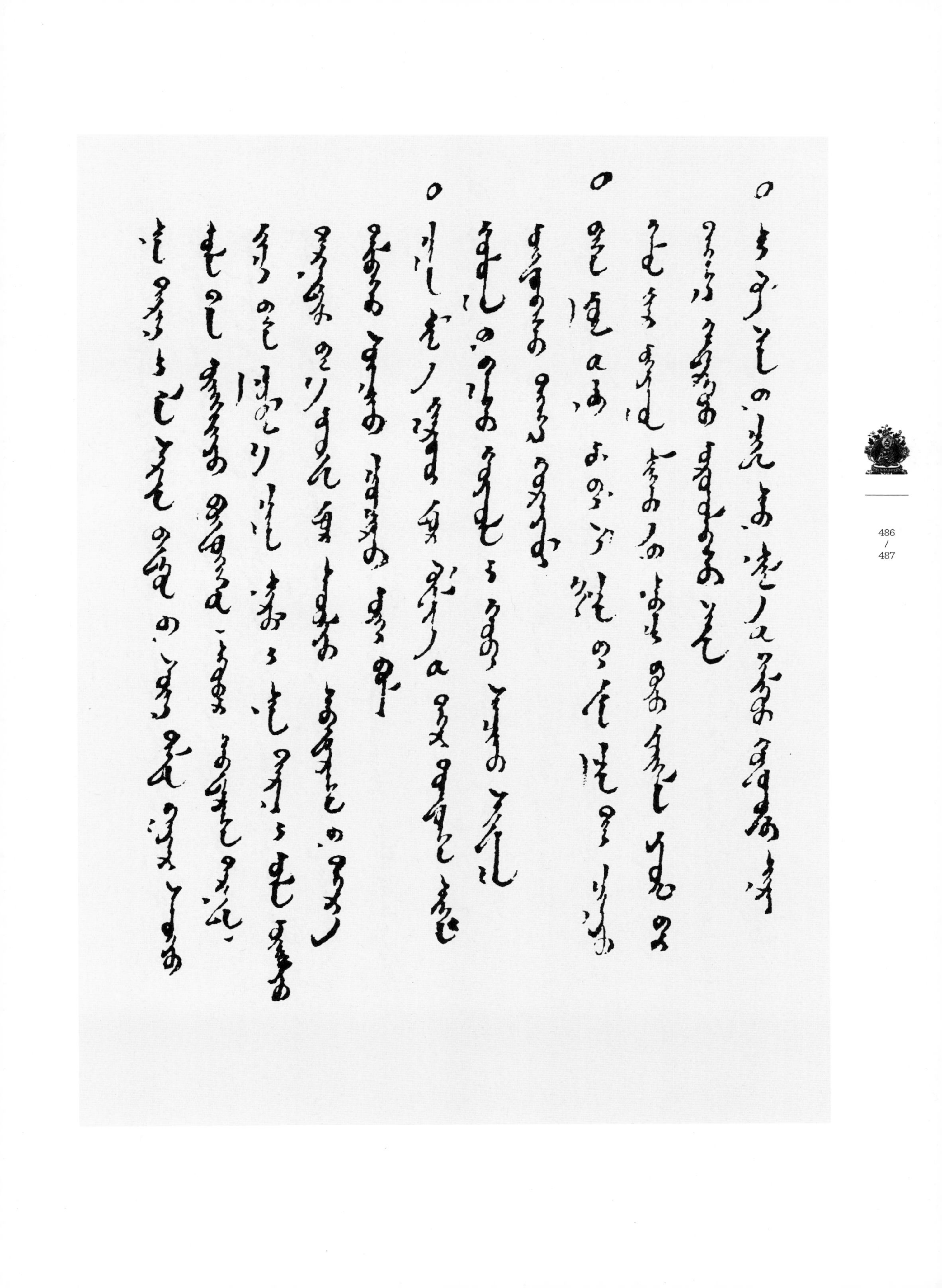

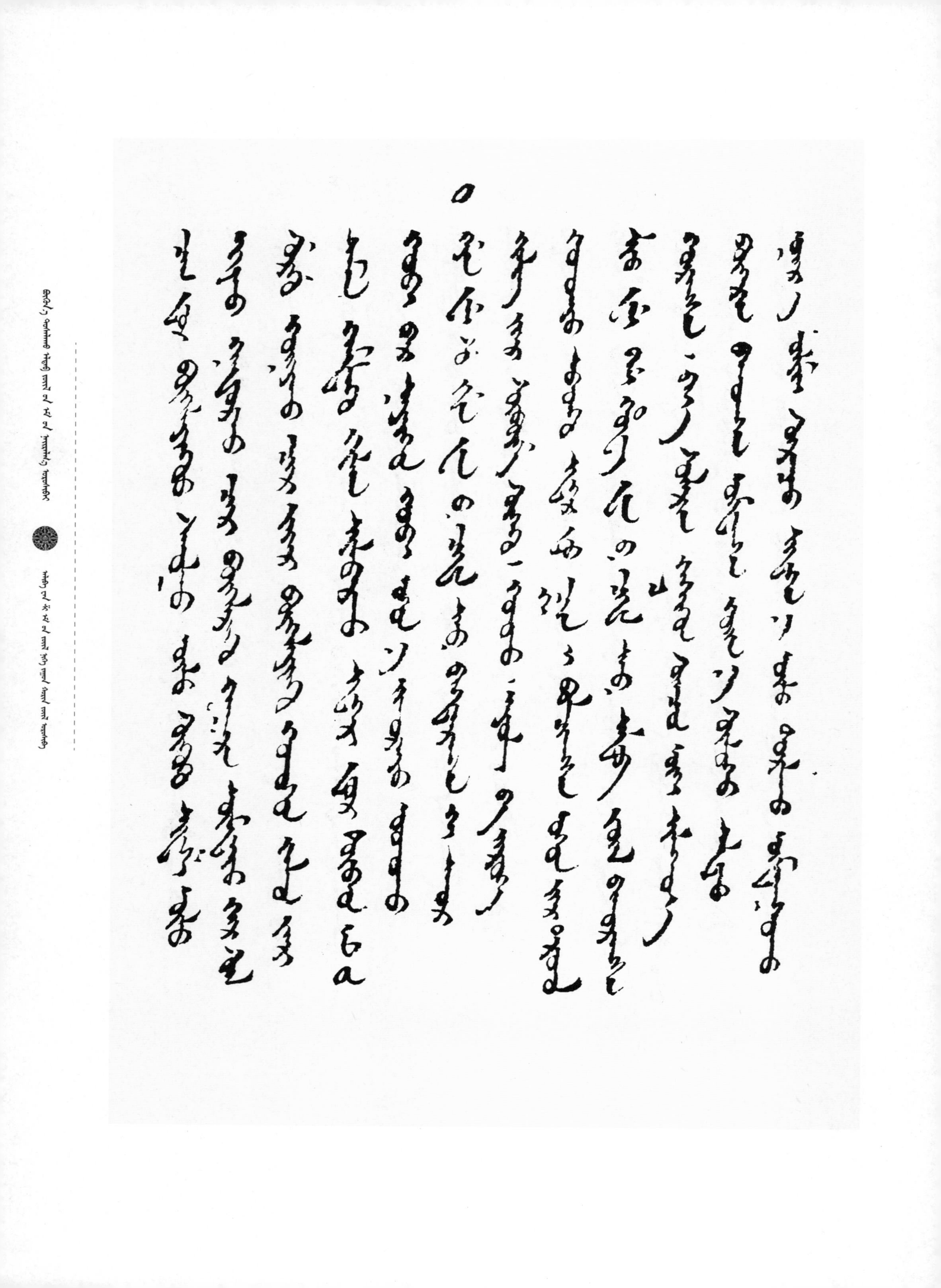

[illegible]

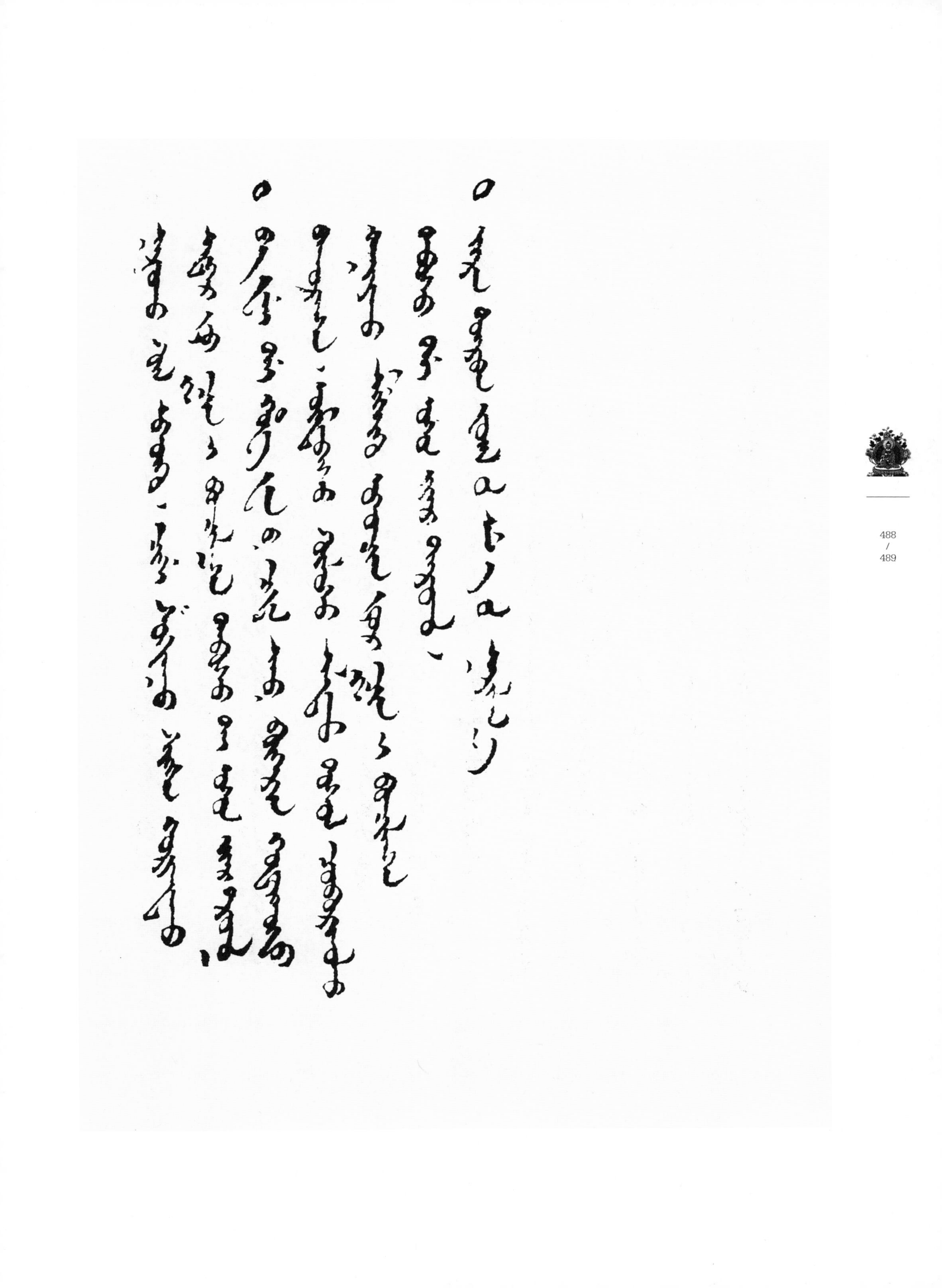

[illegible]

[illegible]

[illegible]

[illegible]

[illegible]

[illegible]

[illegible]

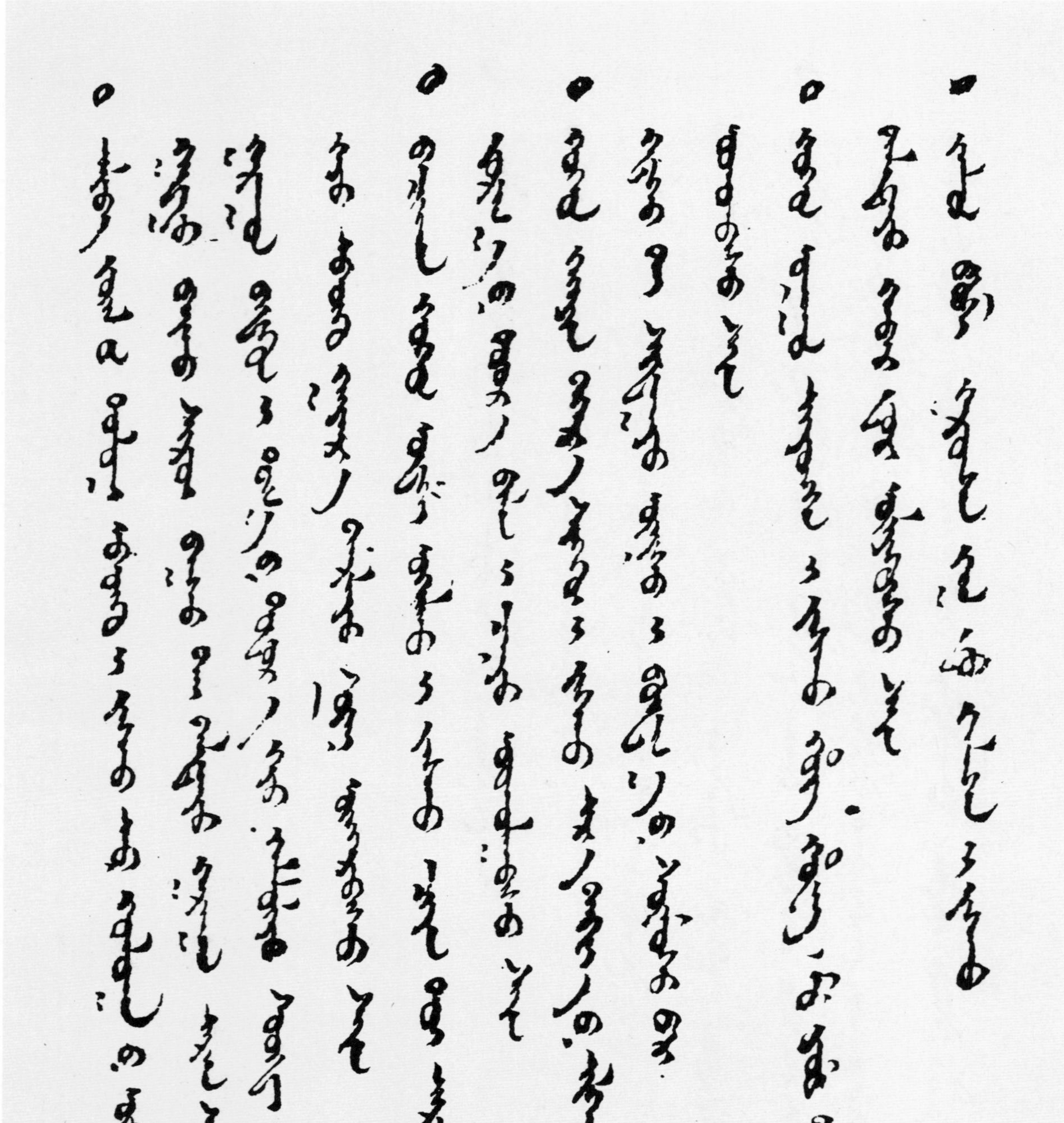

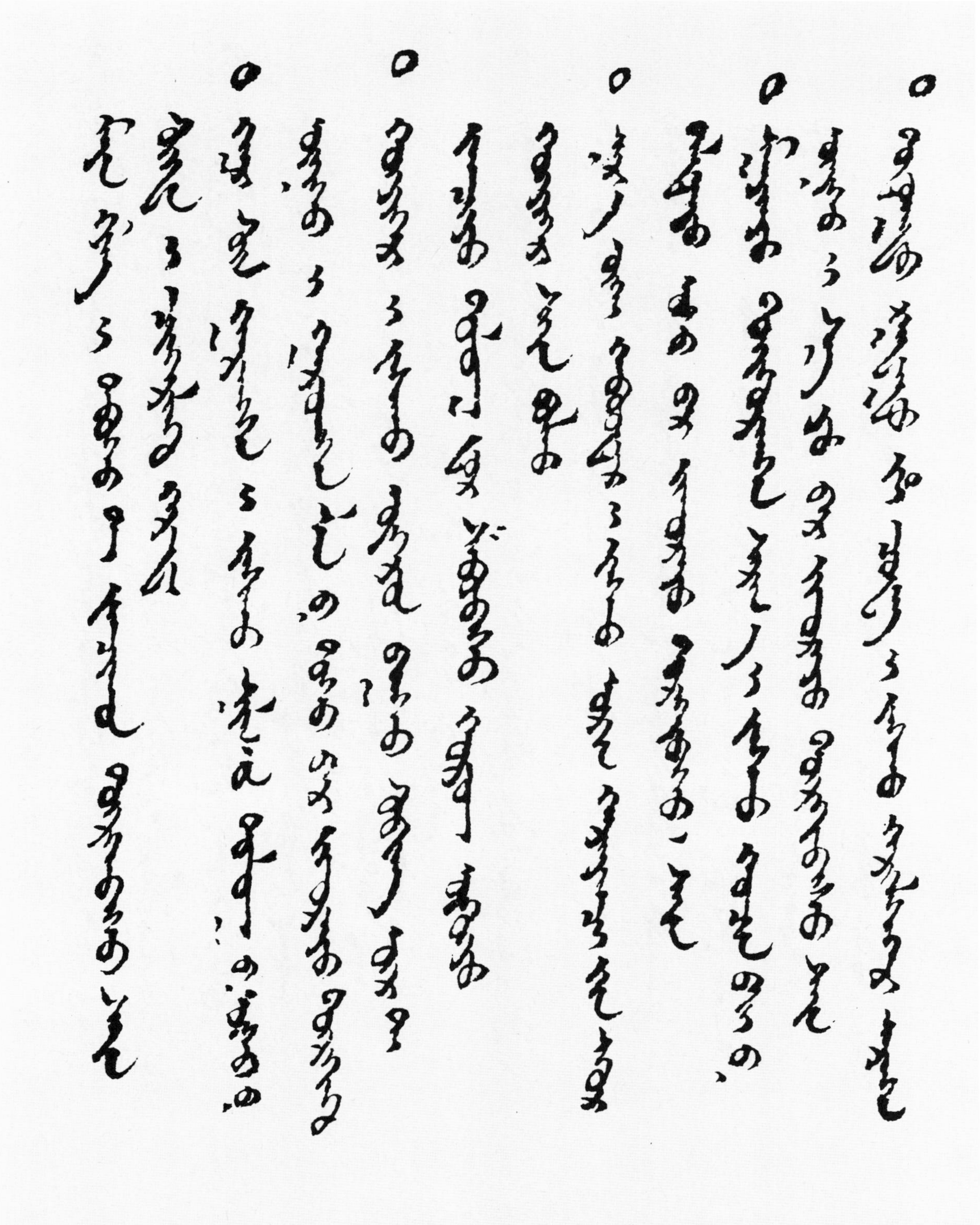

[illegible]

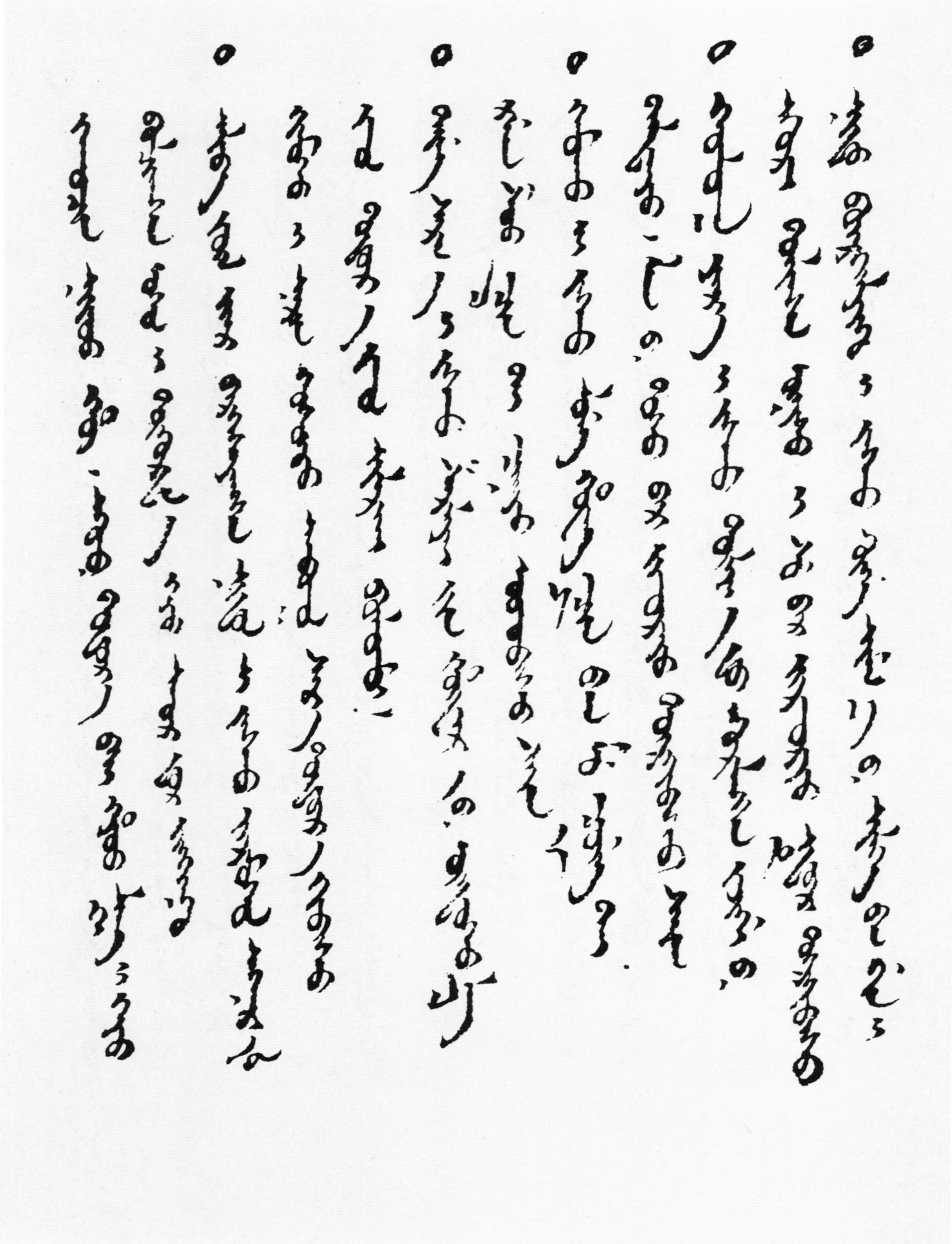

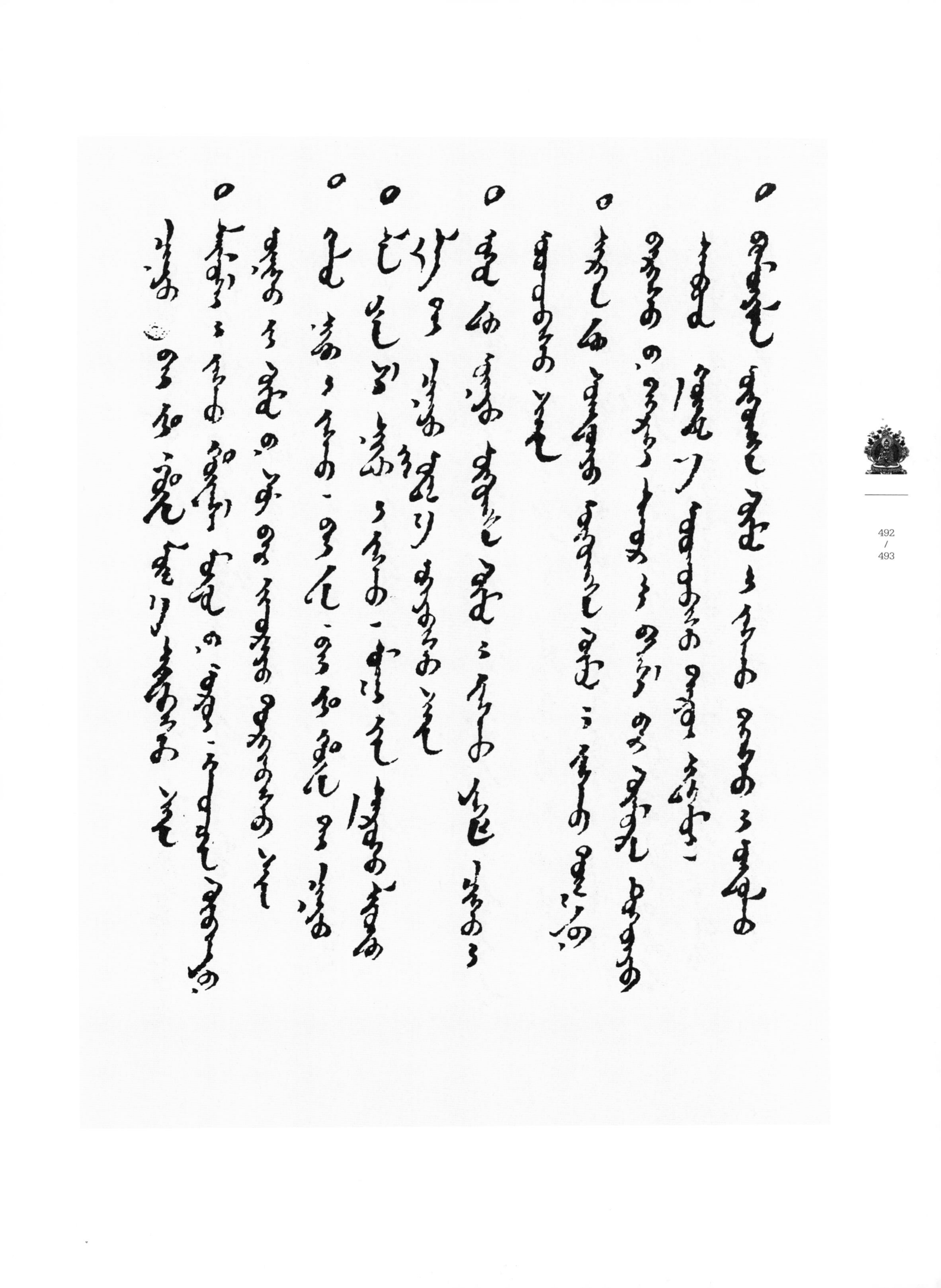

[illegible]

[illegible]

[illegible]

[illegible]

[illegible]

[illegible]

[illegible]

[illegible]

[illegible]

[illegible]

[illegible]

[illegible]

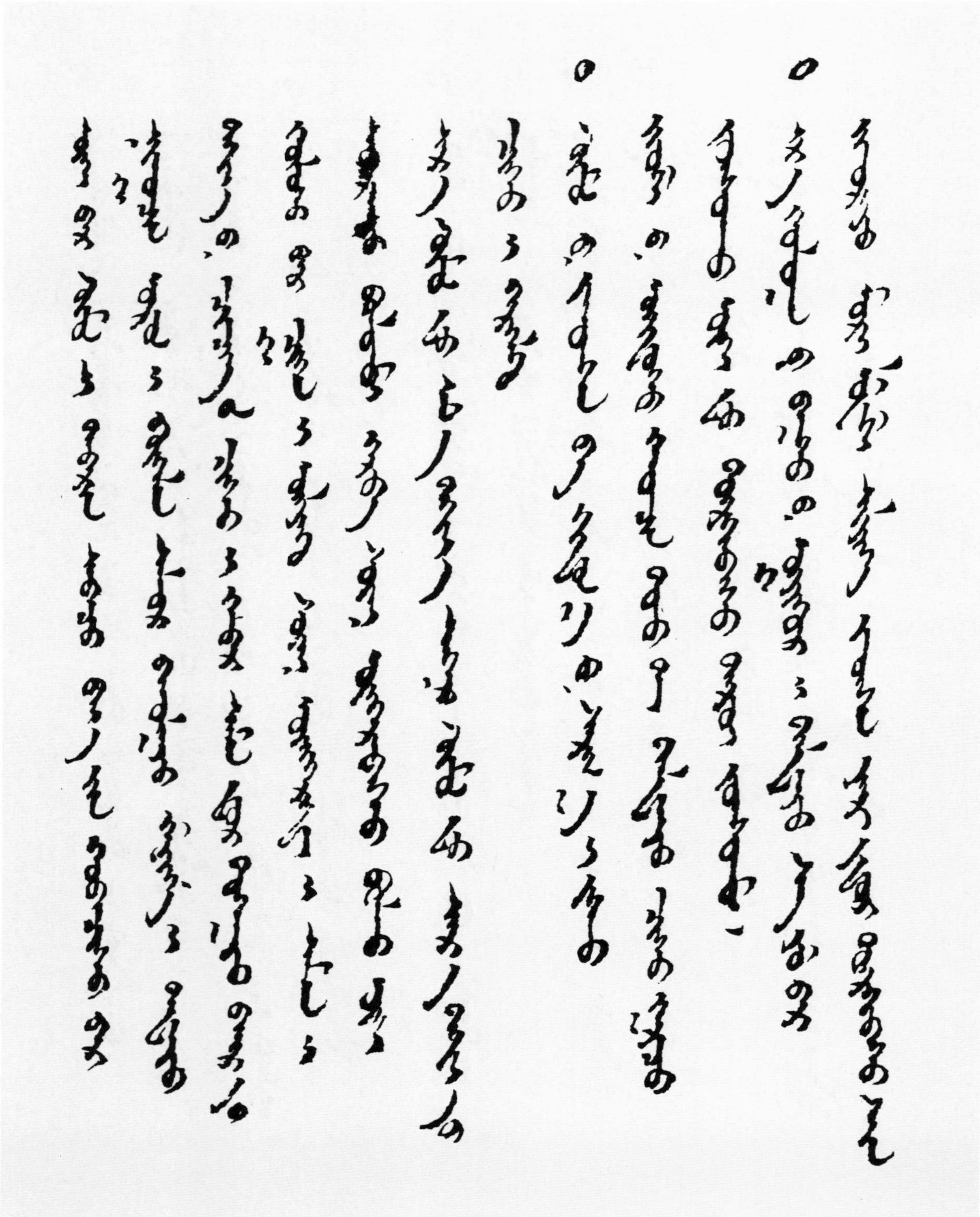

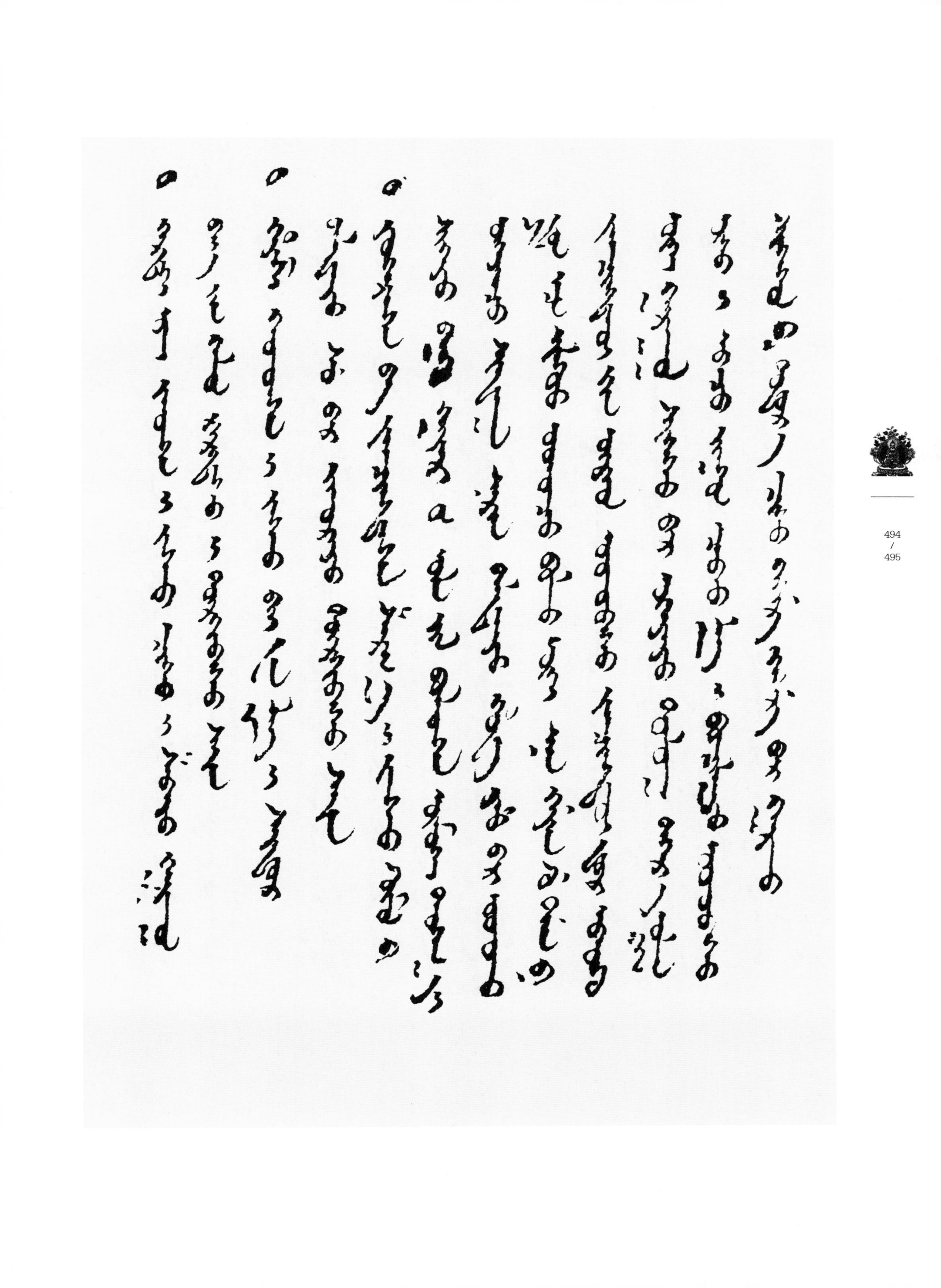

[illegible]

[illegible]

[illegible]

[illegible]

[illegible]

[illegible]

[illegible]

[illegible]

[illegible]

[illegible]

[illegible]

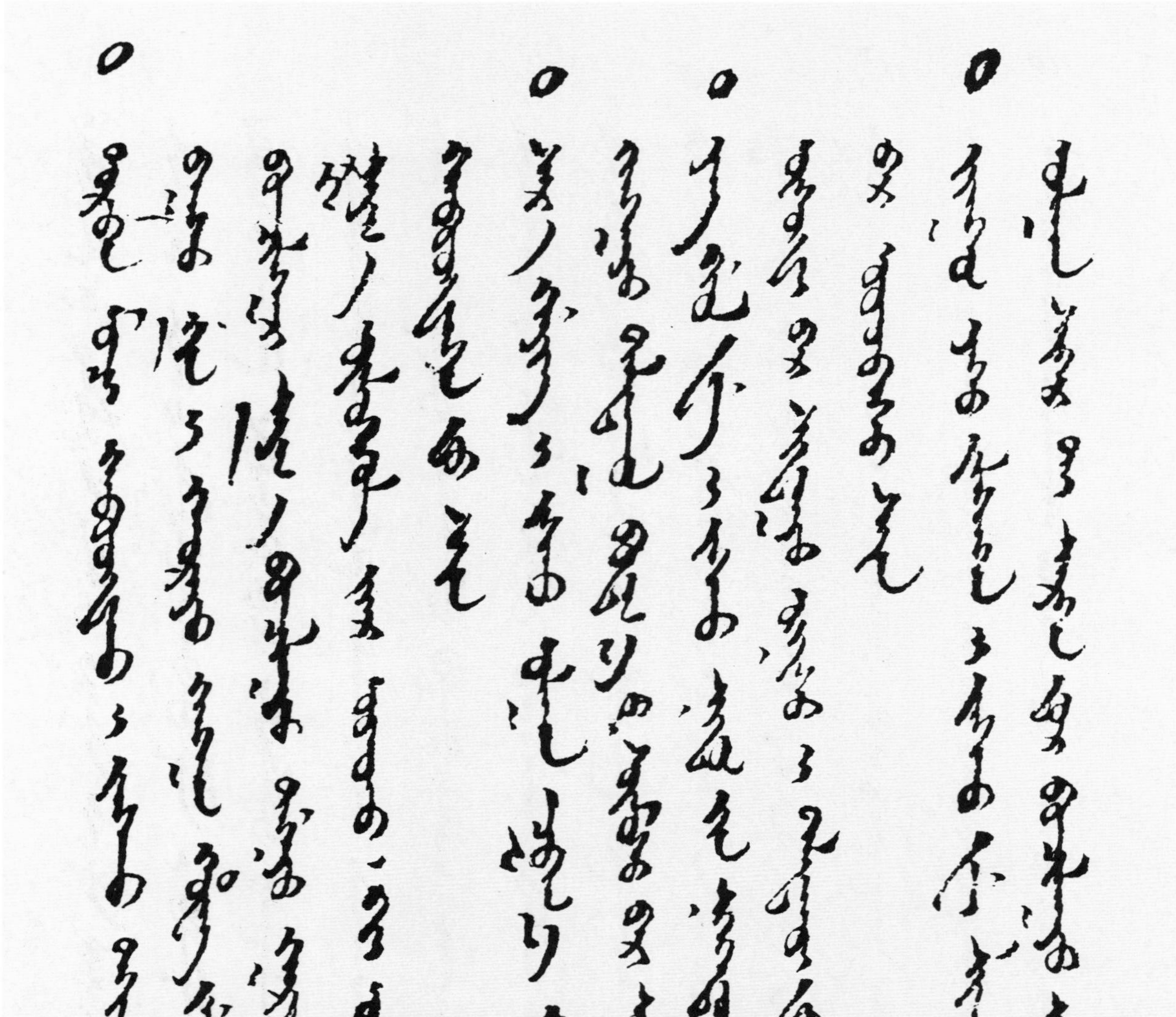

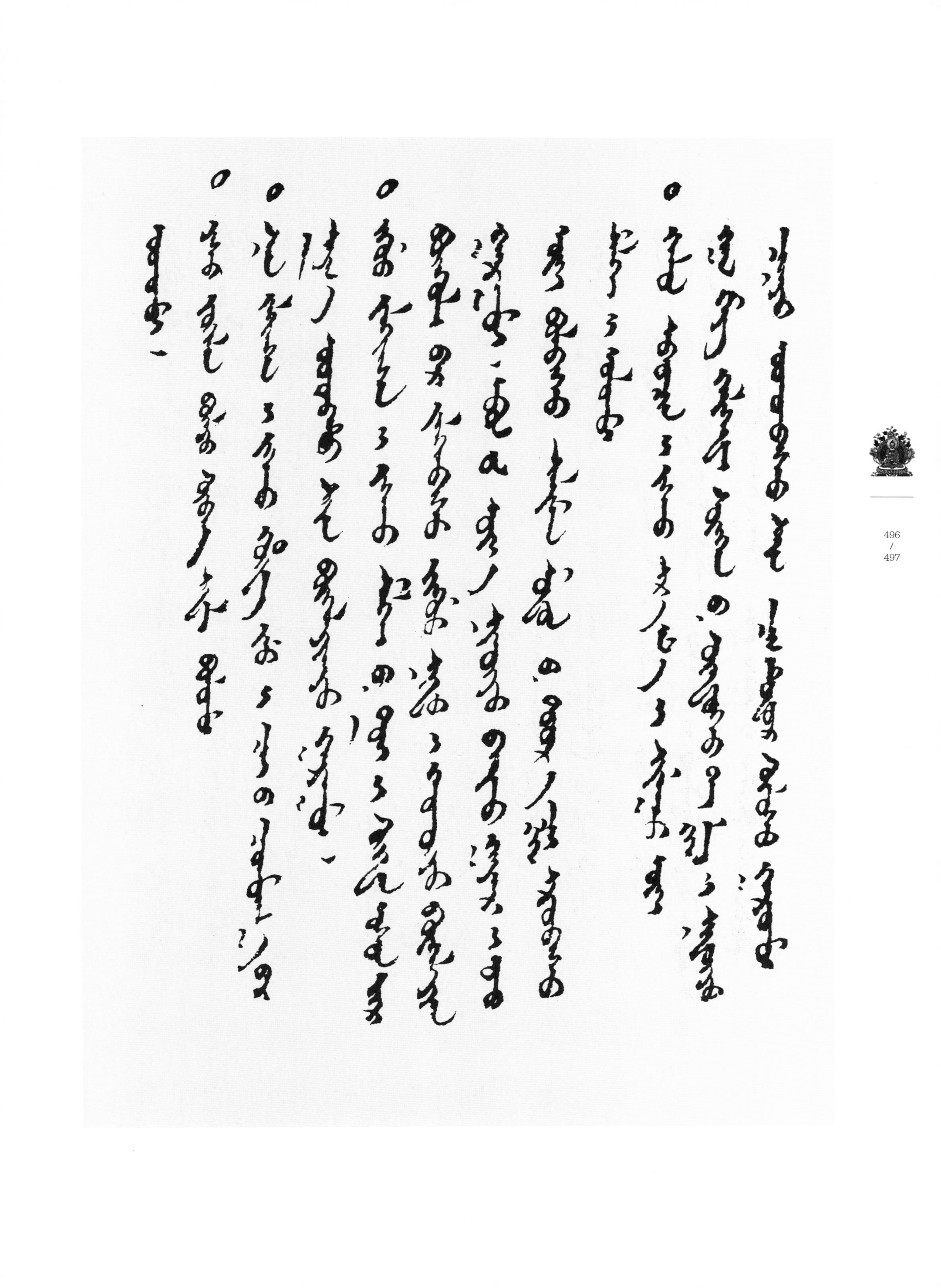

[illegible]

[illegible]

[illegible]

[illegible]

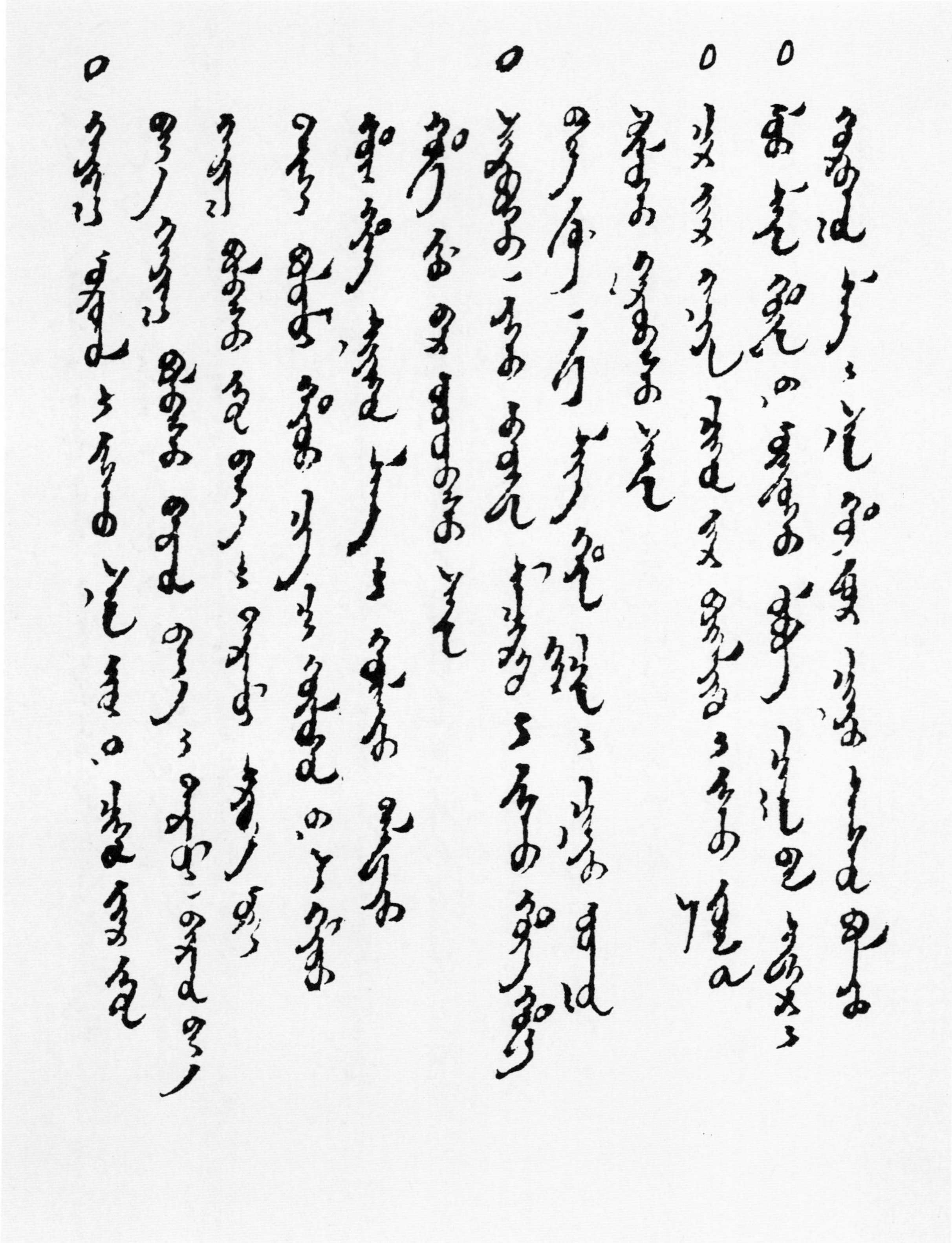

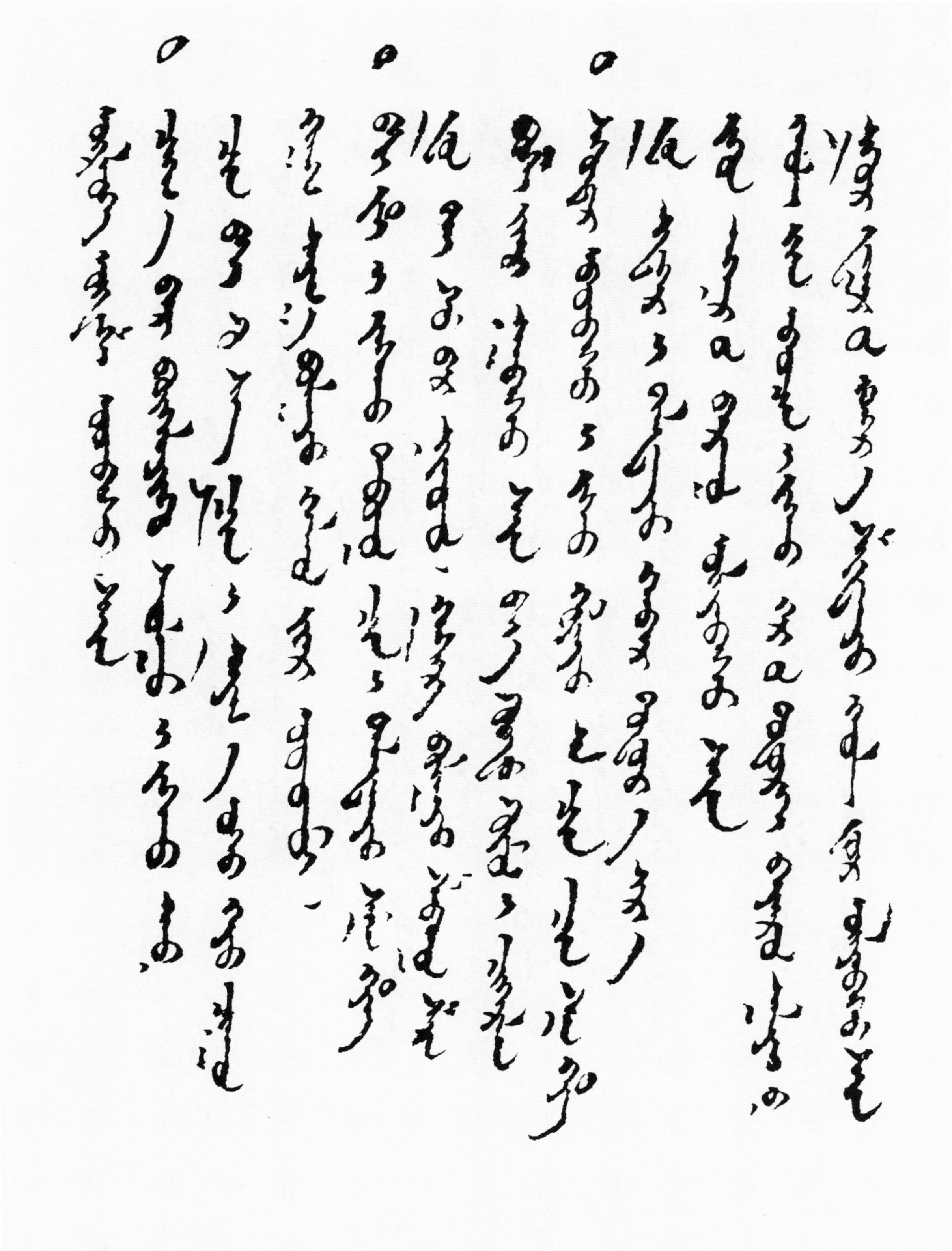

[illegible]

[illegible]

[illegible]

[illegible]

[illegible]

[illegible]

[illegible]

[illegible]

[illegible]

[illegible]

[illegible]

[illegible]

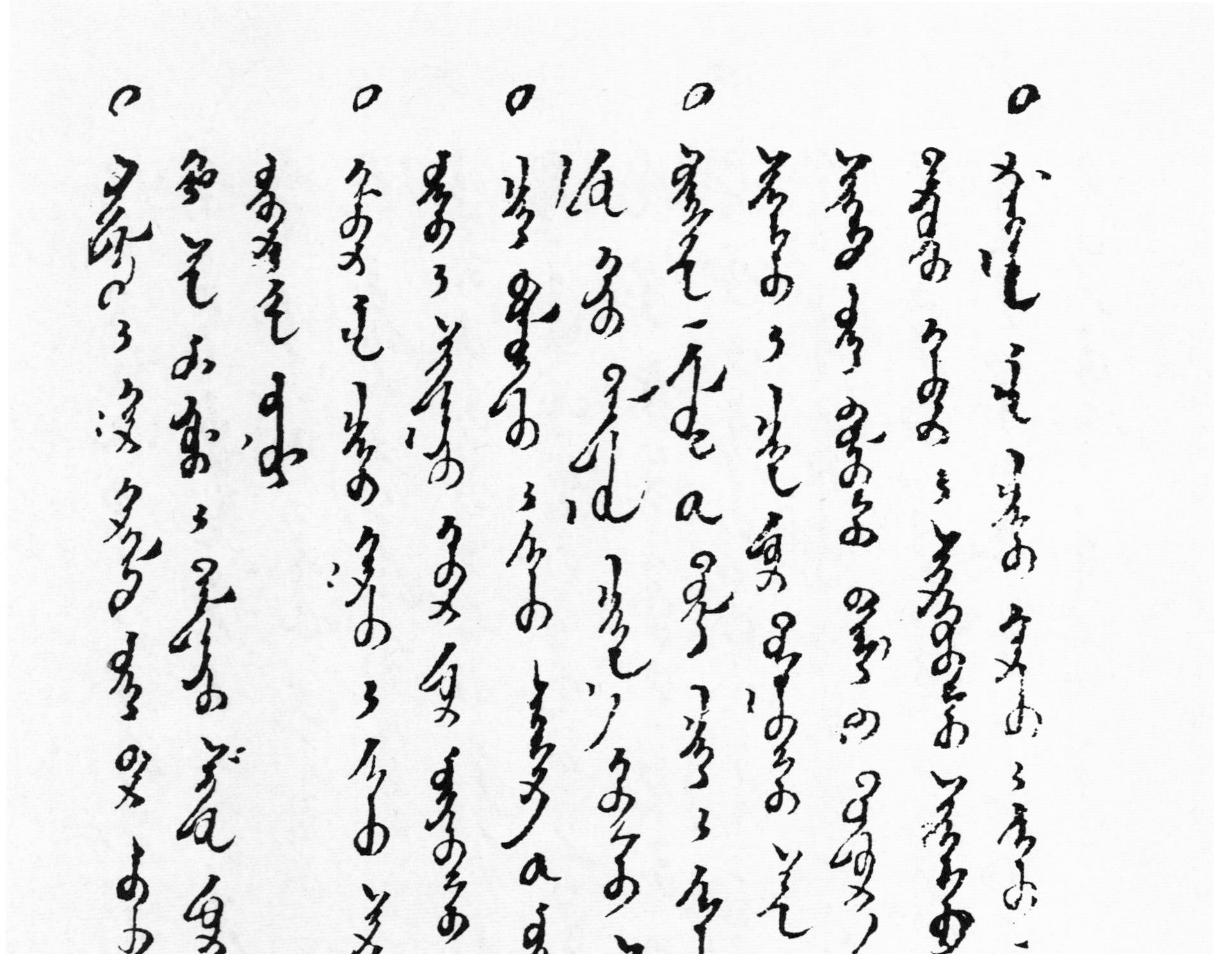

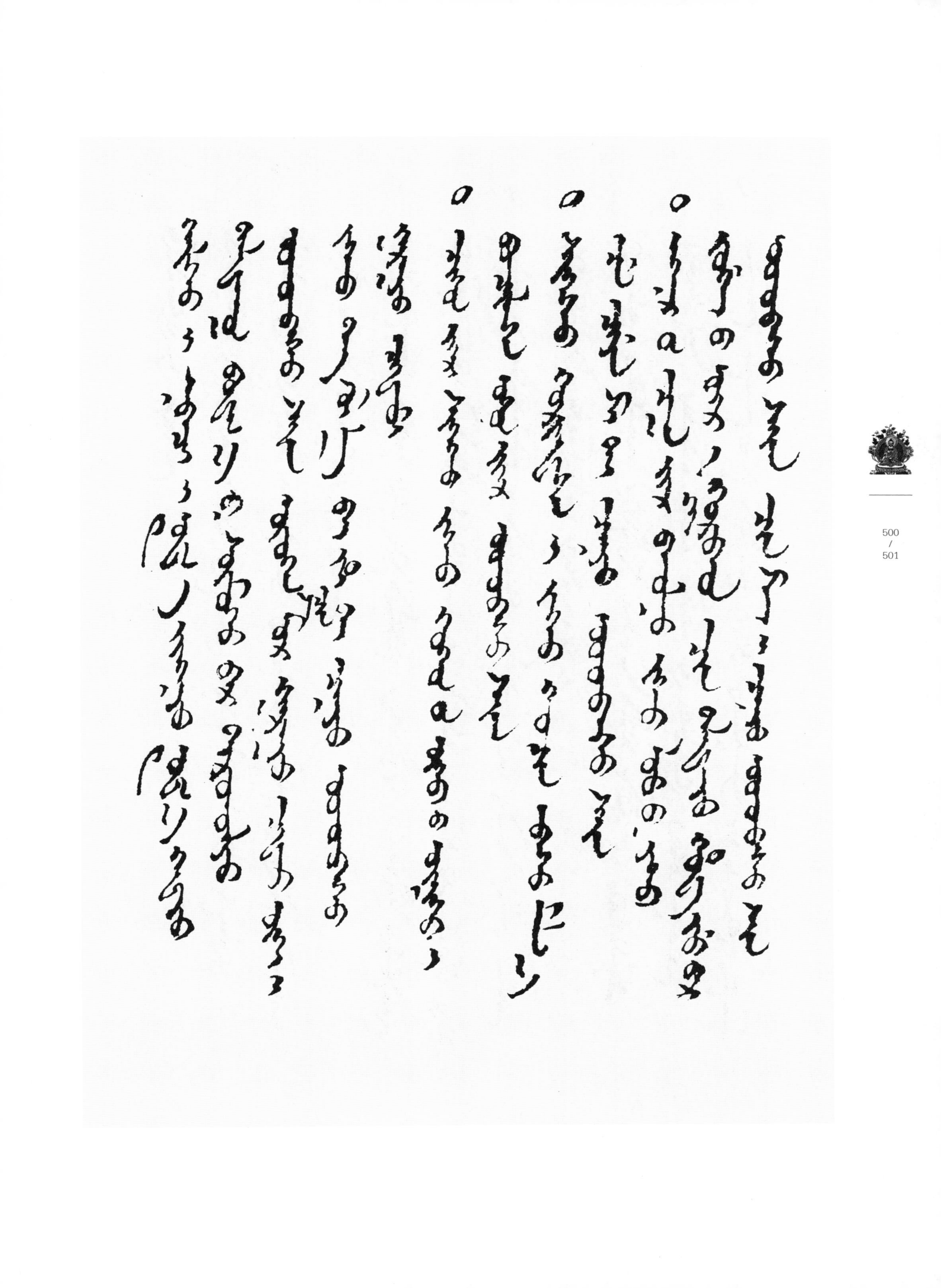

[illegible]

[illegible]

[illegible]

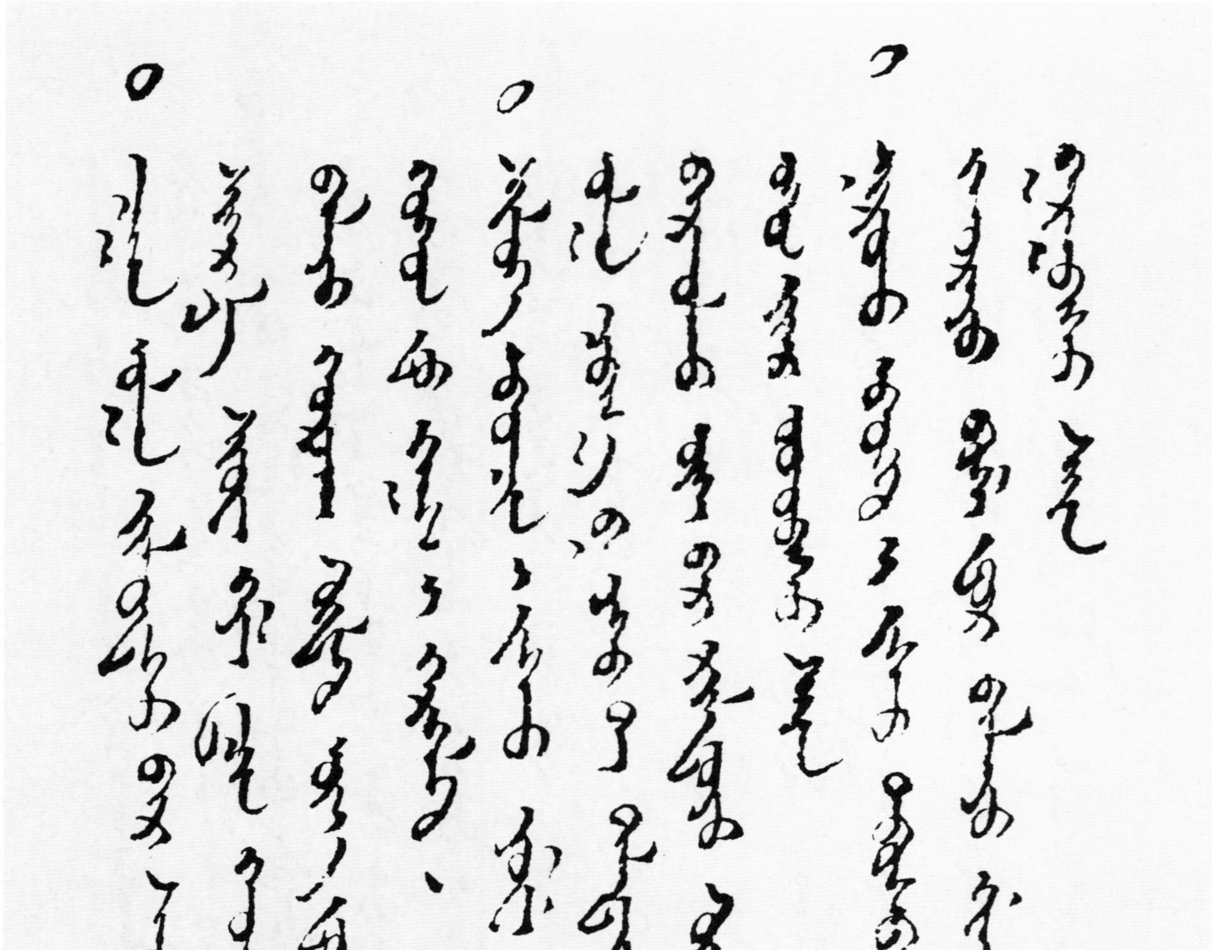

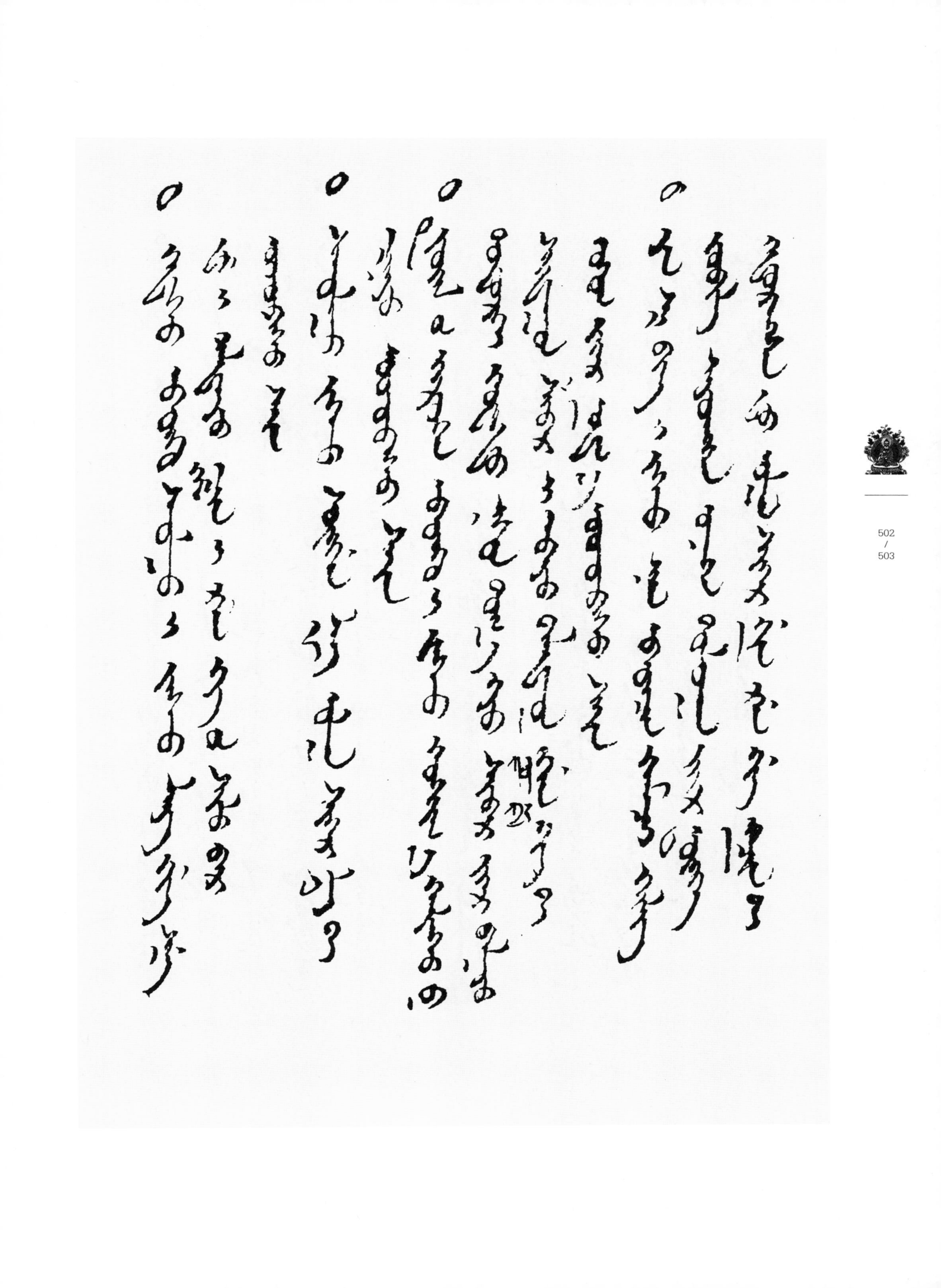

[illegible]

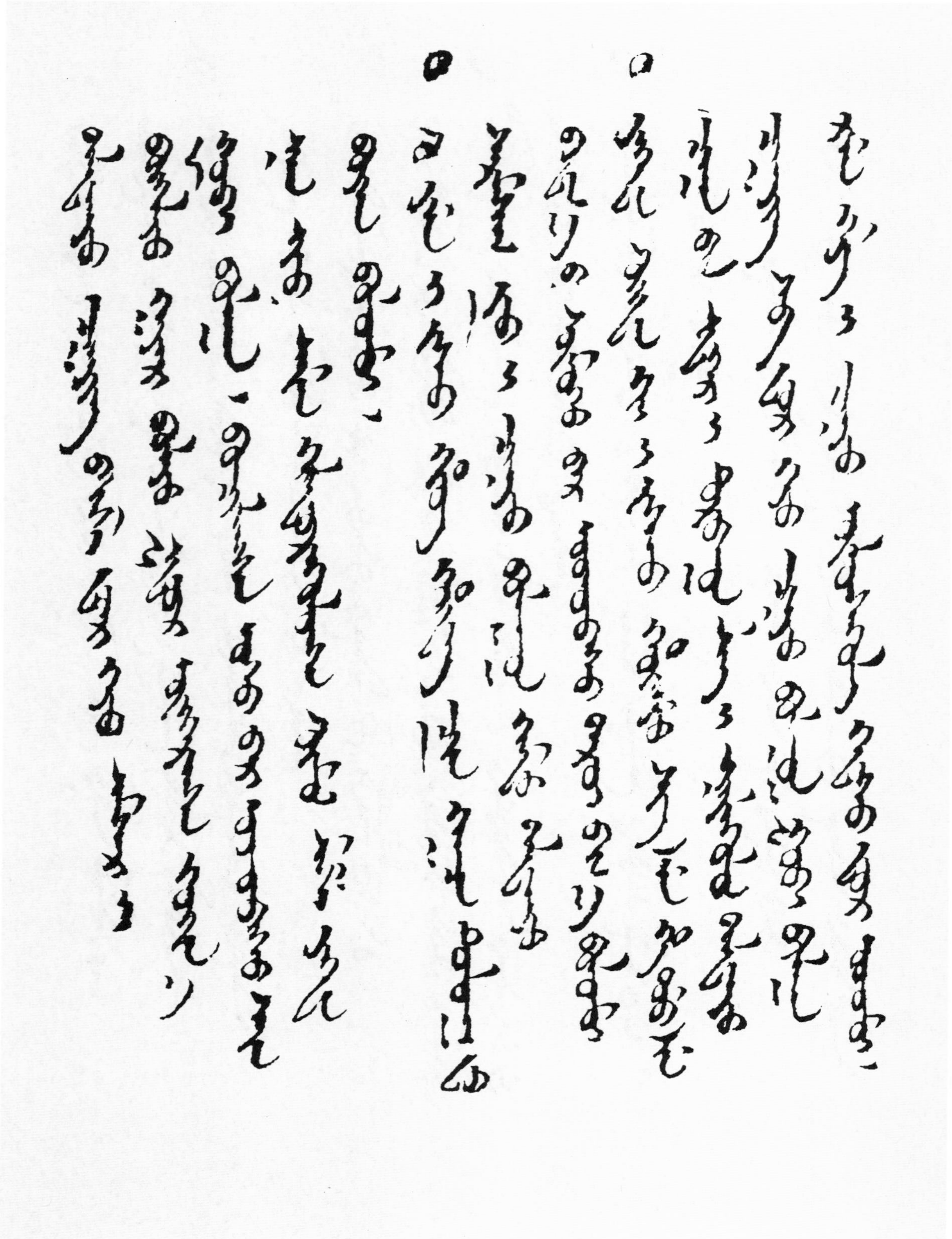

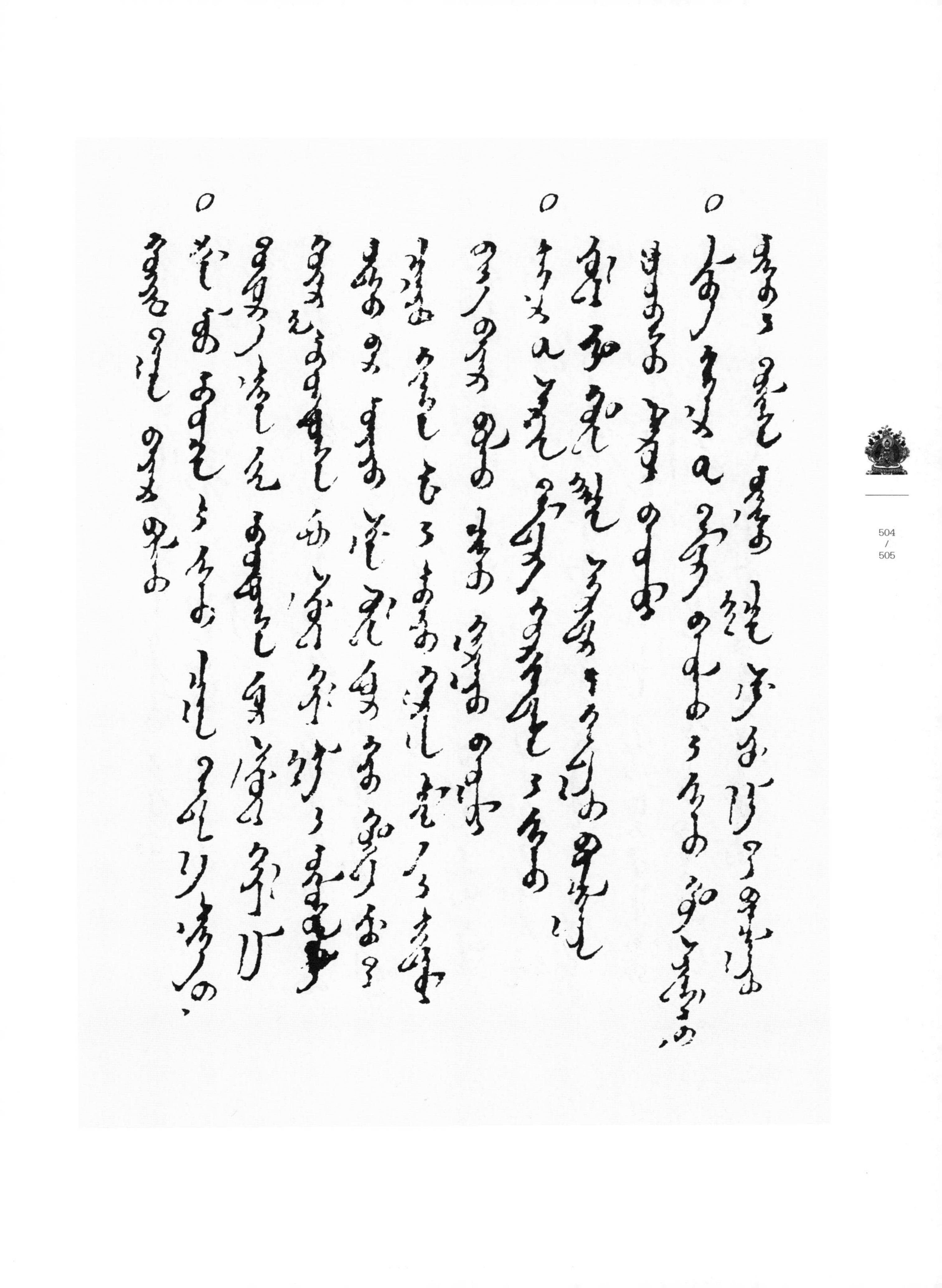

[illegible]

[illegible]

[illegible]

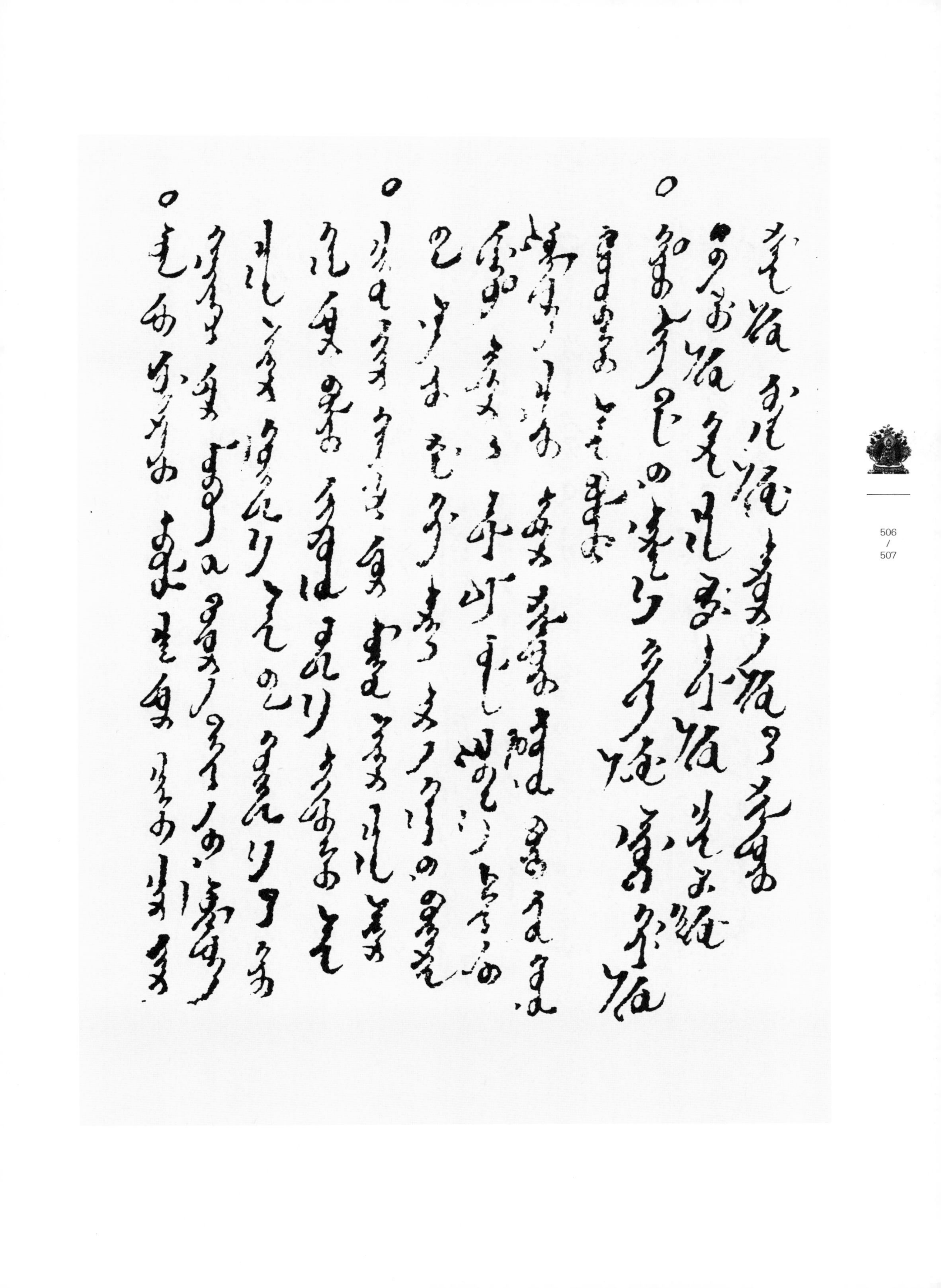

[illegible]
[illegible]
[illegible]
[illegible]
[illegible]
[illegible]
[illegible]
[illegible]
[illegible]

[illegible]
[illegible]

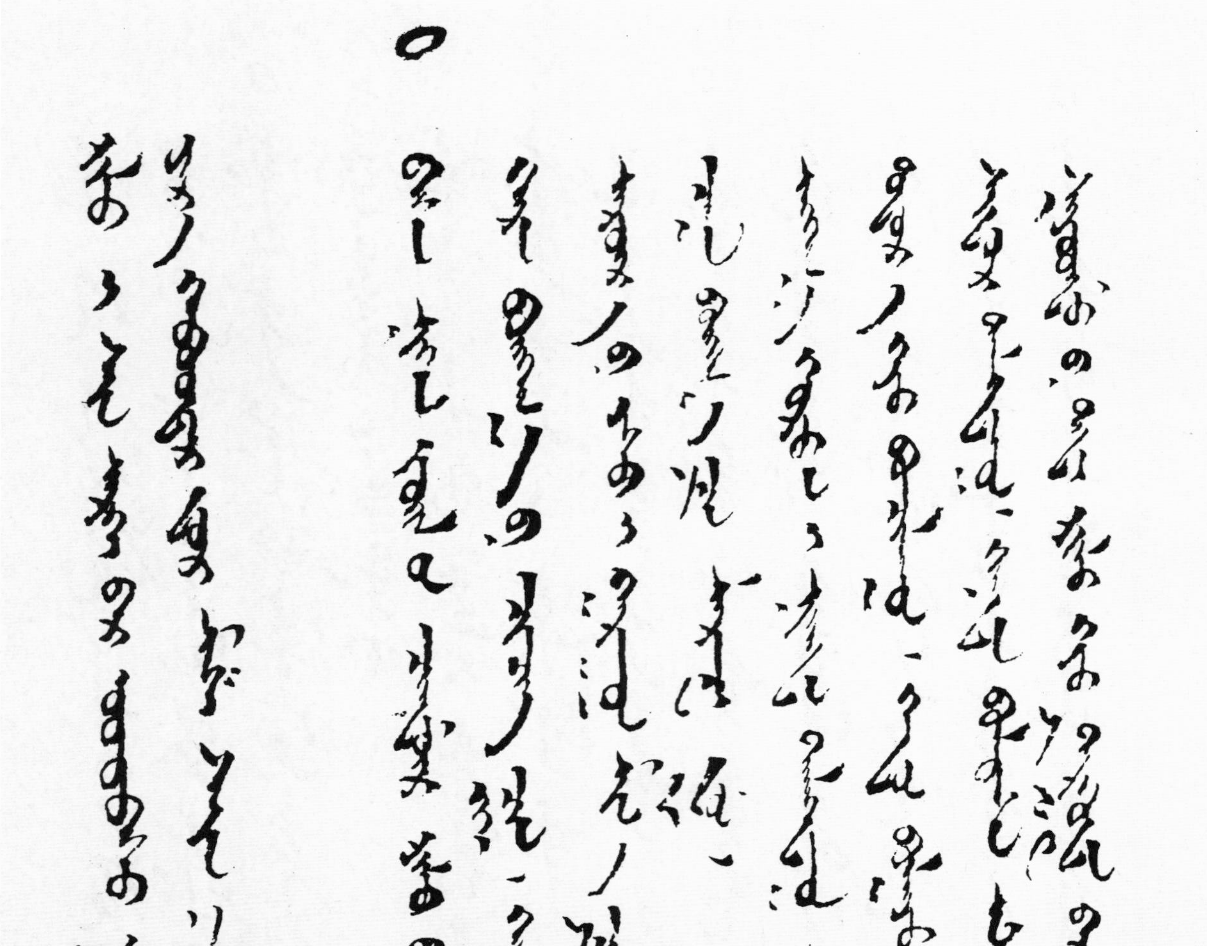

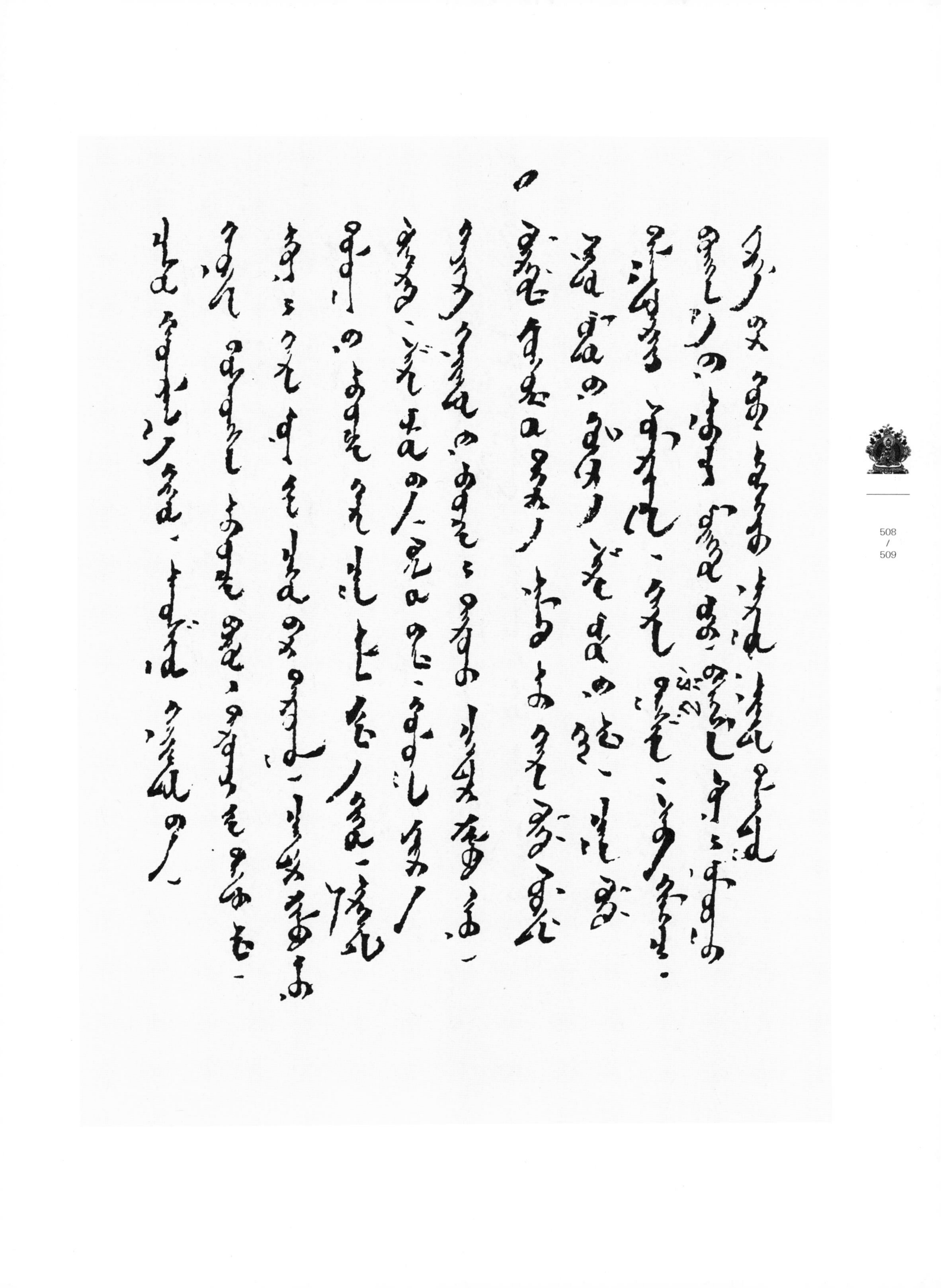

[illegible]
[illegible]
[illegible]
[illegible]
[illegible]
[illegible]
[illegible]
[illegible]
[illegible]
[illegible]
[illegible]

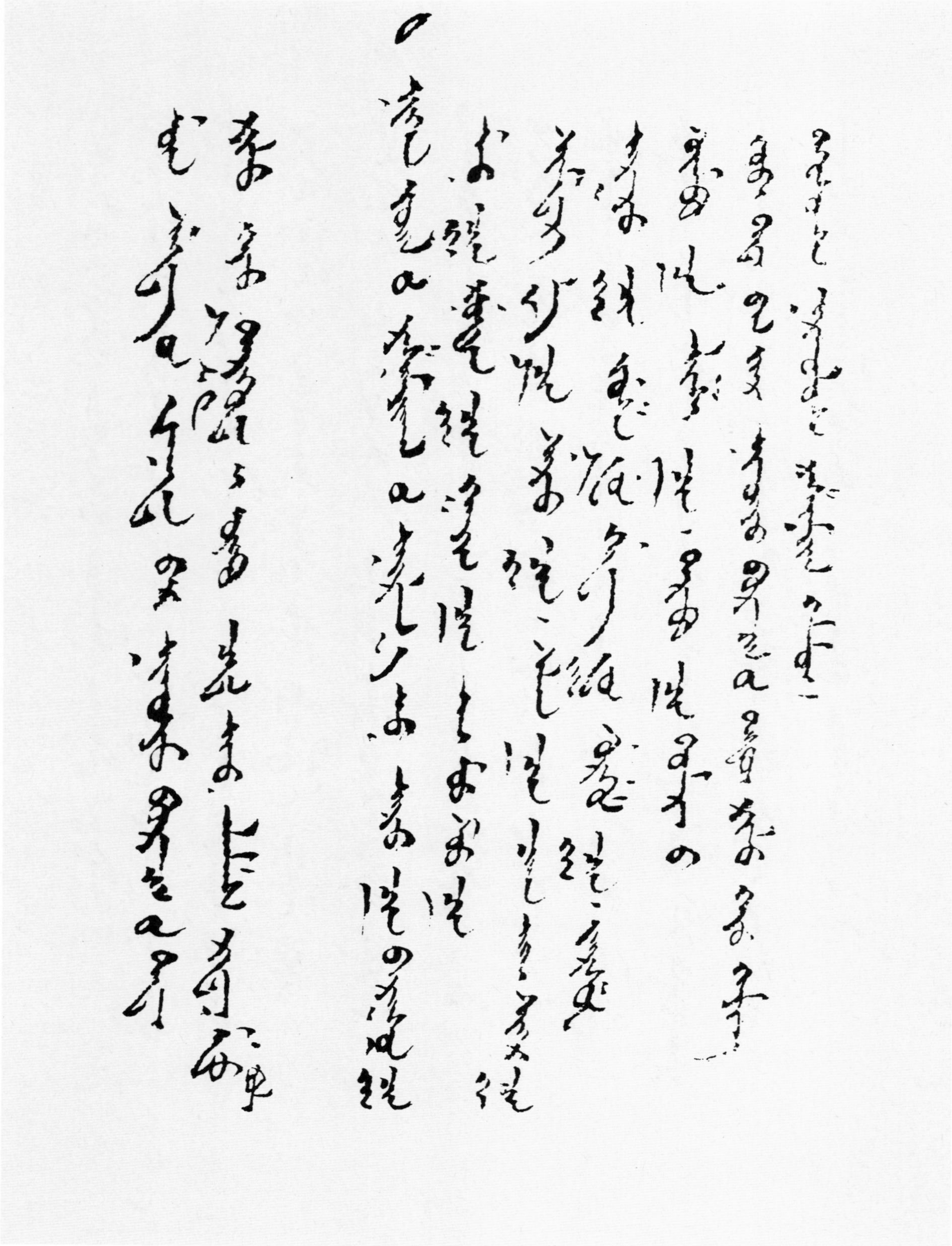

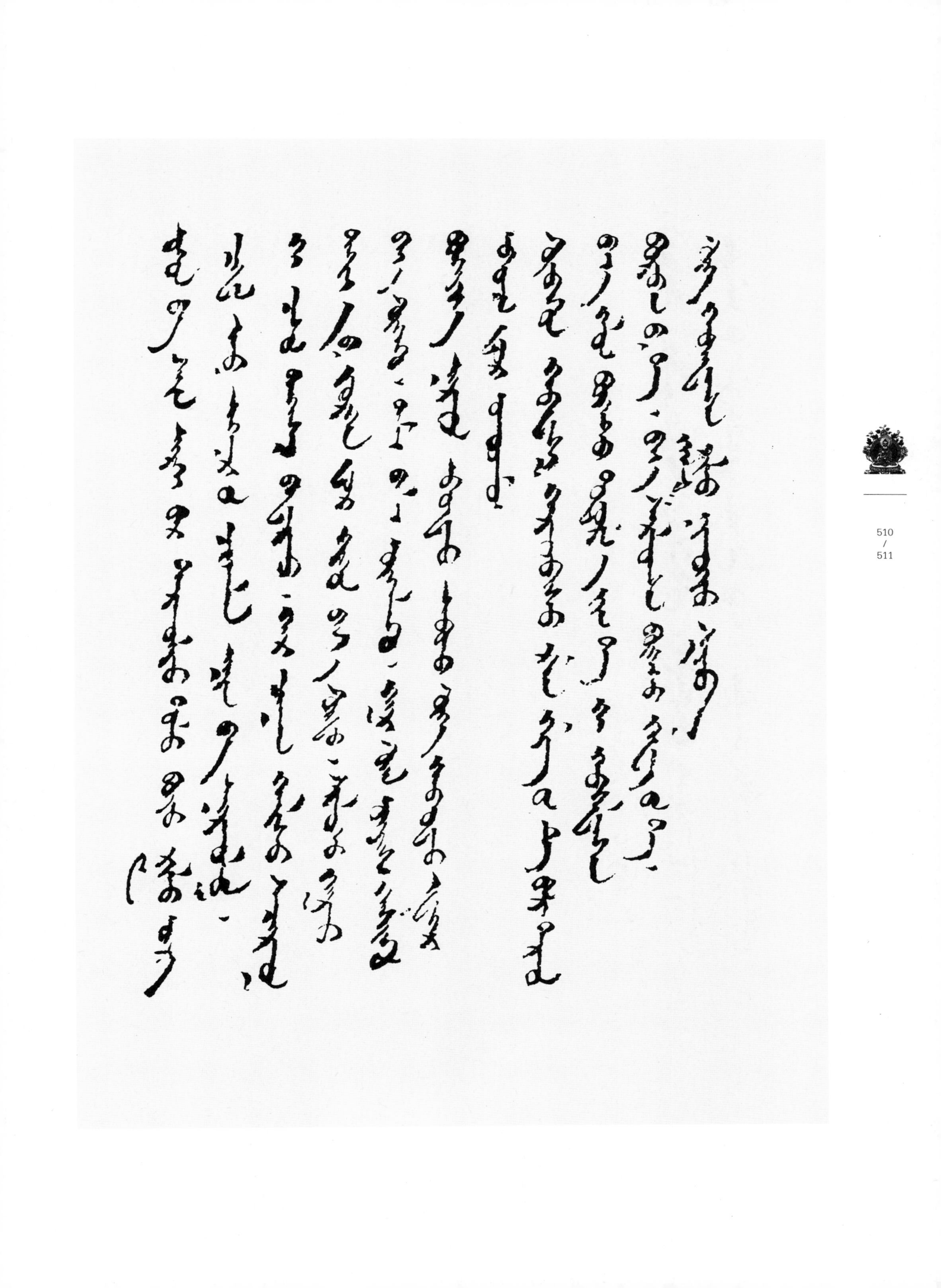

[illegible]

[illegible]

[illegible]

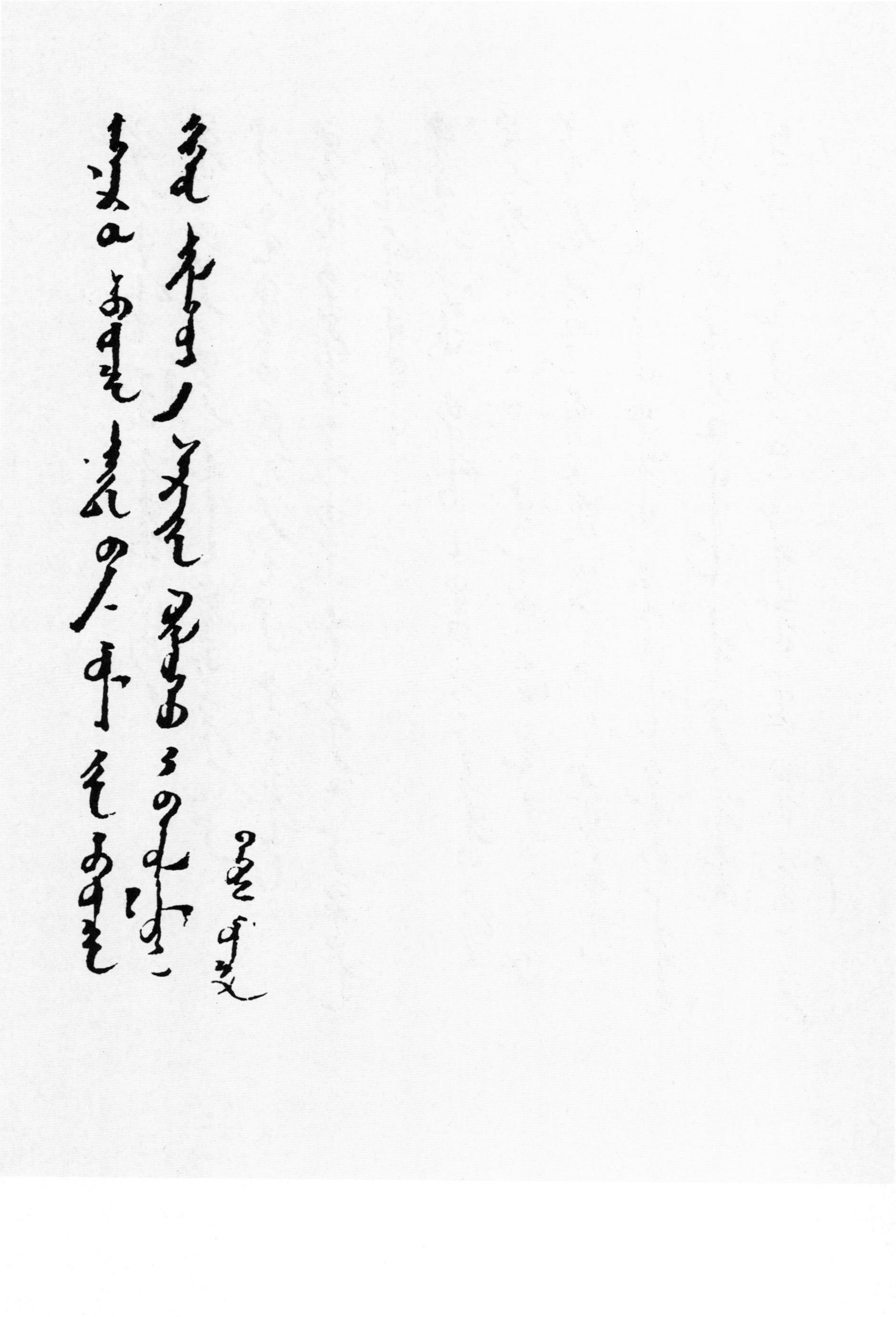

[illegible]

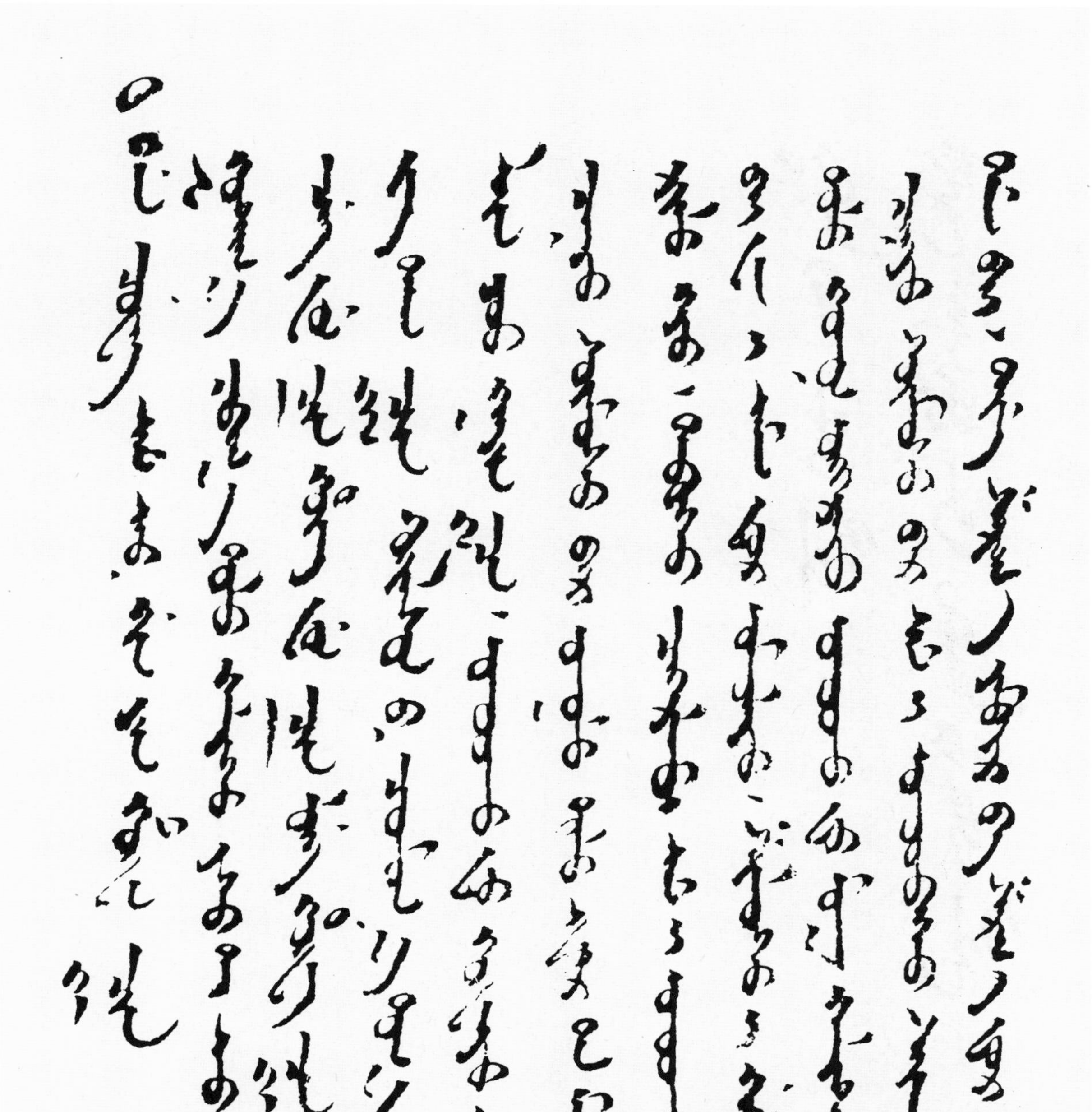

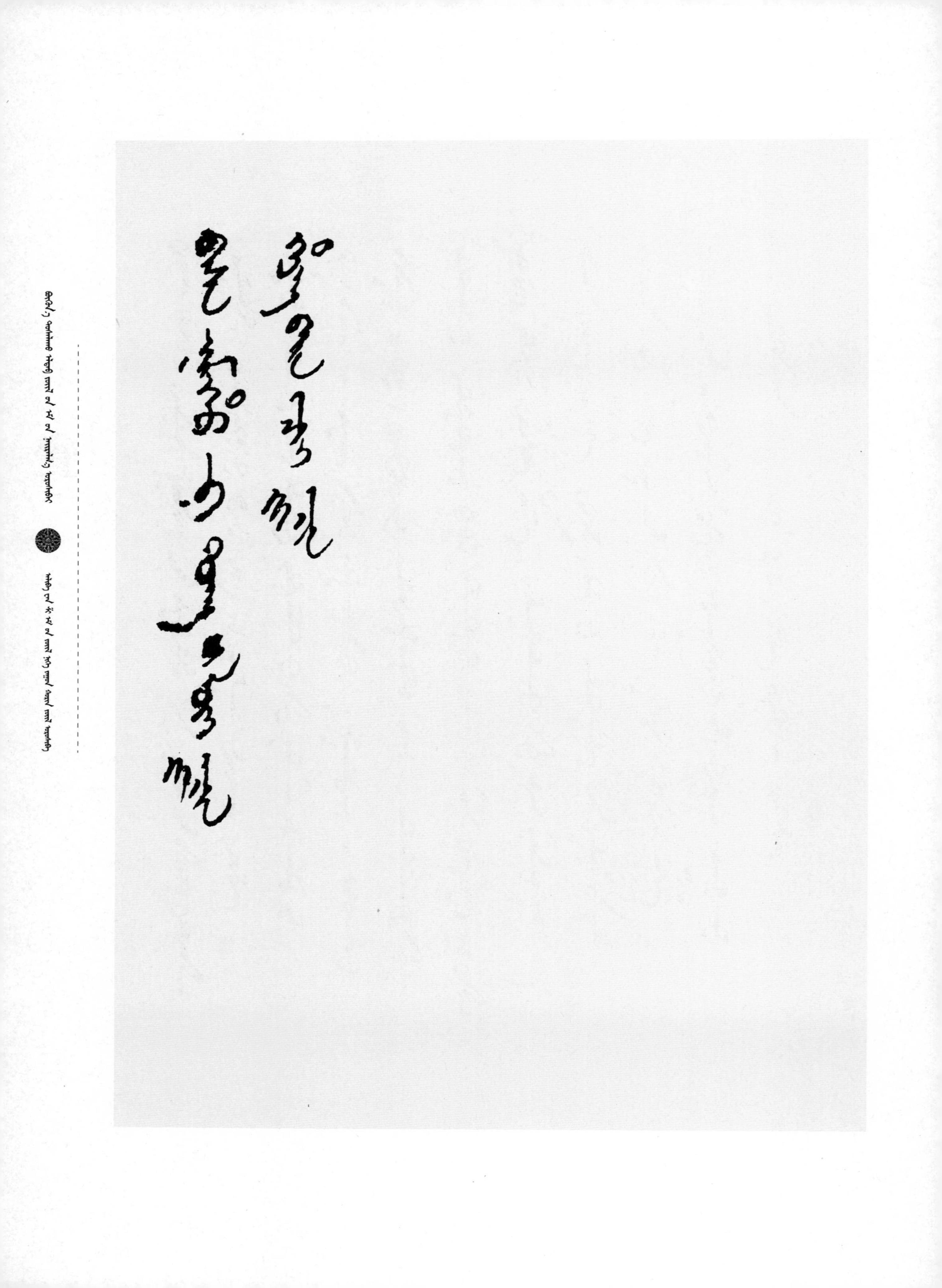

[illegible] [illegible] [illegible] [illegible]

[illegible] [illegible] [illegible] [illegible] [illegible] [illegible]

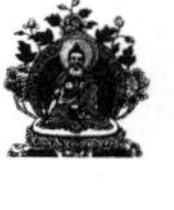

[illegible]

[illegible]

[illegible]

[illegible]

[illegible]

[illegible]

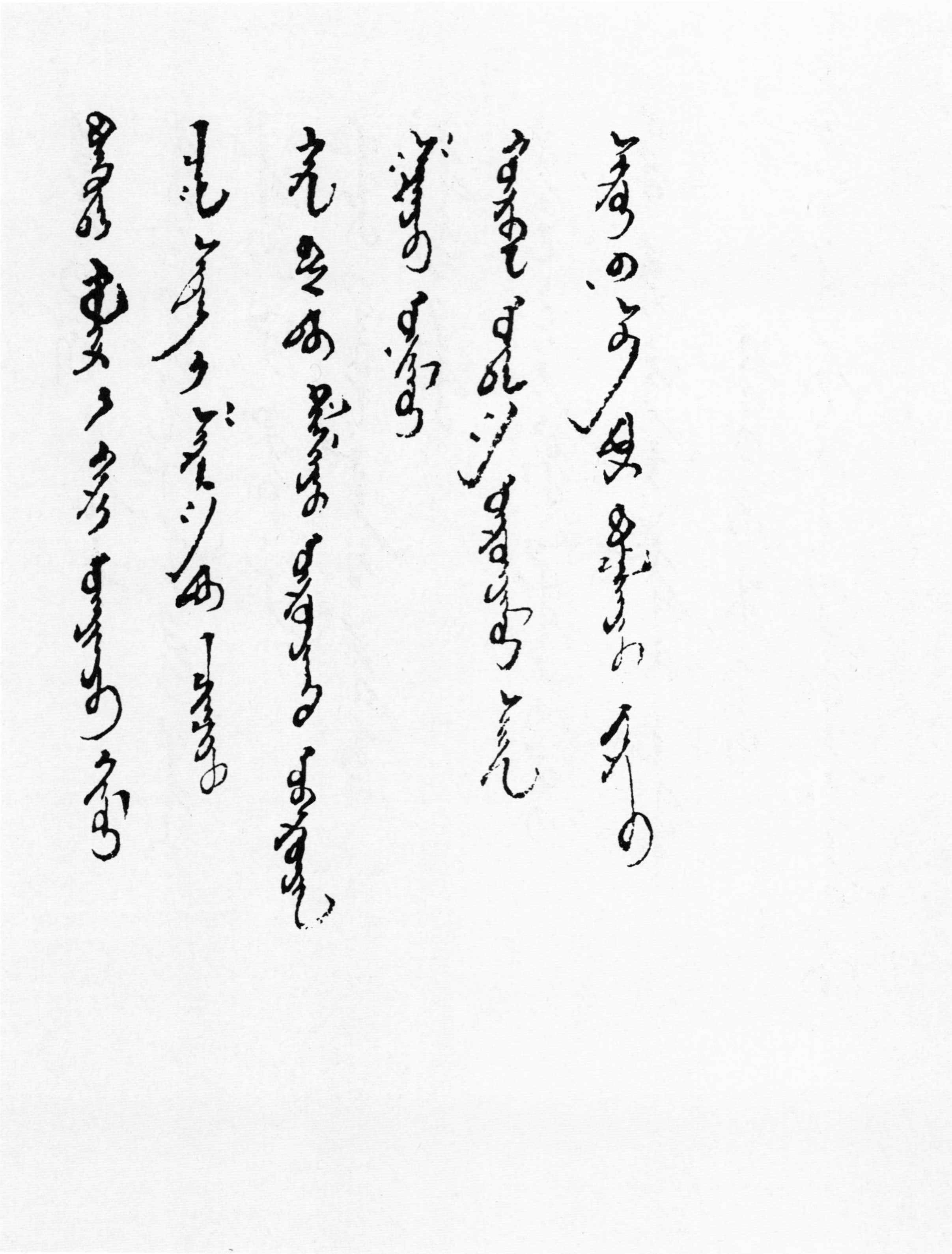

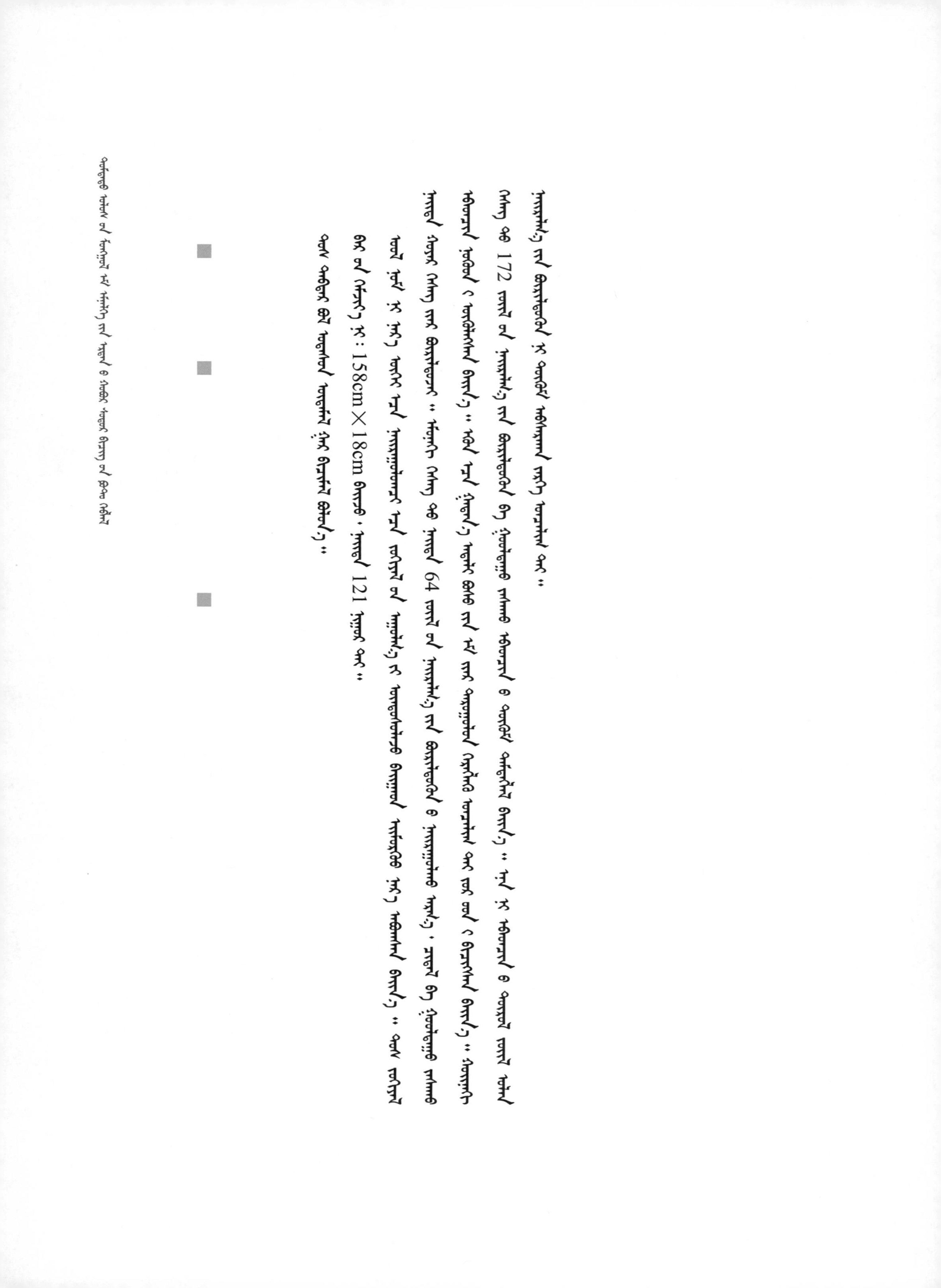

... 158cm×18cm ... 121 ... ::

... 172 ... 64 ...

Prescriptions

药方

10

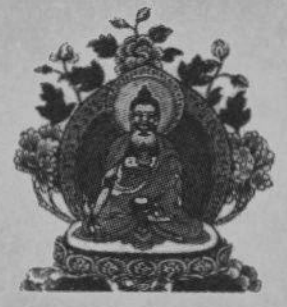

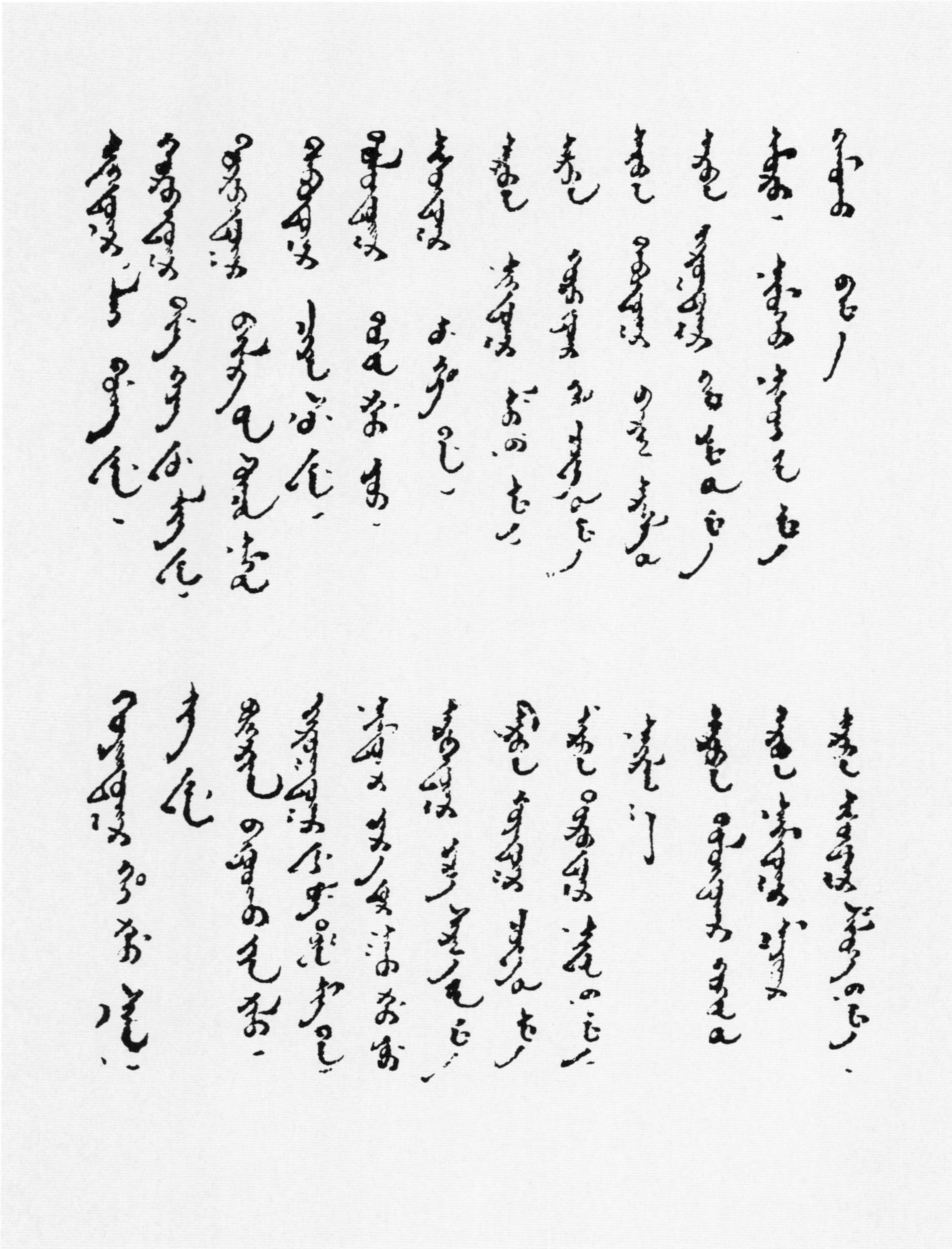

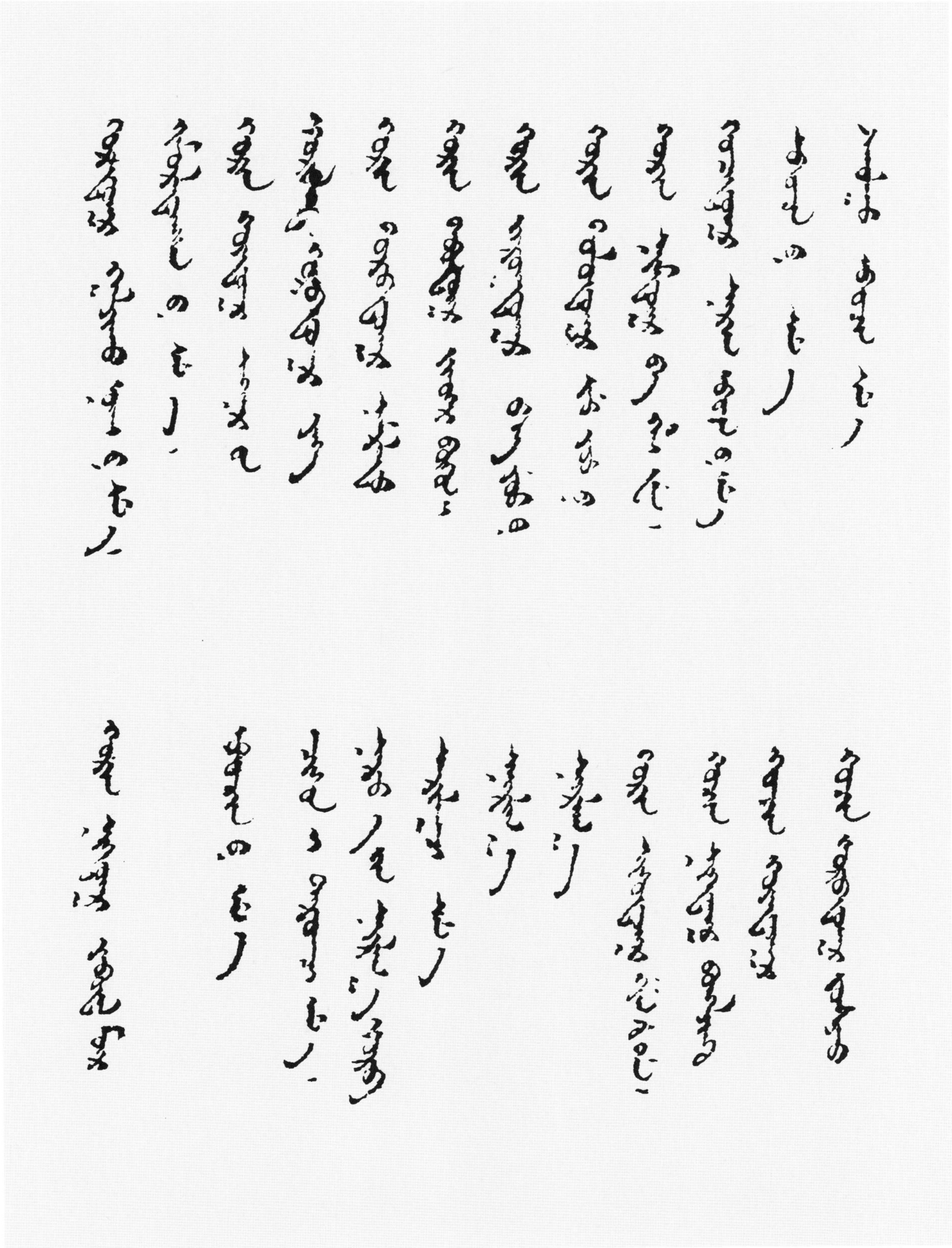

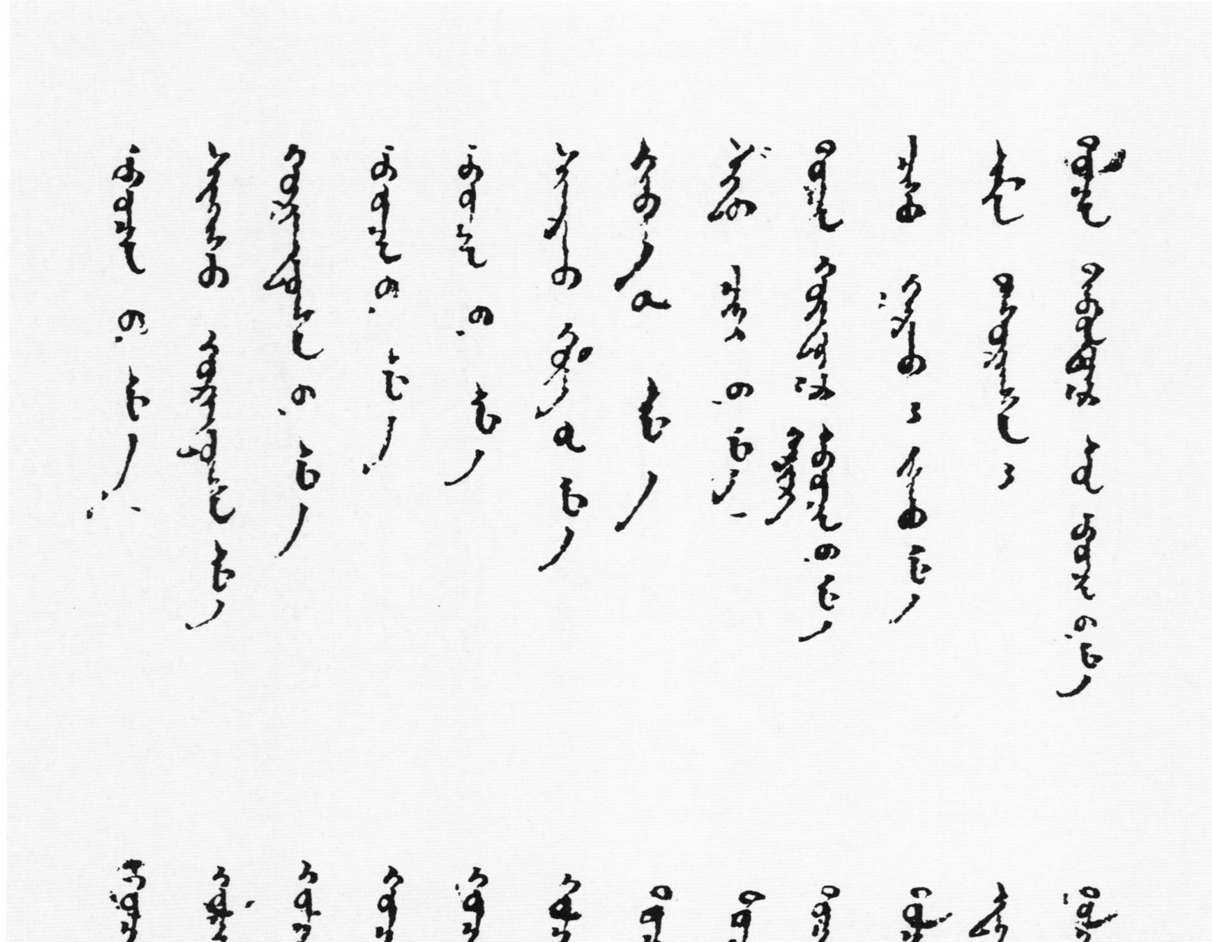

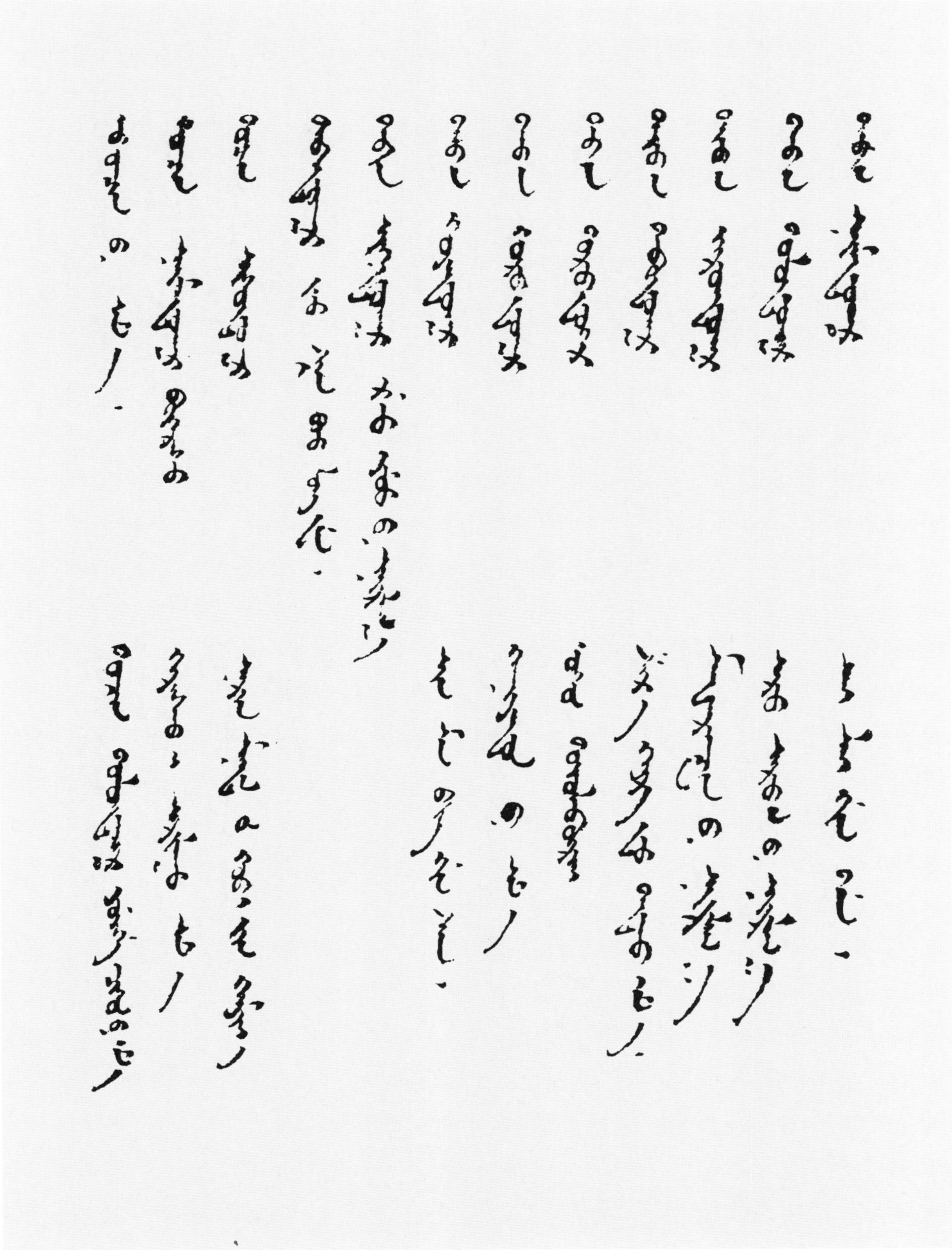

[illegible]

[illegible]

[illegible]

[illegible]

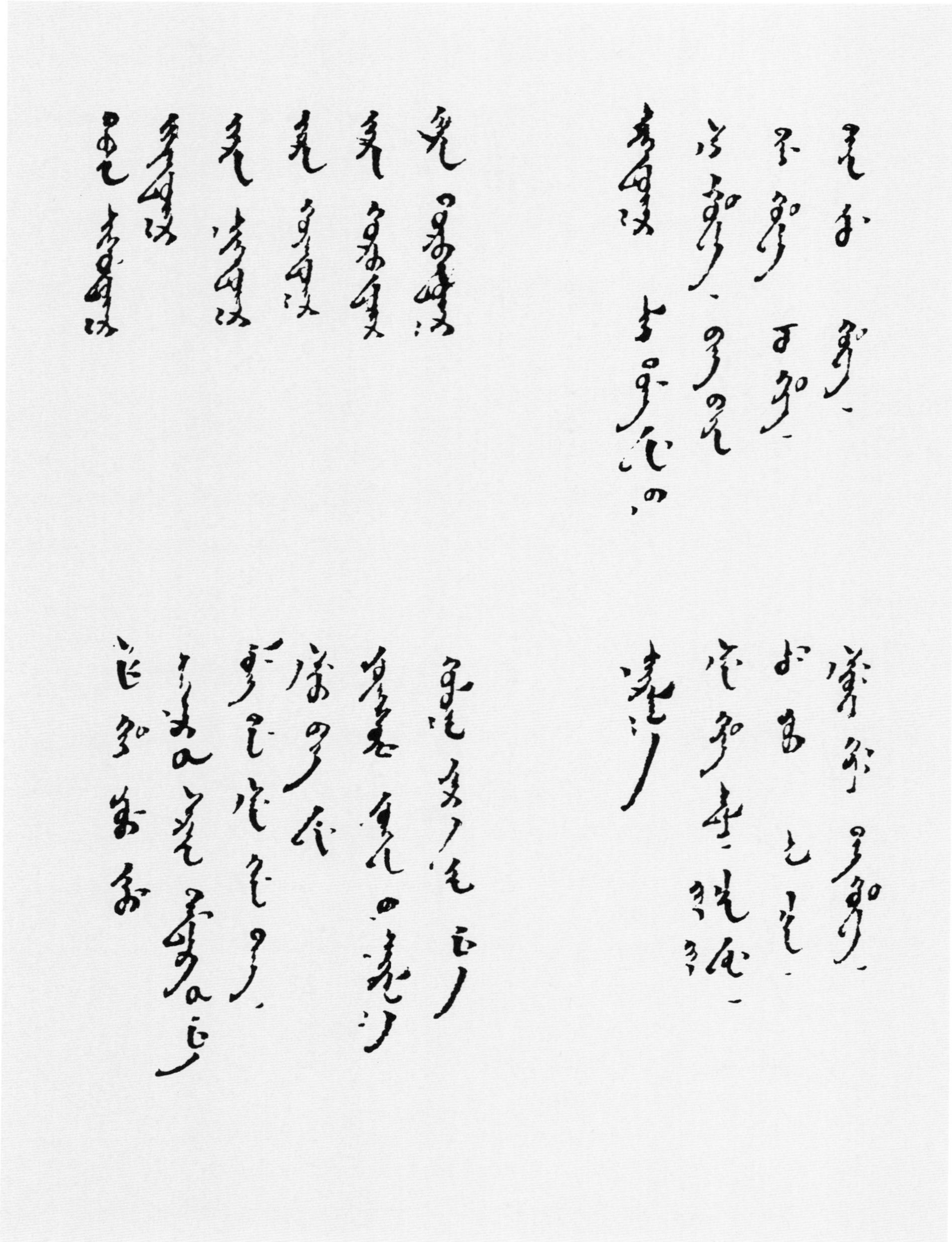

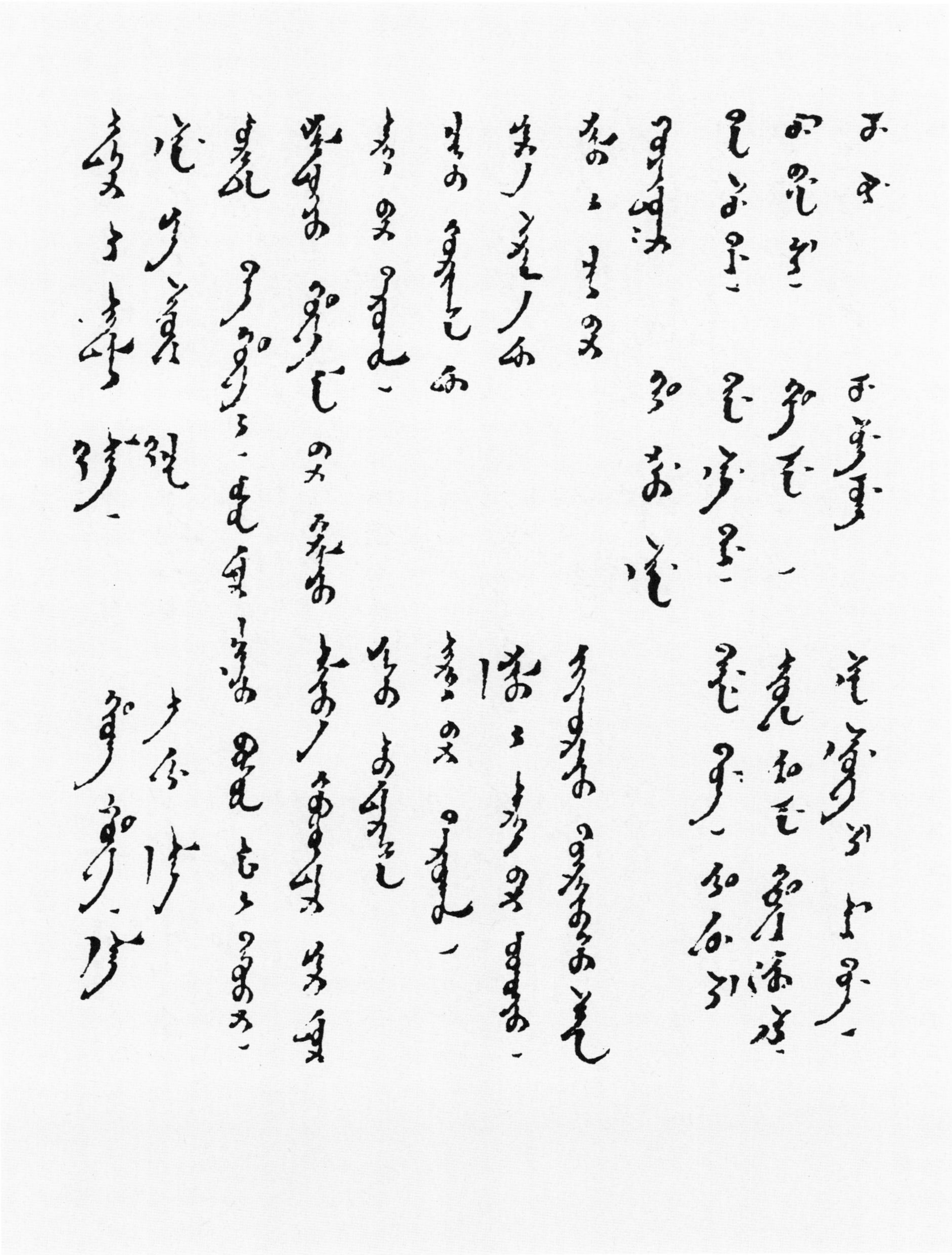

[illegible]

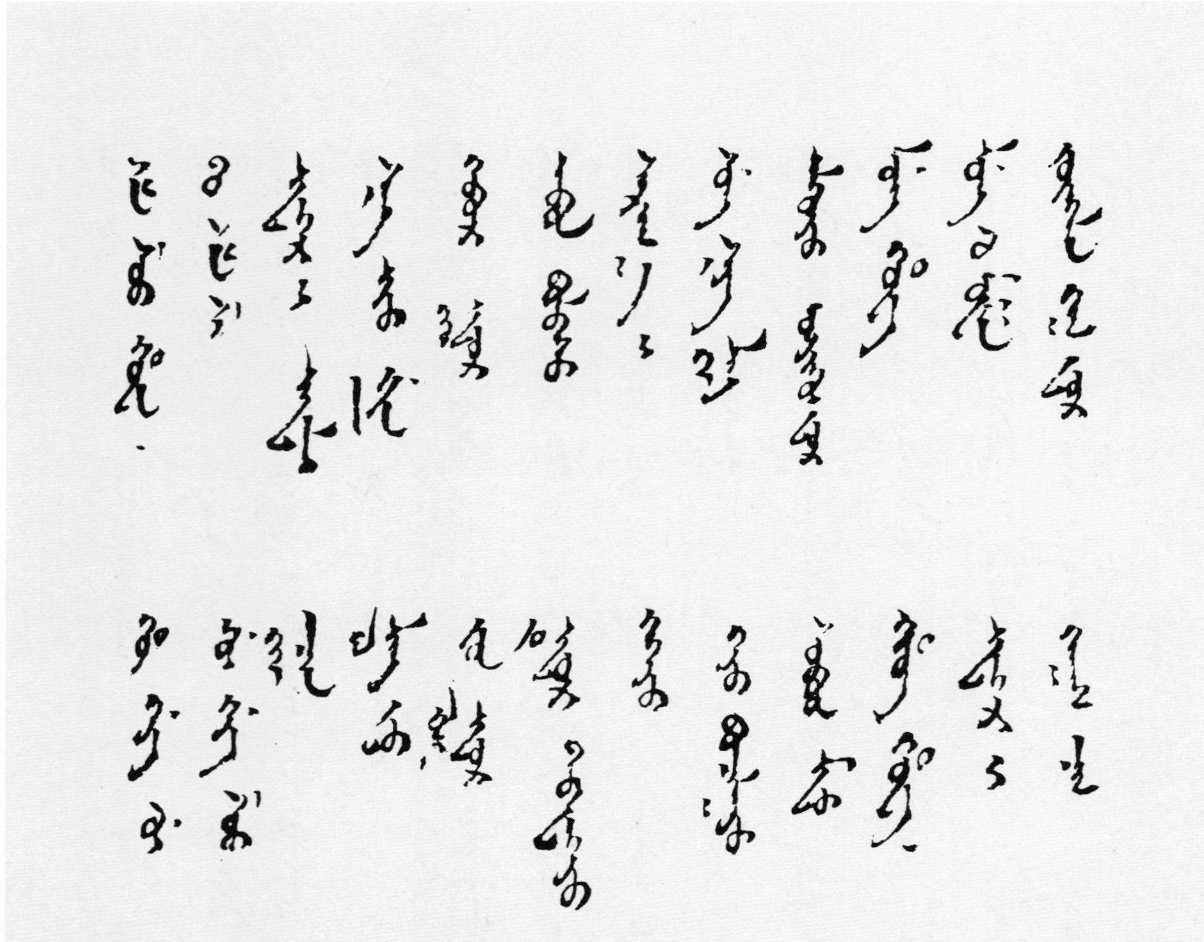

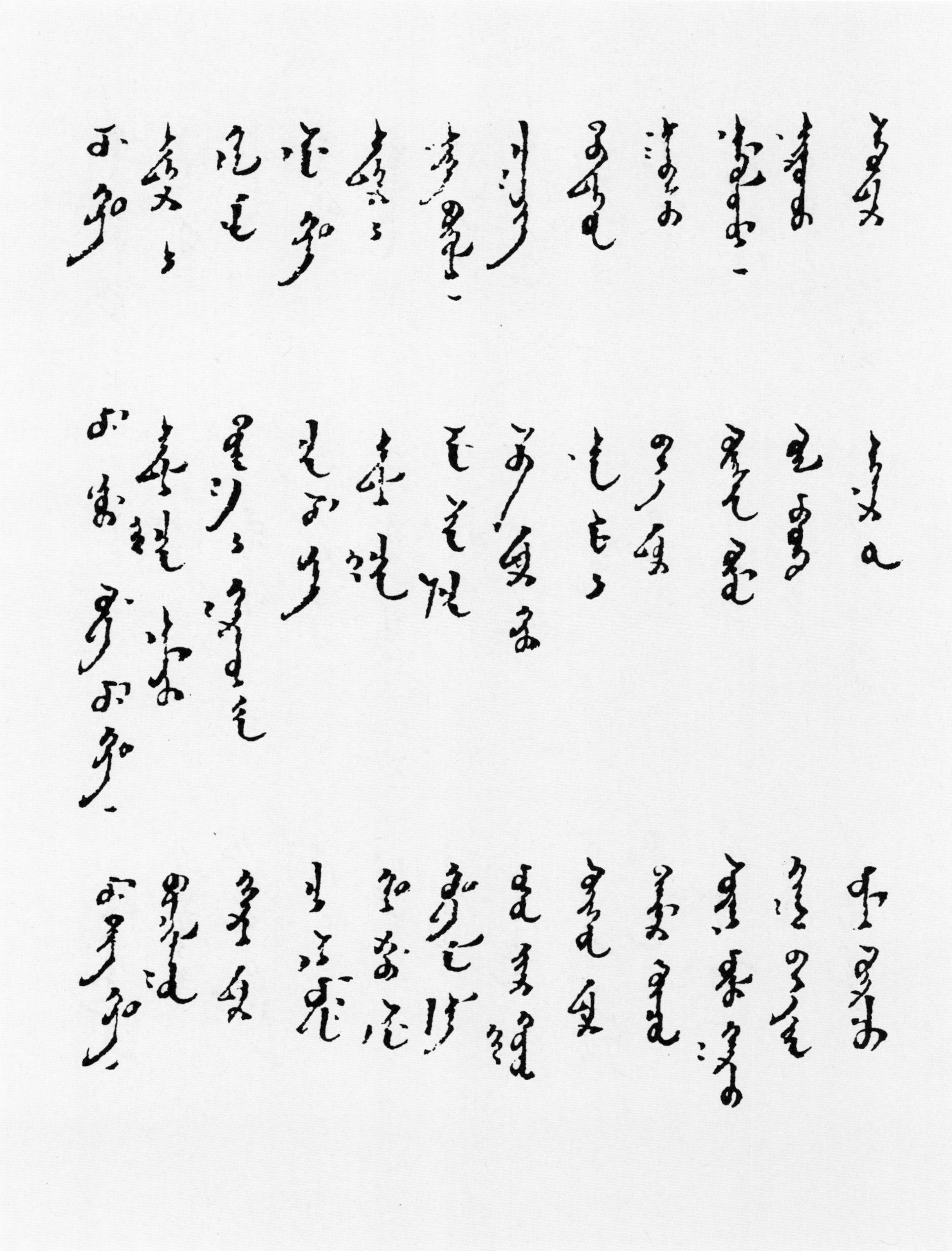

[illegible]

[illegible]

[illegible]

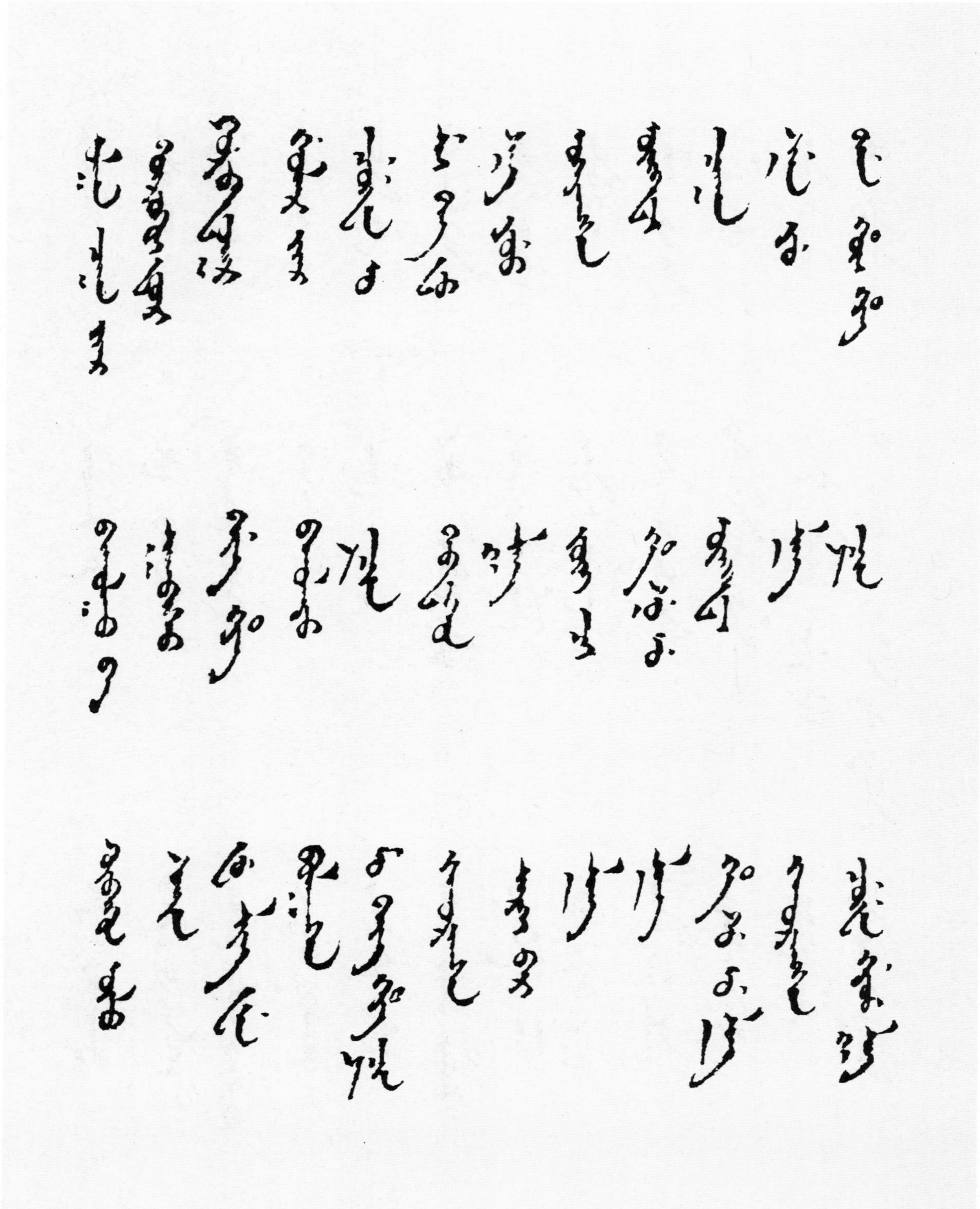

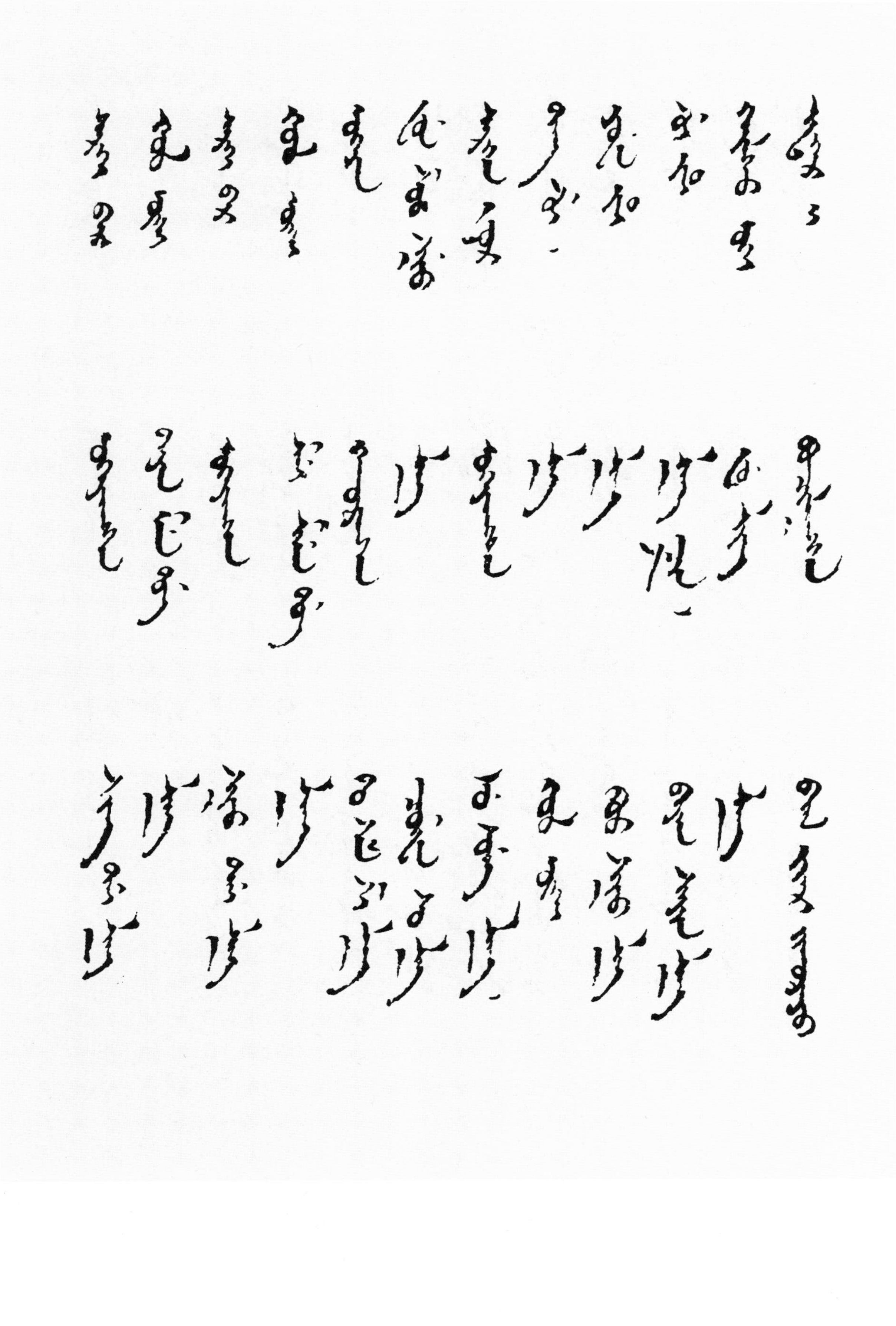

[illegible]

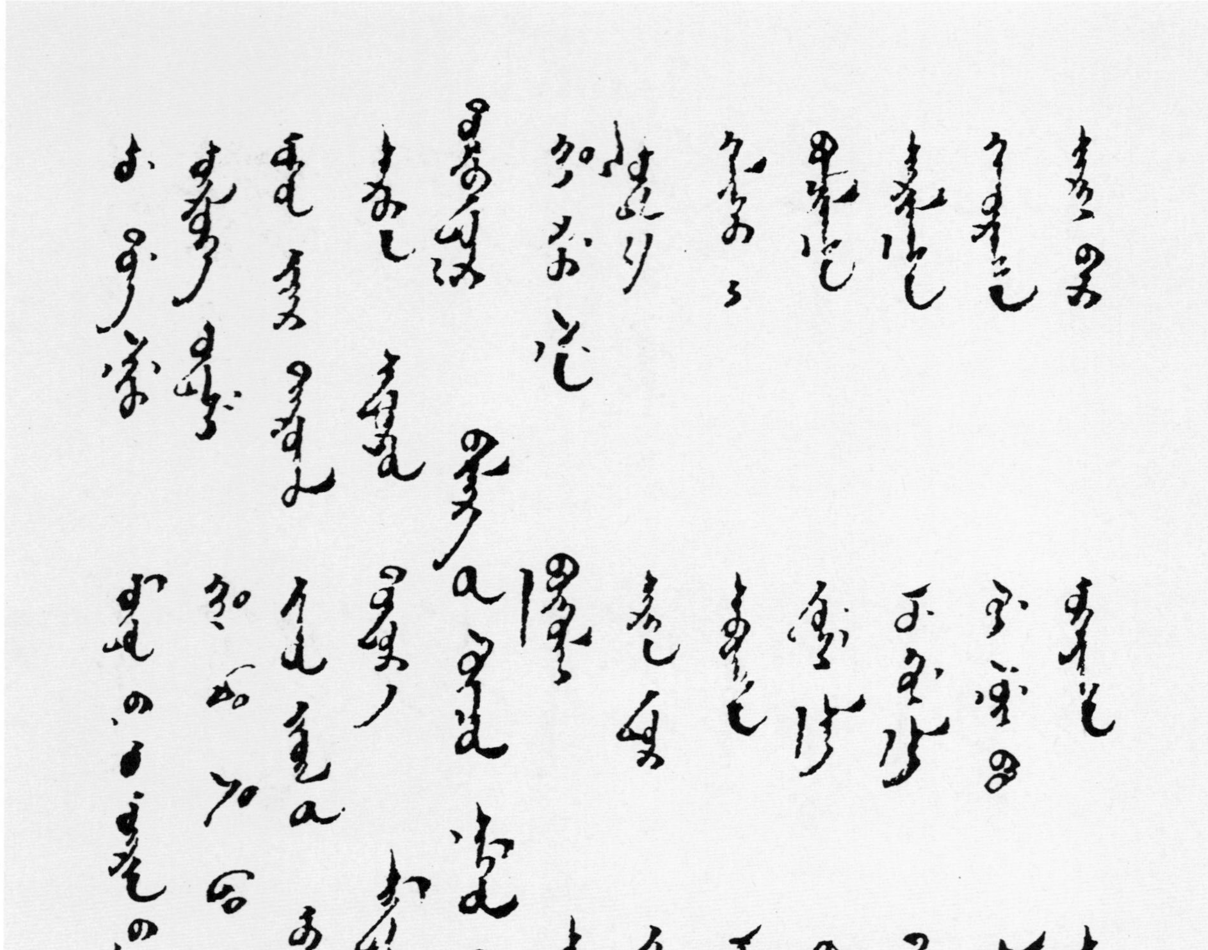

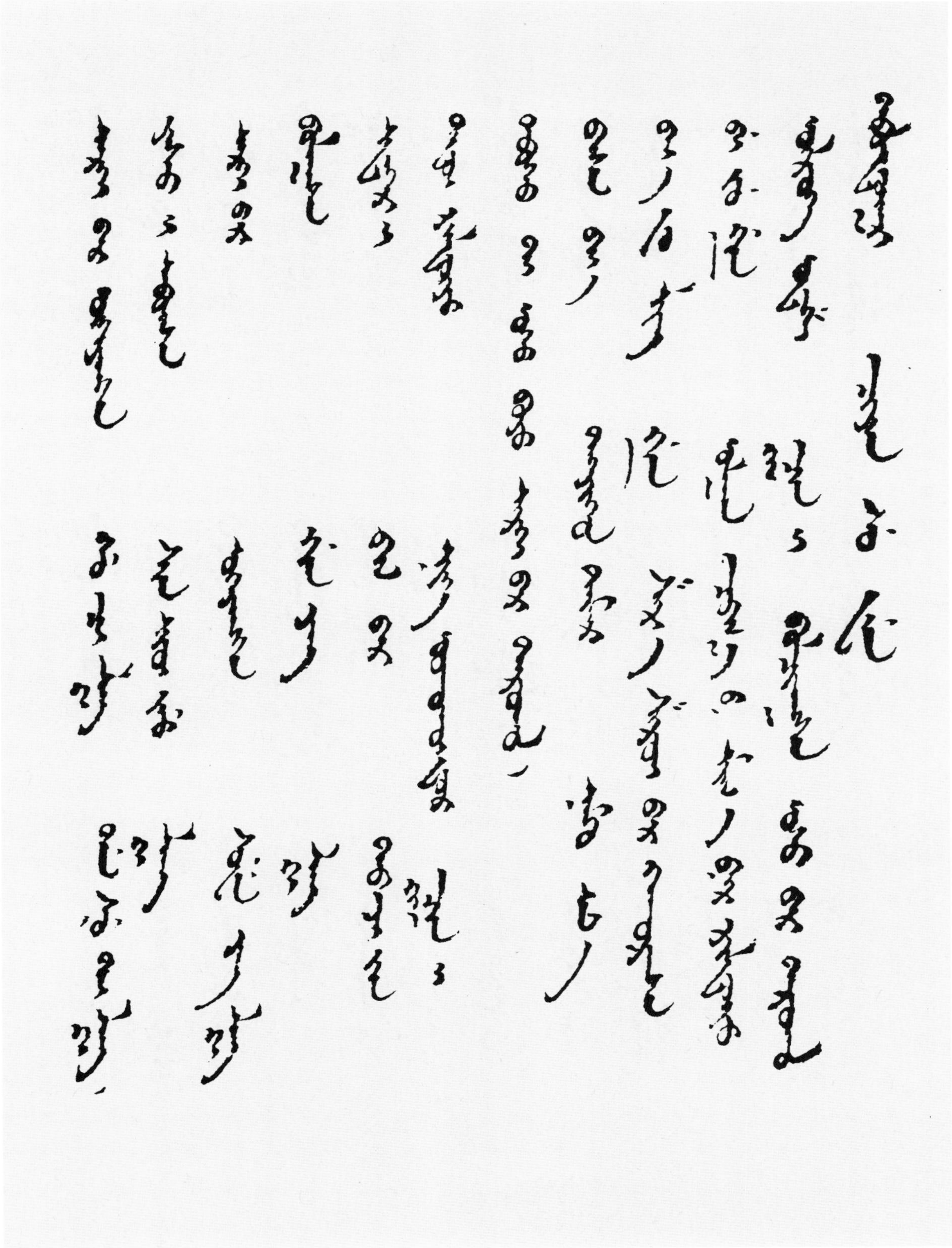

[illegible]

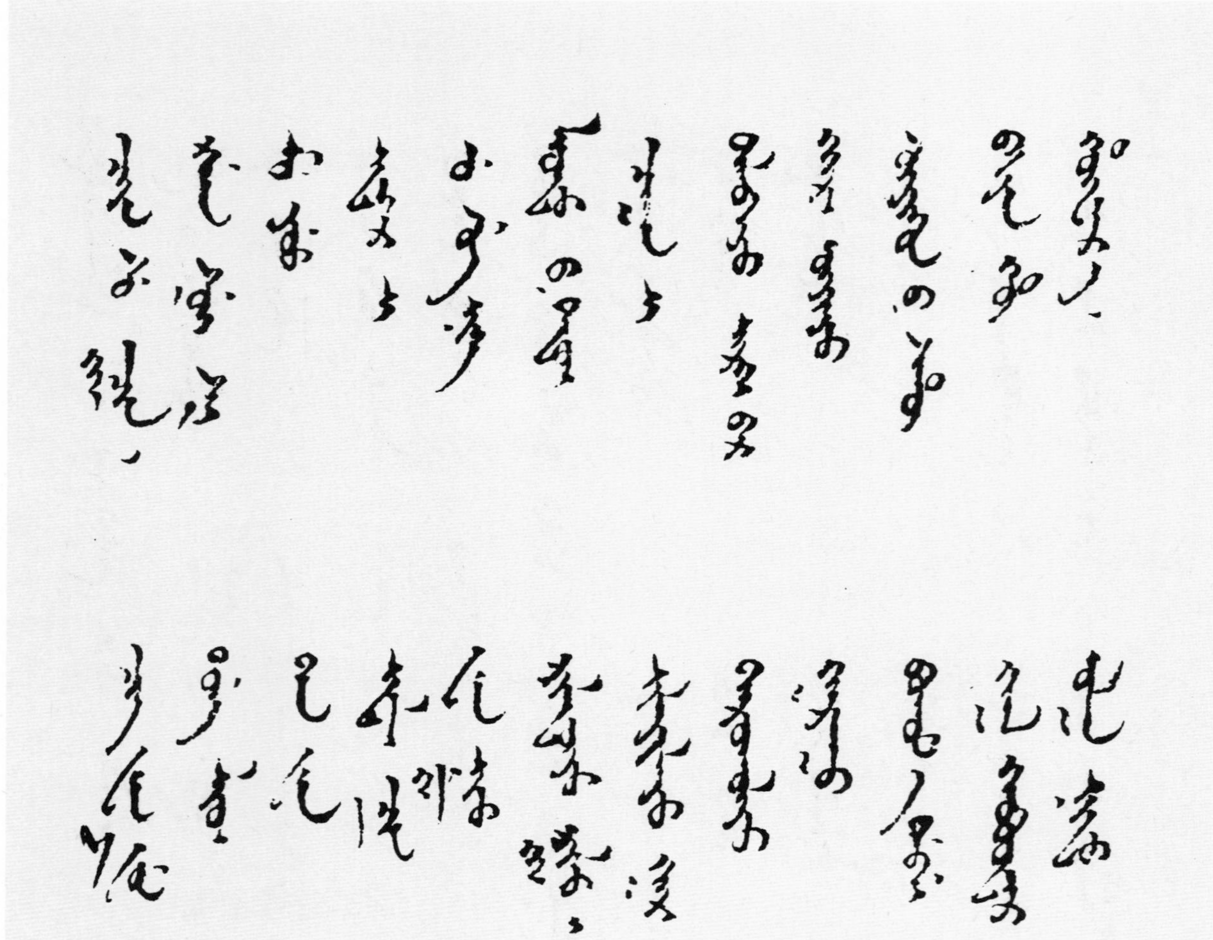

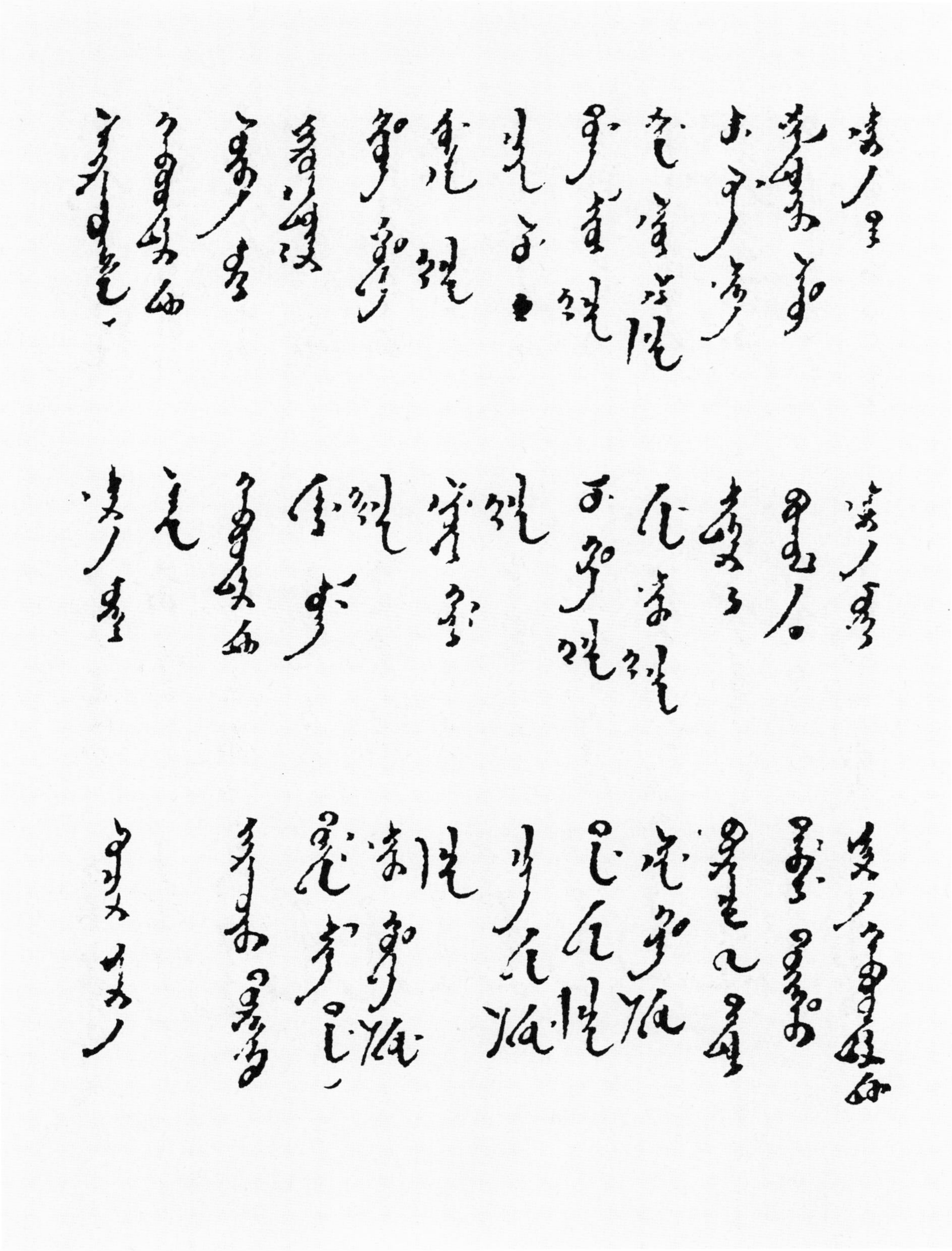

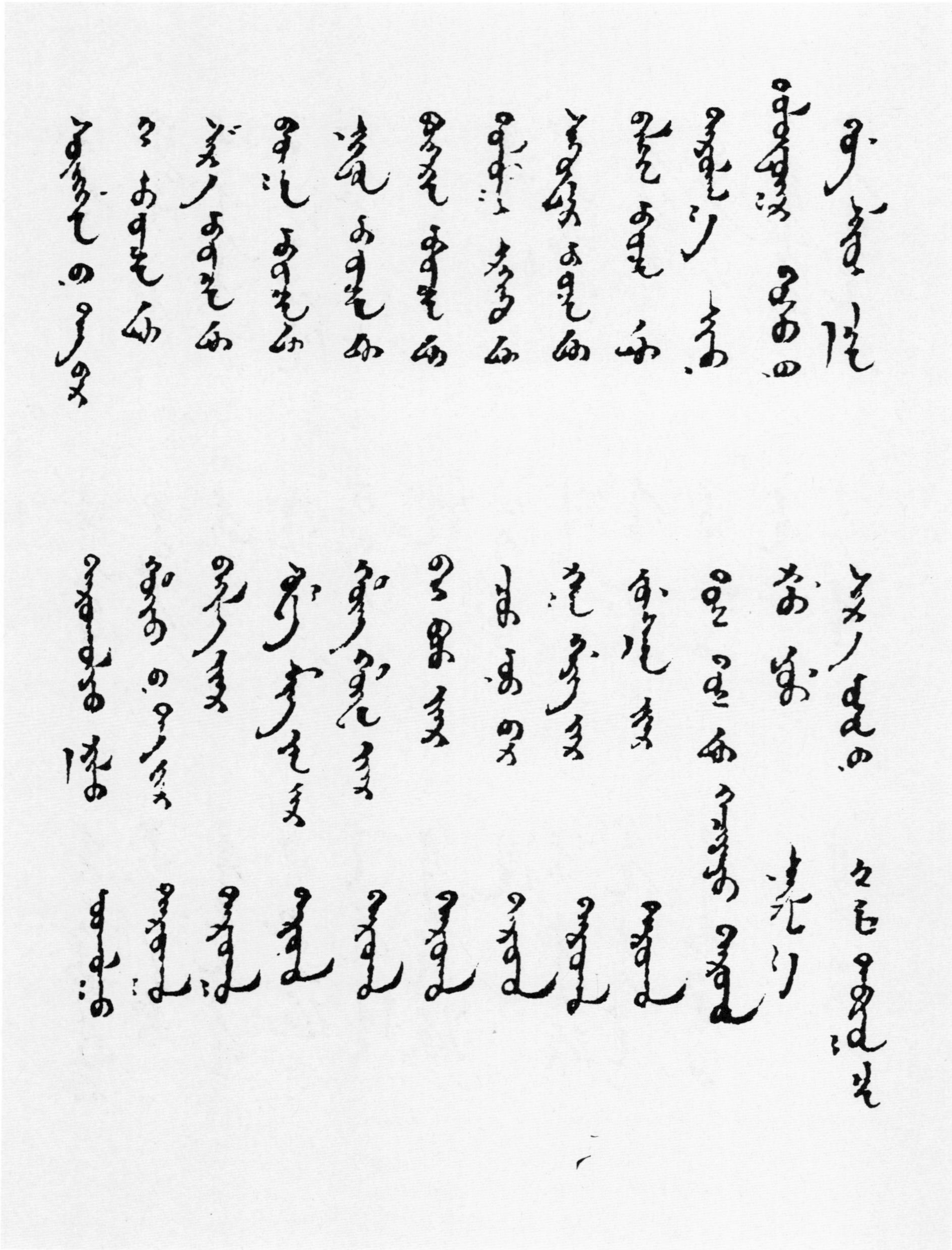

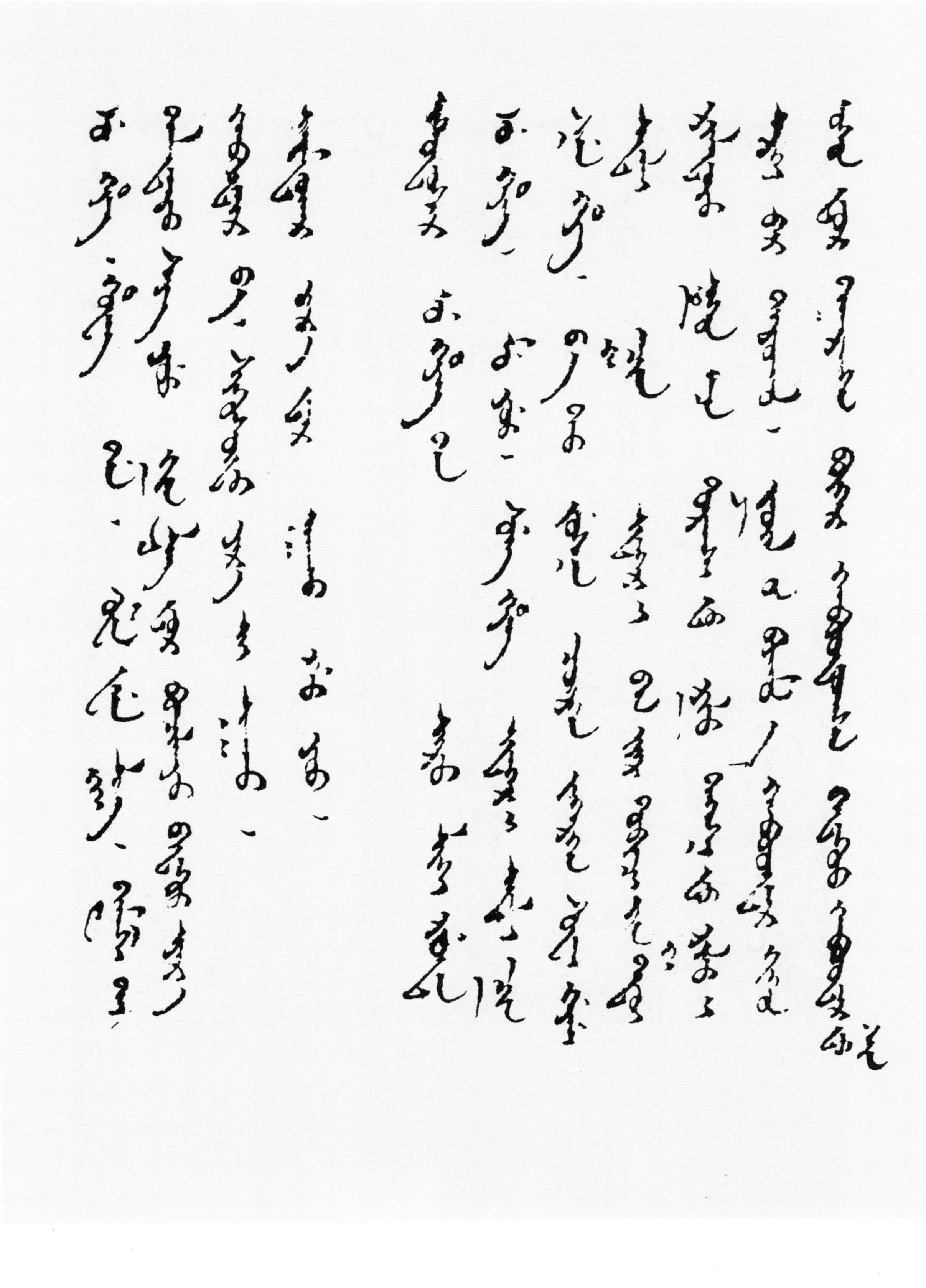

[illegible]

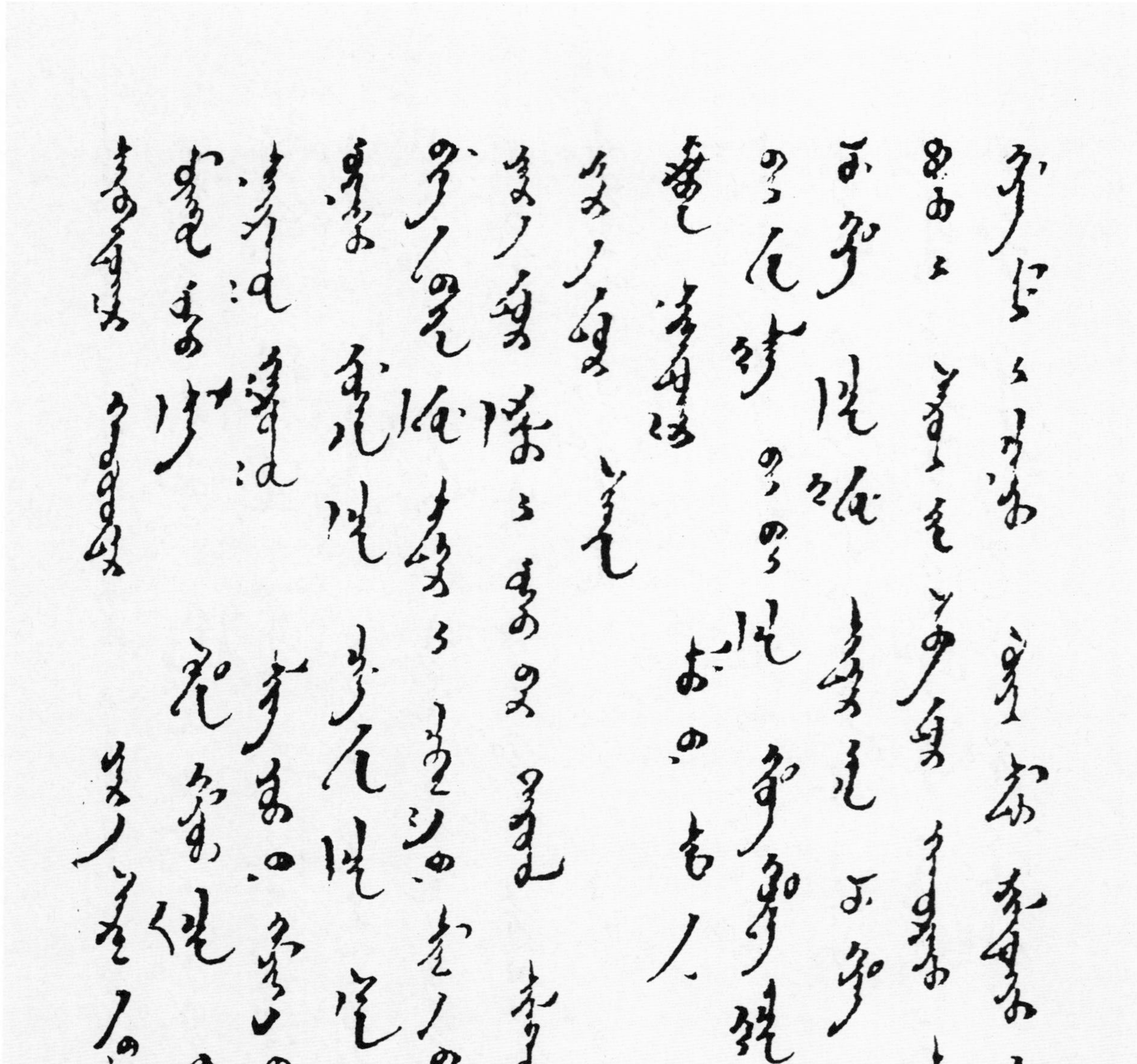

[illegible]

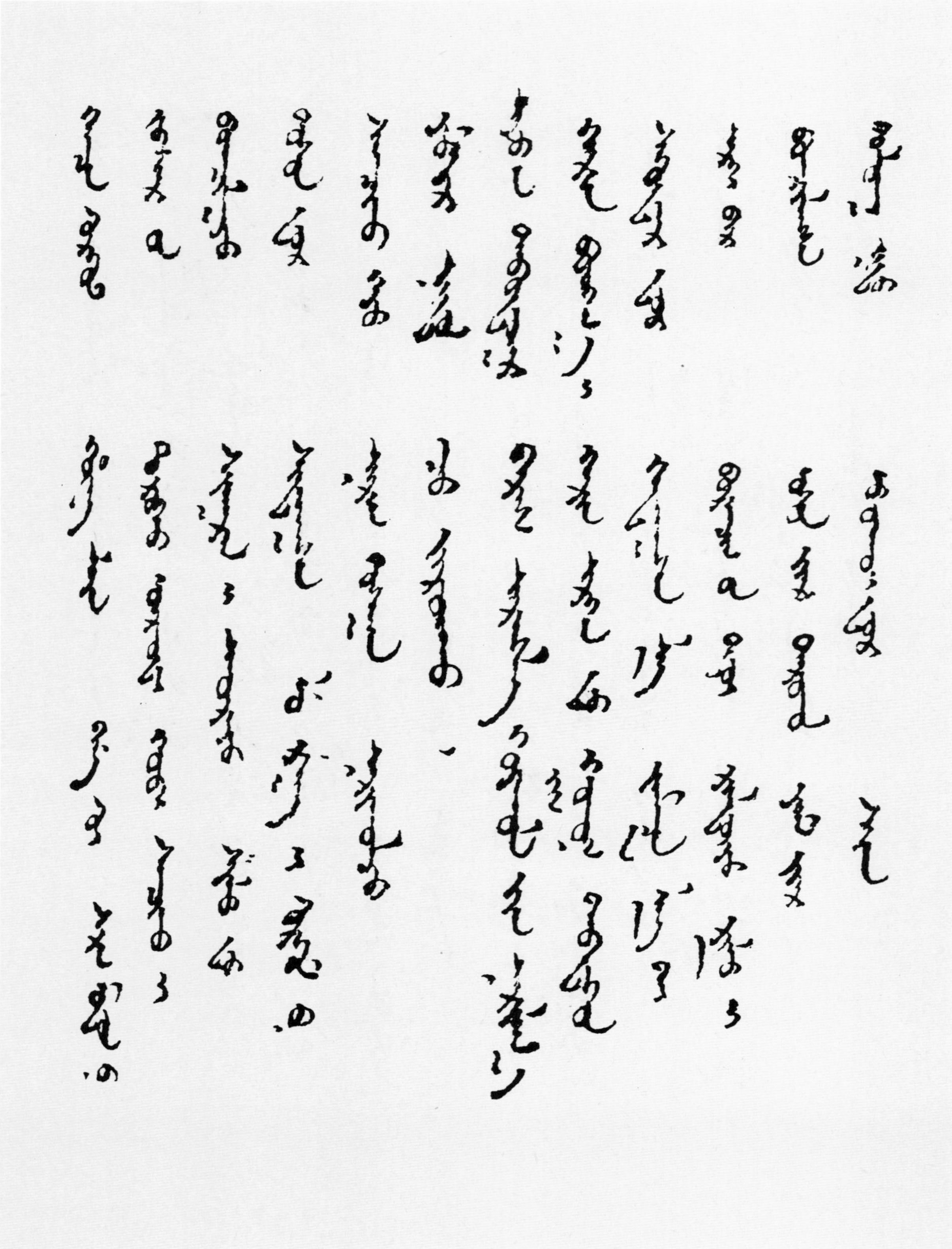

[illegible]

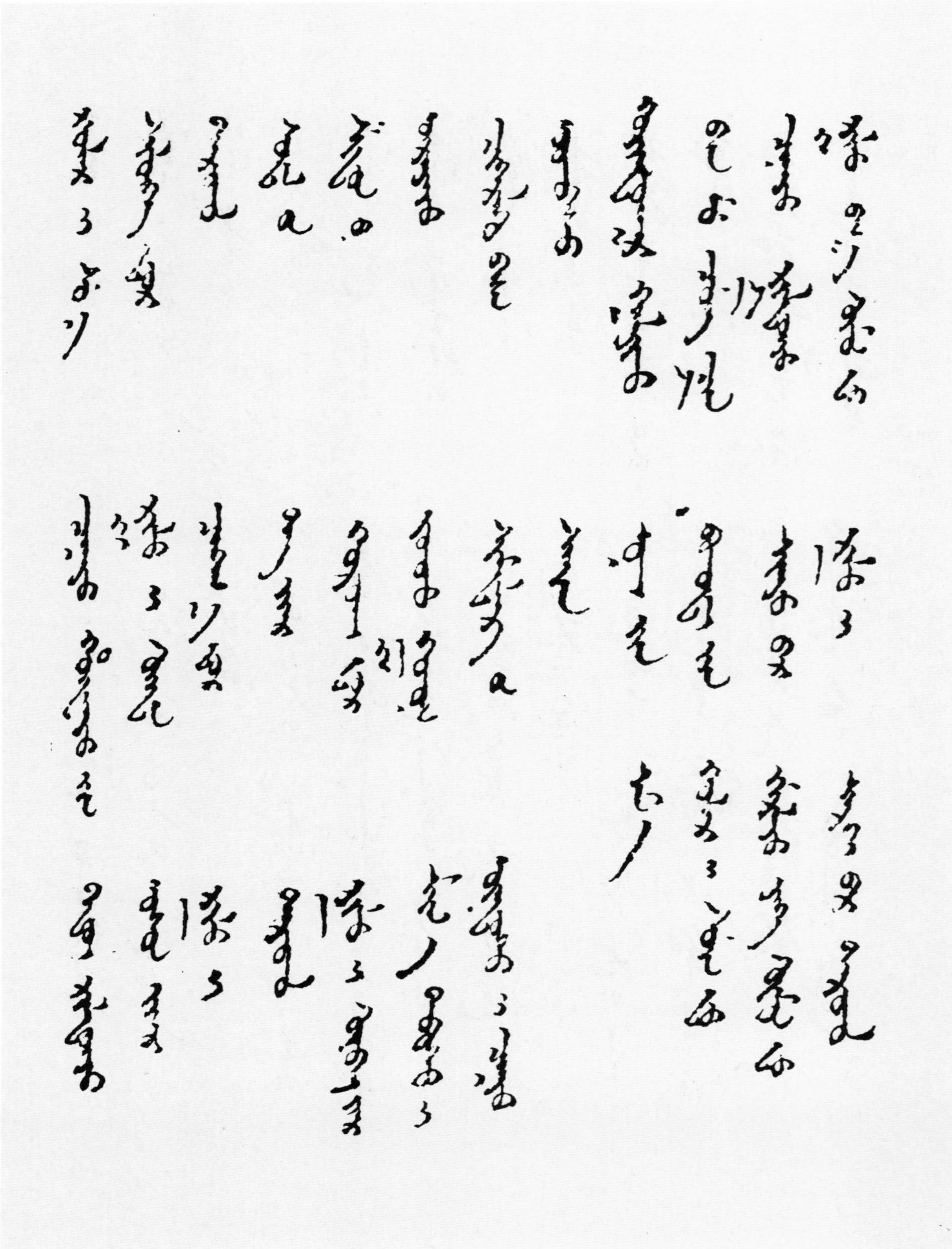

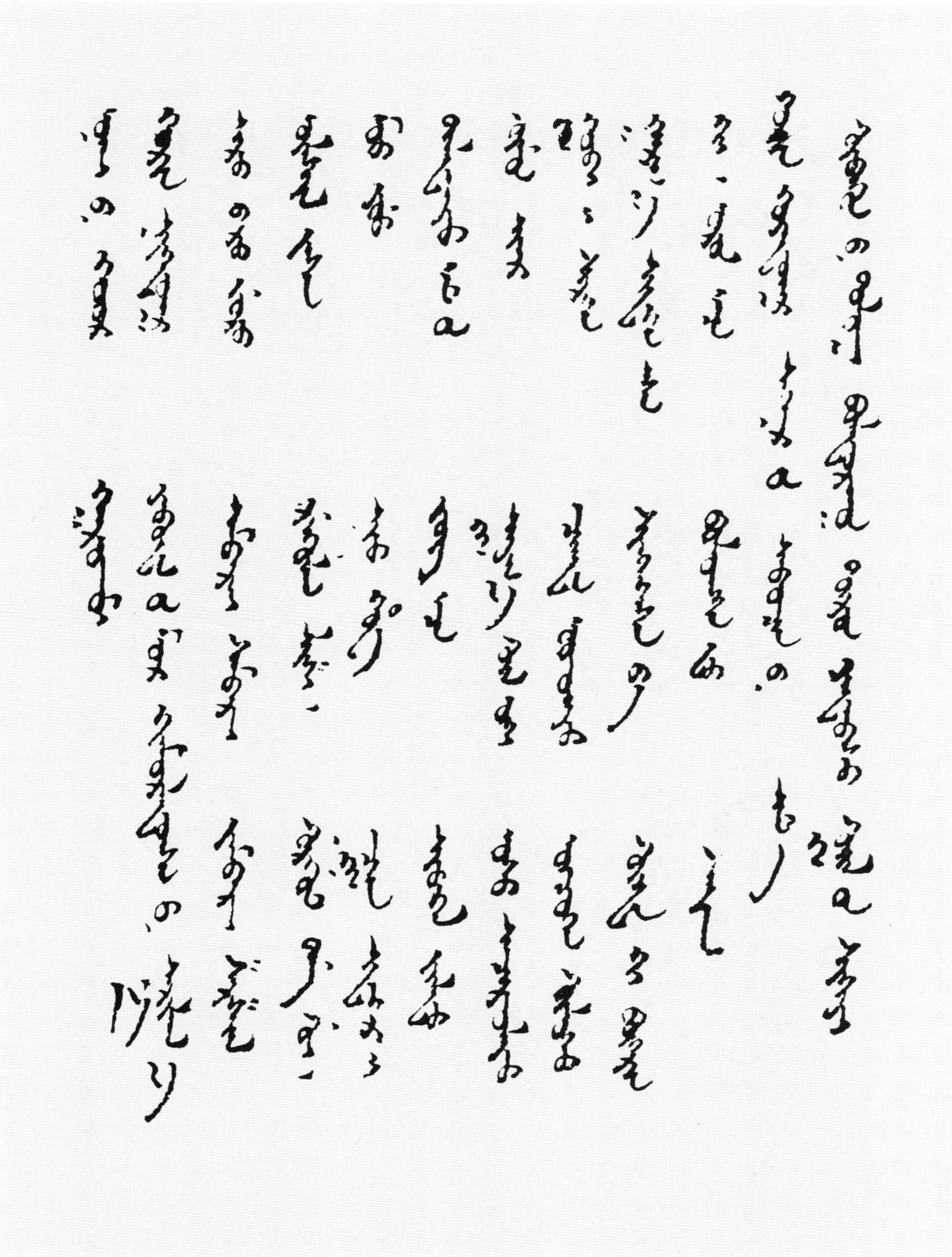

[illegible]

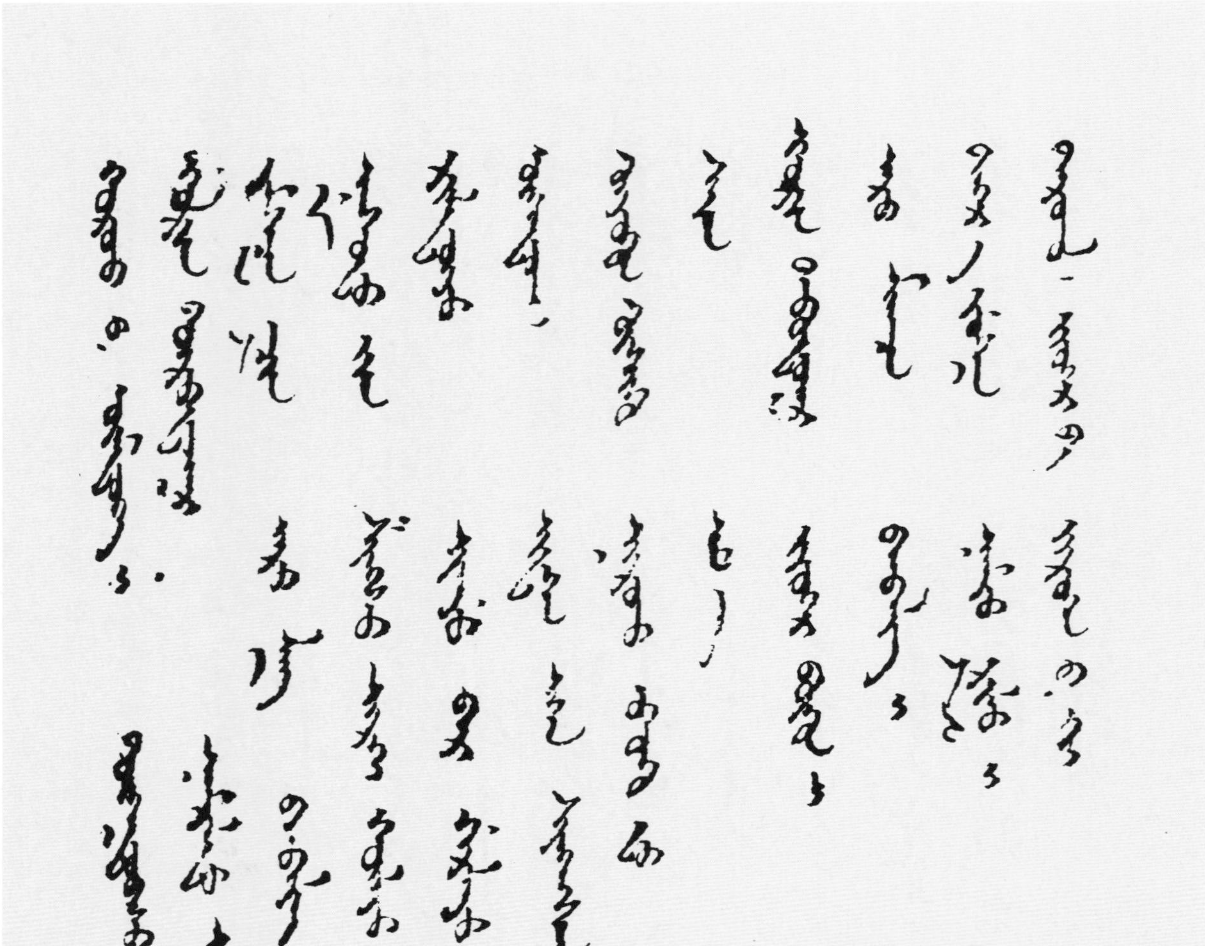

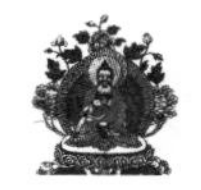

[illegible]

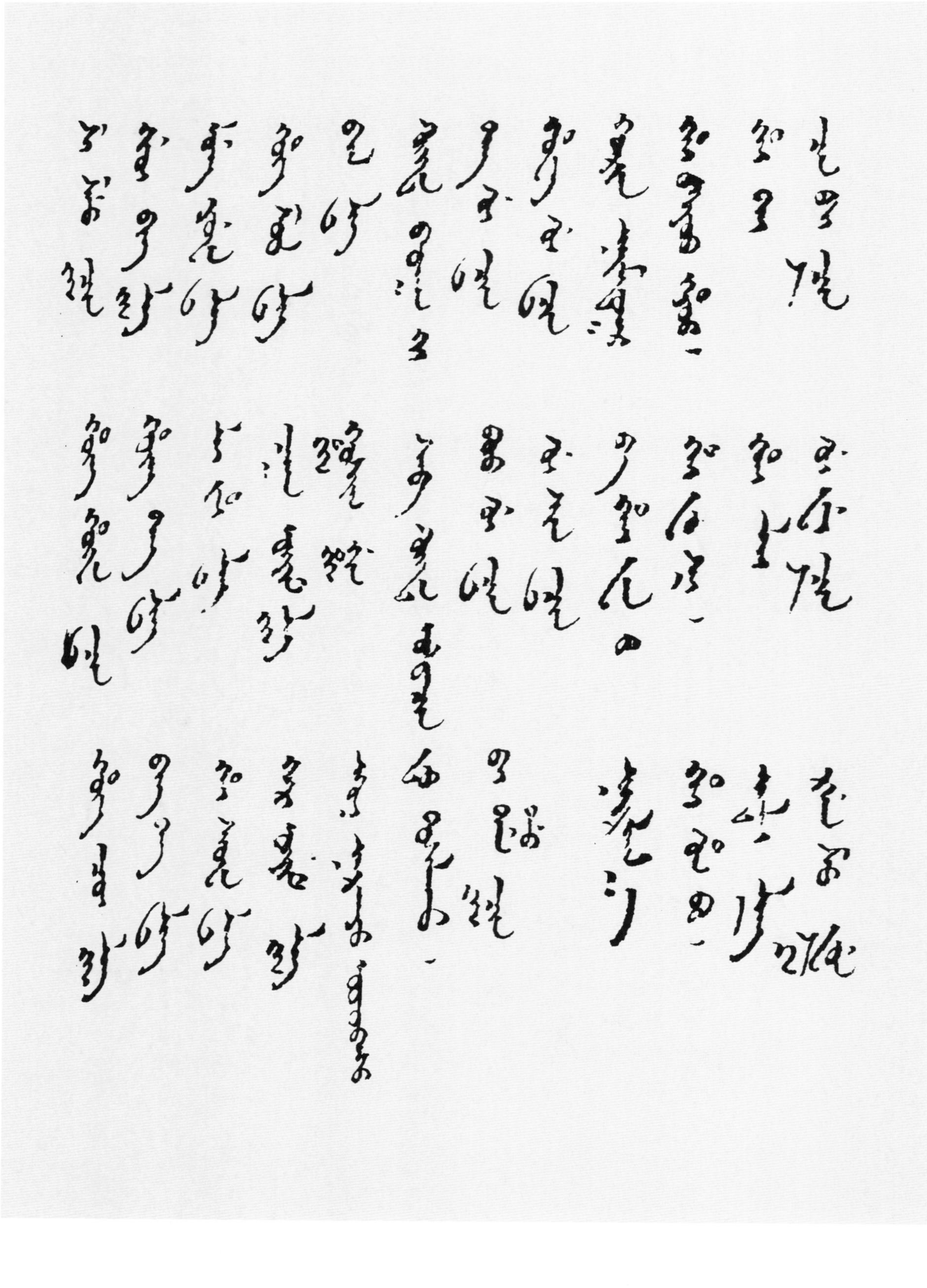

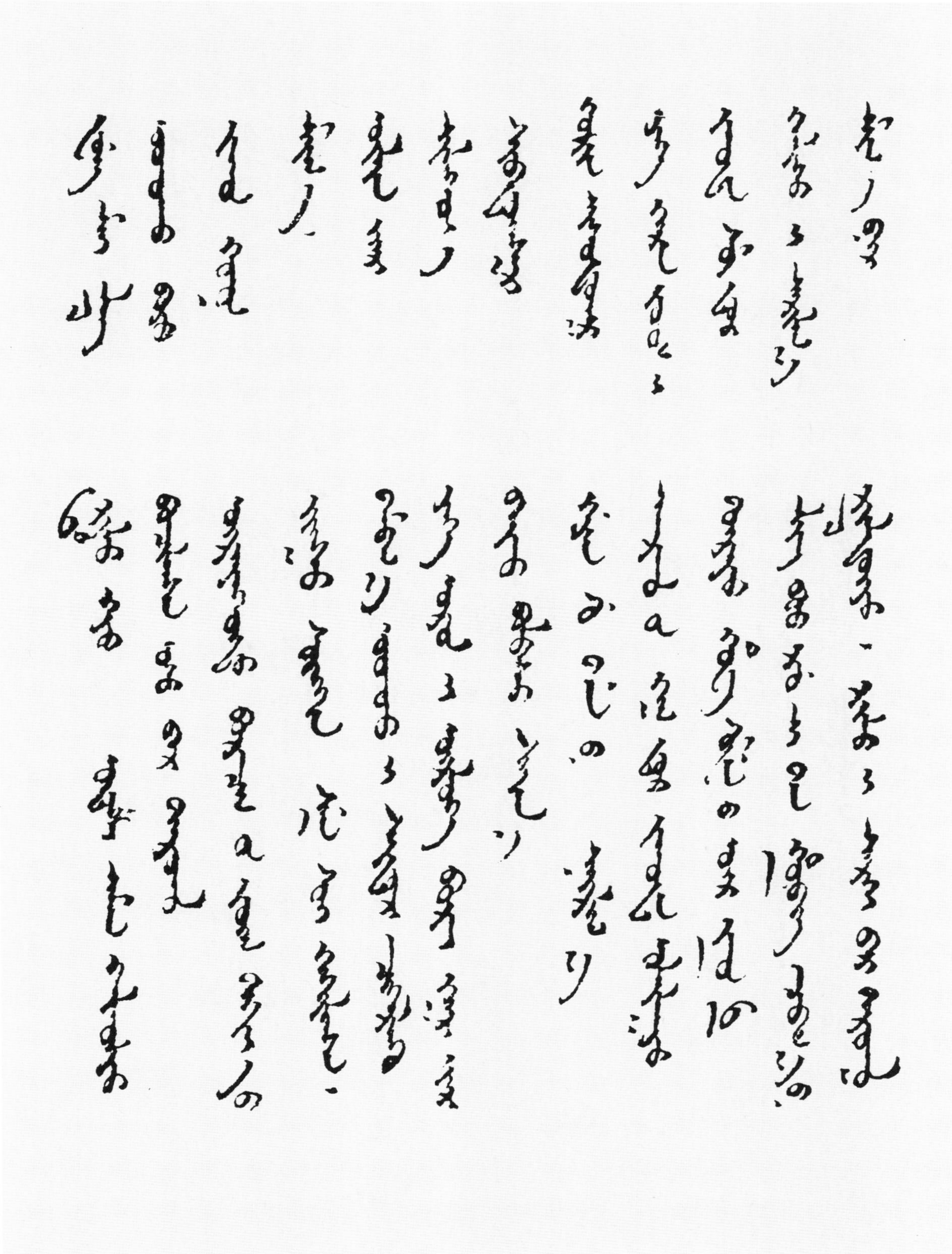

[illegible]

[illegible]

[illegible]

[illegible]

[illegible]

[illegible]

[illegible]

[illegible]

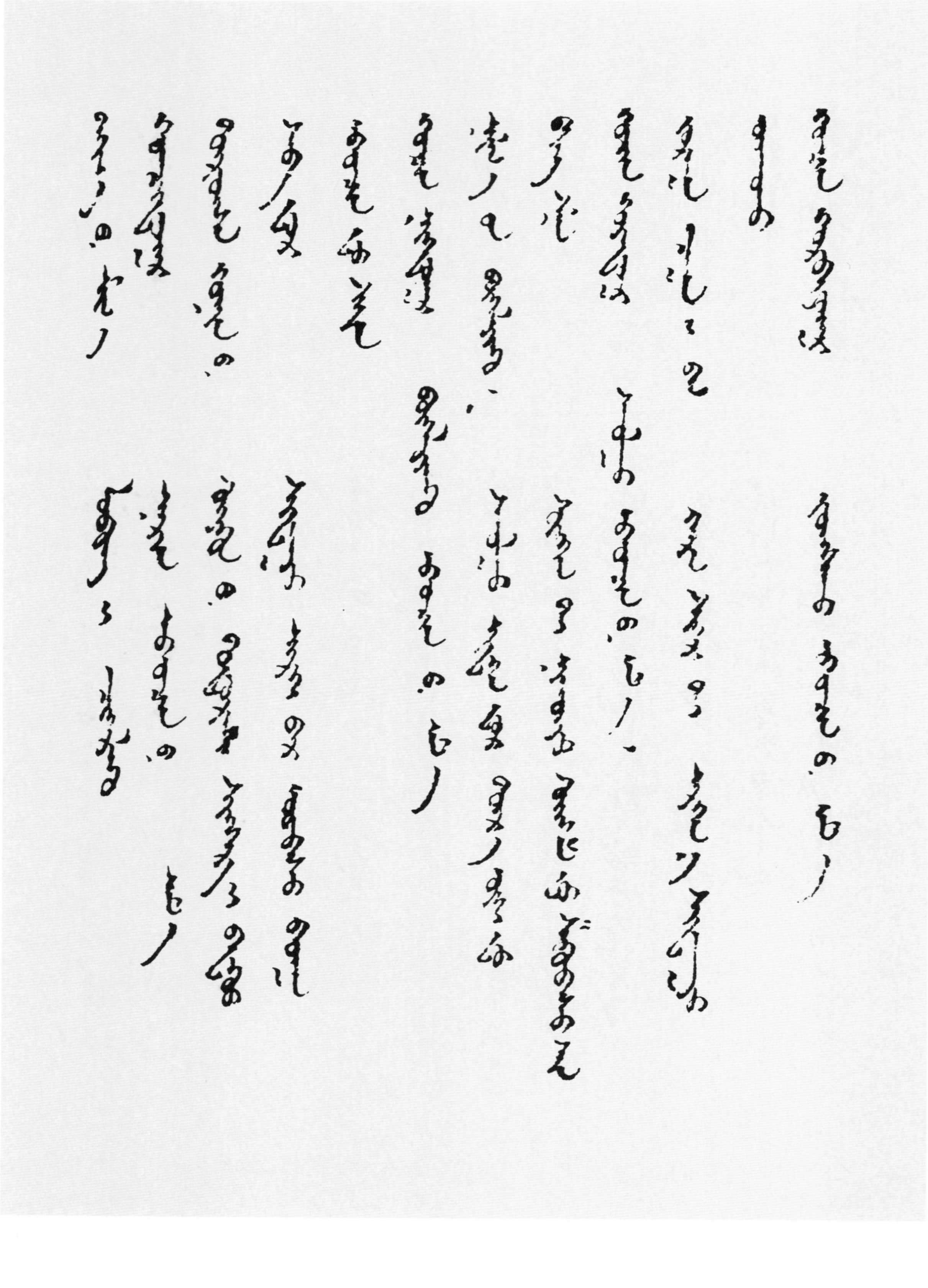

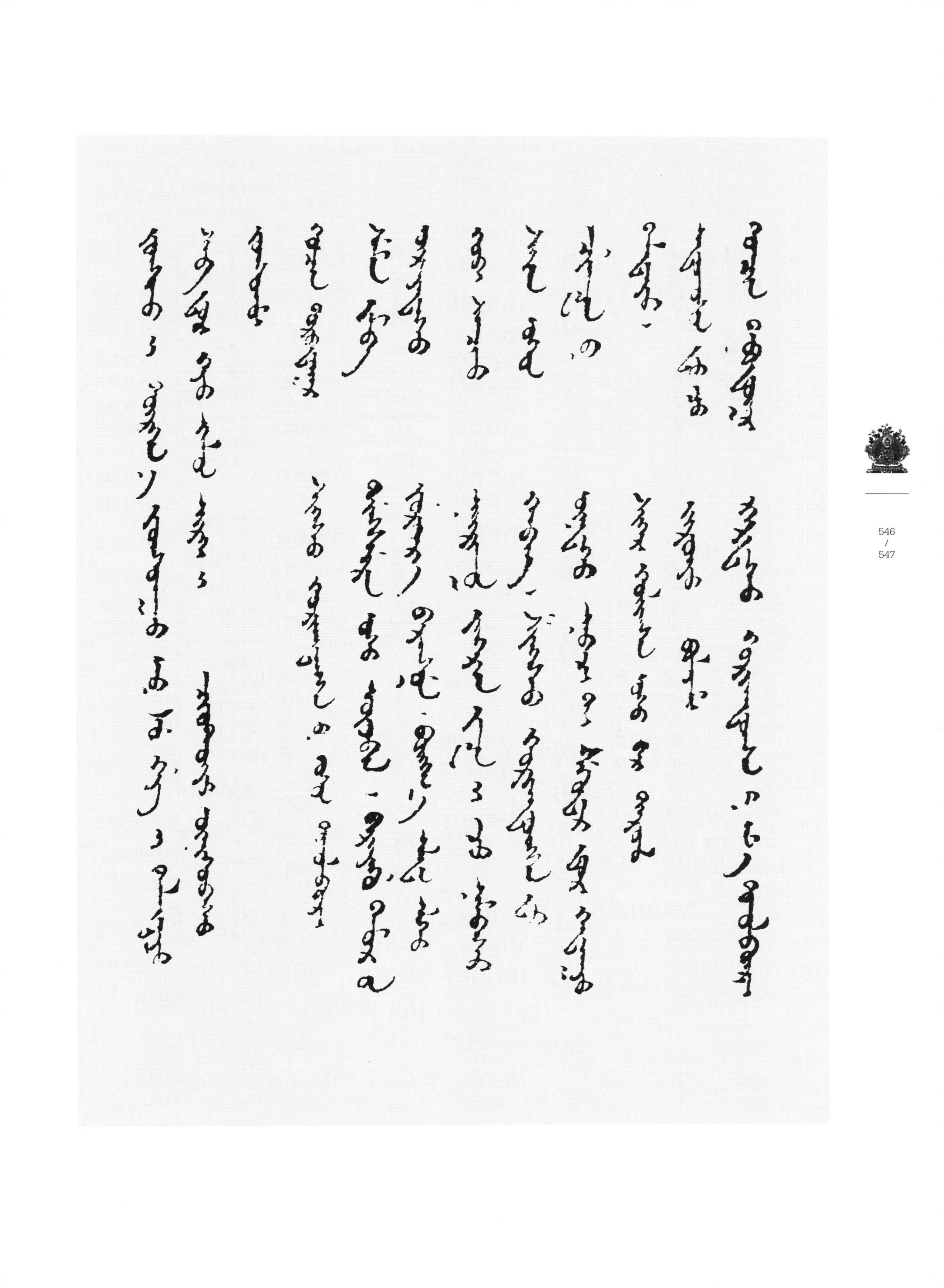

[illegible]

[illegible]

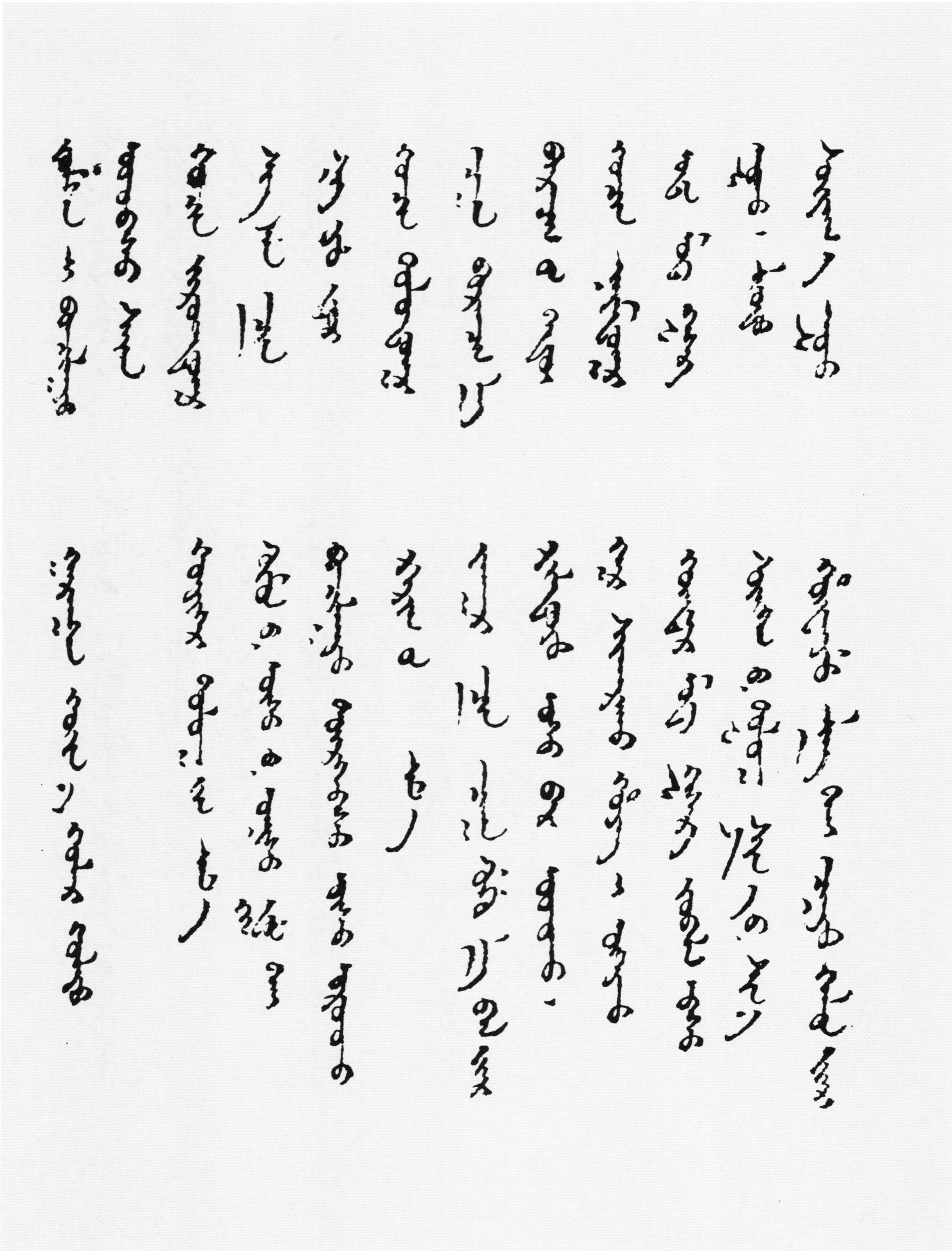

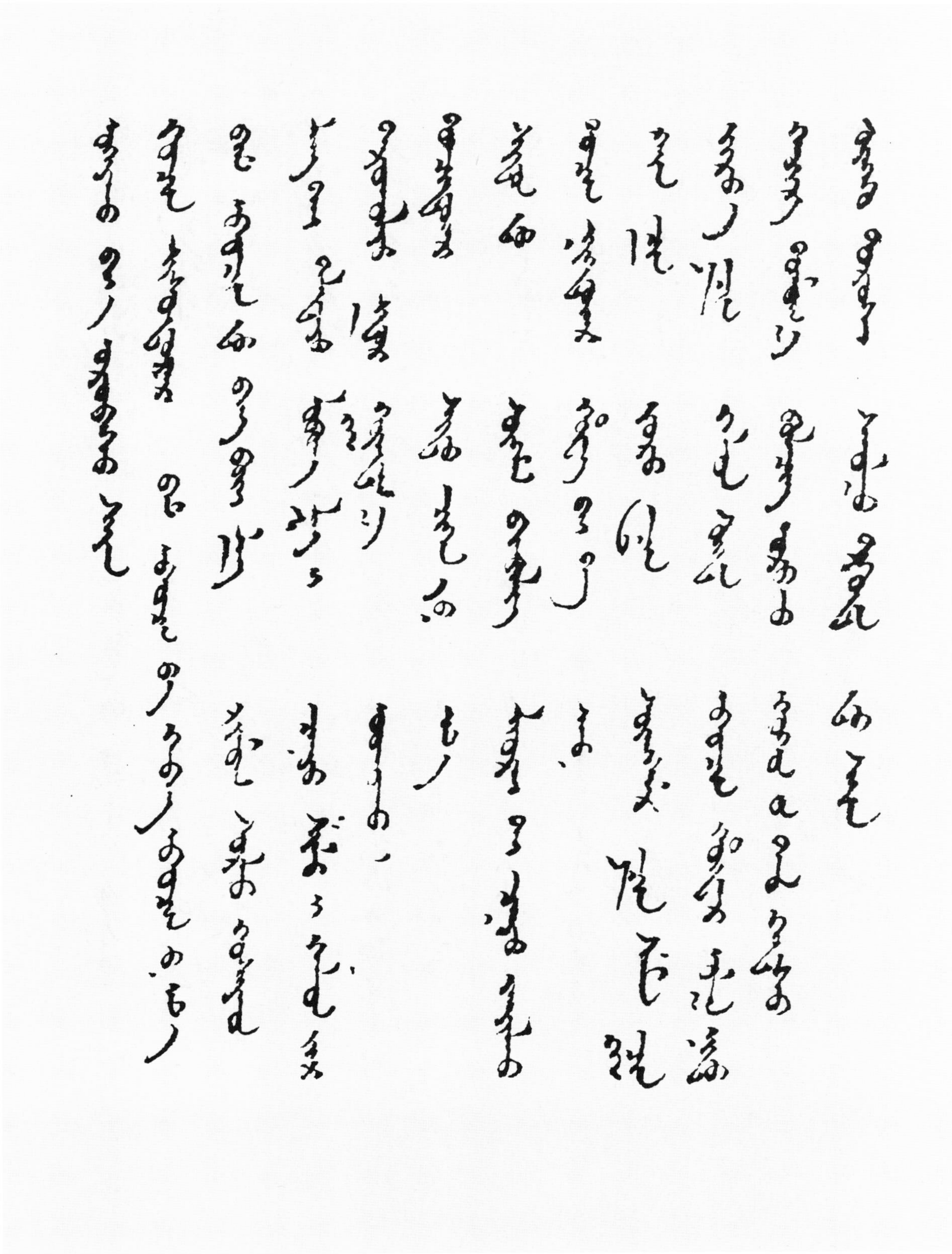

[illegible]

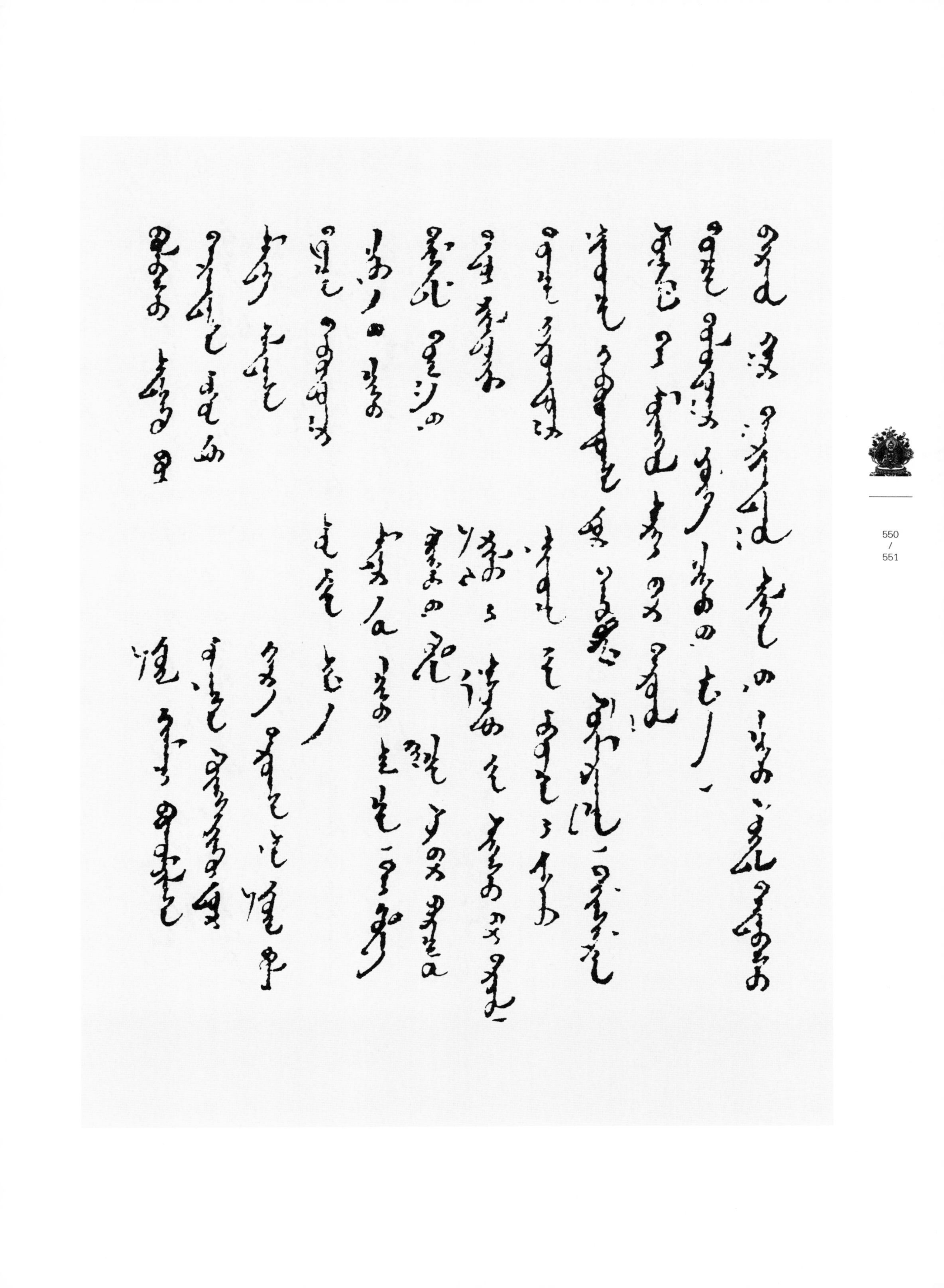

[illegible]

[illegible]

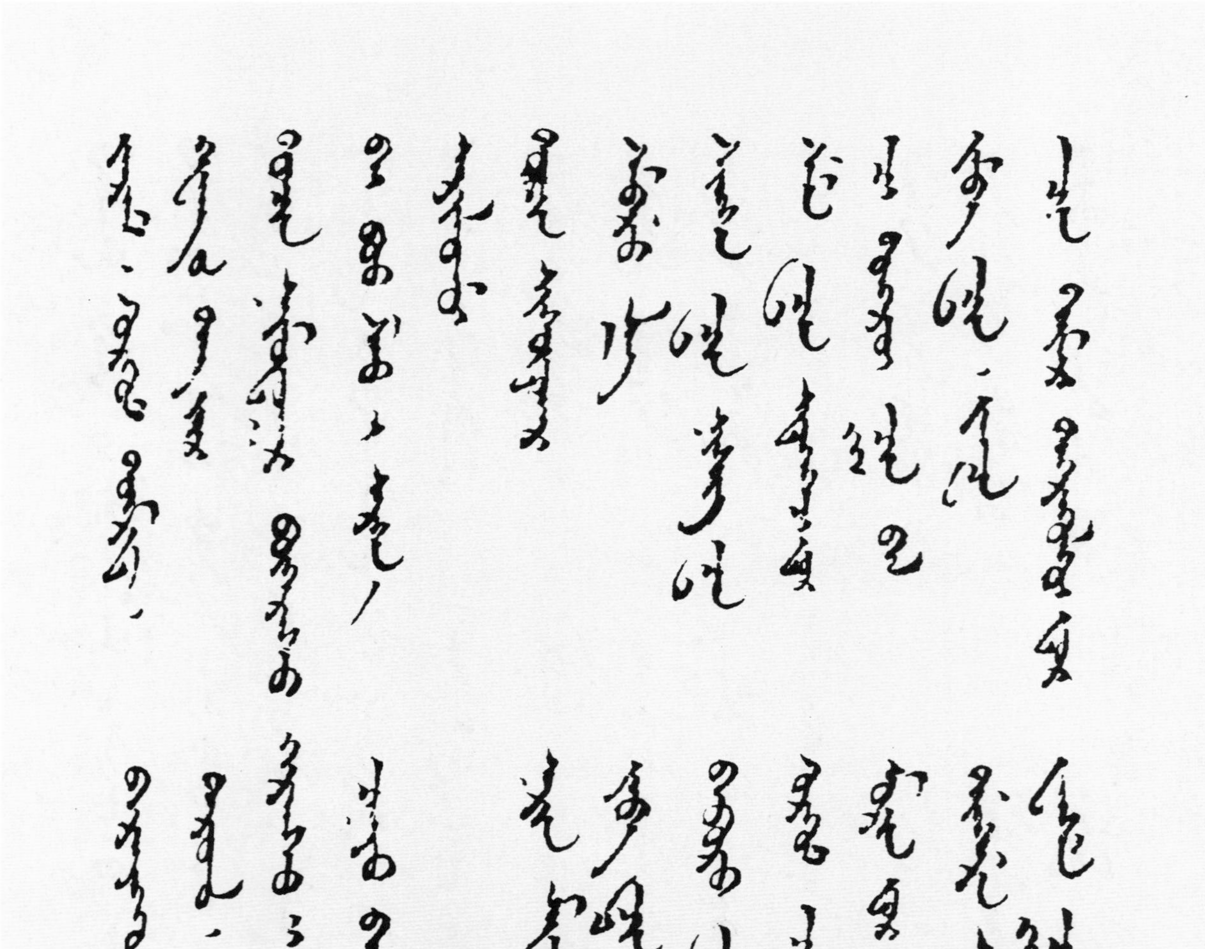

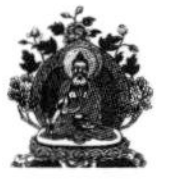

[illegible]

[illegible]

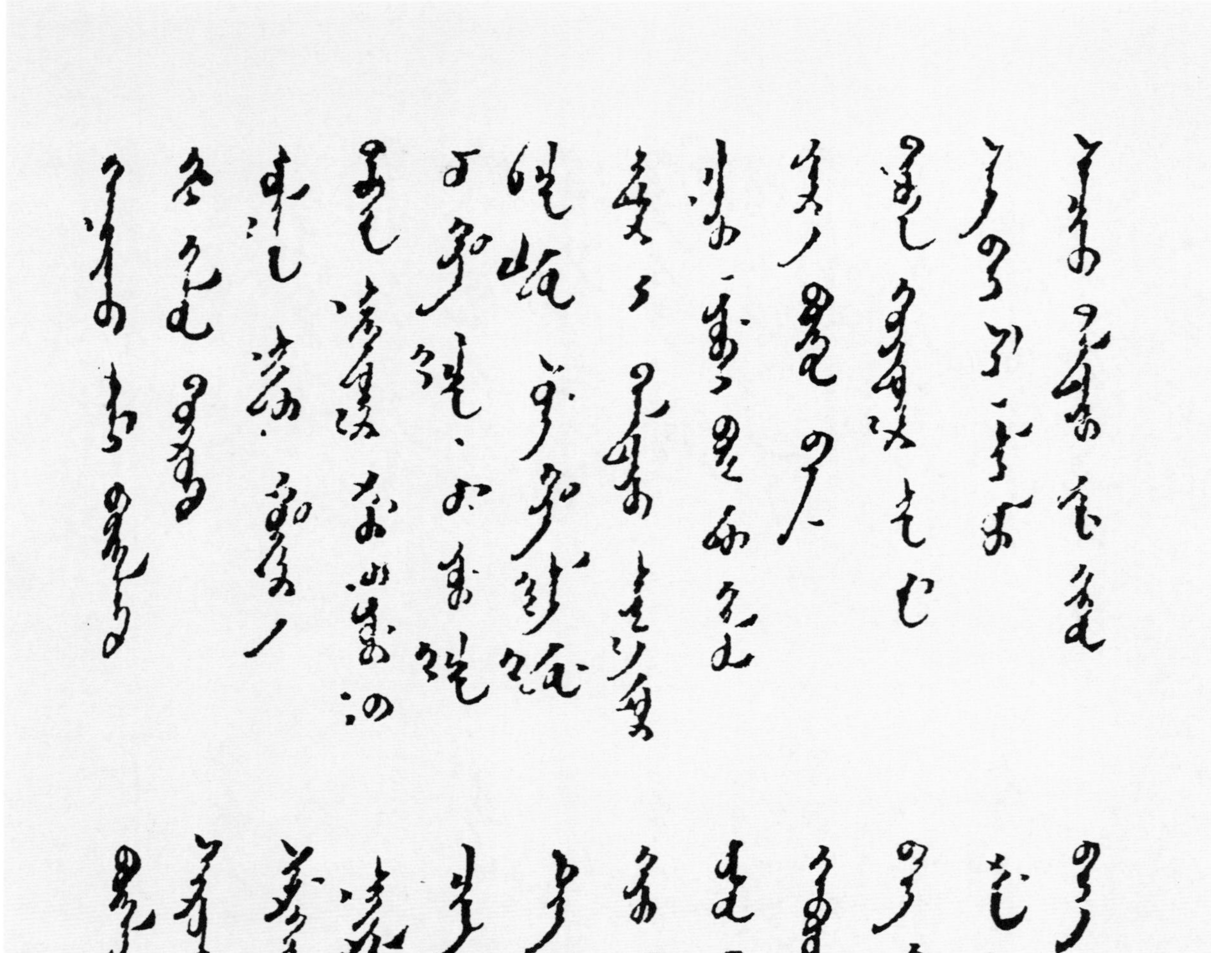

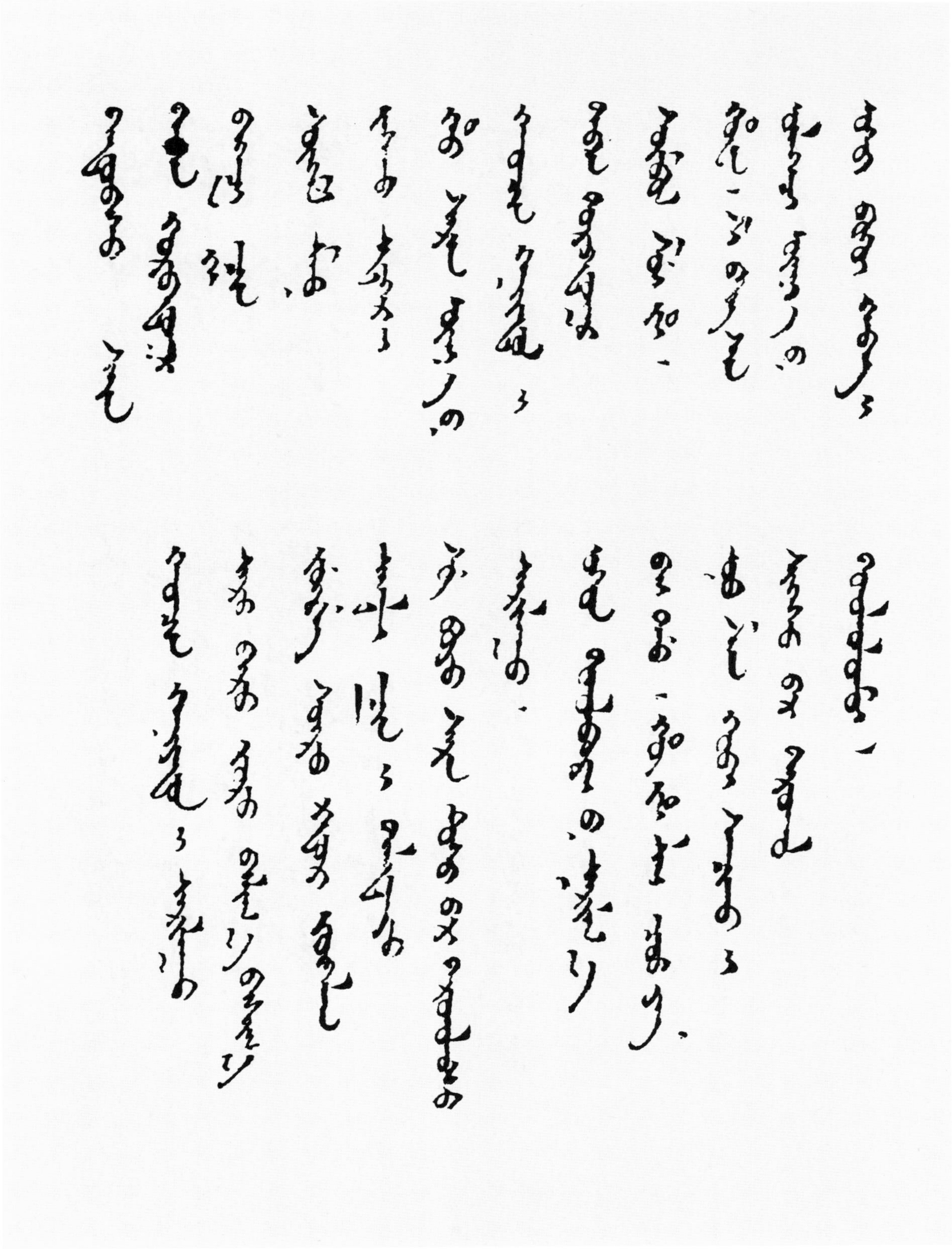

[illegible]

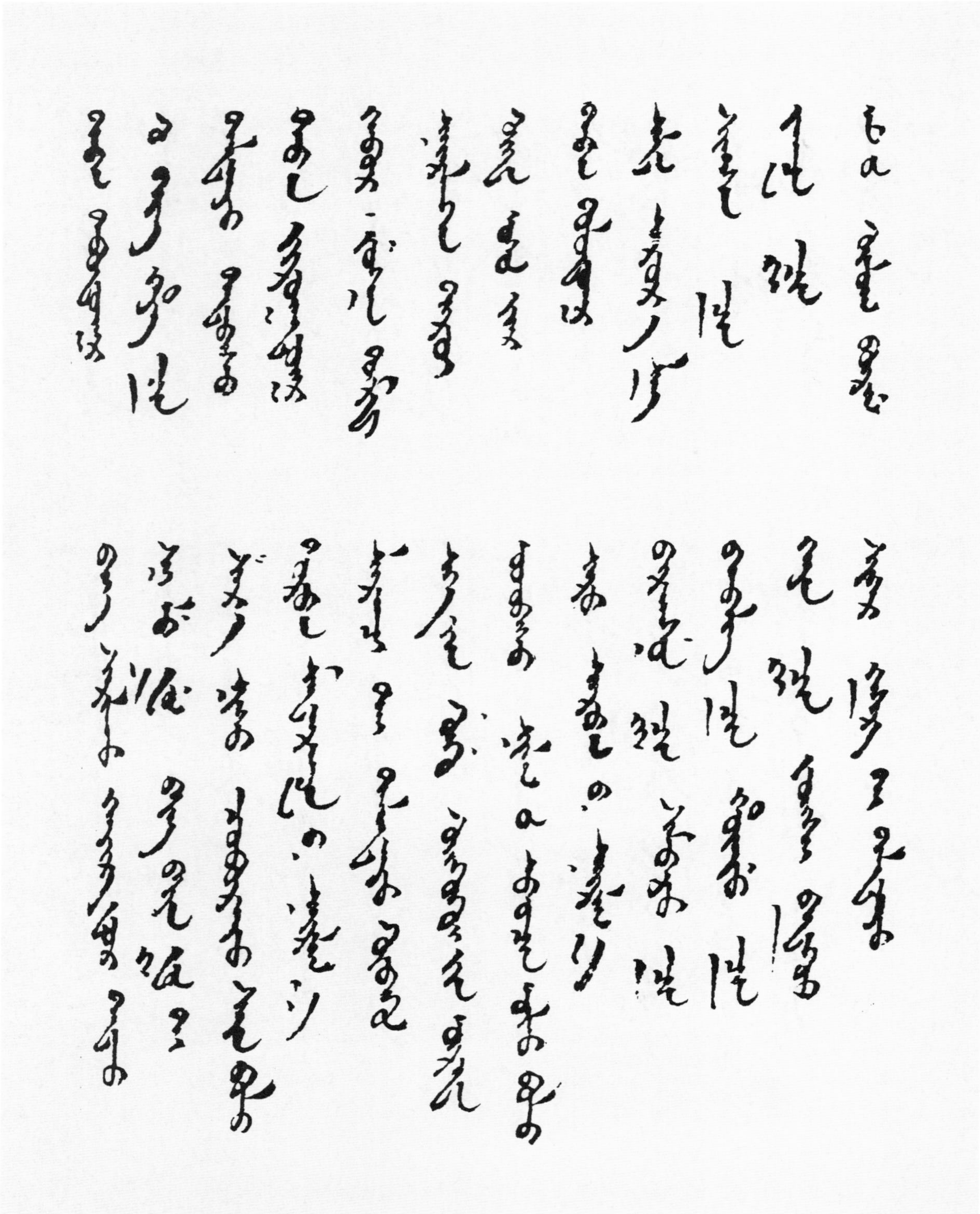

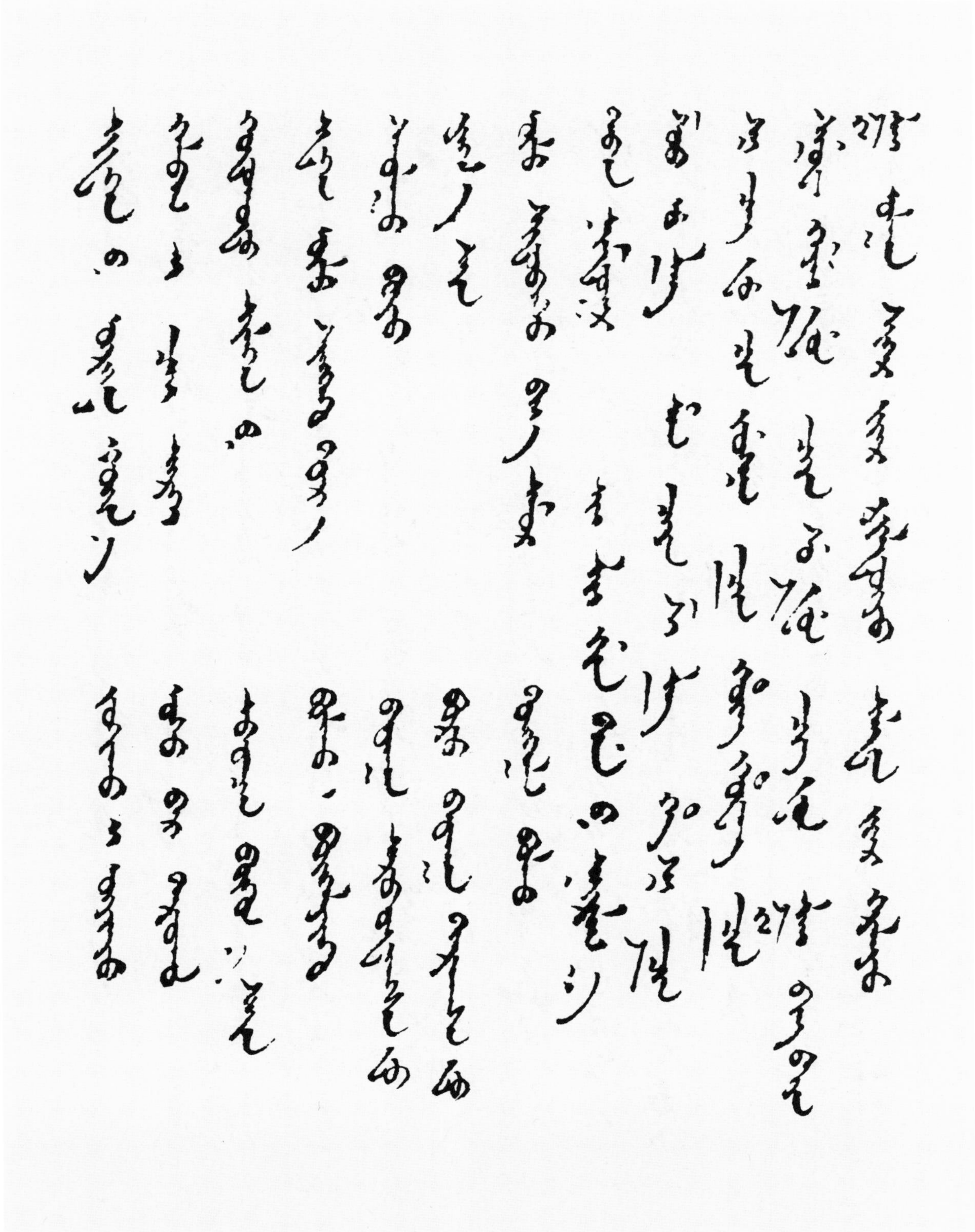

[illegible]

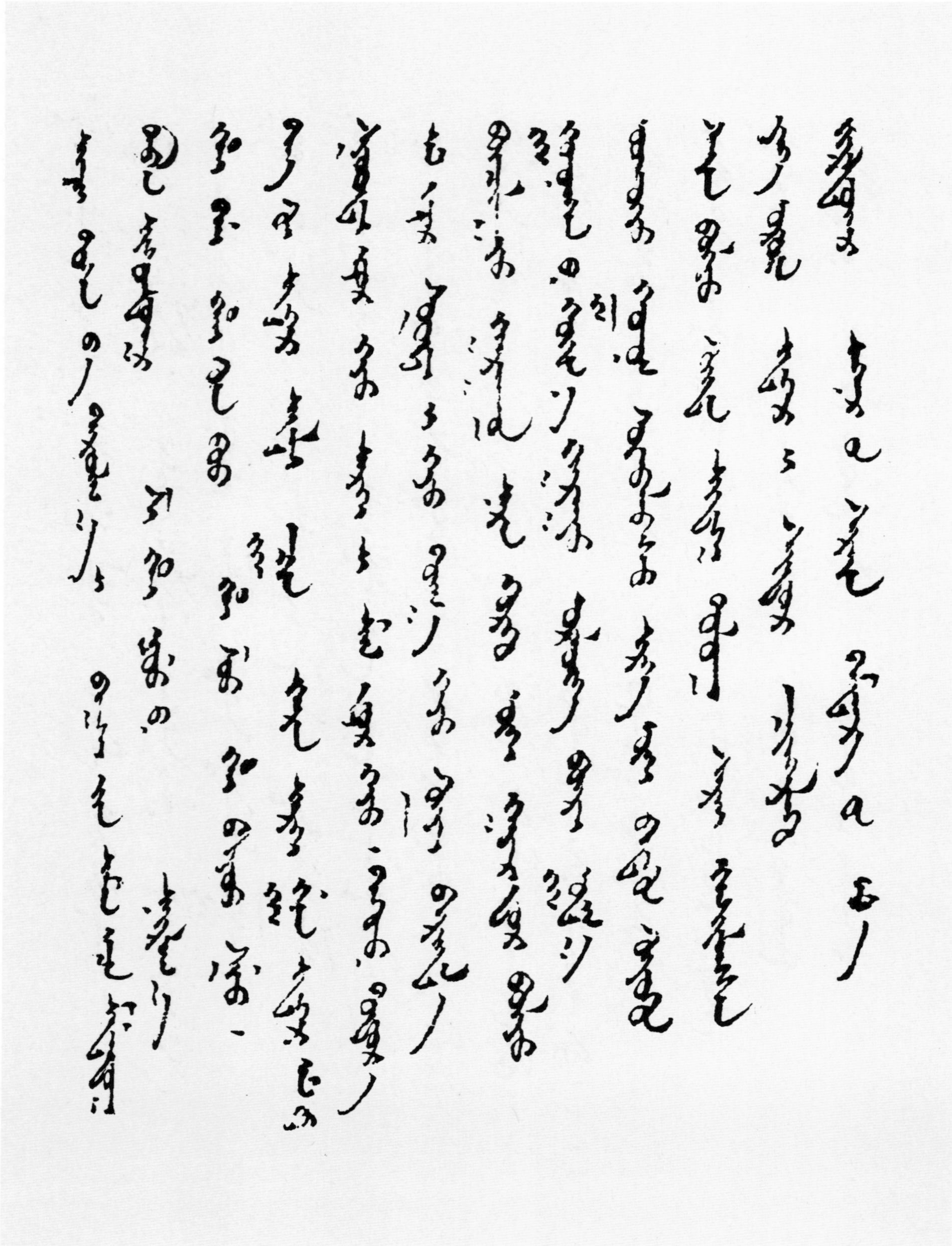

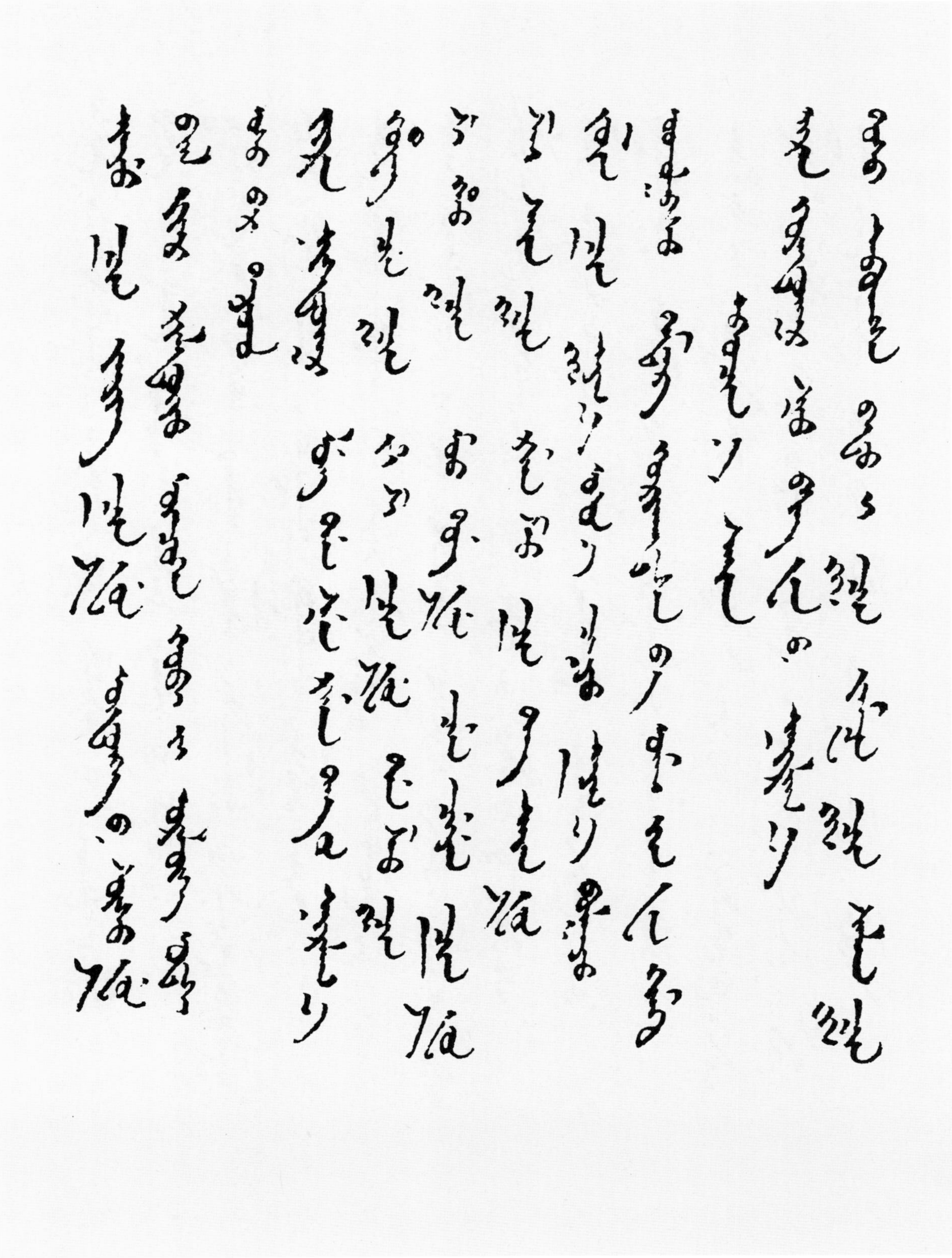

[illegible]

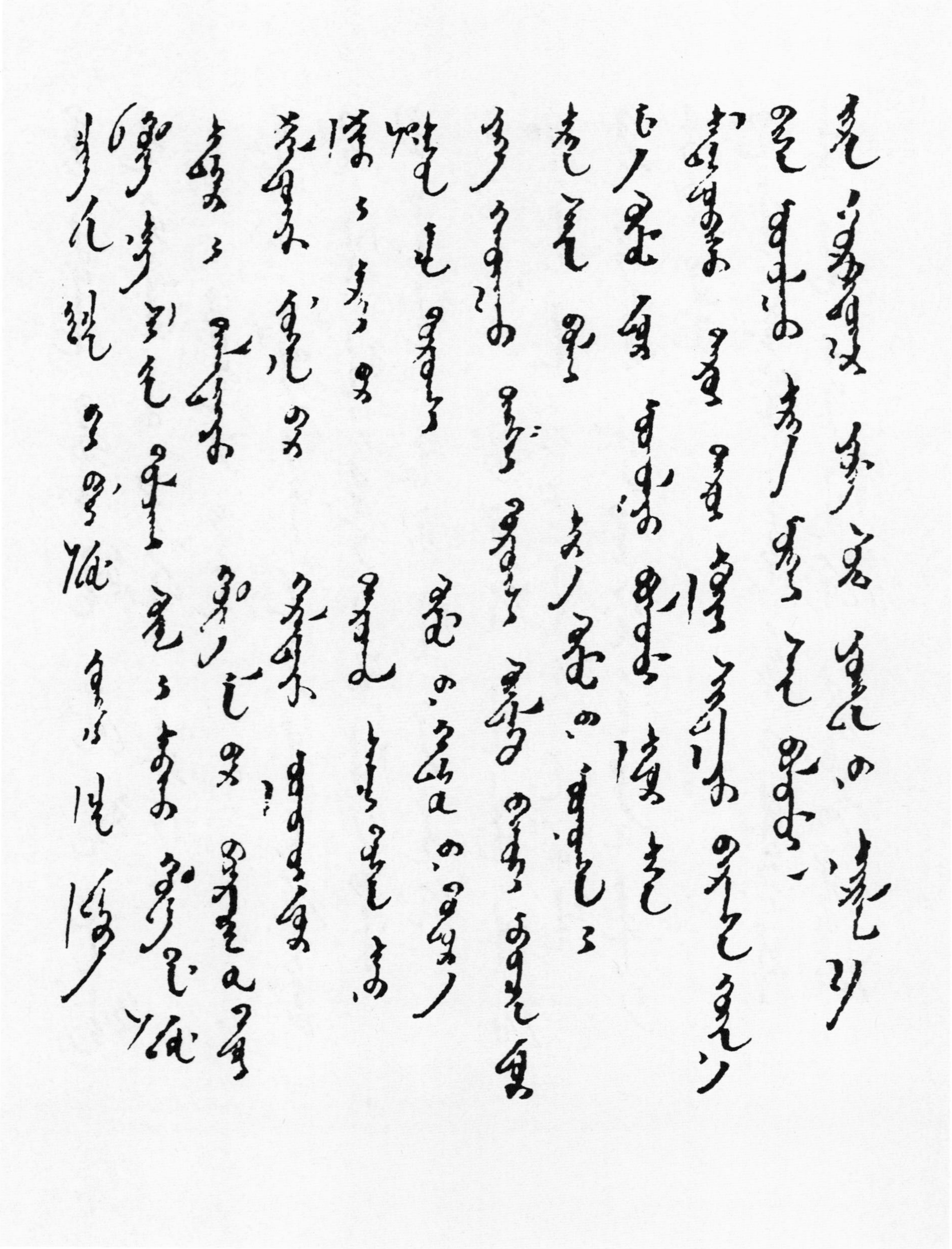

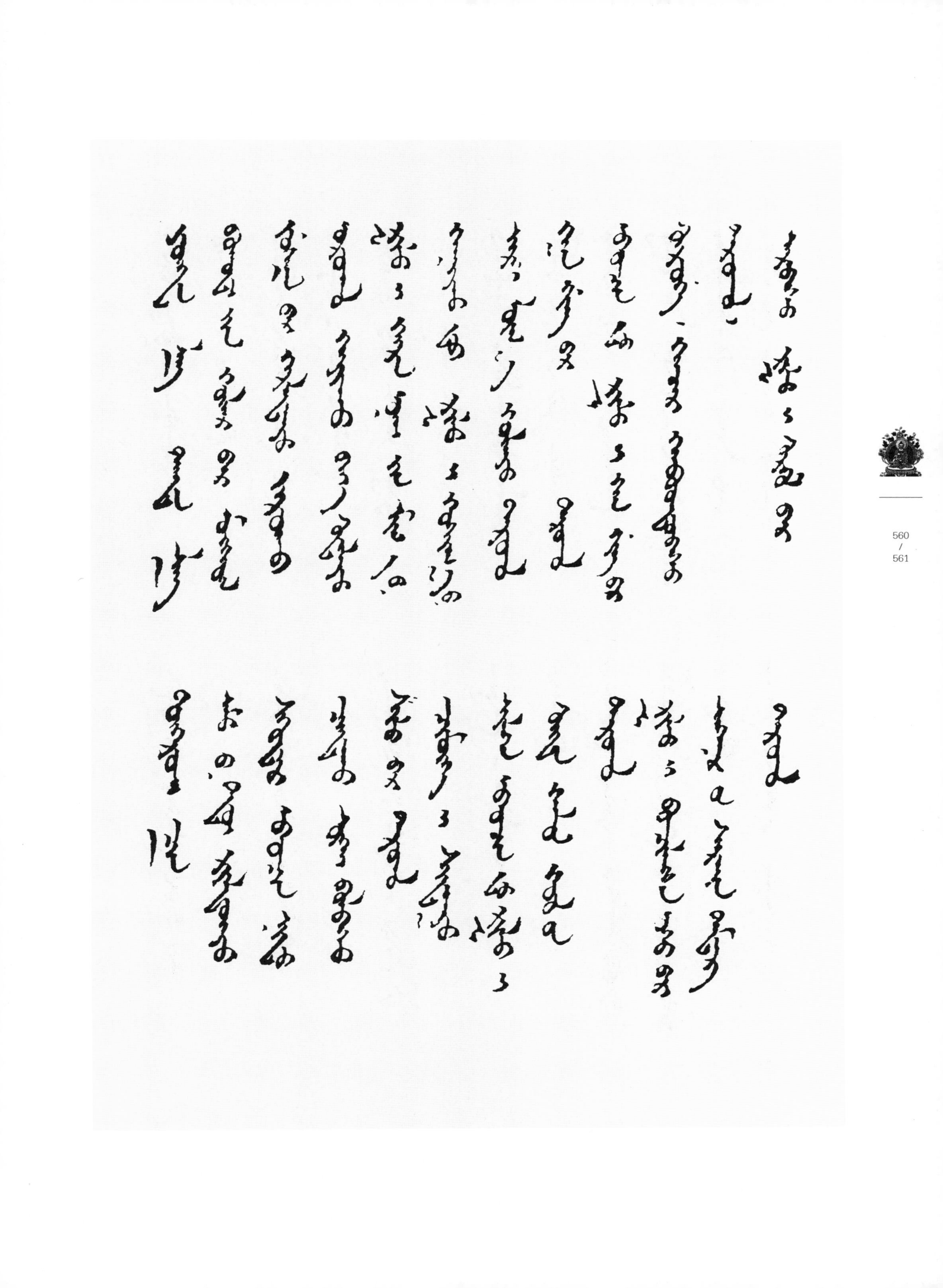

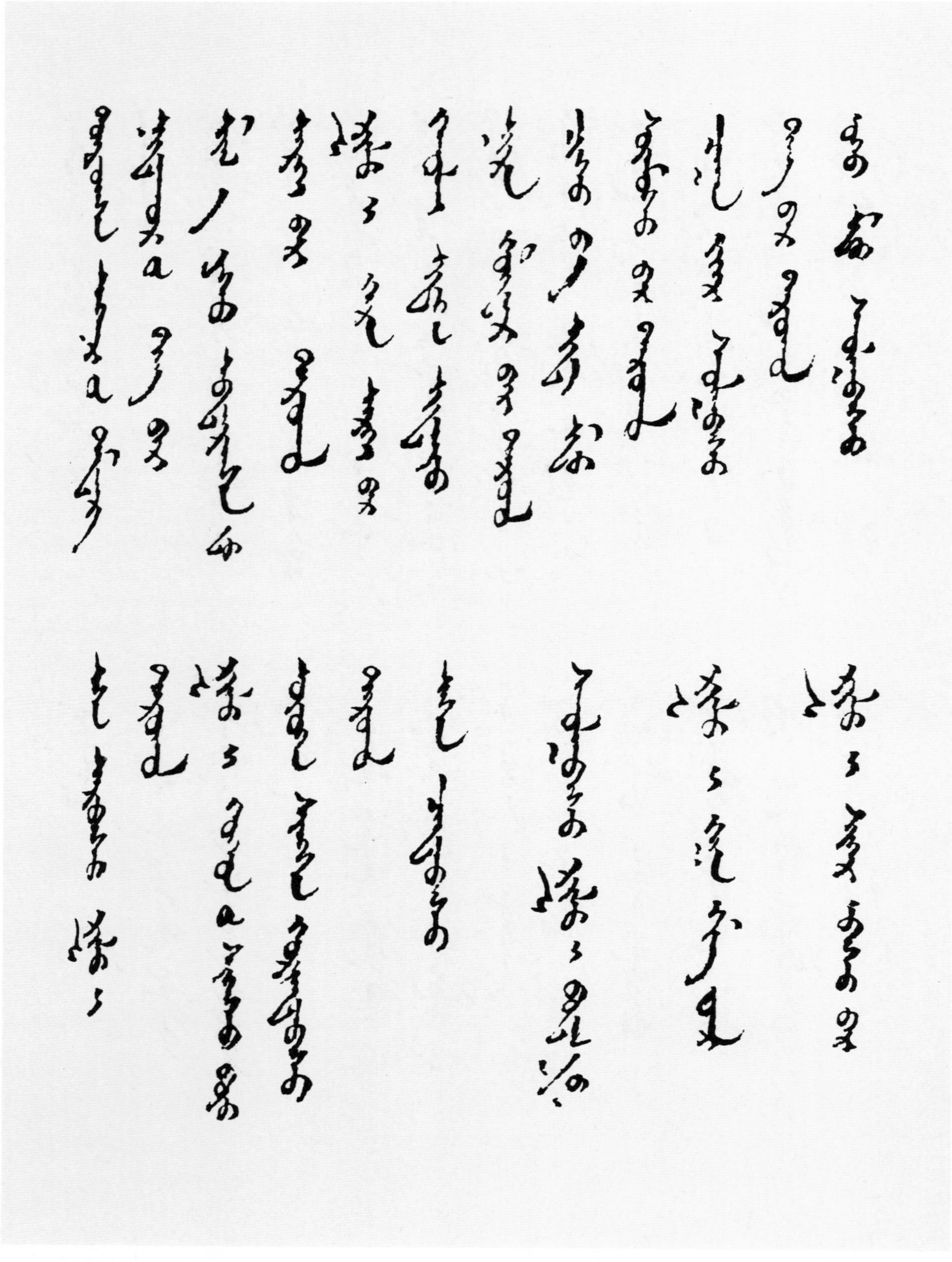

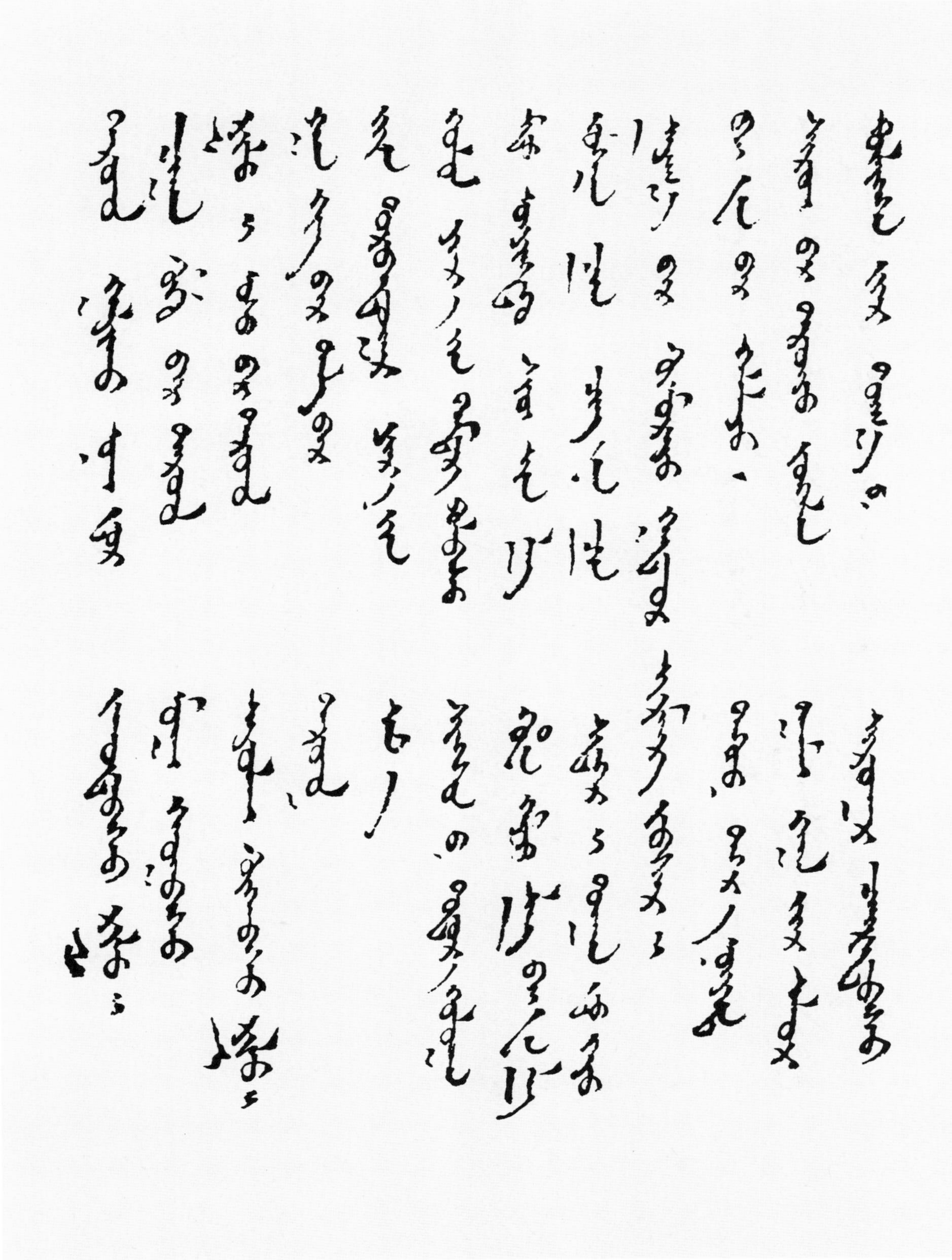

[illegible]

[illegible]

[illegible]

[illegible]

[illegible]

[illegible]

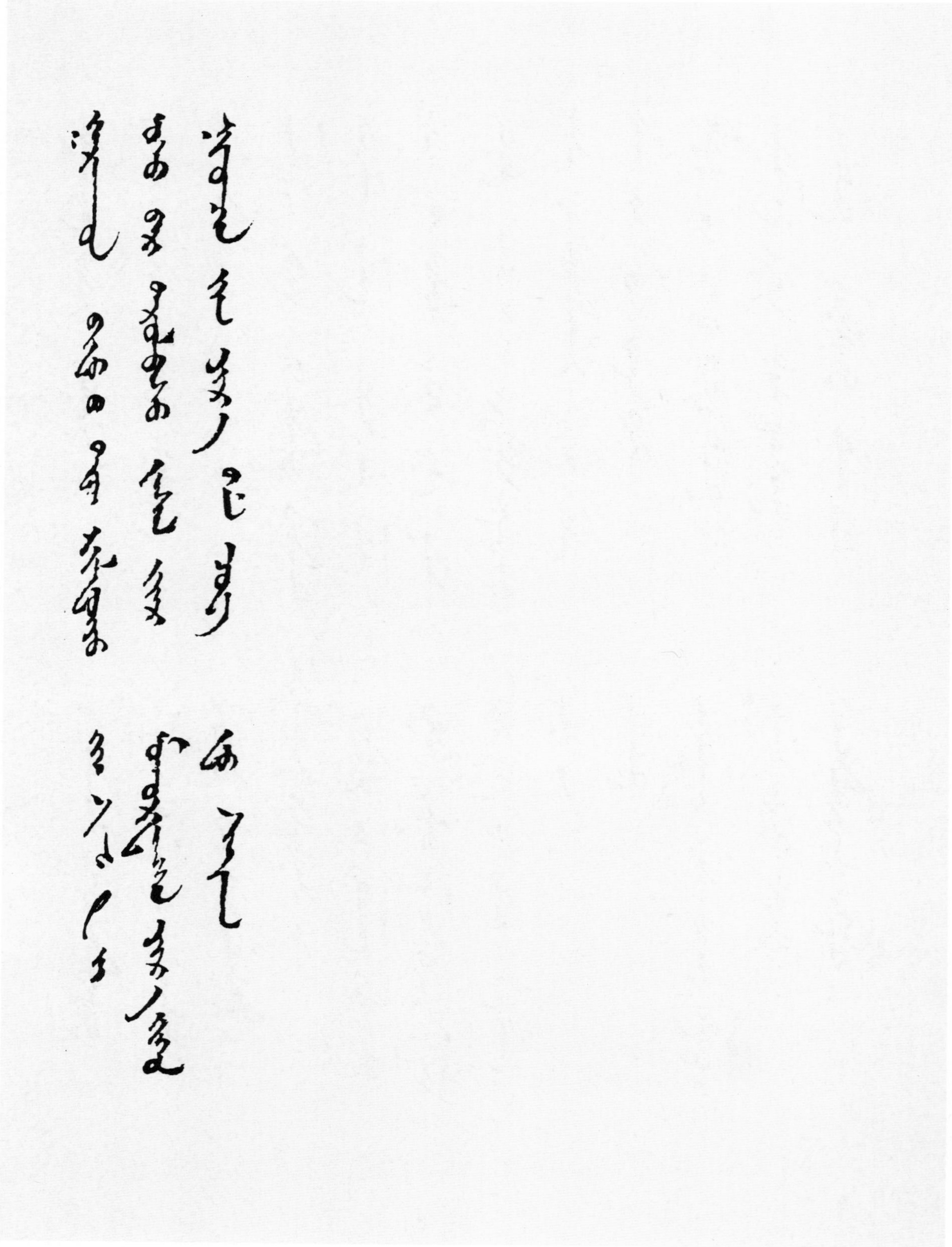

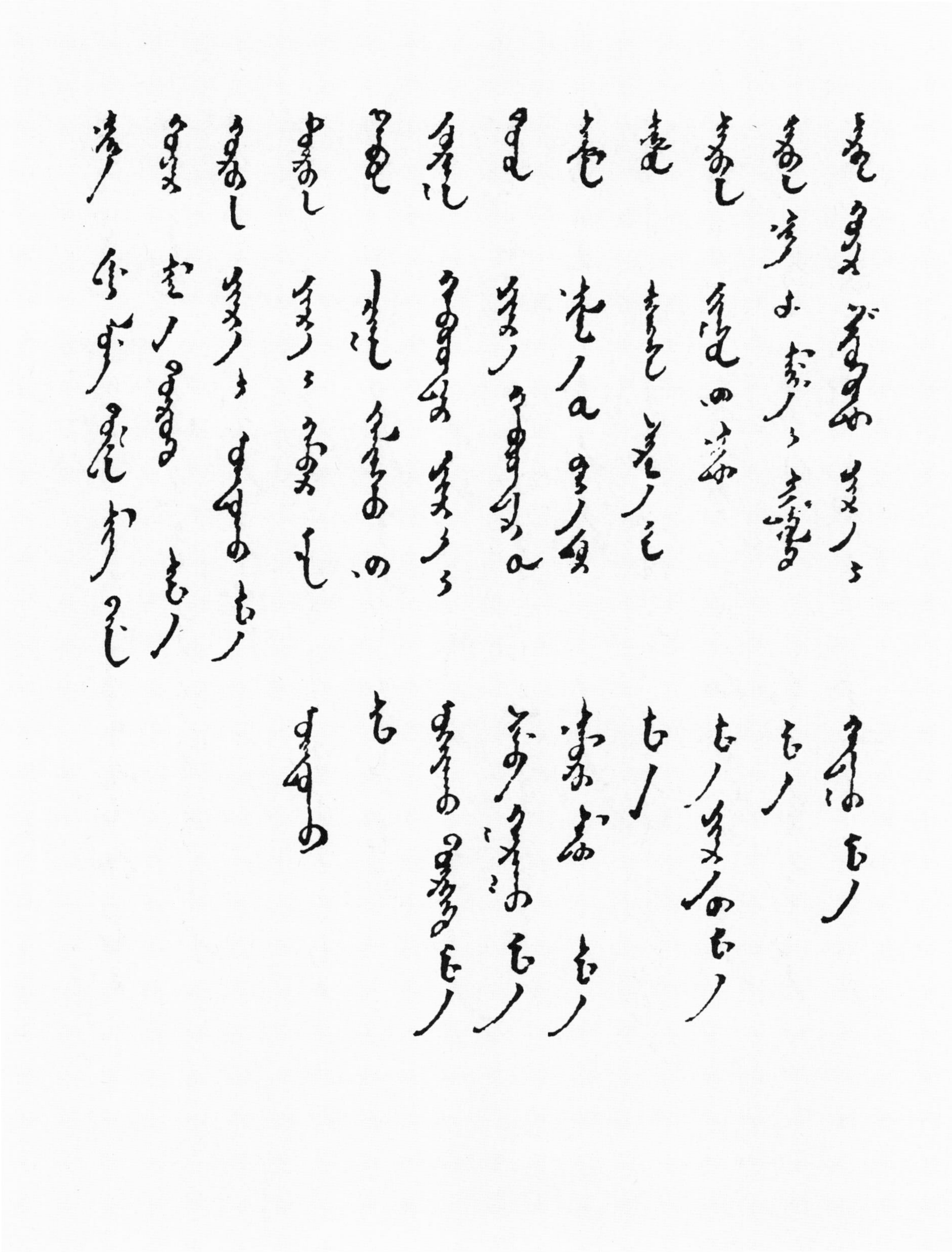

[illegible]

[illegible]

[illegible]

[illegible]

[illegible]

[illegible]

[illegible]

[illegible]

[illegible]

[illegible]

[illegible]

[illegible]

[illegible]

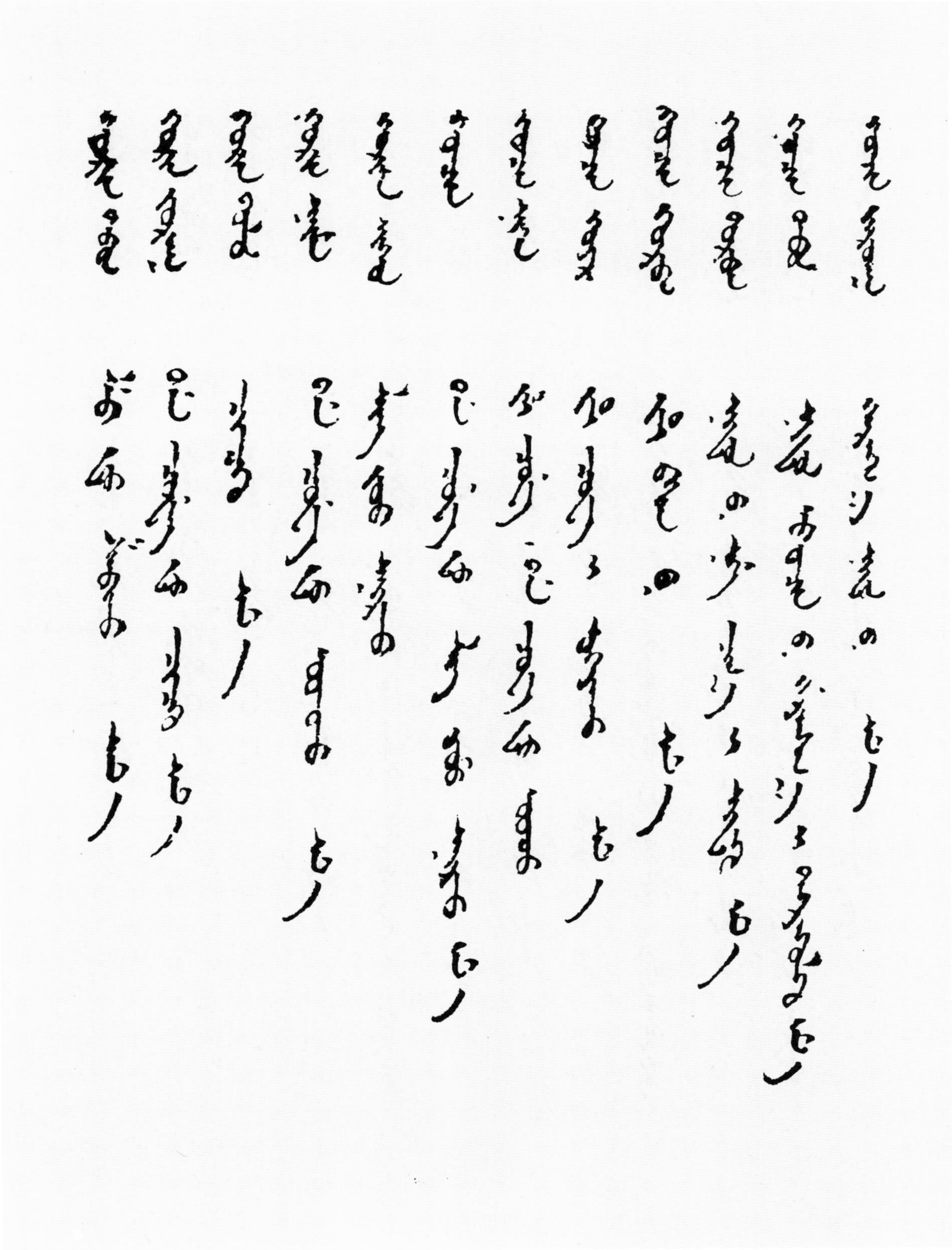

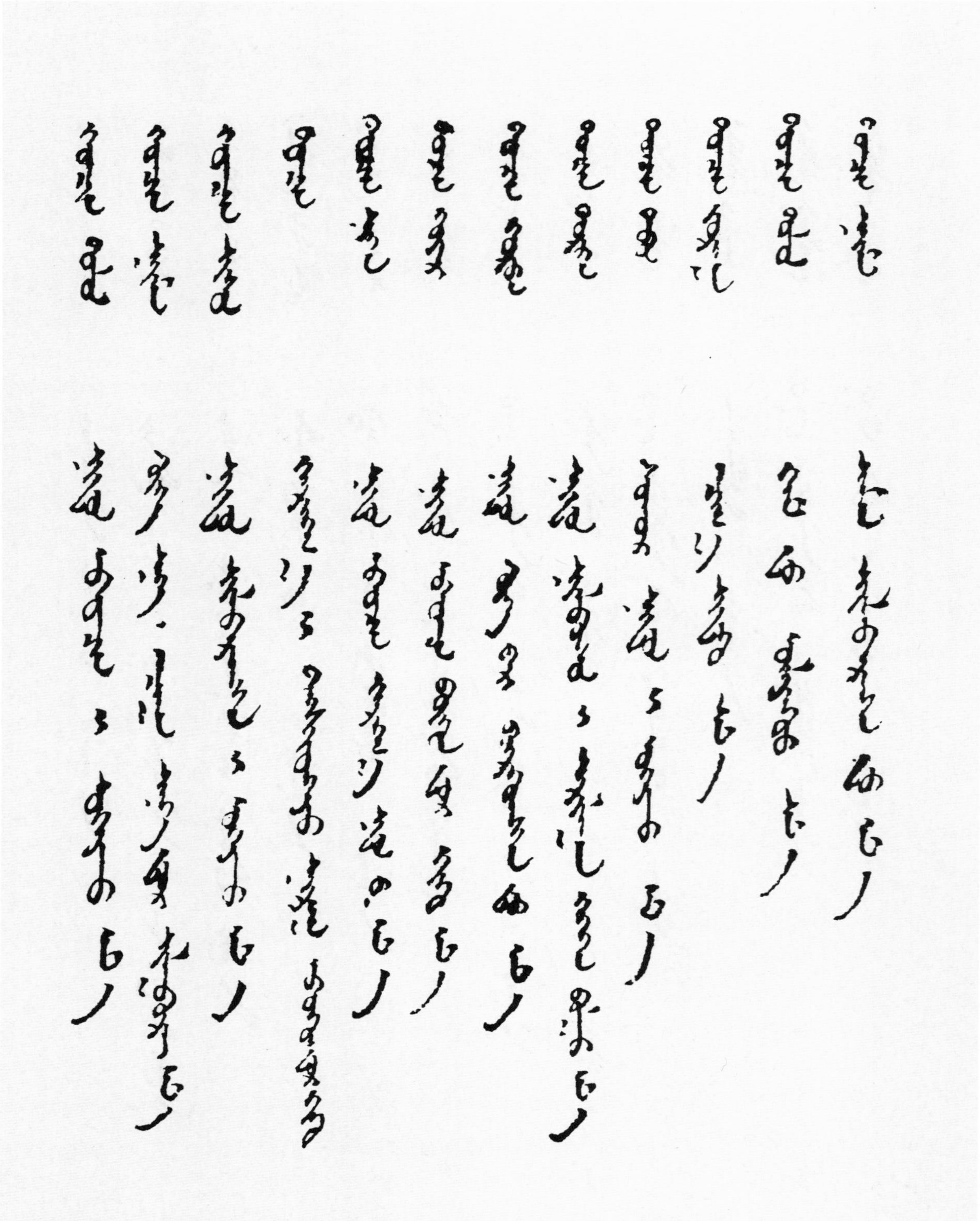

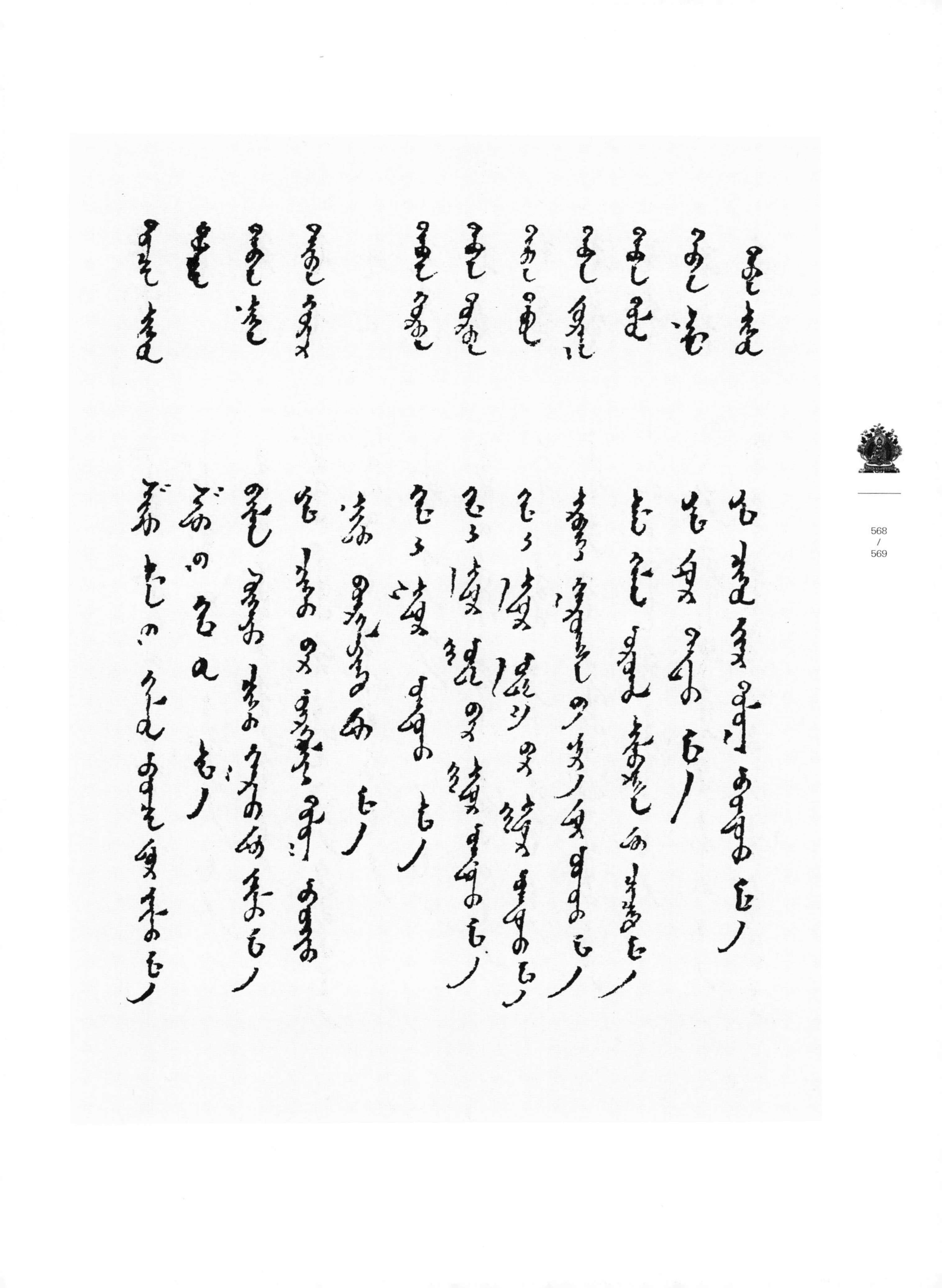

[illegible]

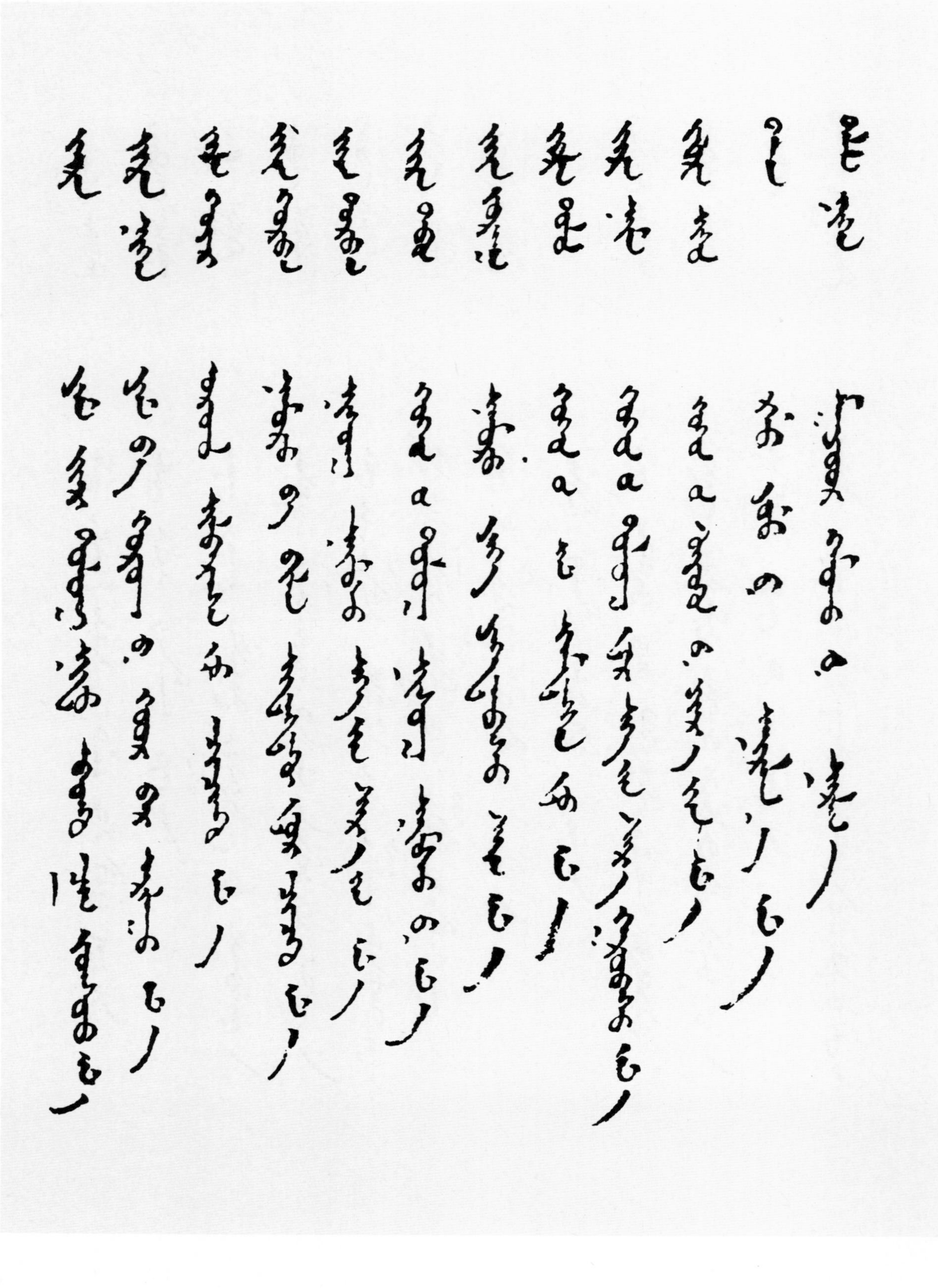

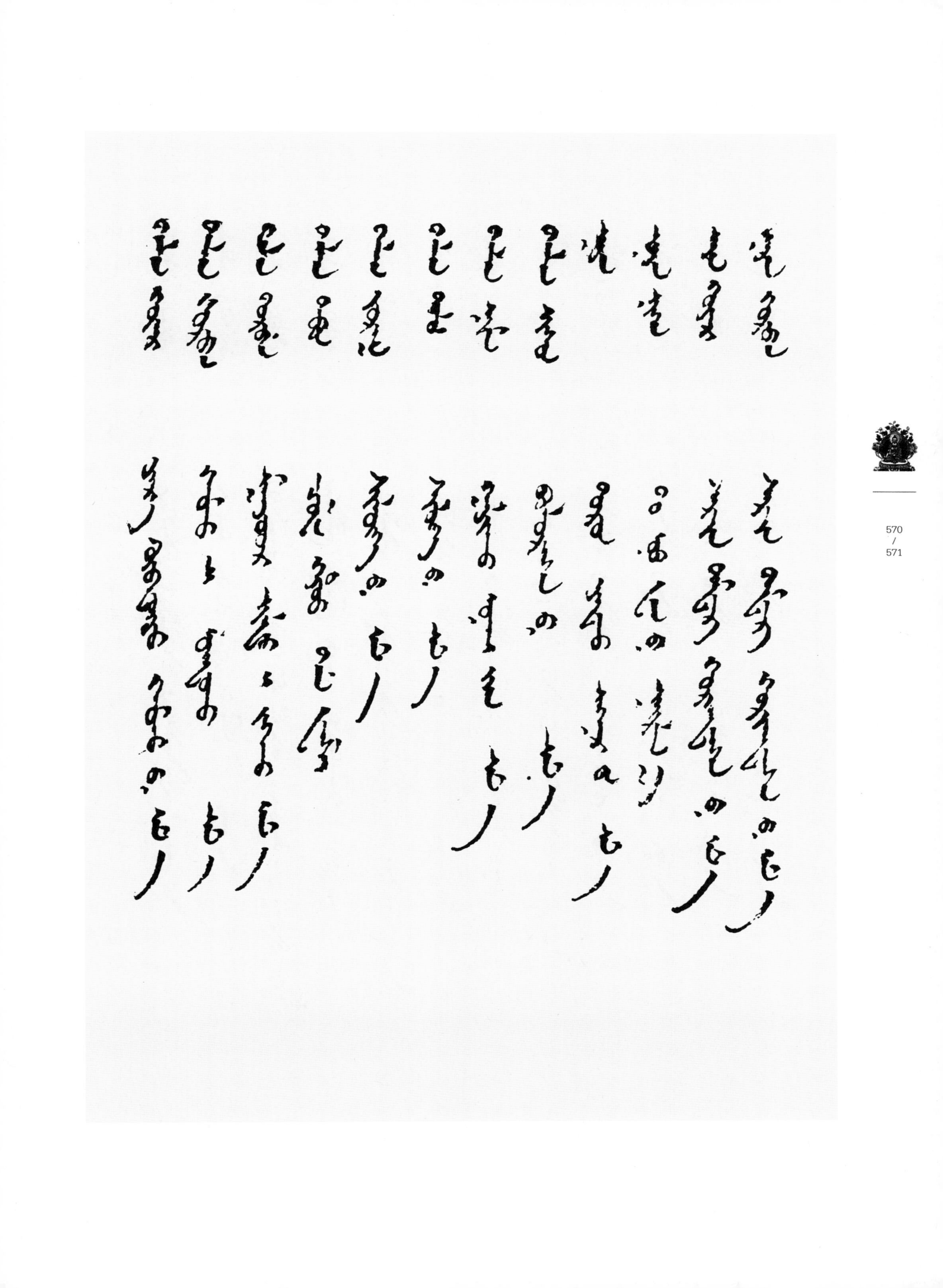

[illegible]

[illegible]

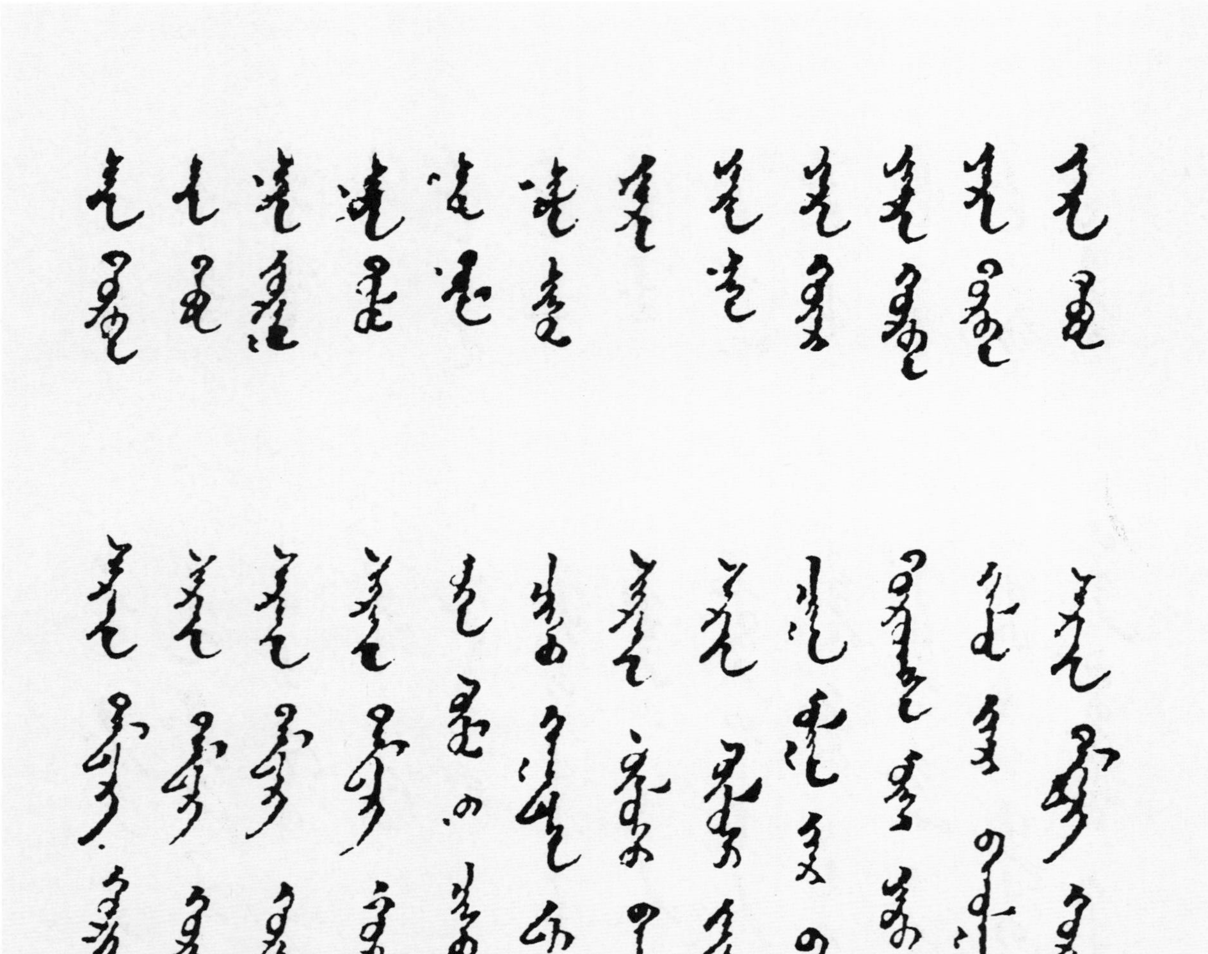

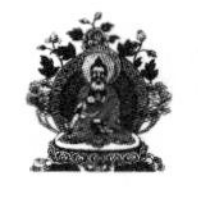

[illegible]

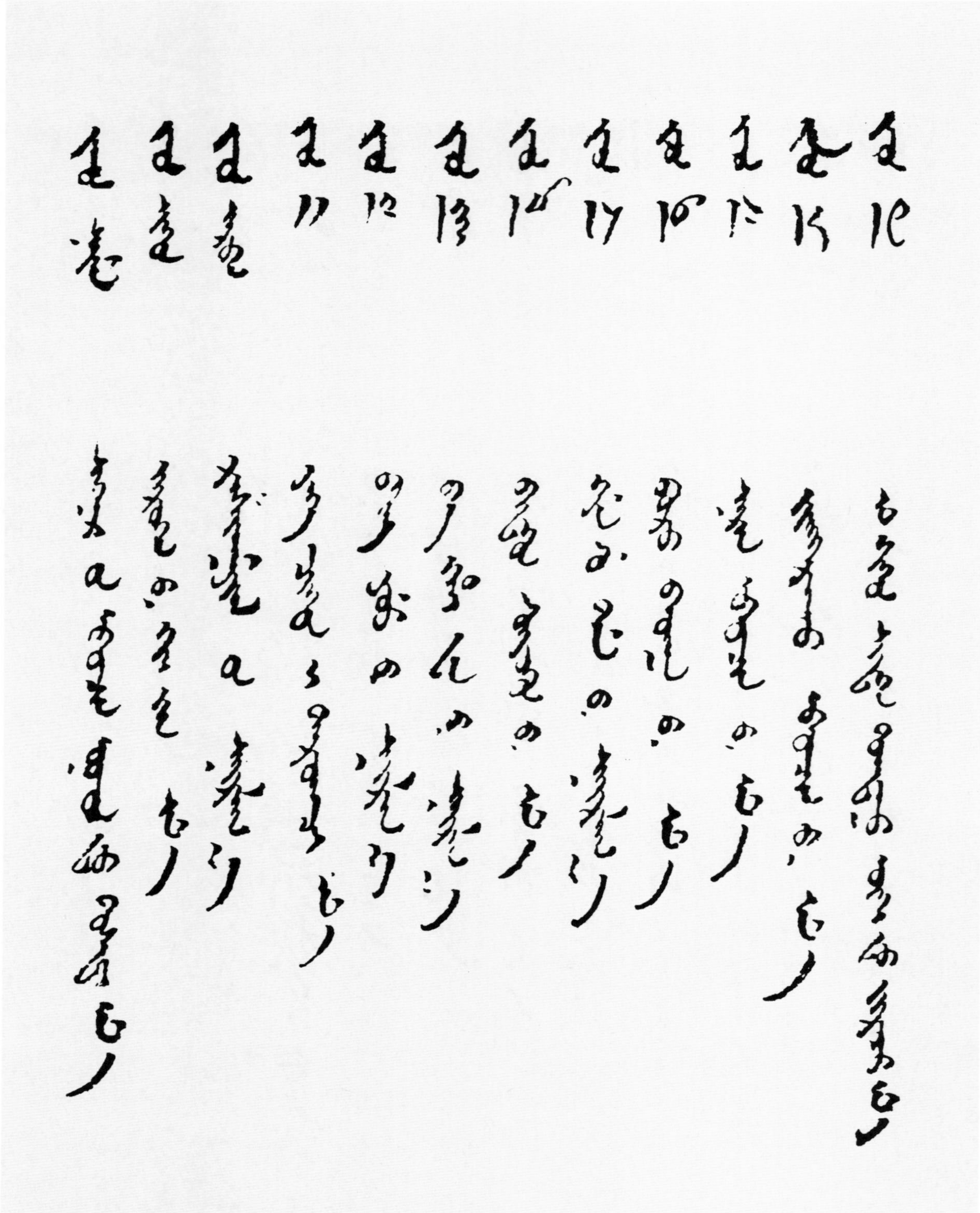

᠒᠐ ᠒᠑ ᠒᠒ ᠒᠓ ᠒᠔ ᠒᠕ ᠒᠖ ᠒᠗ ᠒᠘ ᠒᠙ ᠓᠐ ᠓᠑

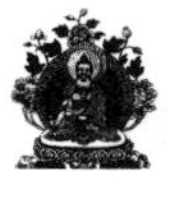

[illegible]

[illegible]

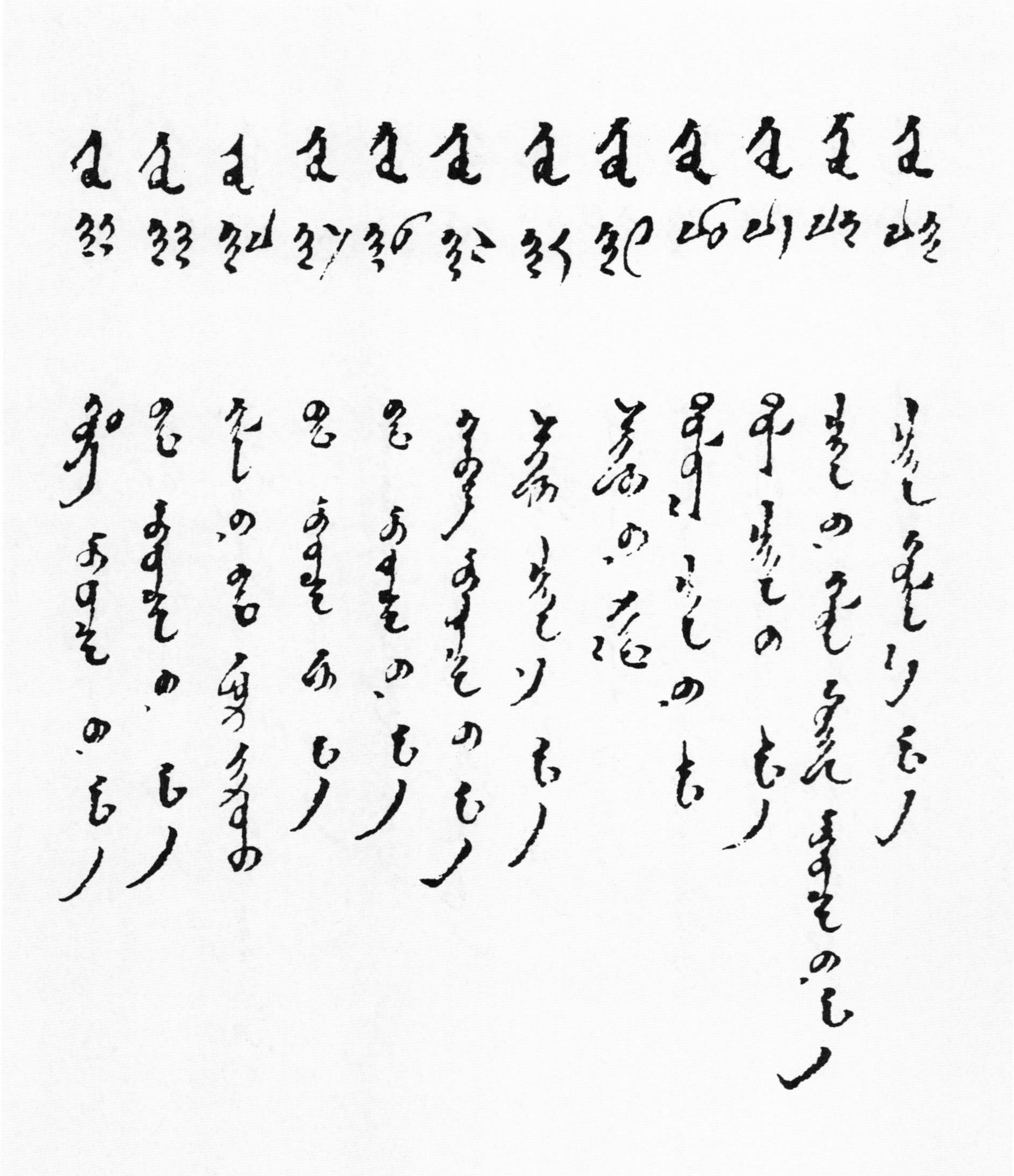

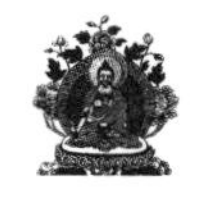

[illegible]

[illegible]

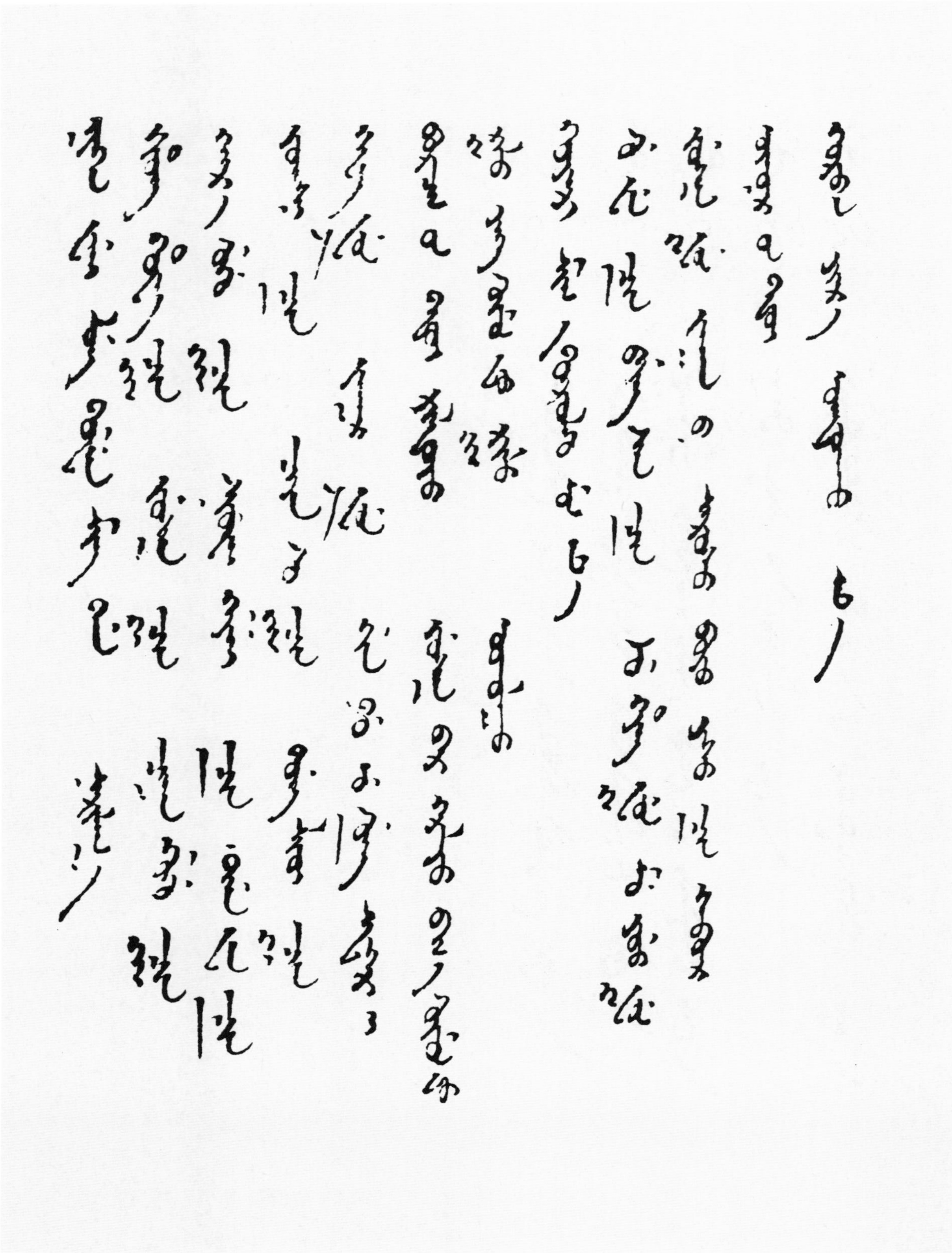

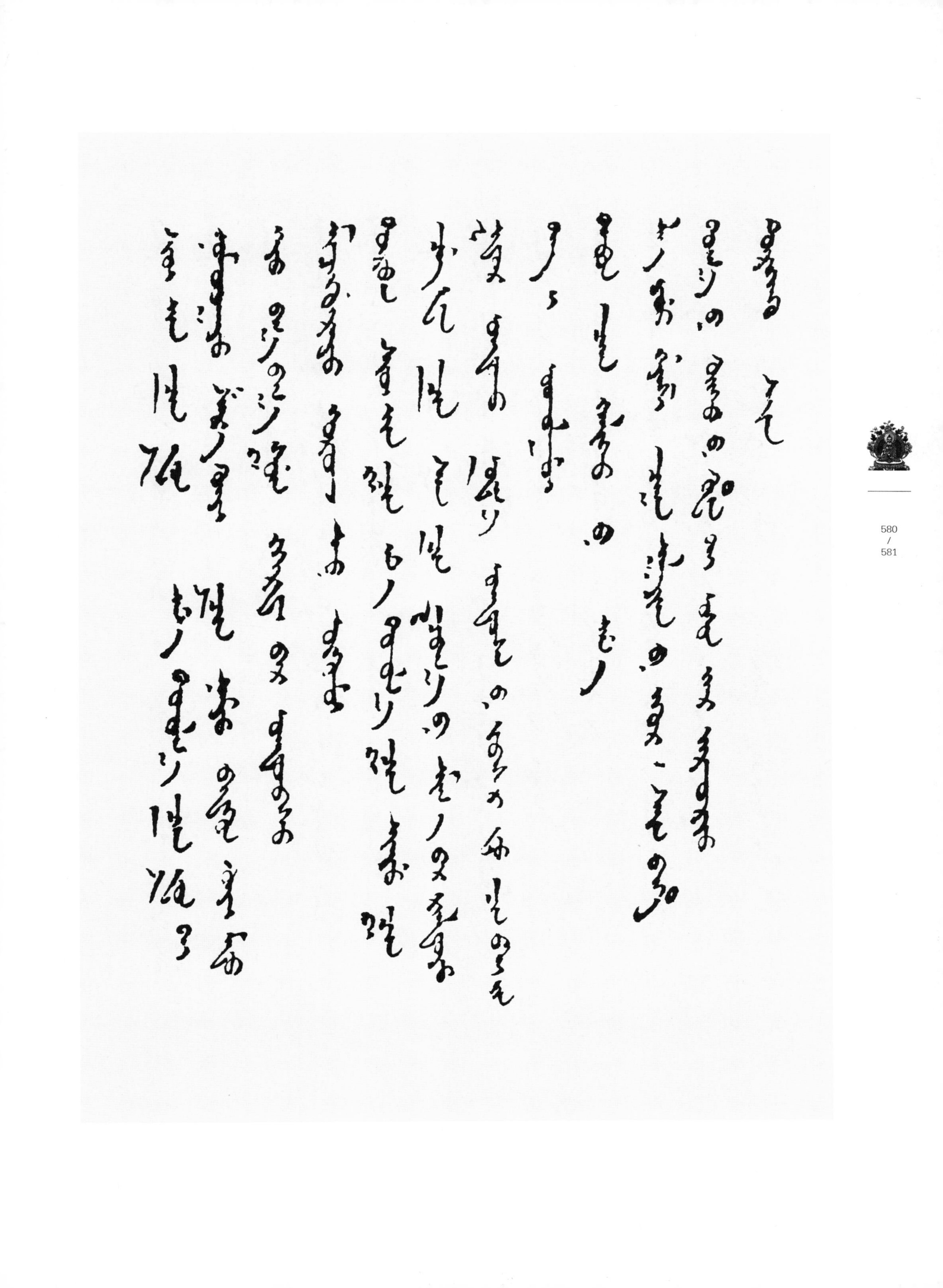

[illegible]

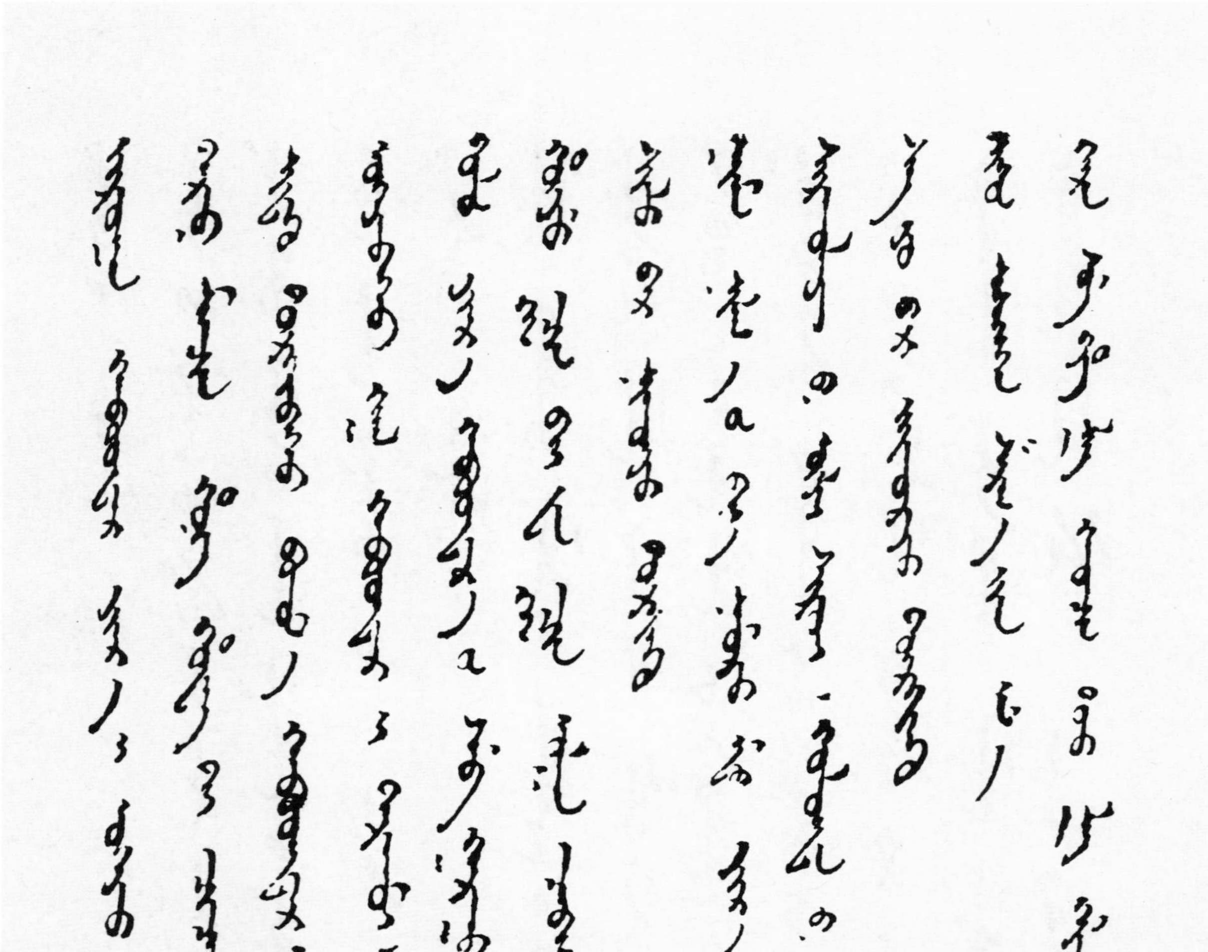

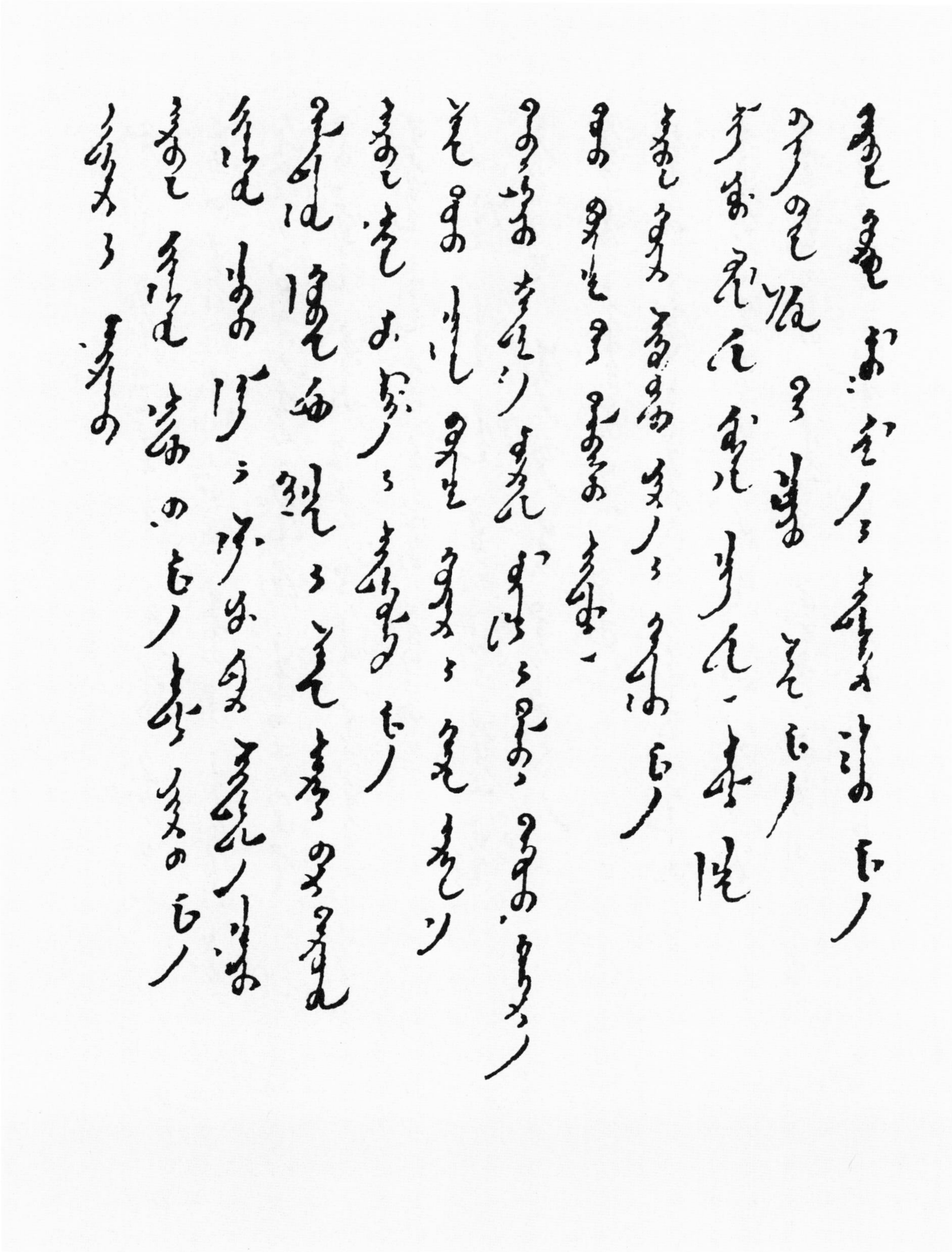

[illegible]

[illegible]

[illegible]

[illegible]

[illegible]

[illegible]

[illegible]

[illegible]

[illegible]

[illegible]

[illegible]

[illegible]

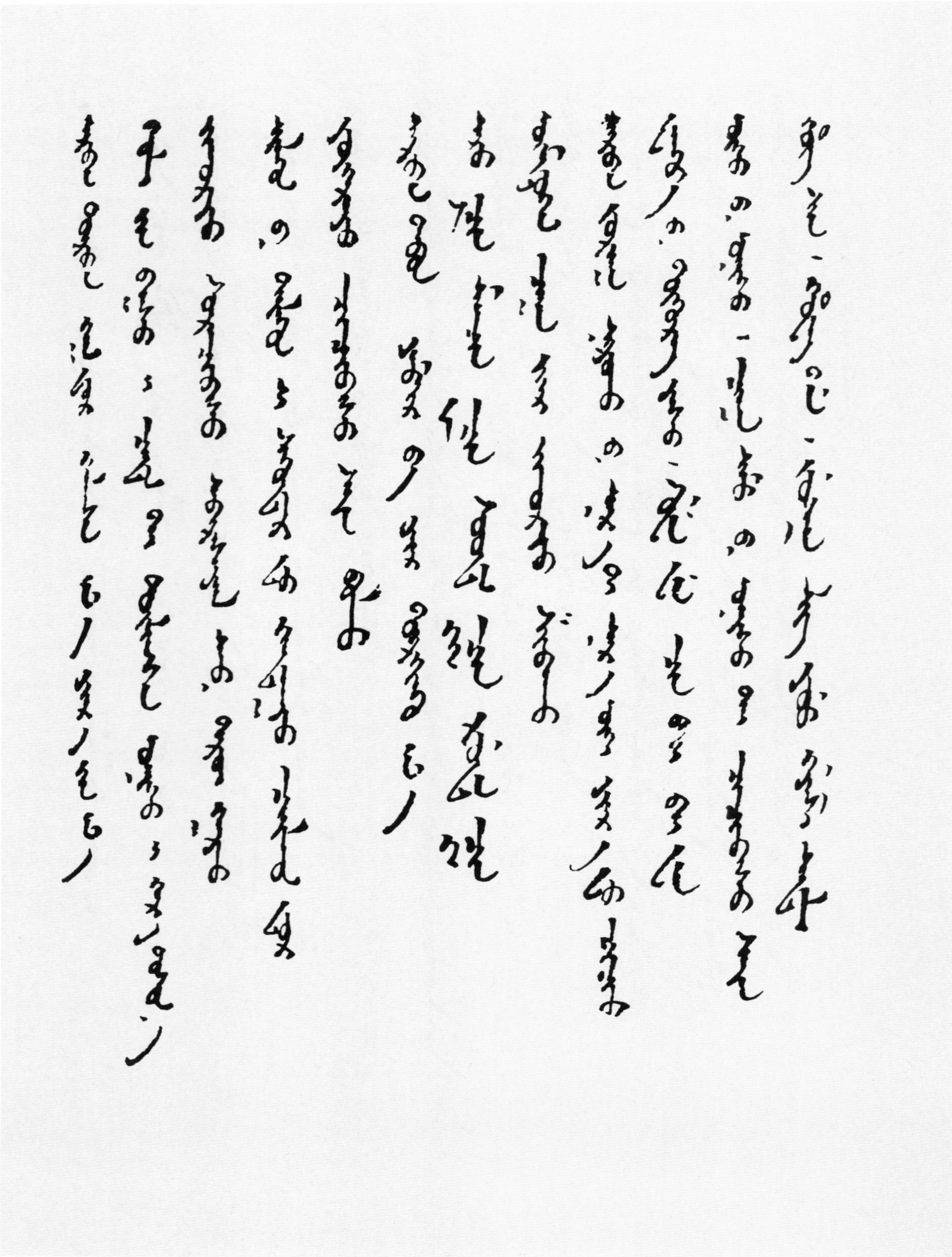

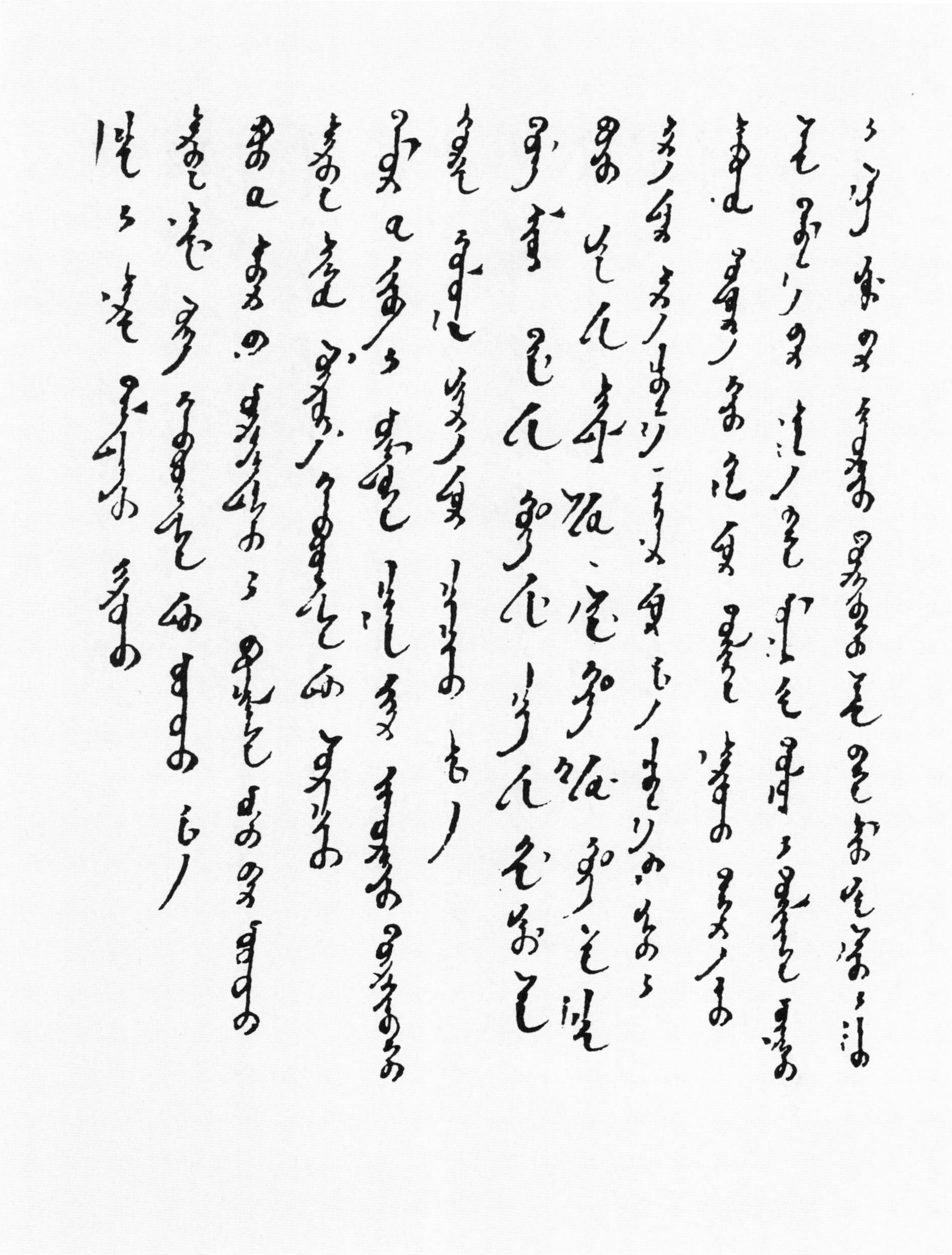

[illegible]
[illegible]
[illegible]
[illegible]
[illegible]
[illegible]
[illegible]
[illegible]
[illegible]
[illegible]
[illegible]

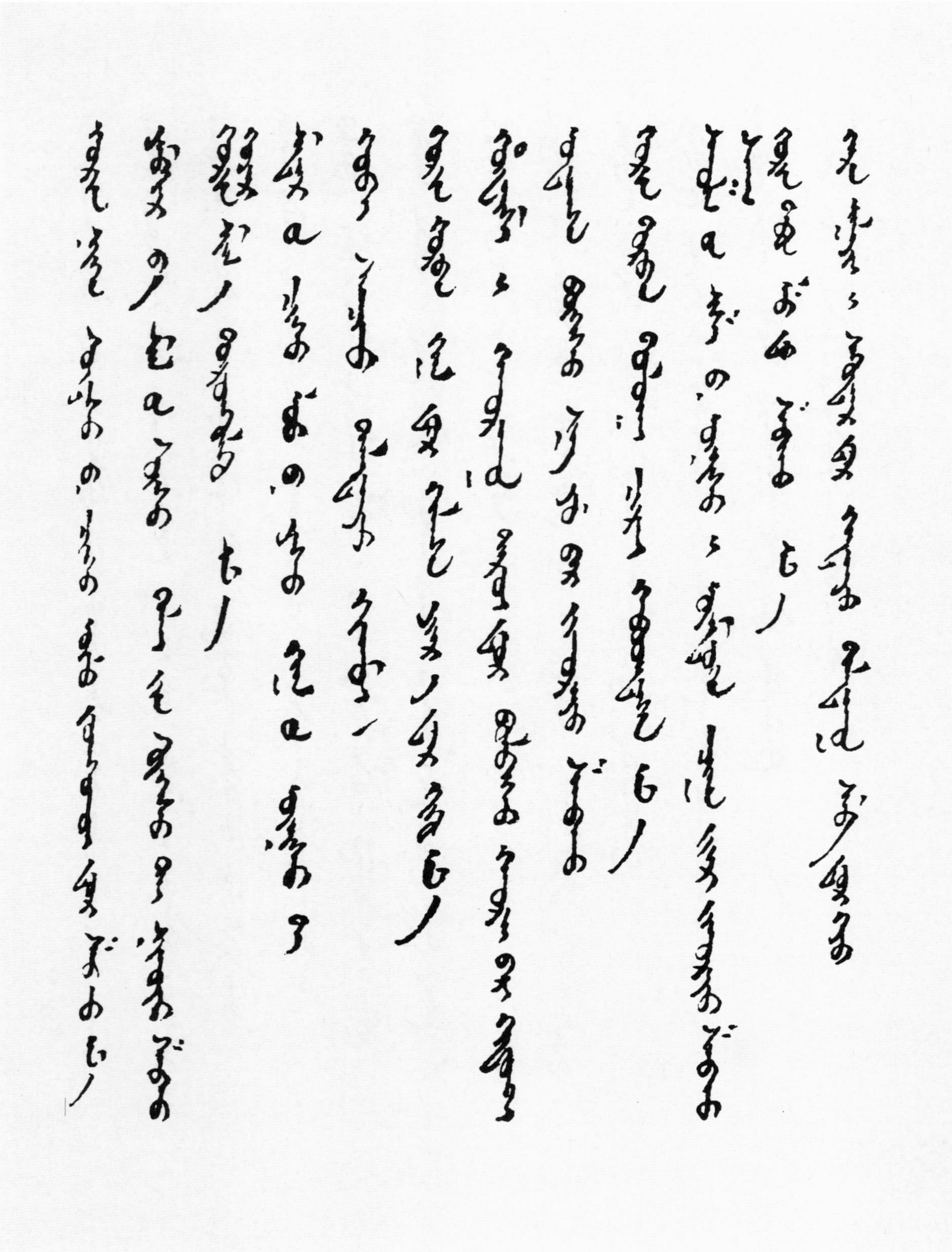

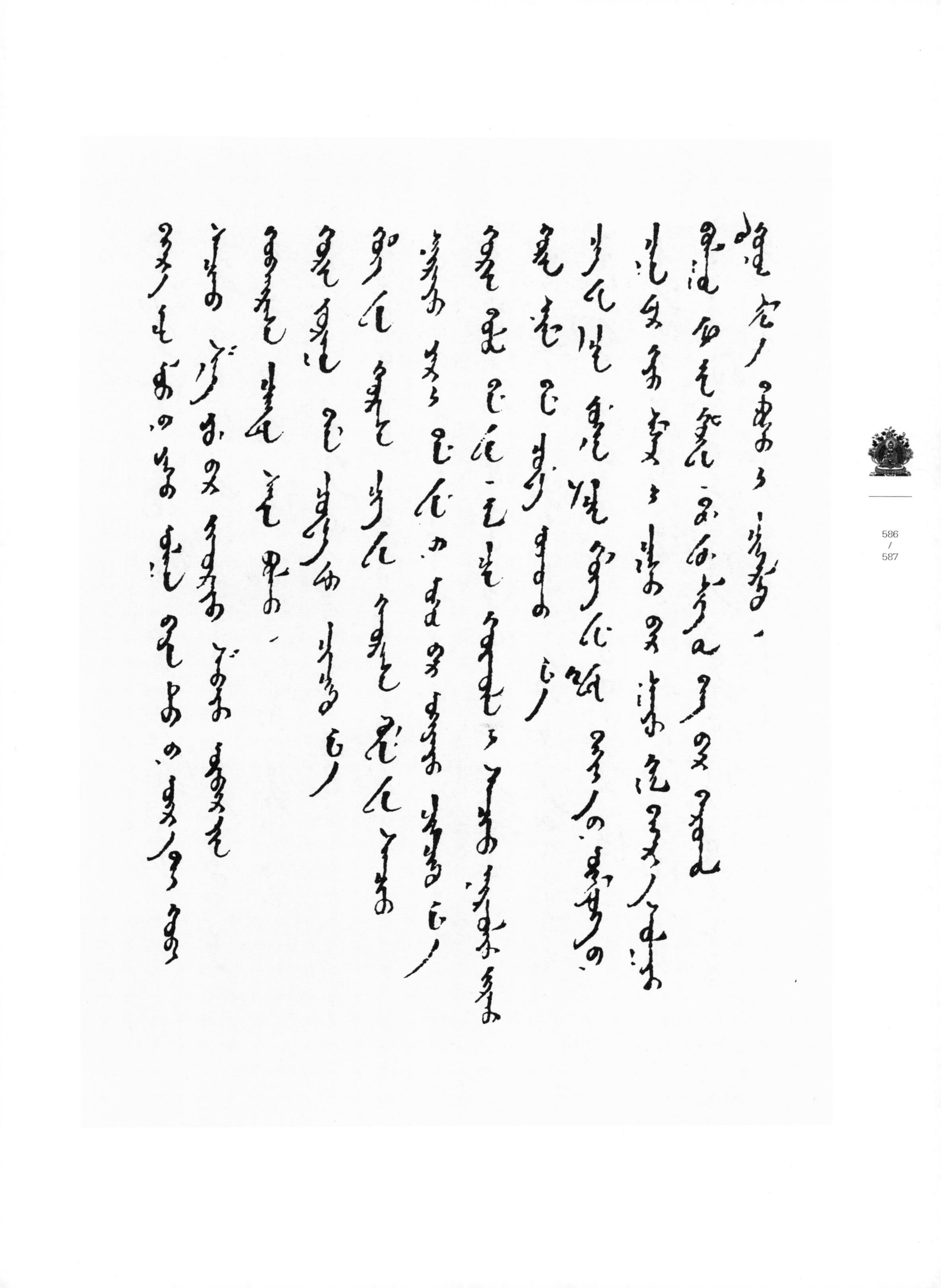

[illegible]

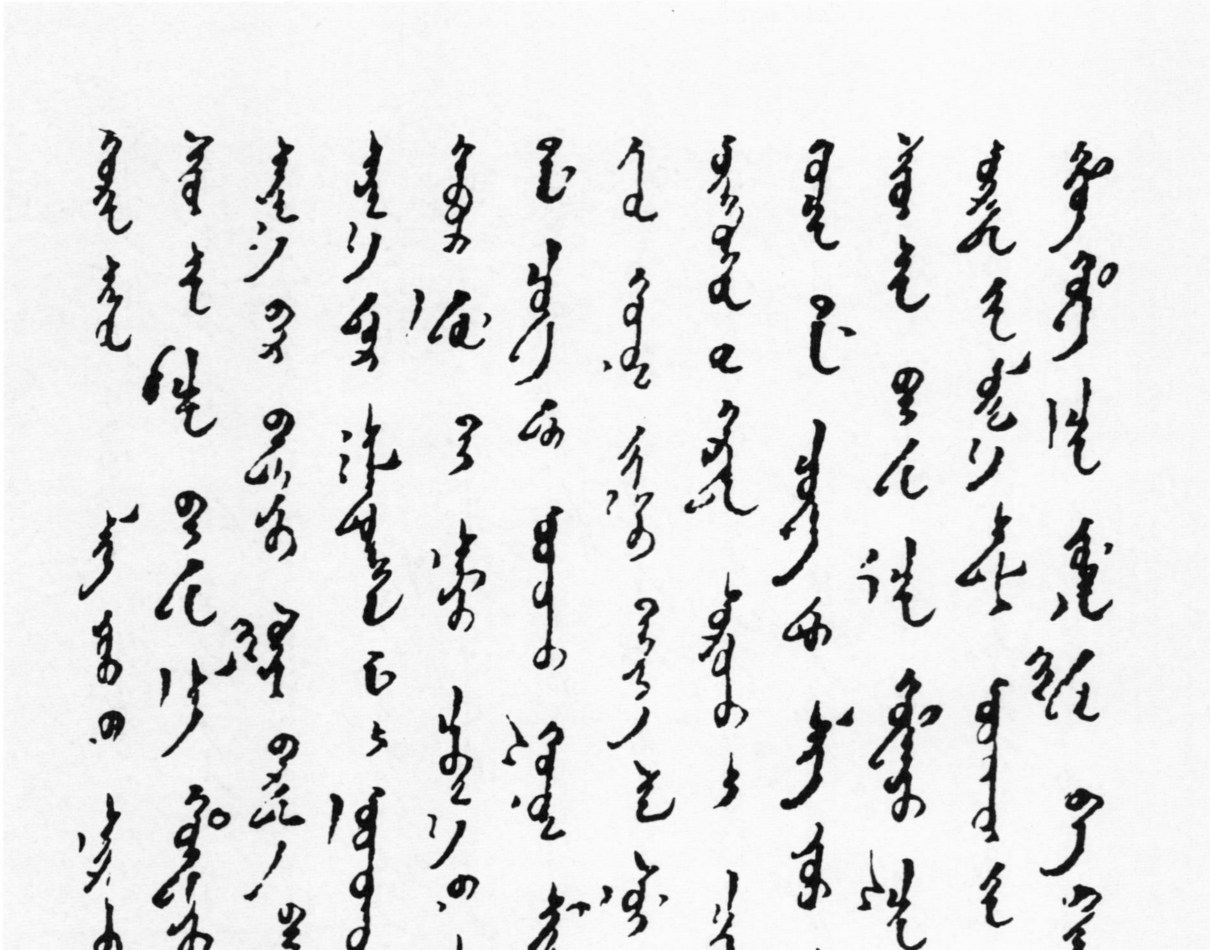

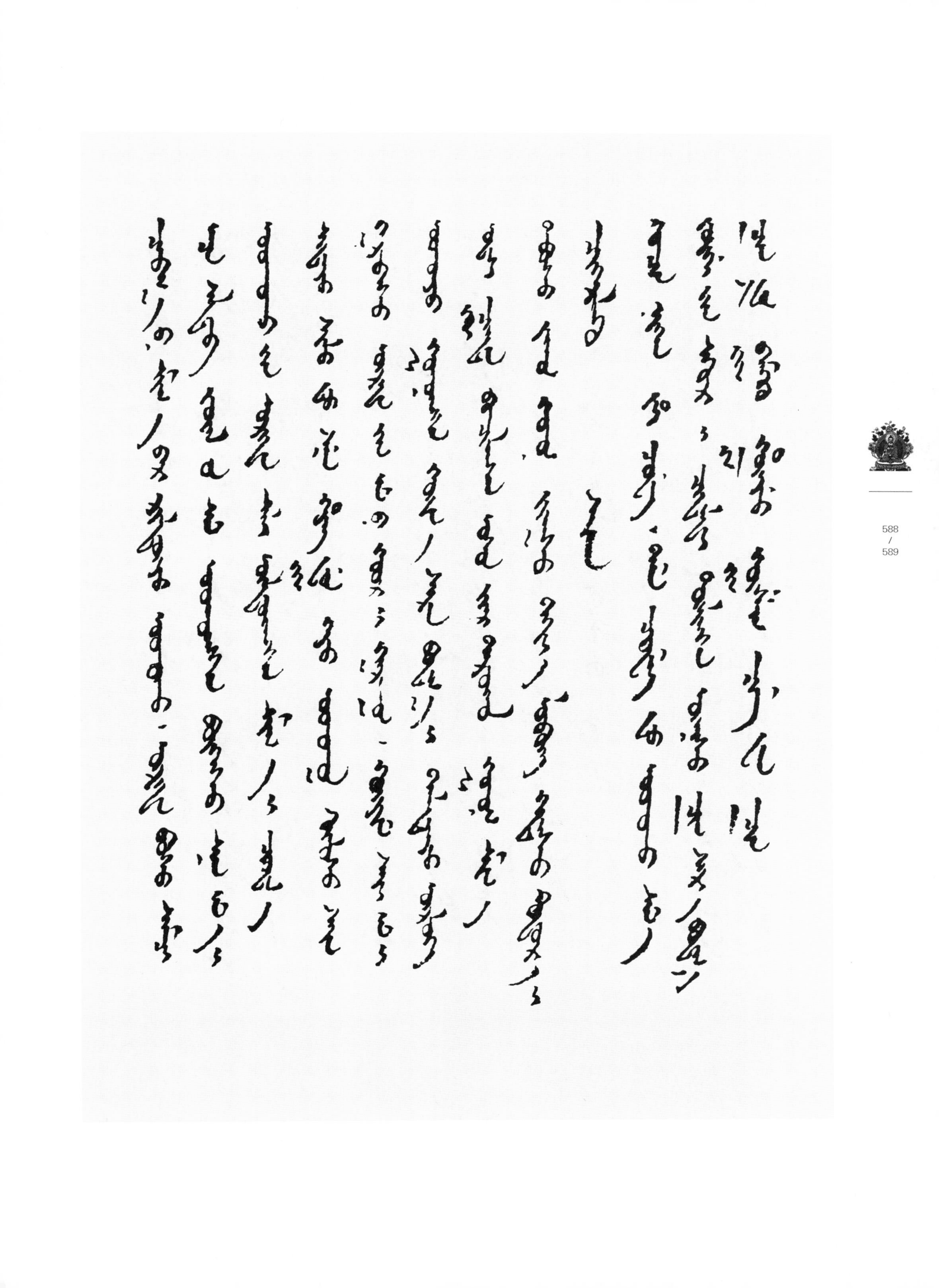

[illegible]

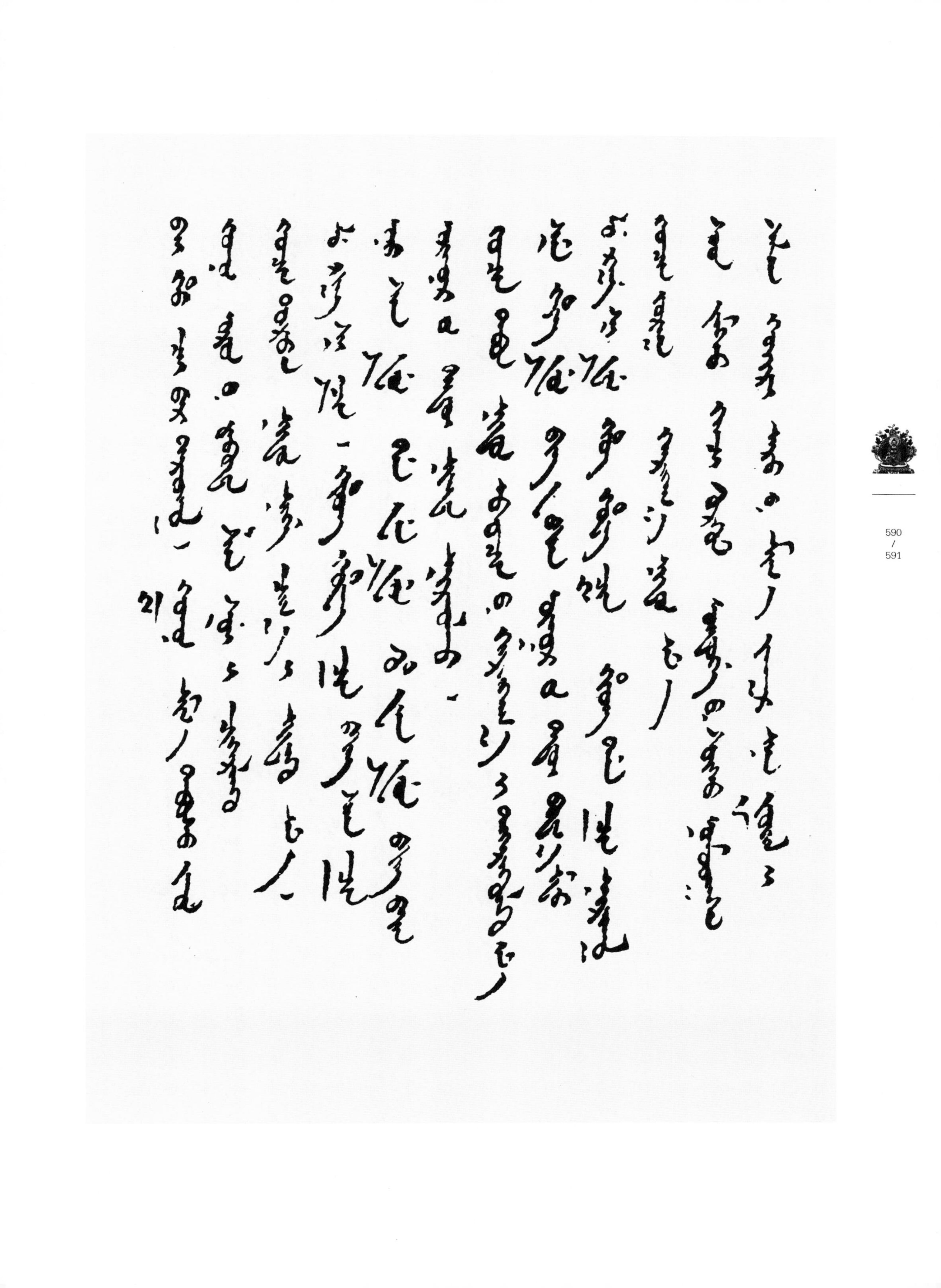

21

[illegible]

[illegible]

[illegible]

[illegible]

[illegible]

[illegible]

[illegible]

[illegible]

[illegible]

[illegible]

[illegible]

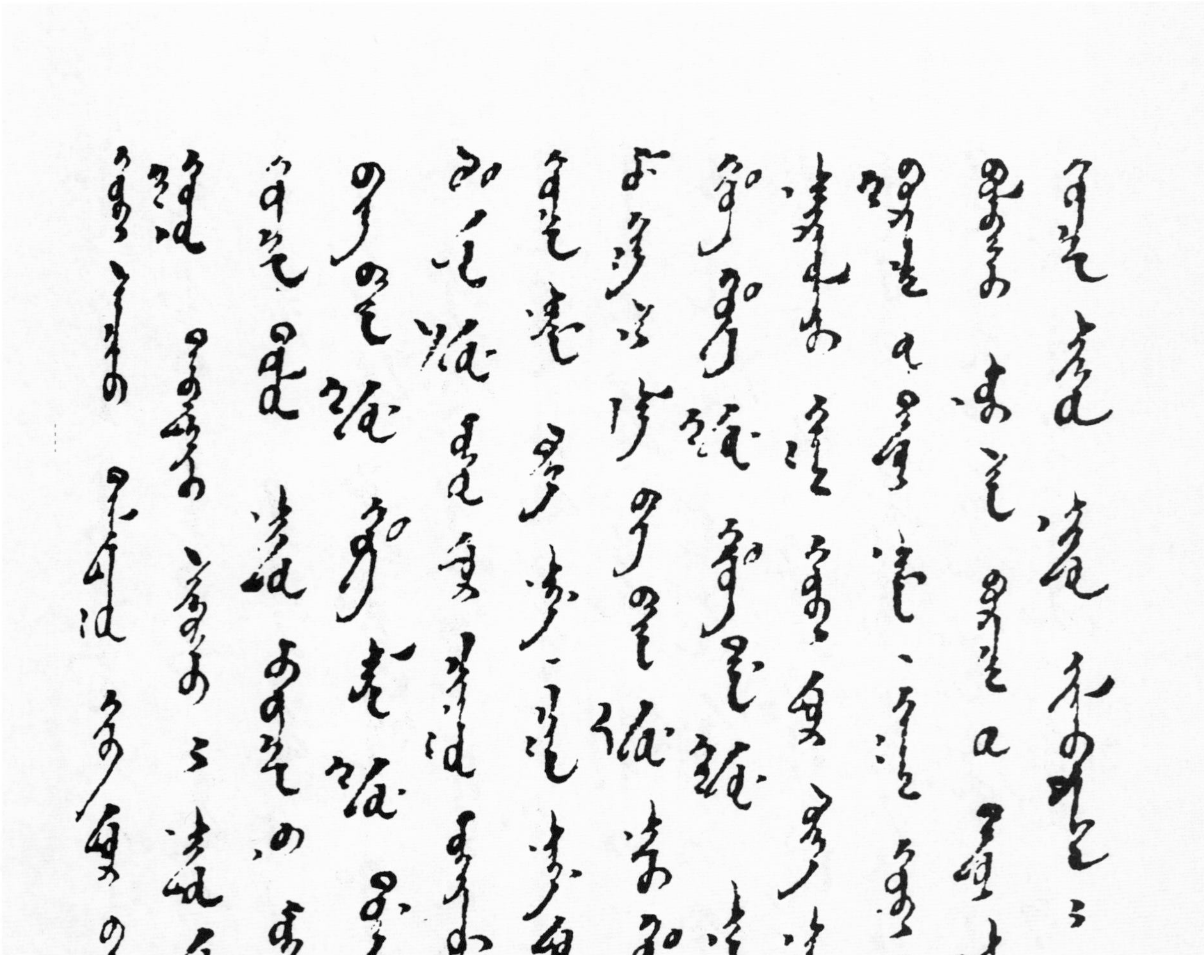

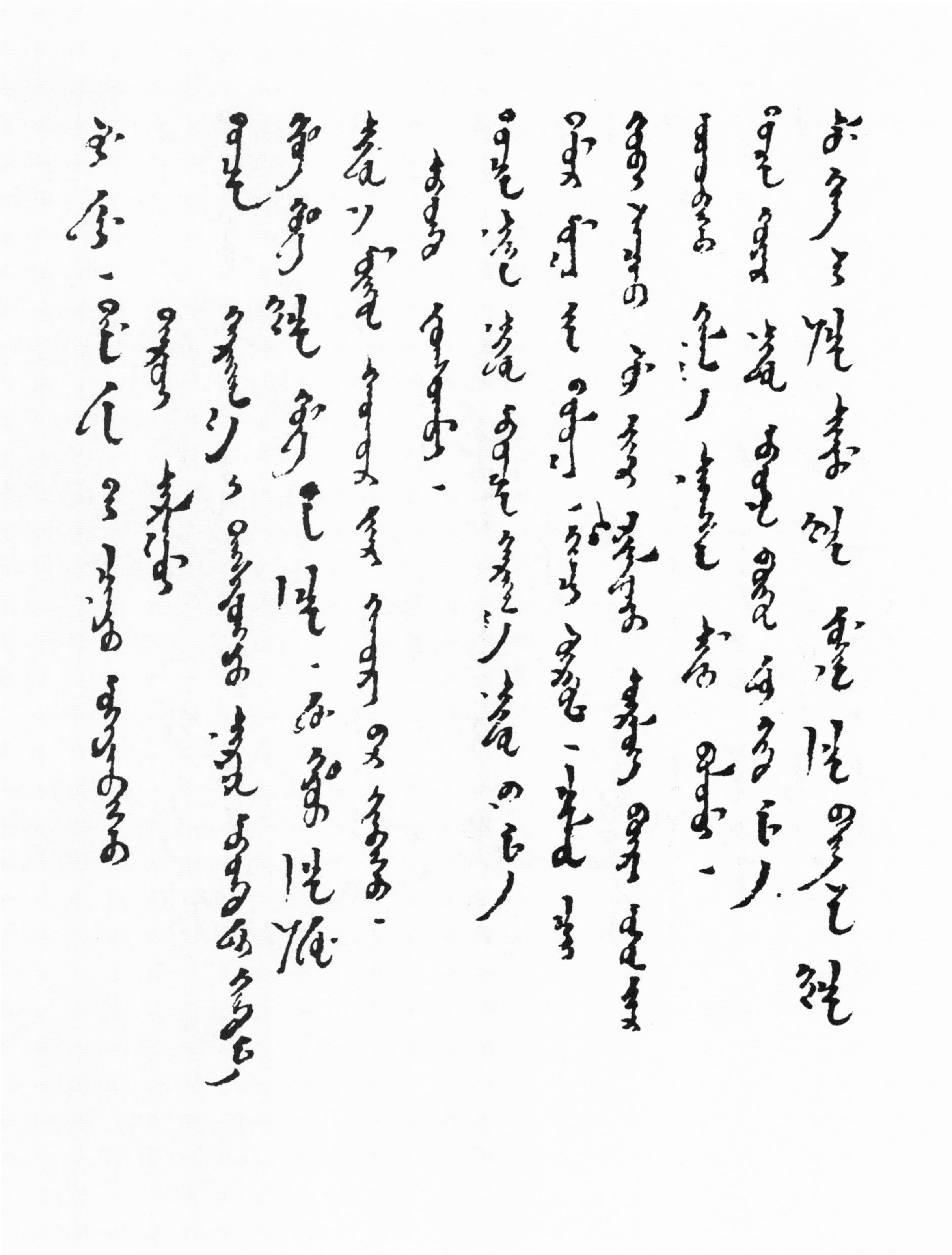

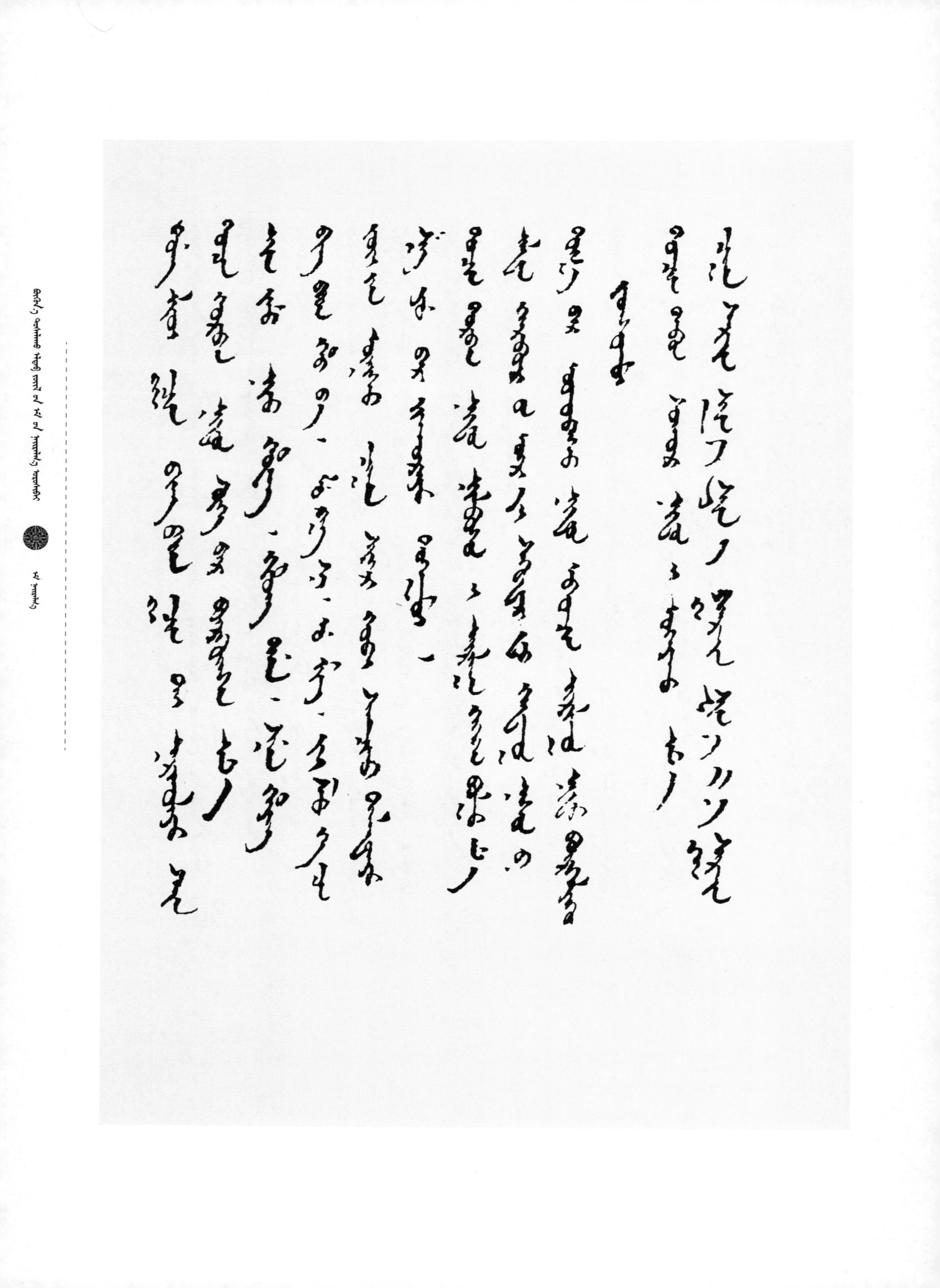

[illegible]

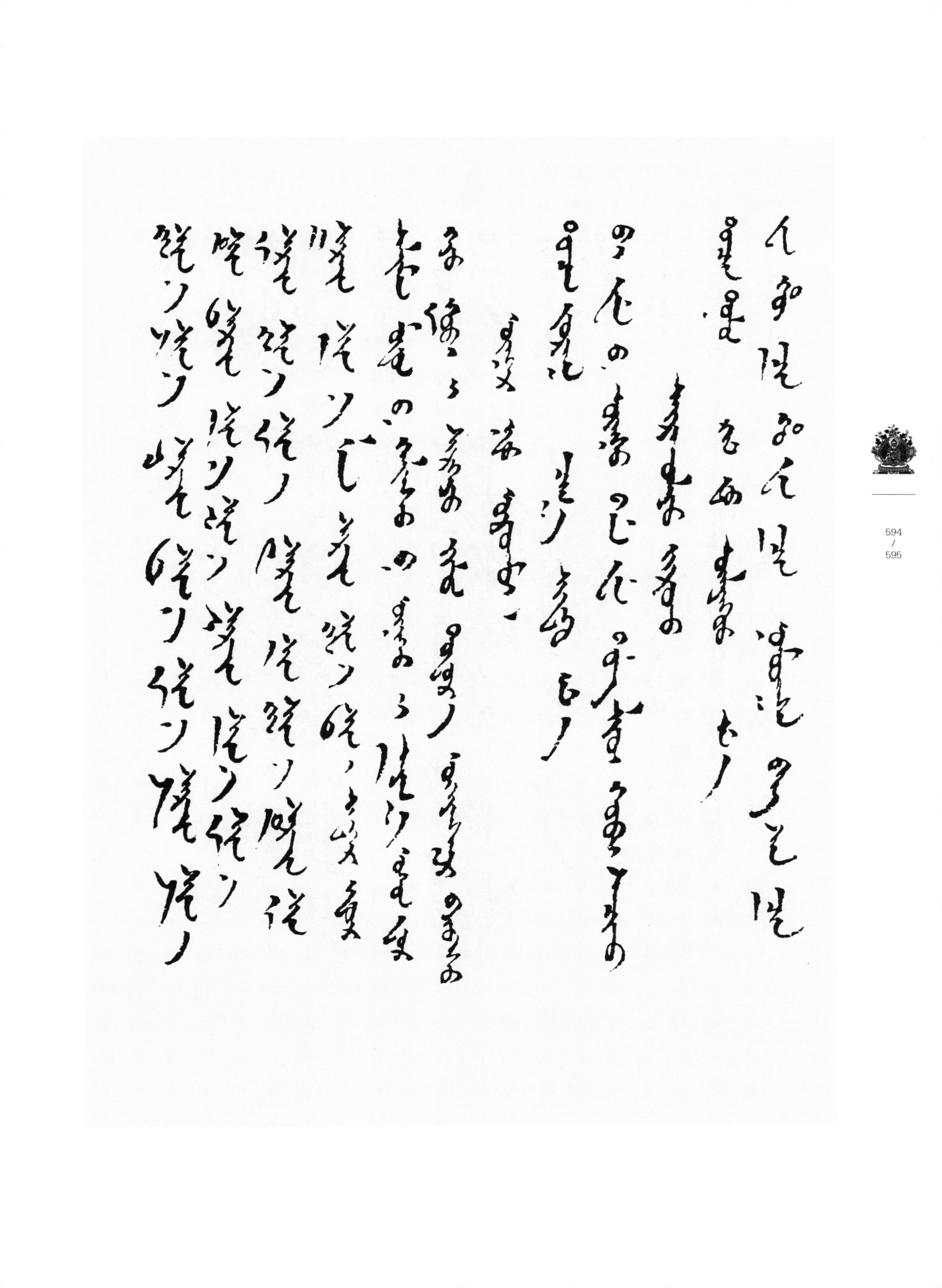

[illegible]
[illegible]
[illegible]
[illegible]
[illegible]
[illegible]
[illegible]
[illegible]
[illegible]
[illegible]
[illegible]
[illegible]

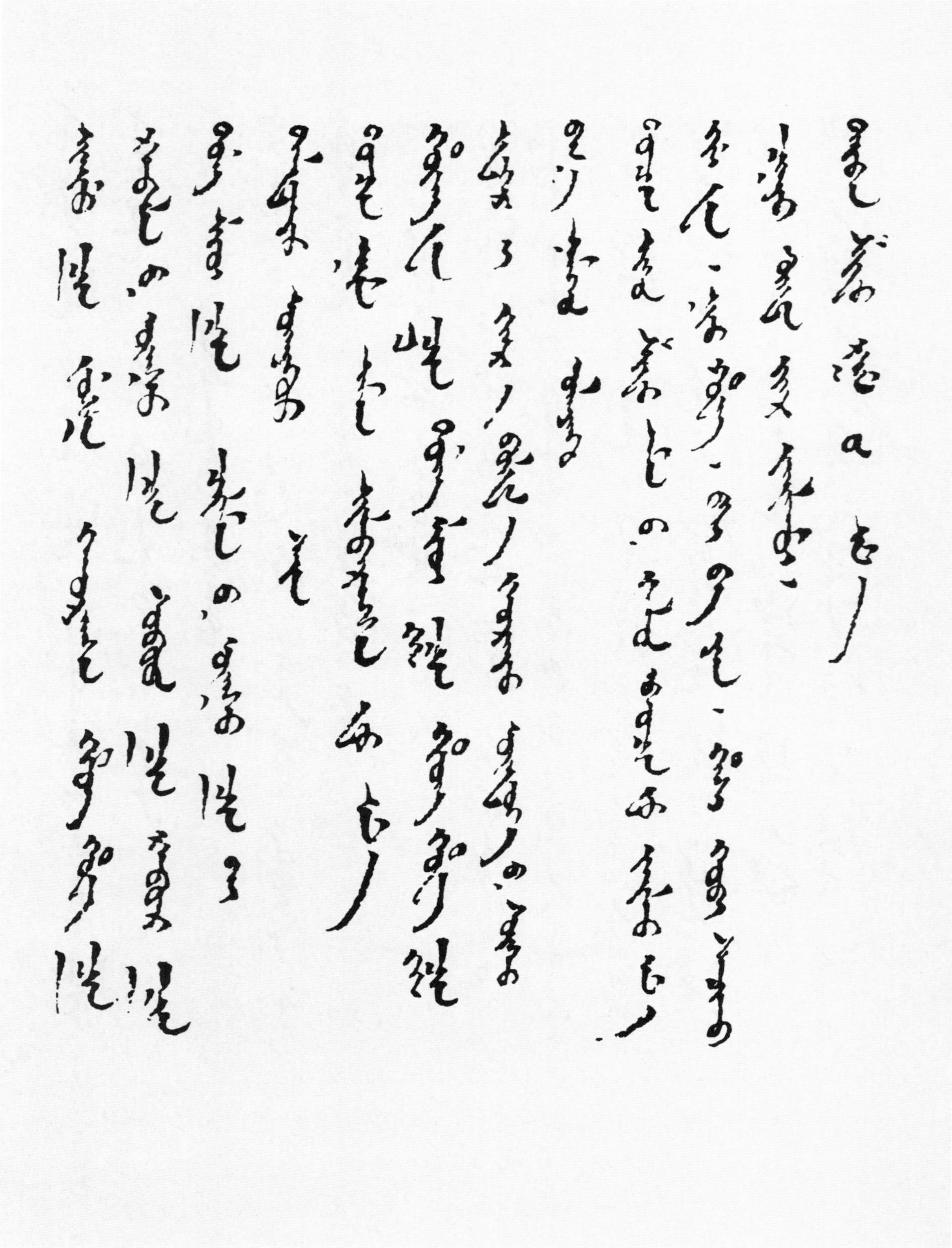

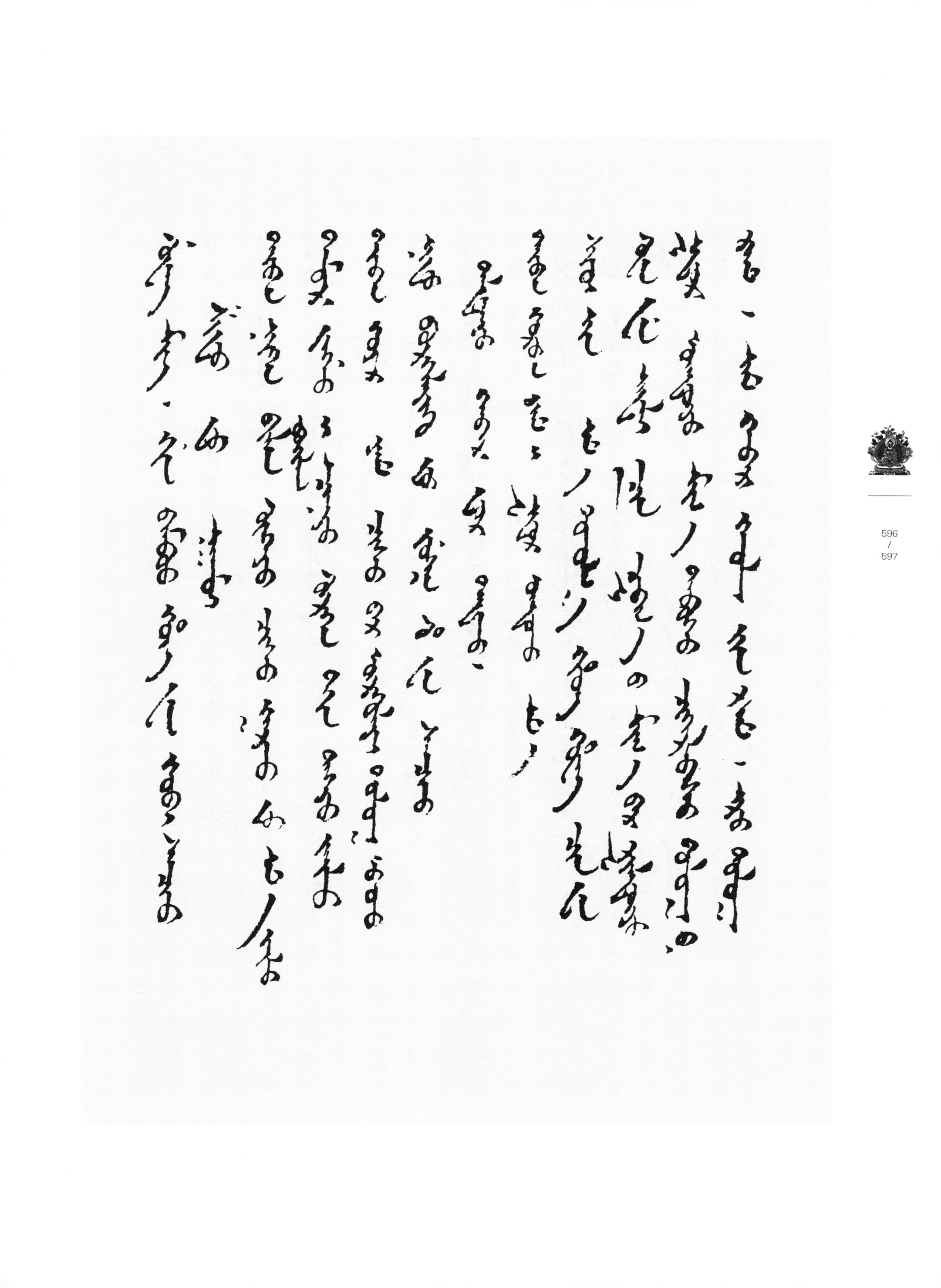

[illegible]

[illegible]

[illegible]

[illegible]

[illegible]

[illegible]

[illegible]

[illegible]

[illegible]

[illegible]

[illegible]

[illegible]

[illegible]

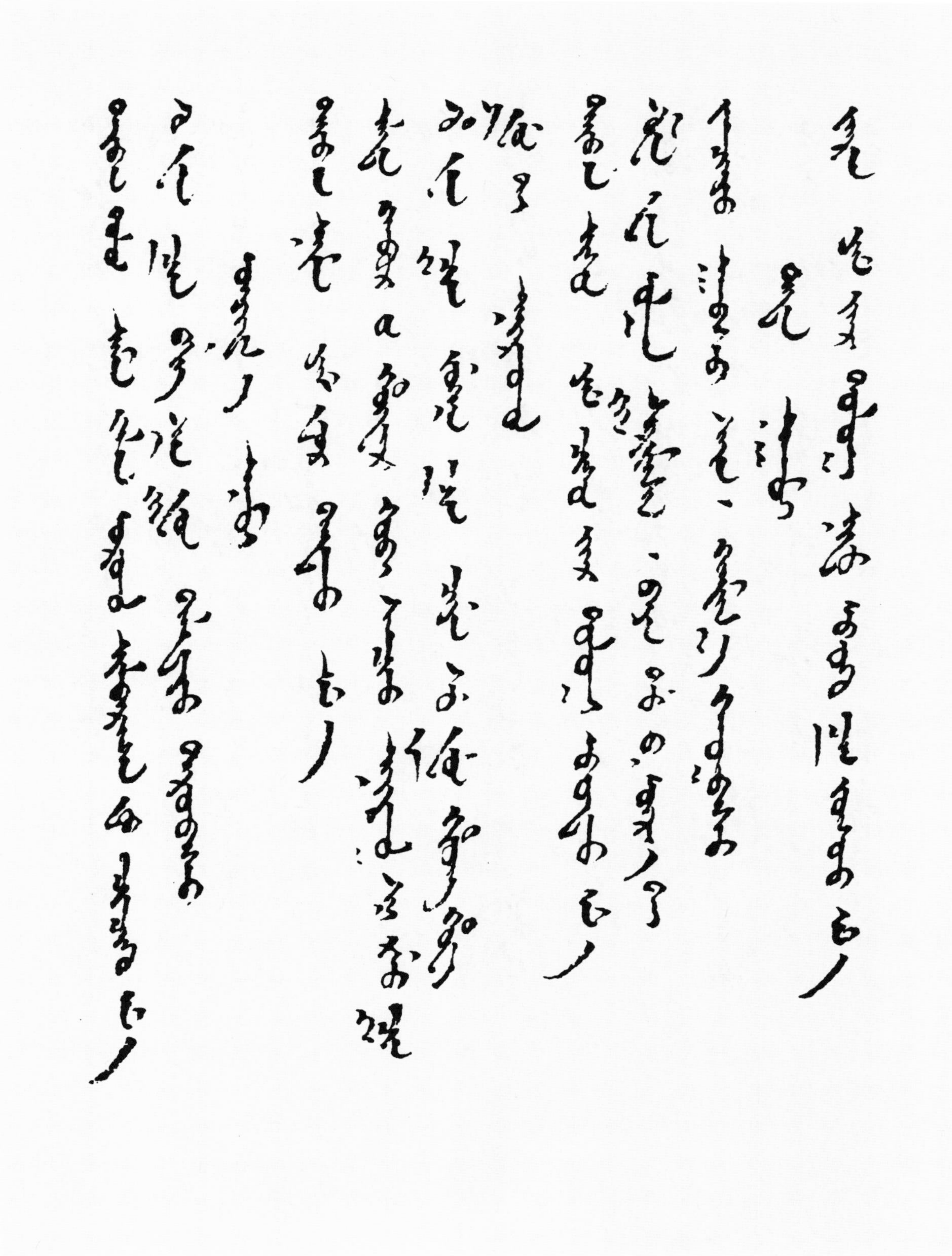

[illegible]
[illegible]
[illegible]
[illegible]
[illegible]
[illegible]
[illegible]
[illegible]
[illegible]
[illegible]
[illegible]
[illegible]
[illegible]

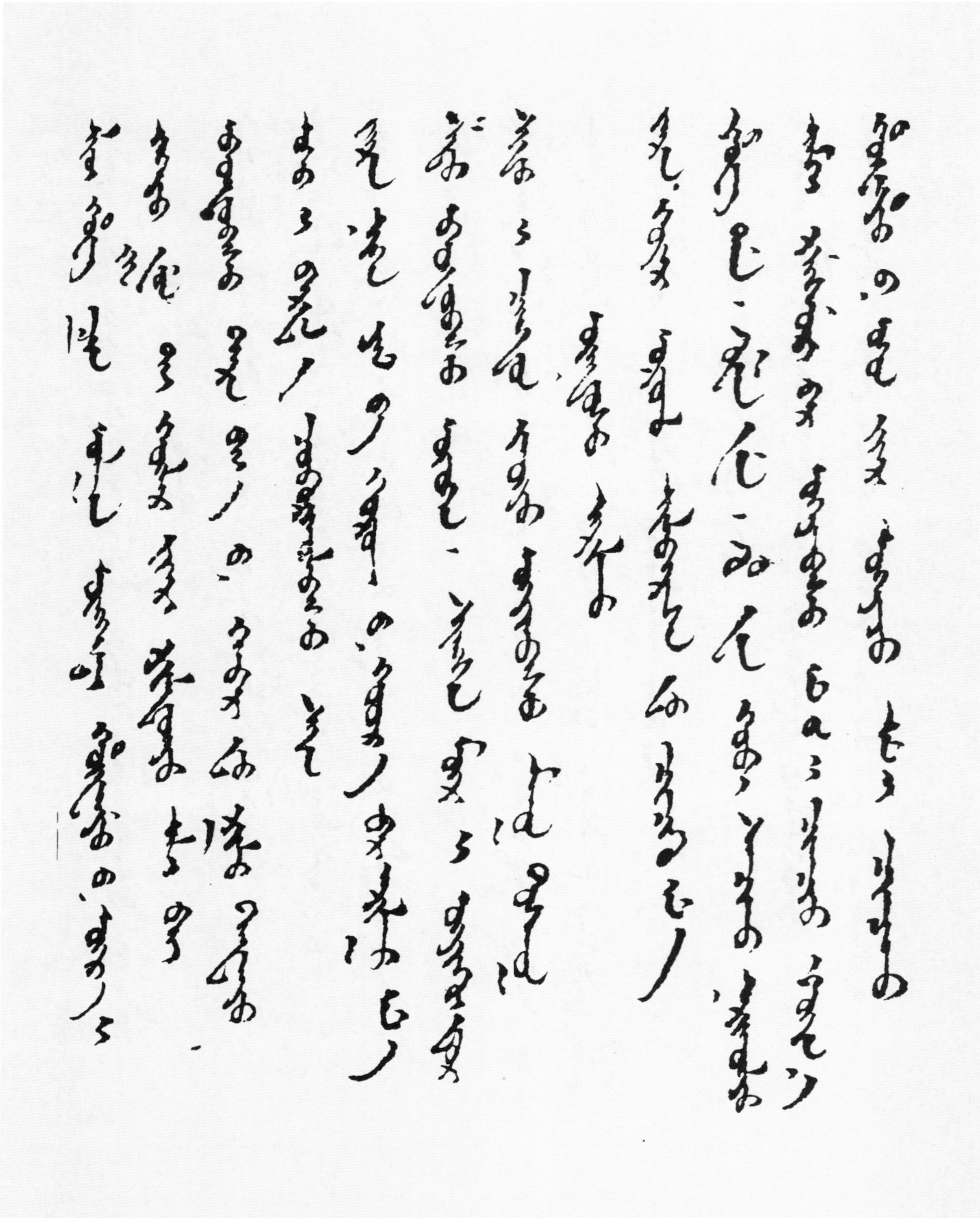

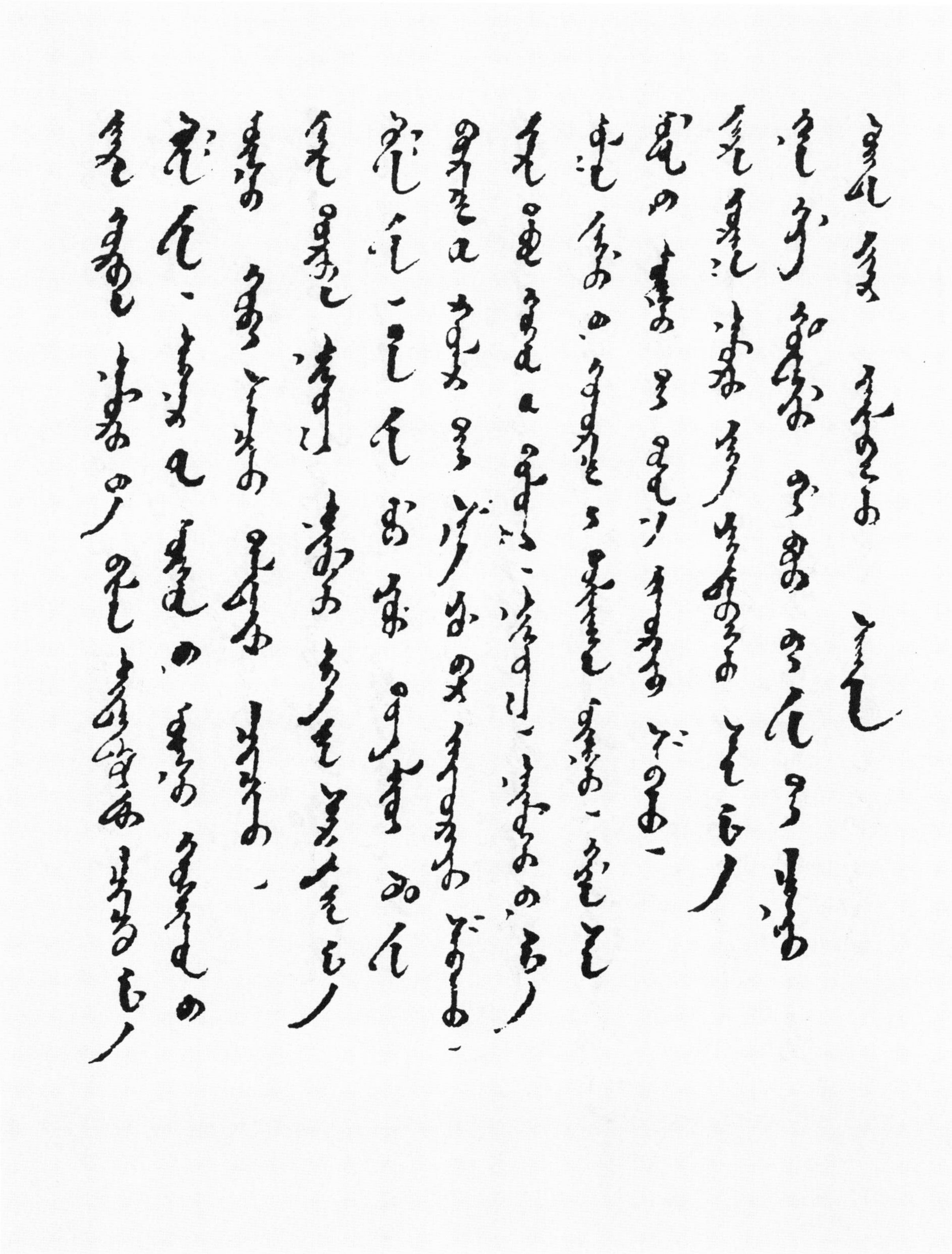

[illegible]

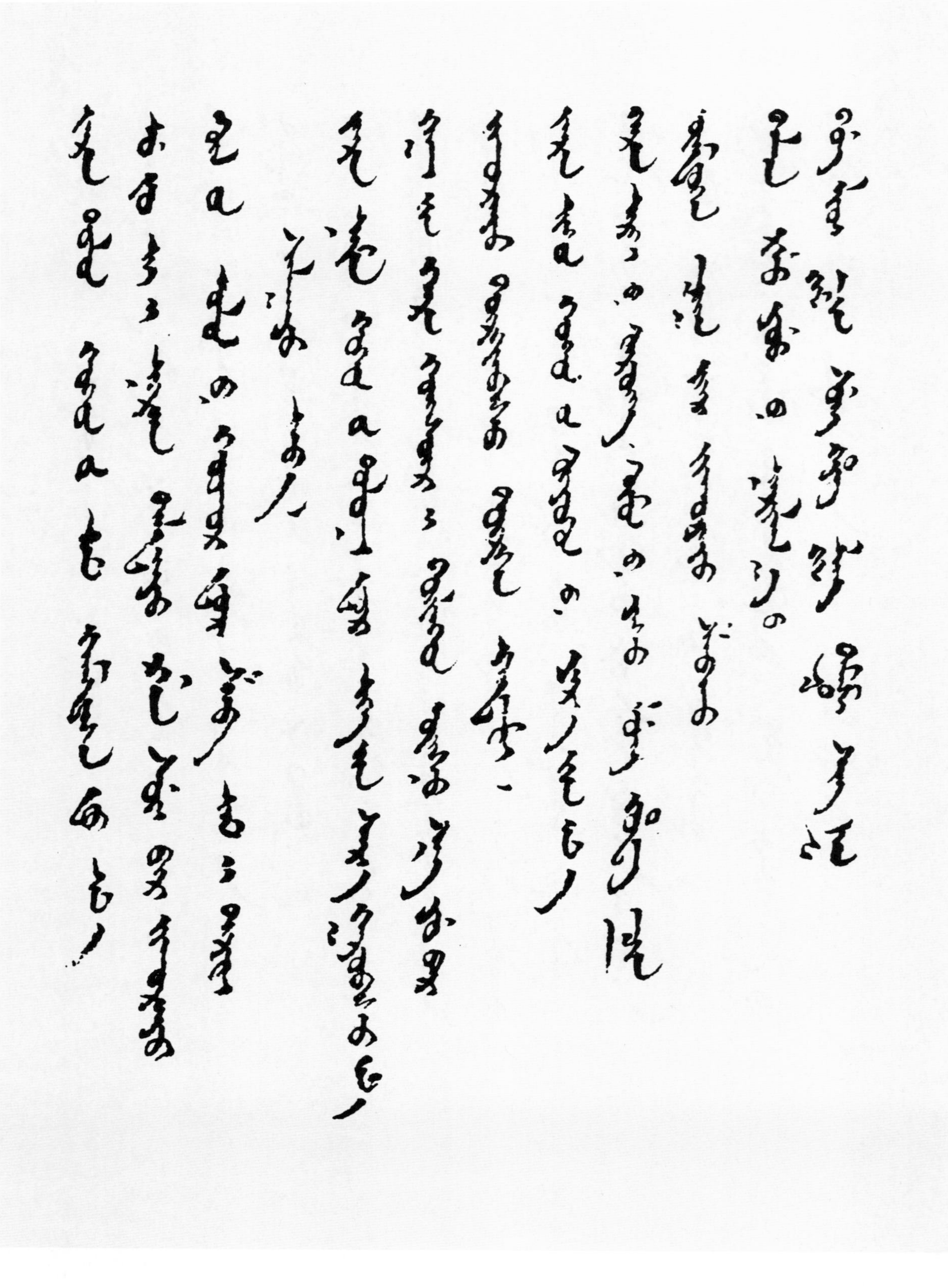

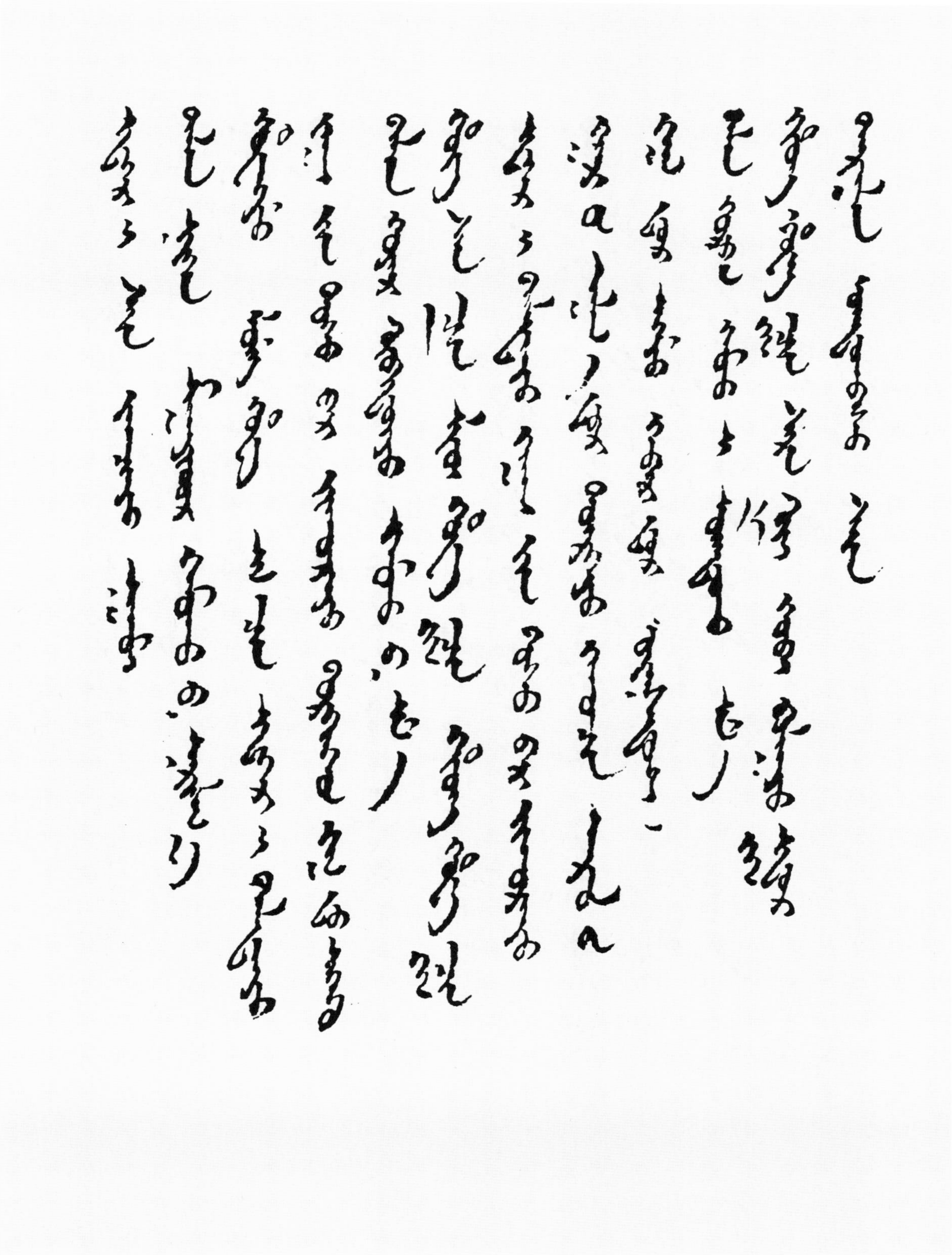

[illegible]
[illegible]
[illegible]
[illegible]
[illegible]
[illegible]
[illegible]
[illegible]
[illegible]
[illegible]
[illegible]
[illegible]

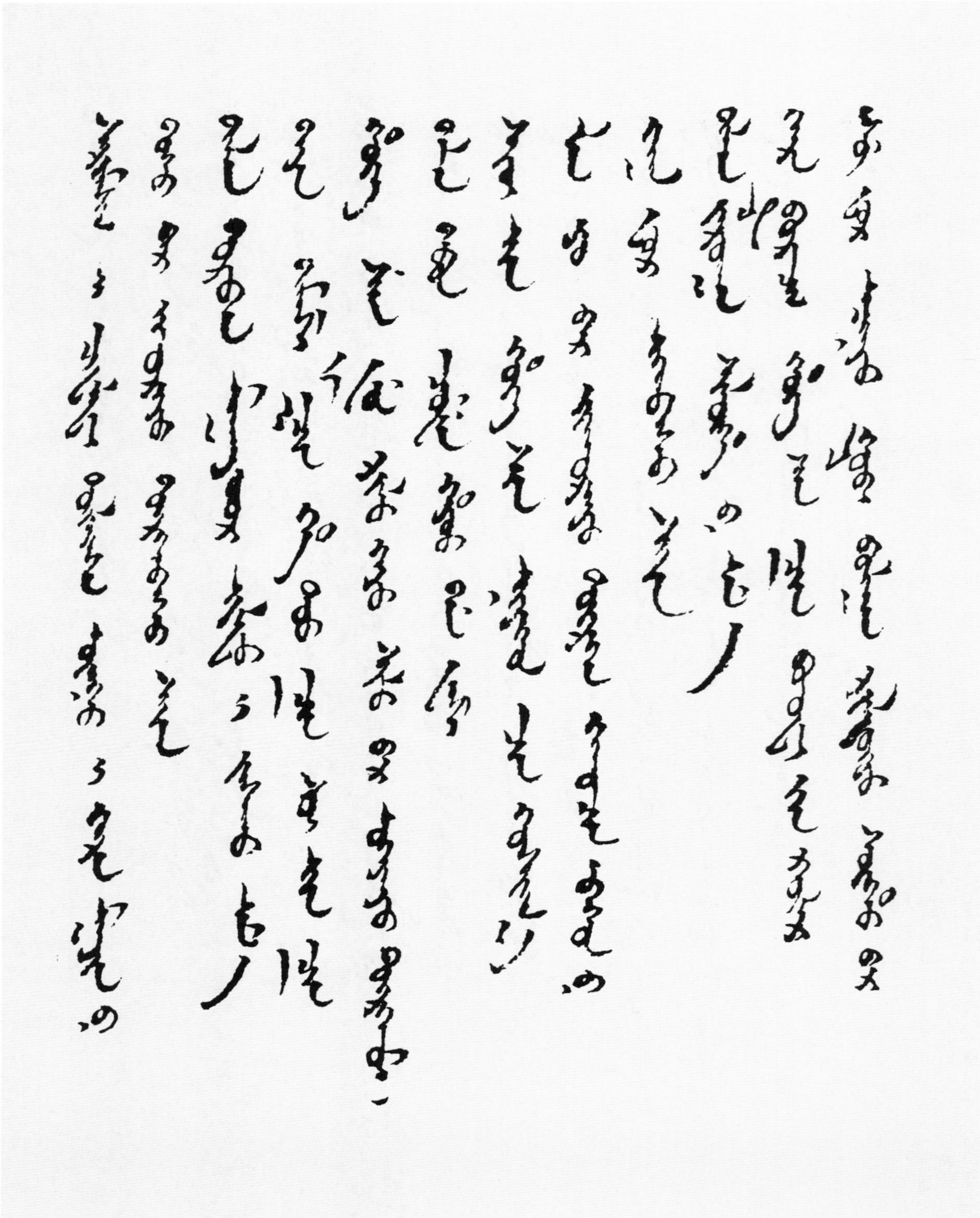

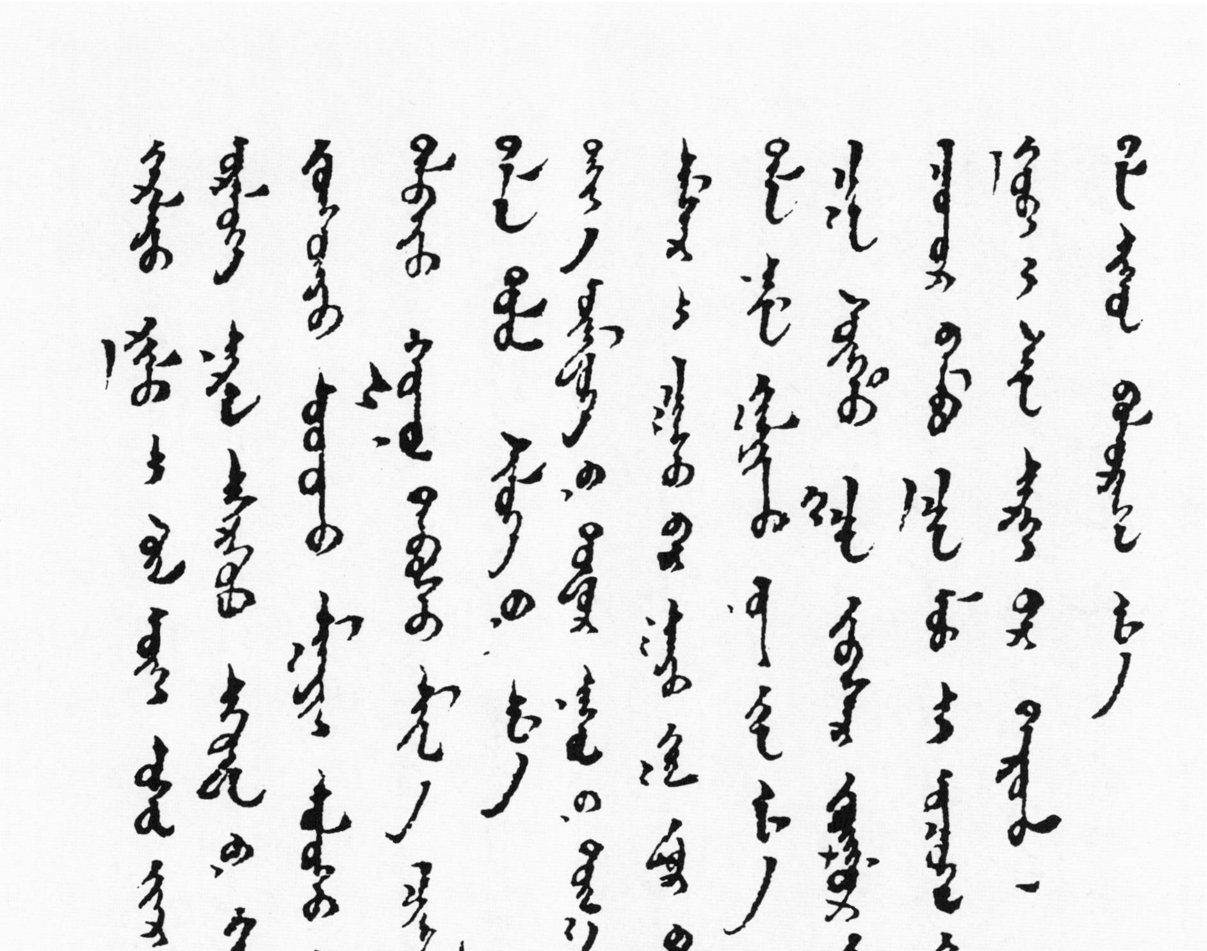

[illegible]
[illegible]
[illegible]
[illegible]
[illegible]
[illegible]
[illegible]
[illegible]
[illegible]
[illegible]
[illegible]
[illegible]
[illegible]
[illegible]

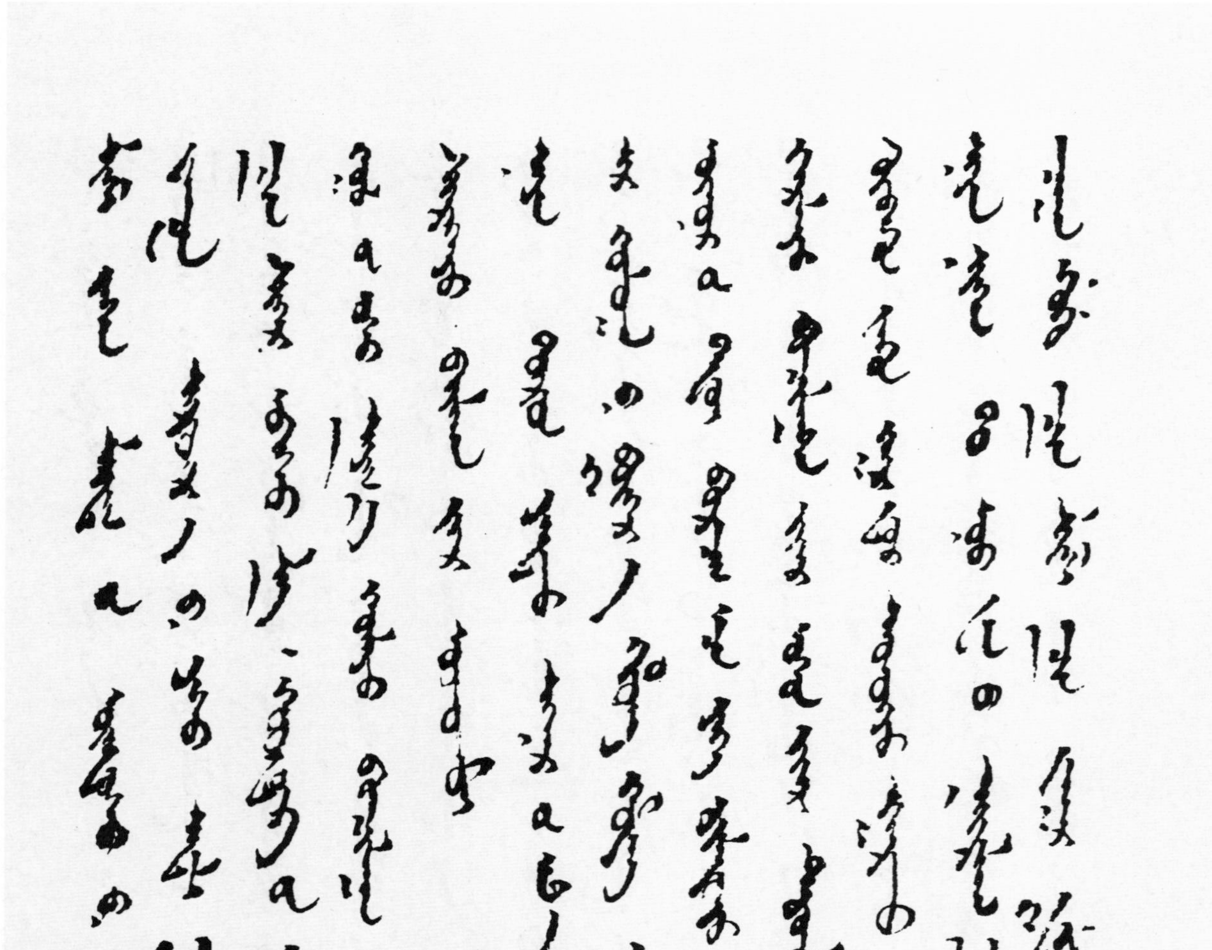

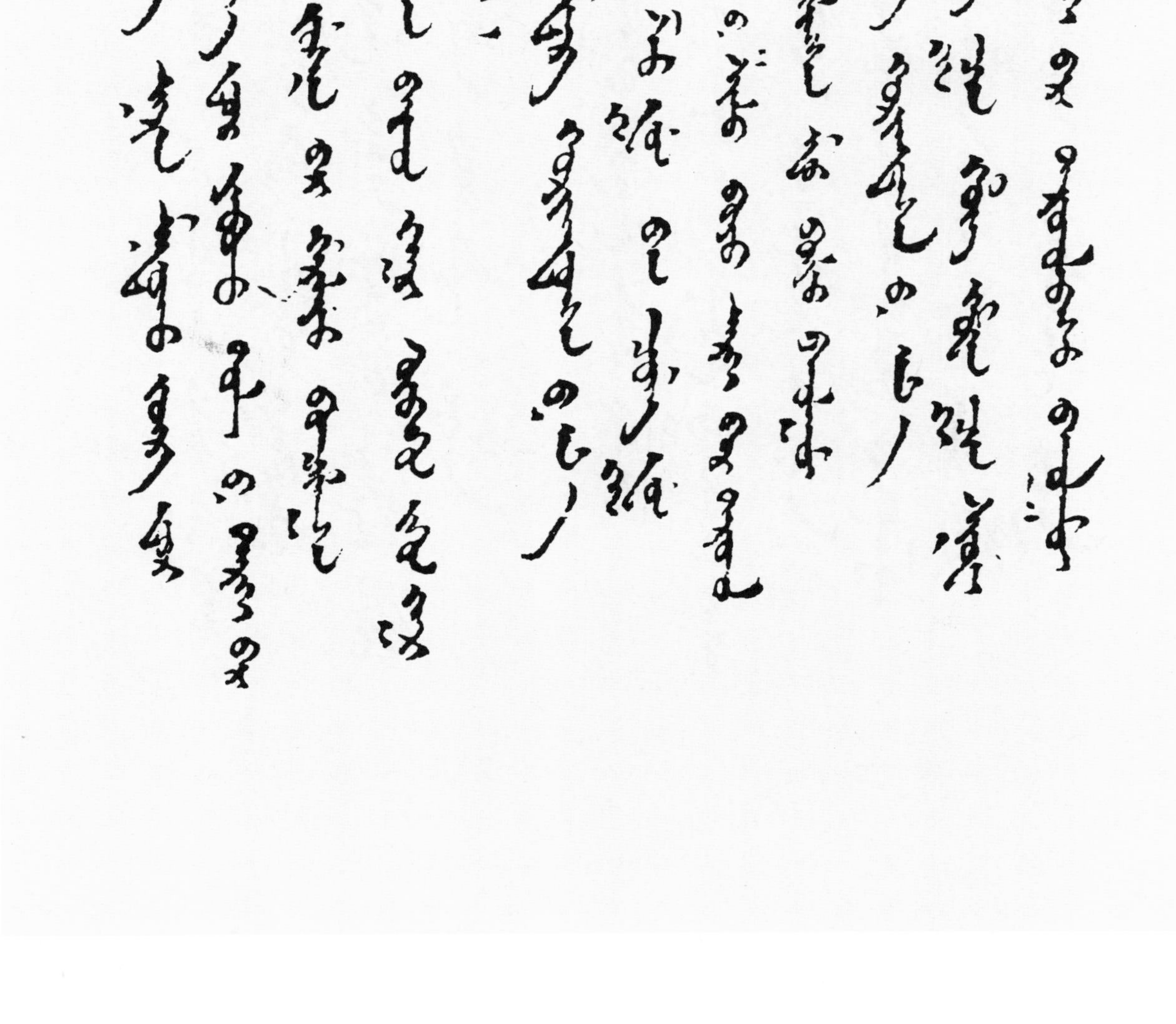

[illegible]
[illegible]
[illegible]
[illegible]
[illegible]
[illegible]
[illegible]
[illegible]
[illegible]
[illegible]
[illegible]
[illegible]

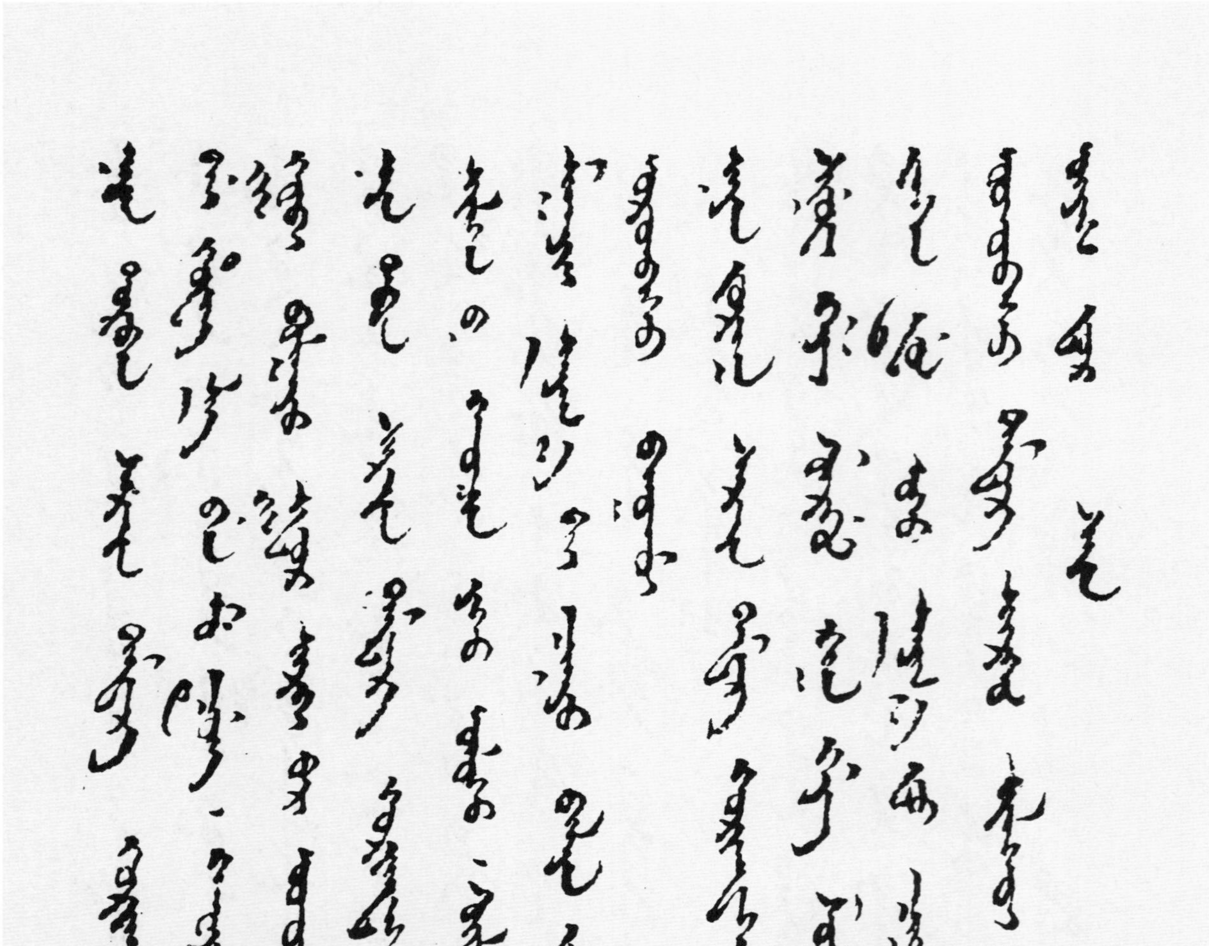

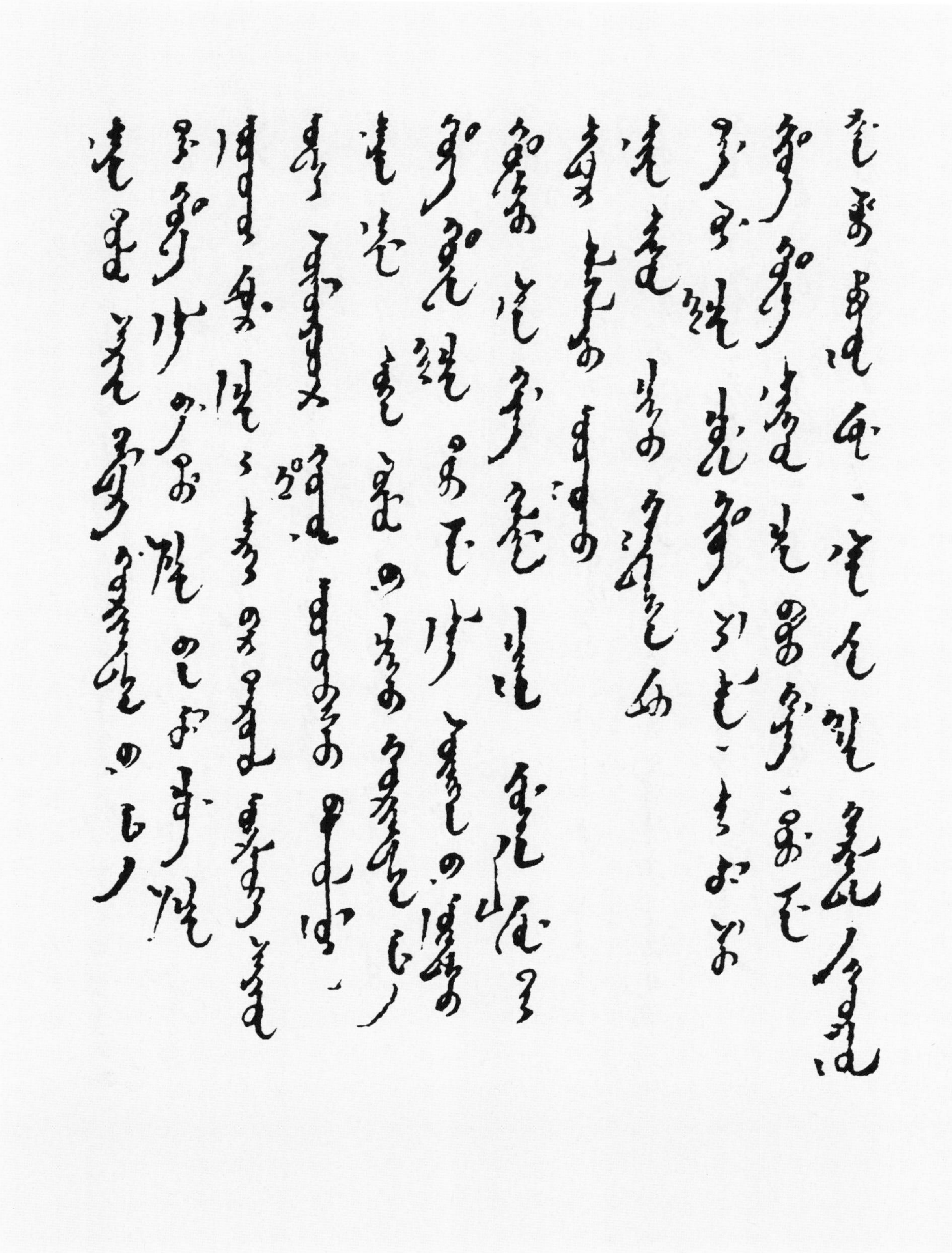

[illegible]

[illegible]

[illegible]

[illegible]

[illegible]

[illegible]

[illegible]

[illegible]

[illegible]

[illegible]

[illegible]

[illegible]

[illegible]

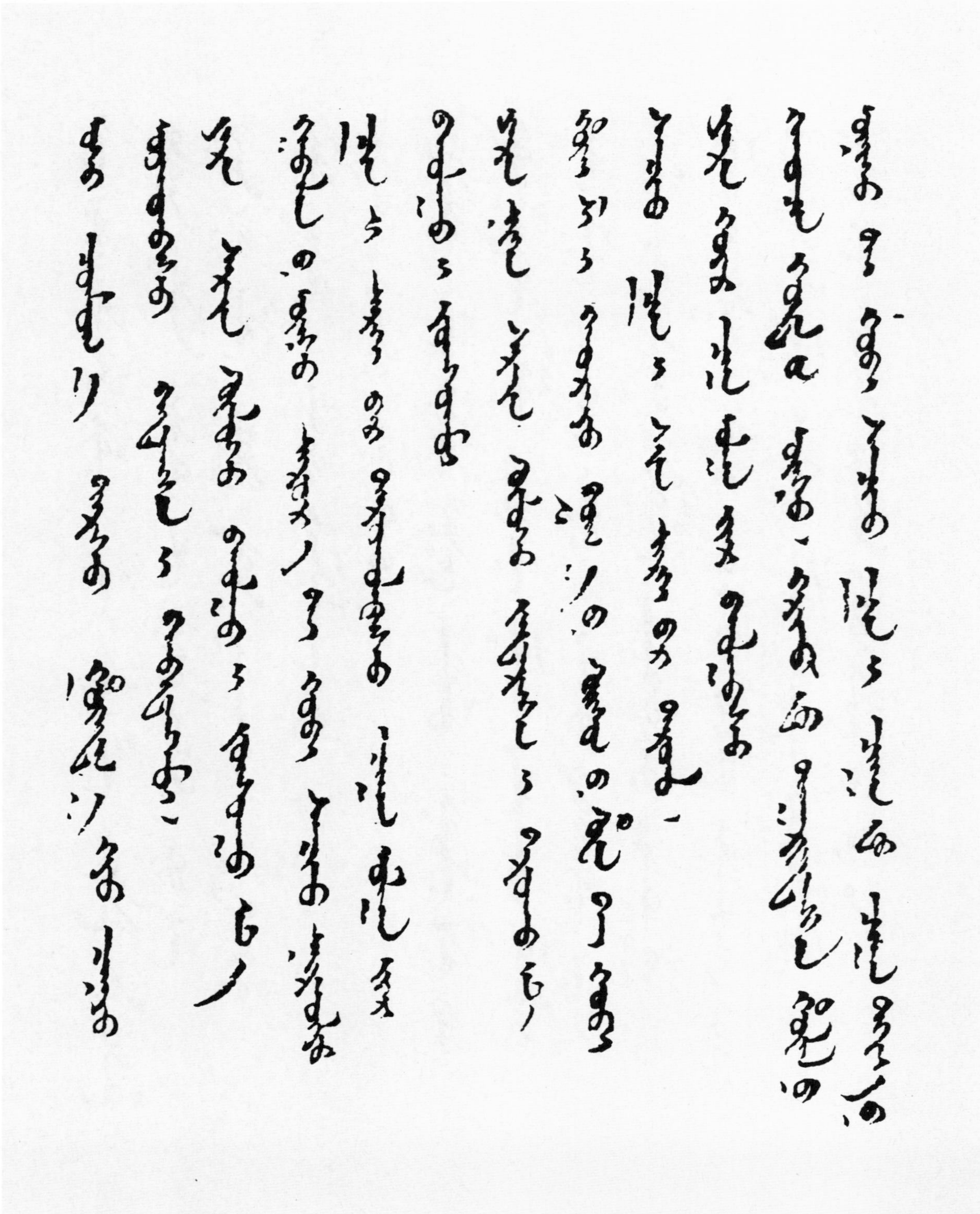

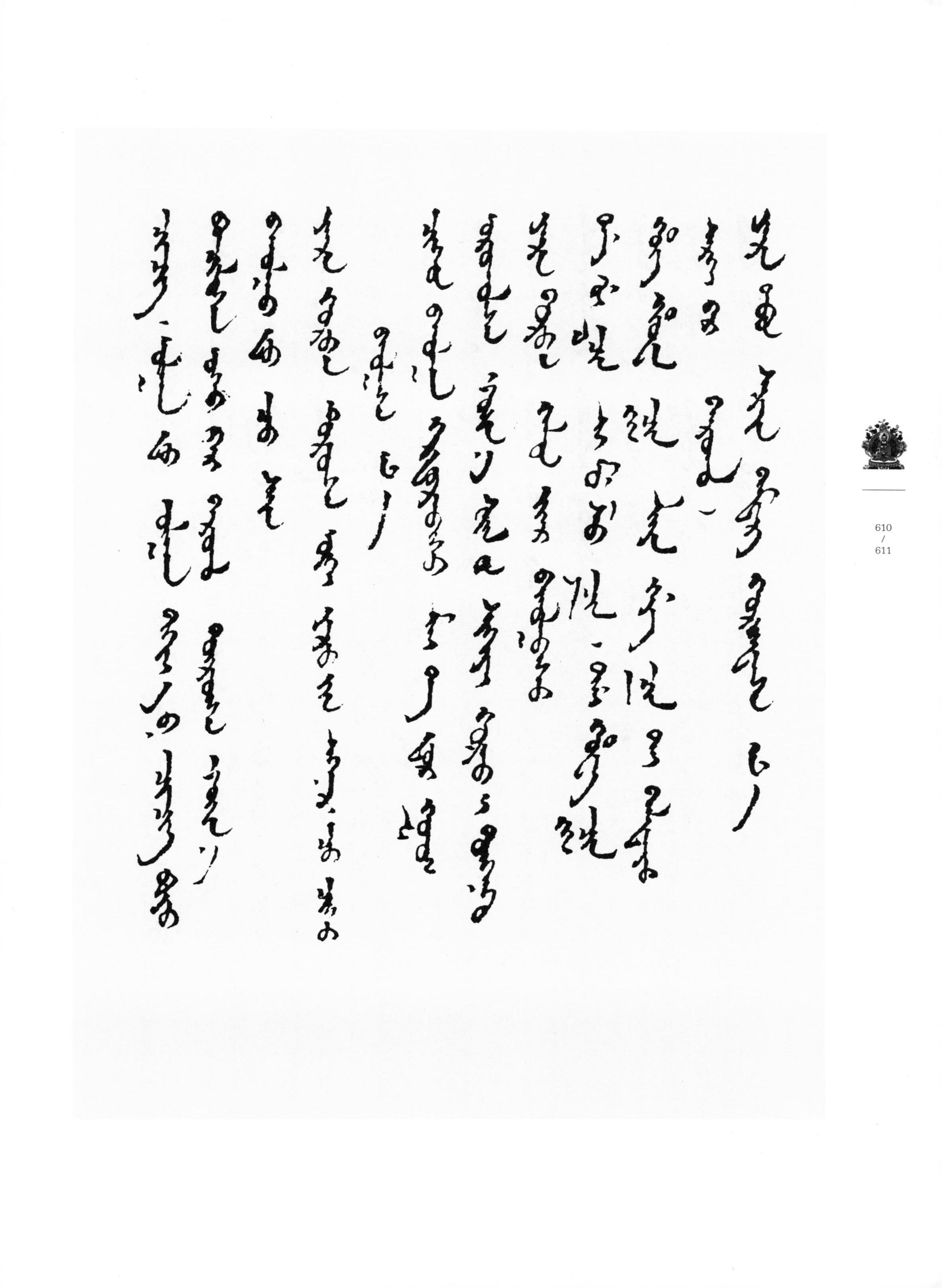

[illegible]
[illegible]
[illegible]
[illegible]
[illegible]
[illegible]
[illegible]
[illegible]
[illegible]
[illegible]
[illegible]
[illegible]

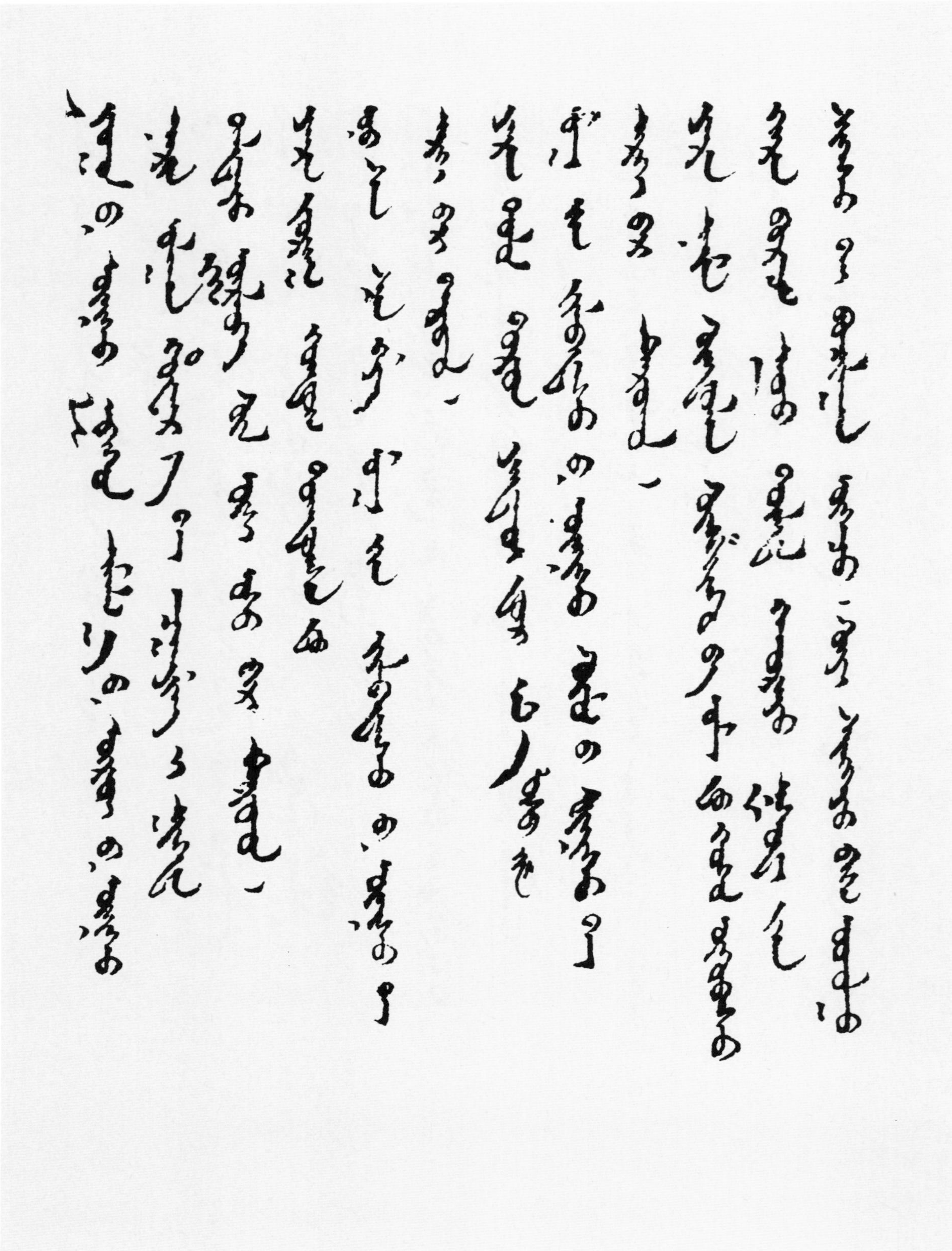

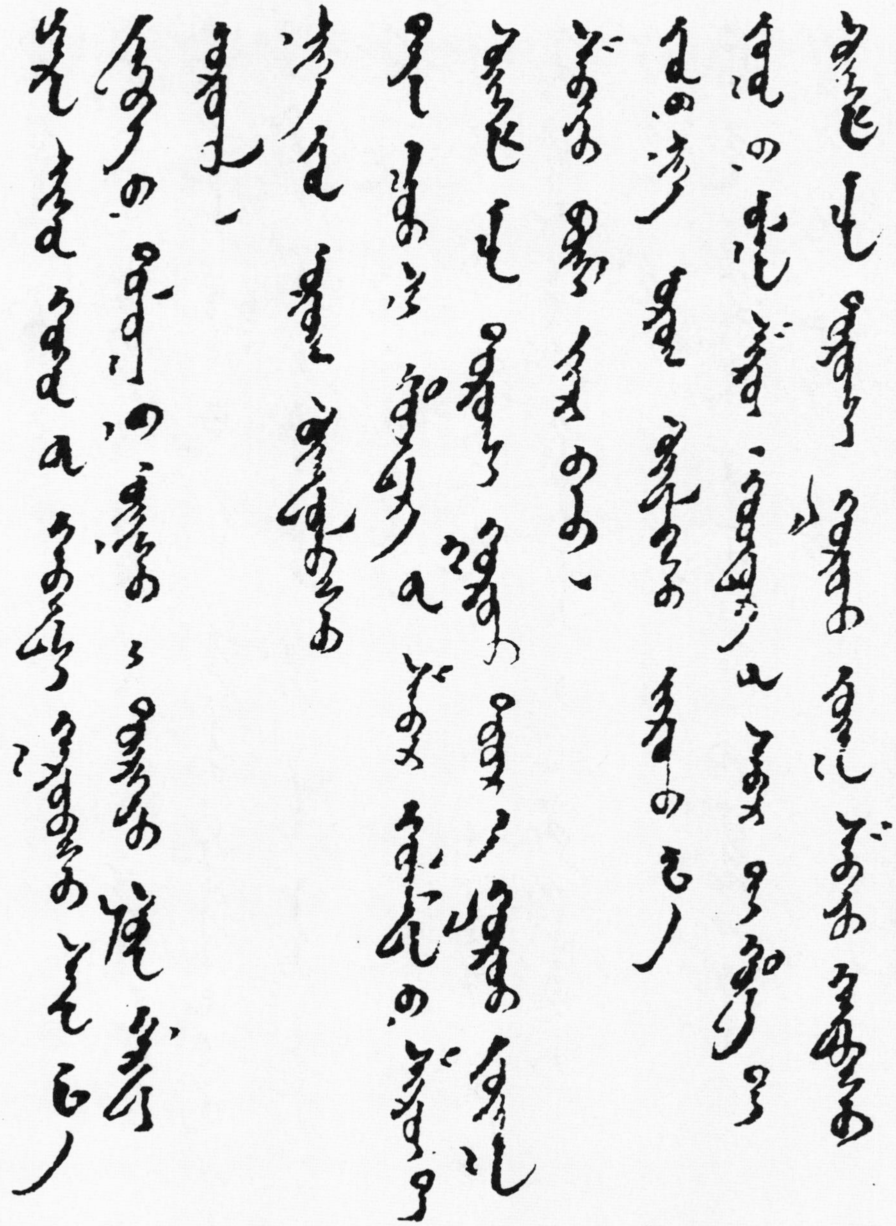

[illegible]
[illegible]
[illegible]
[illegible]
[illegible]
[illegible]
[illegible]
[illegible]
[illegible]
[illegible]
[illegible]
[illegible]

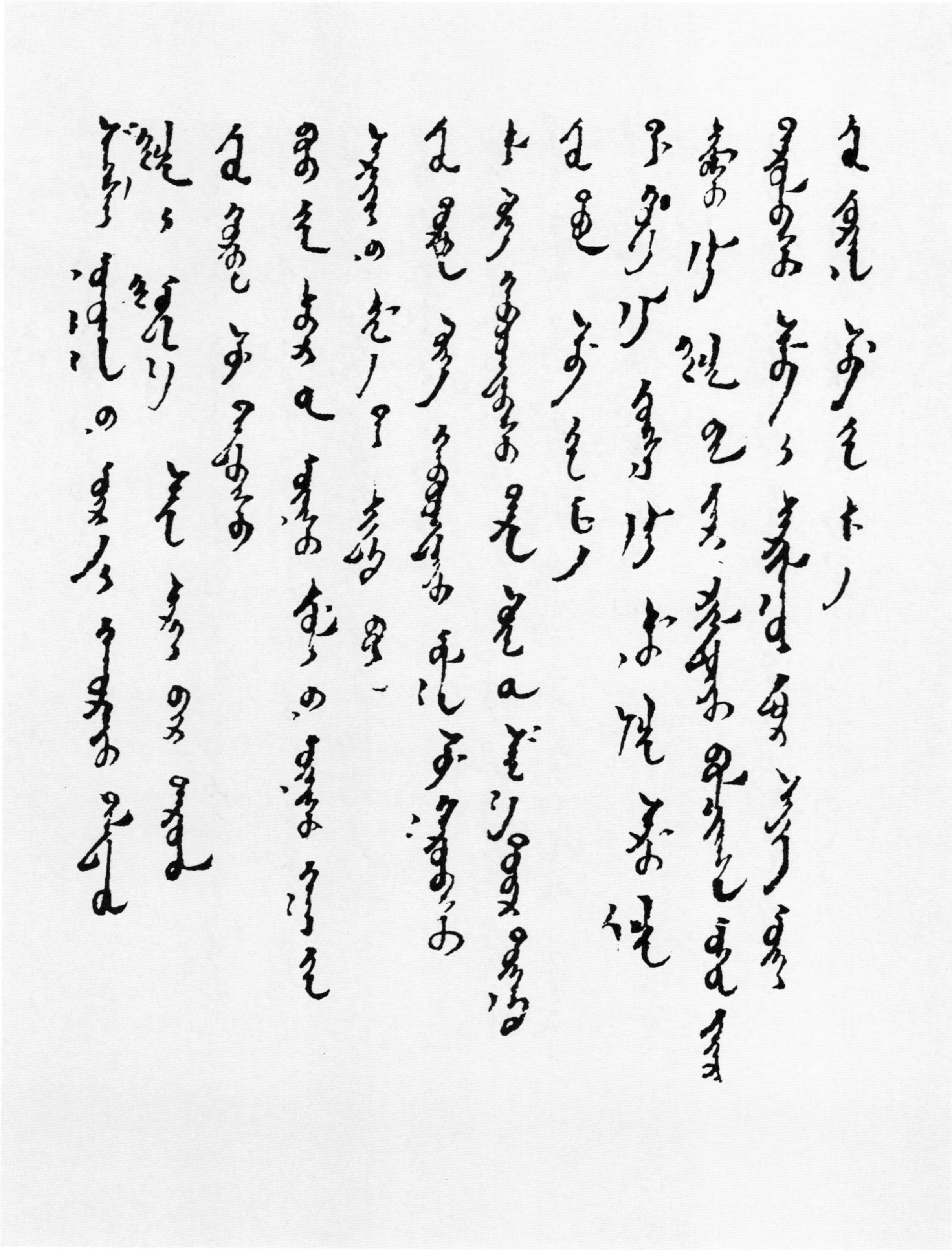

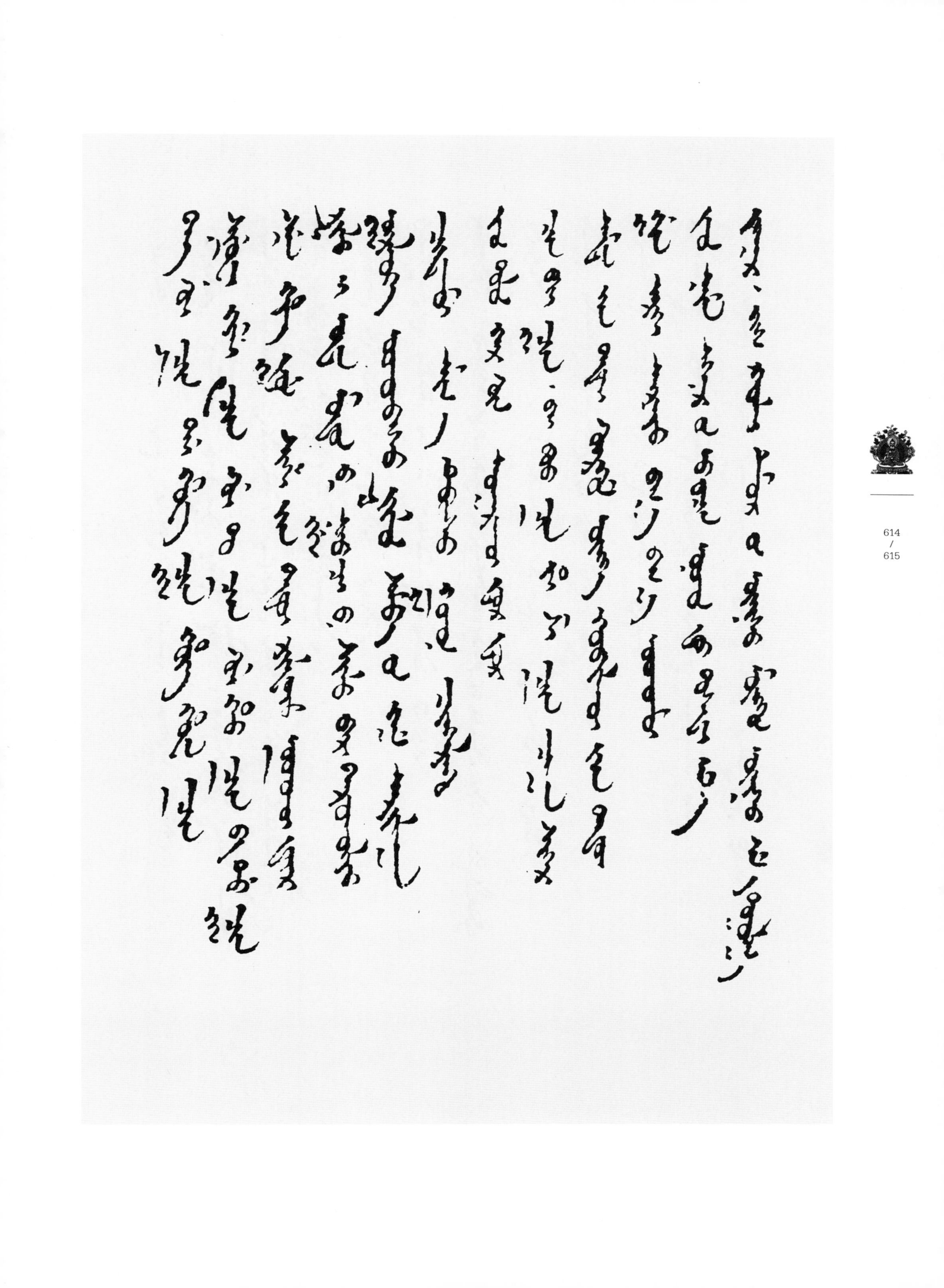

[illegible]

[illegible]

[illegible]

[illegible]

[illegible]

[illegible]

[illegible]

[illegible]

[illegible]

[illegible]

[illegible]

[illegible]

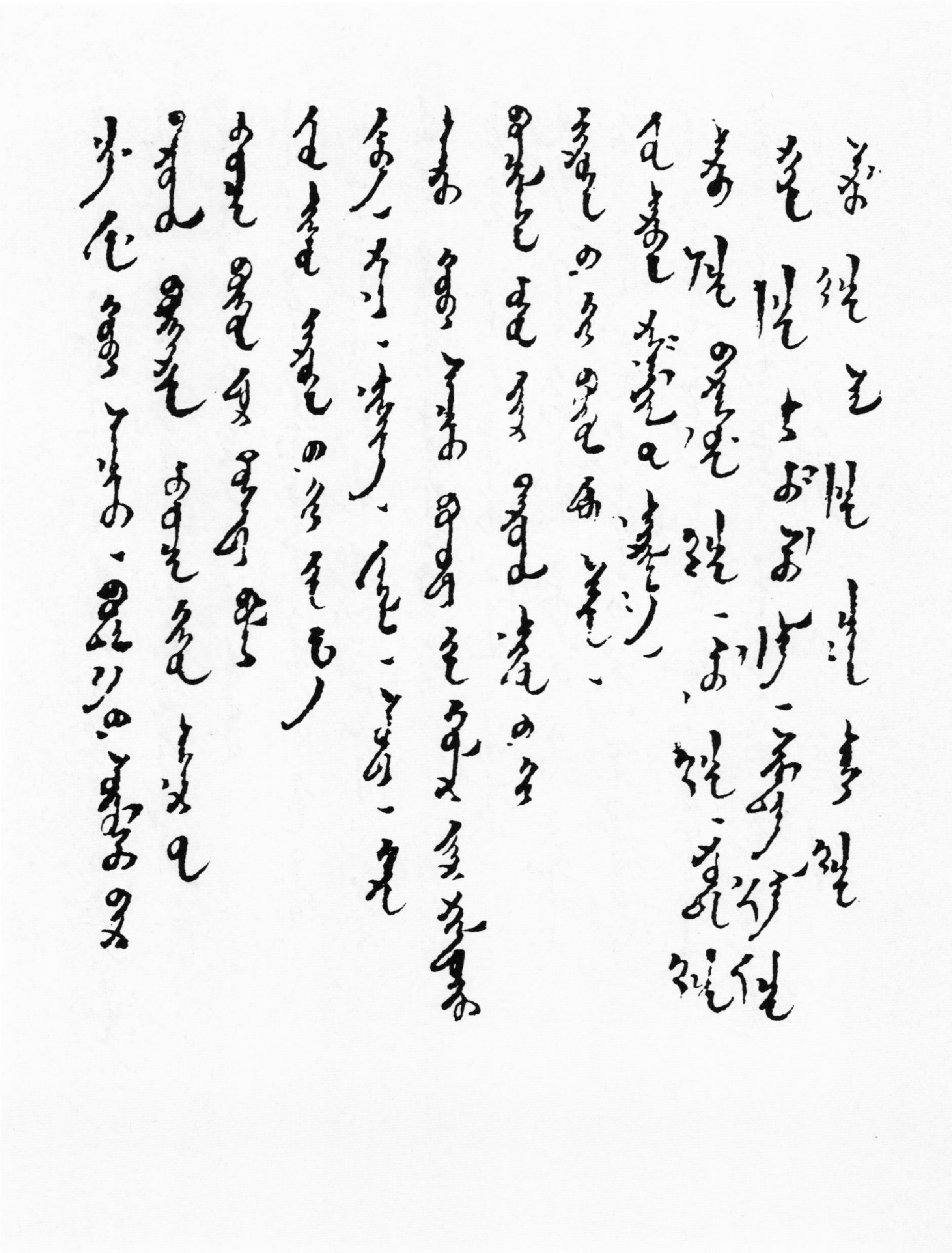

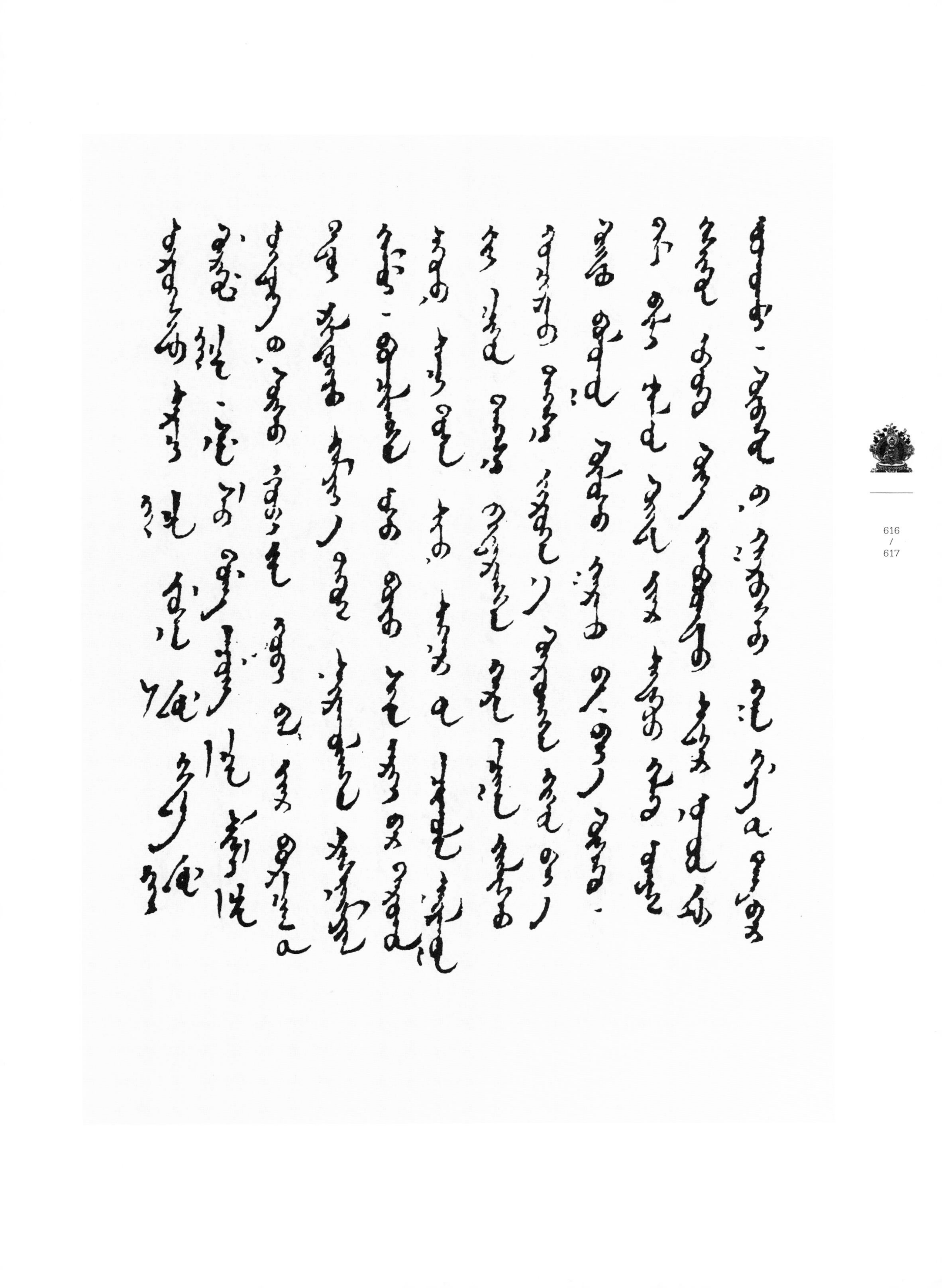

[illegible]
[illegible]
[illegible]
[illegible]
[illegible]
[illegible]
[illegible]
[illegible]
[illegible]
[illegible]
[illegible]
[illegible]
[illegible]

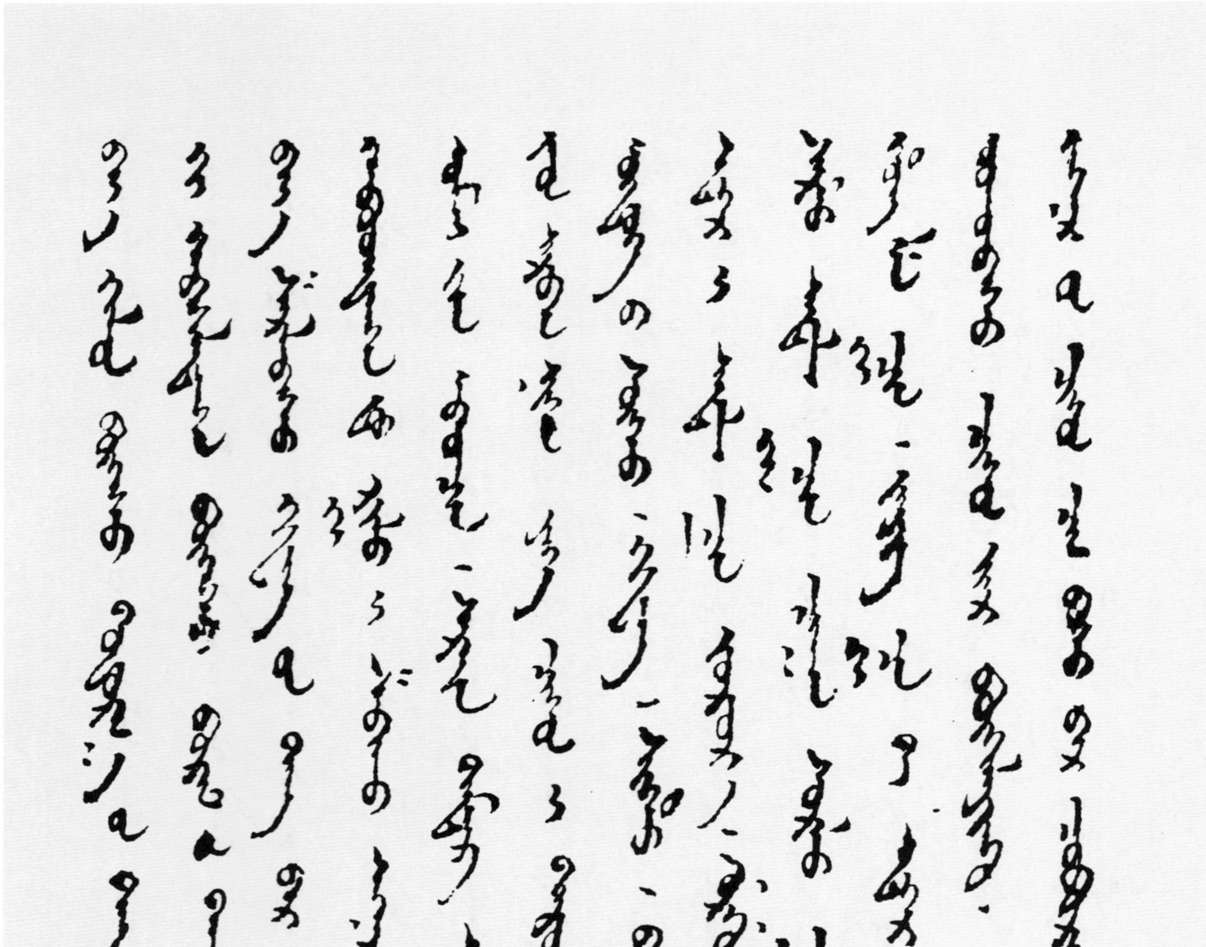

[illegible]

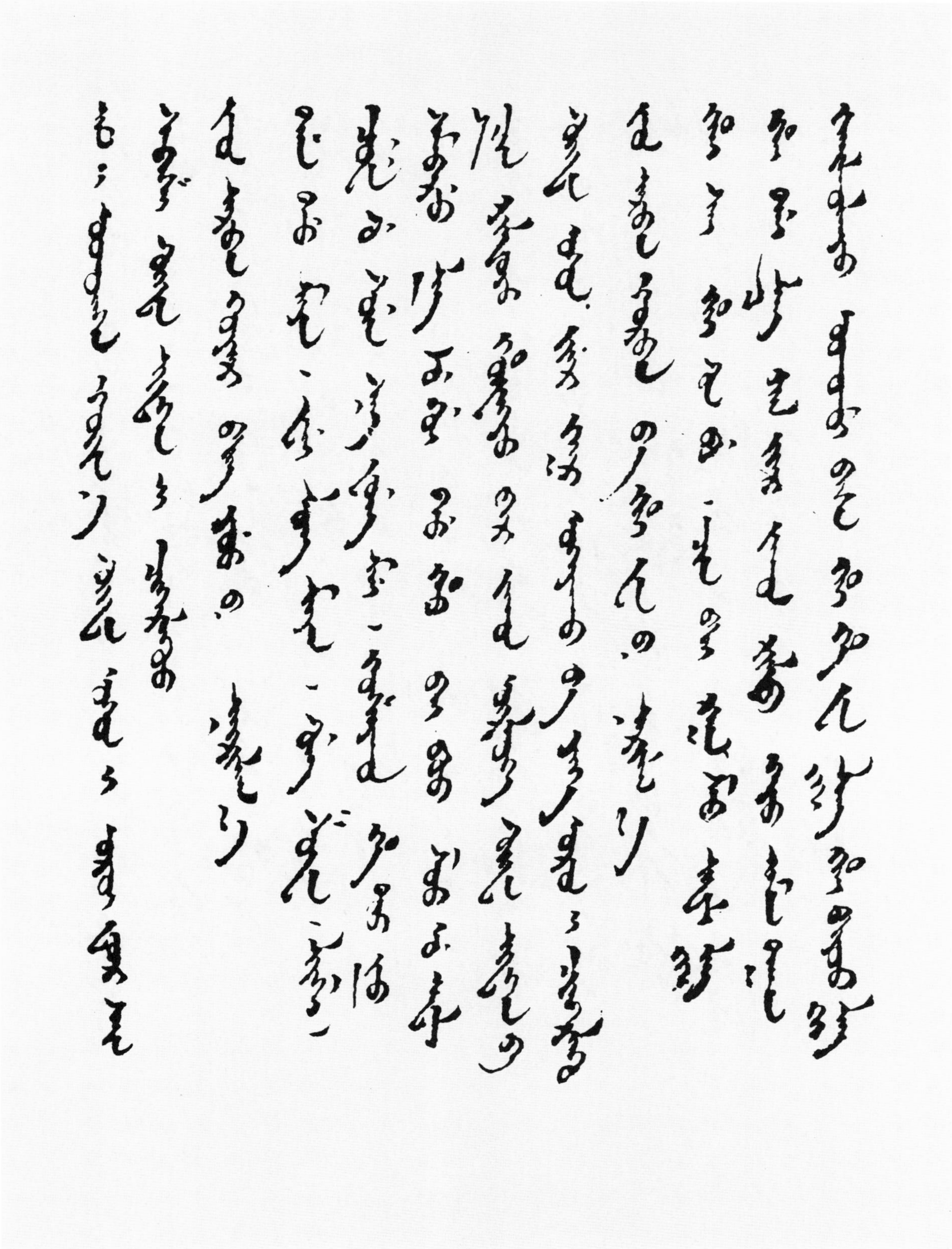

[illegible]

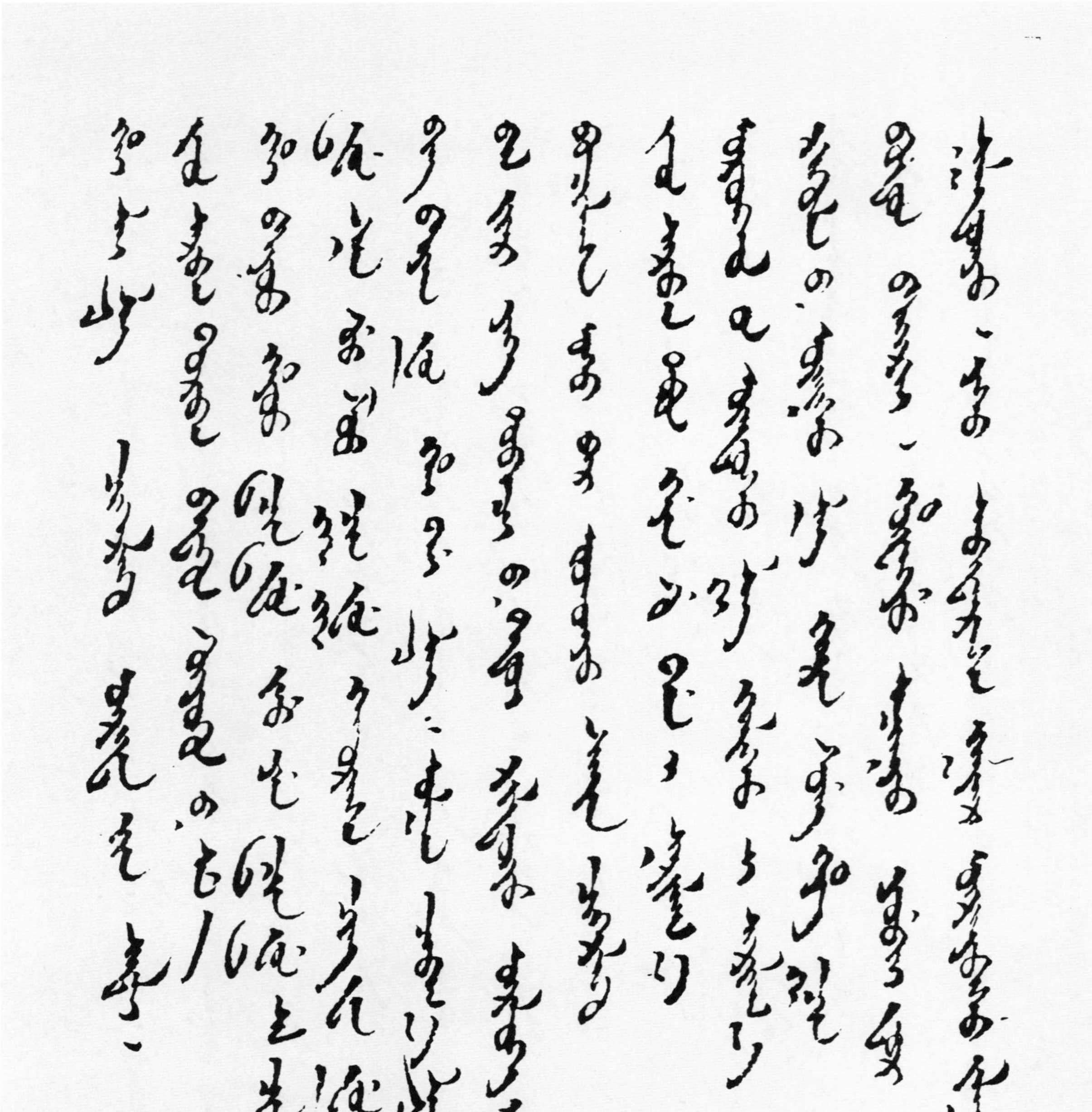

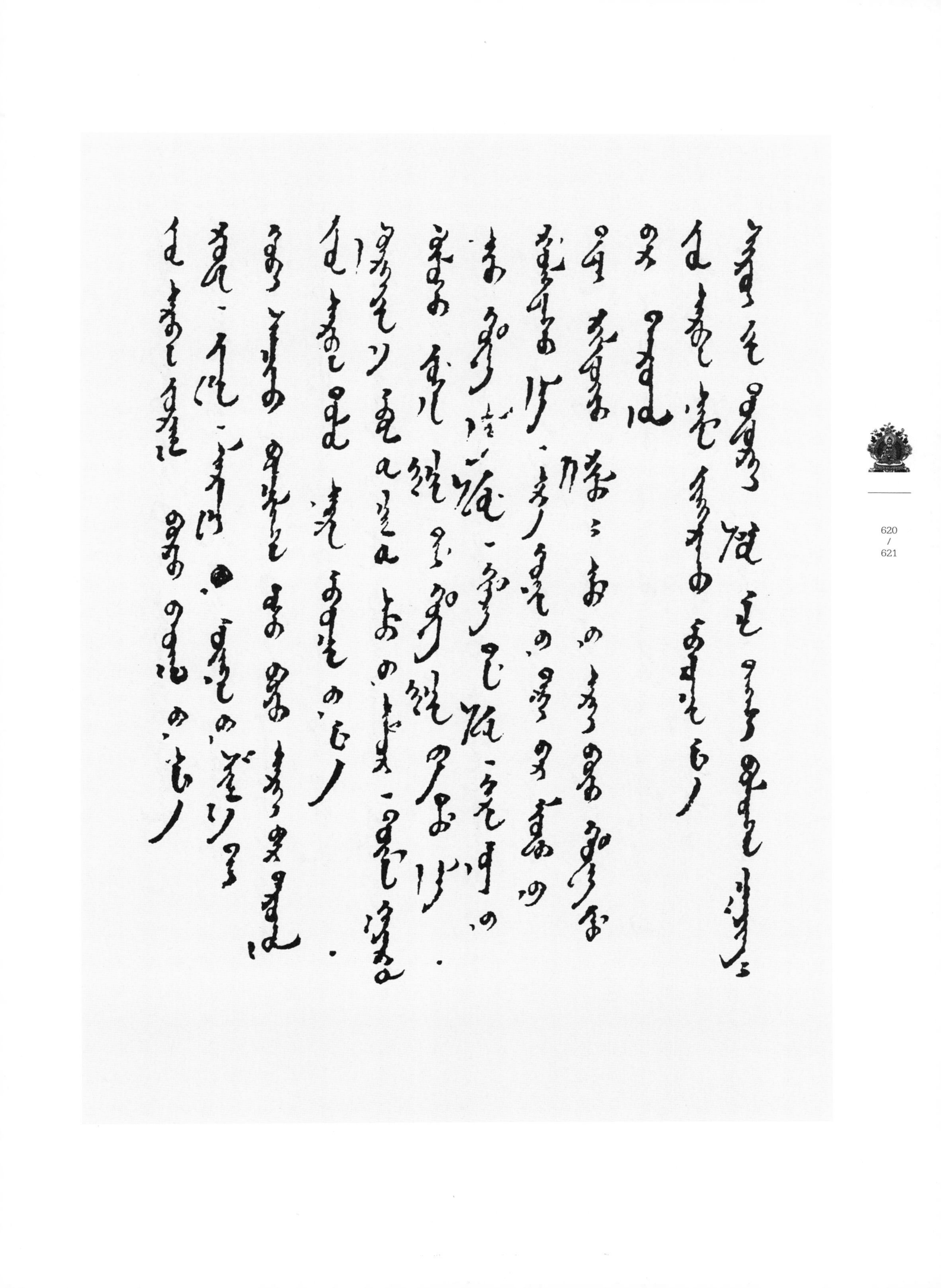

[illegible]
[illegible]
[illegible]
[illegible]
[illegible]
[illegible]
[illegible]
[illegible]
[illegible]
[illegible]
[illegible]
[illegible]

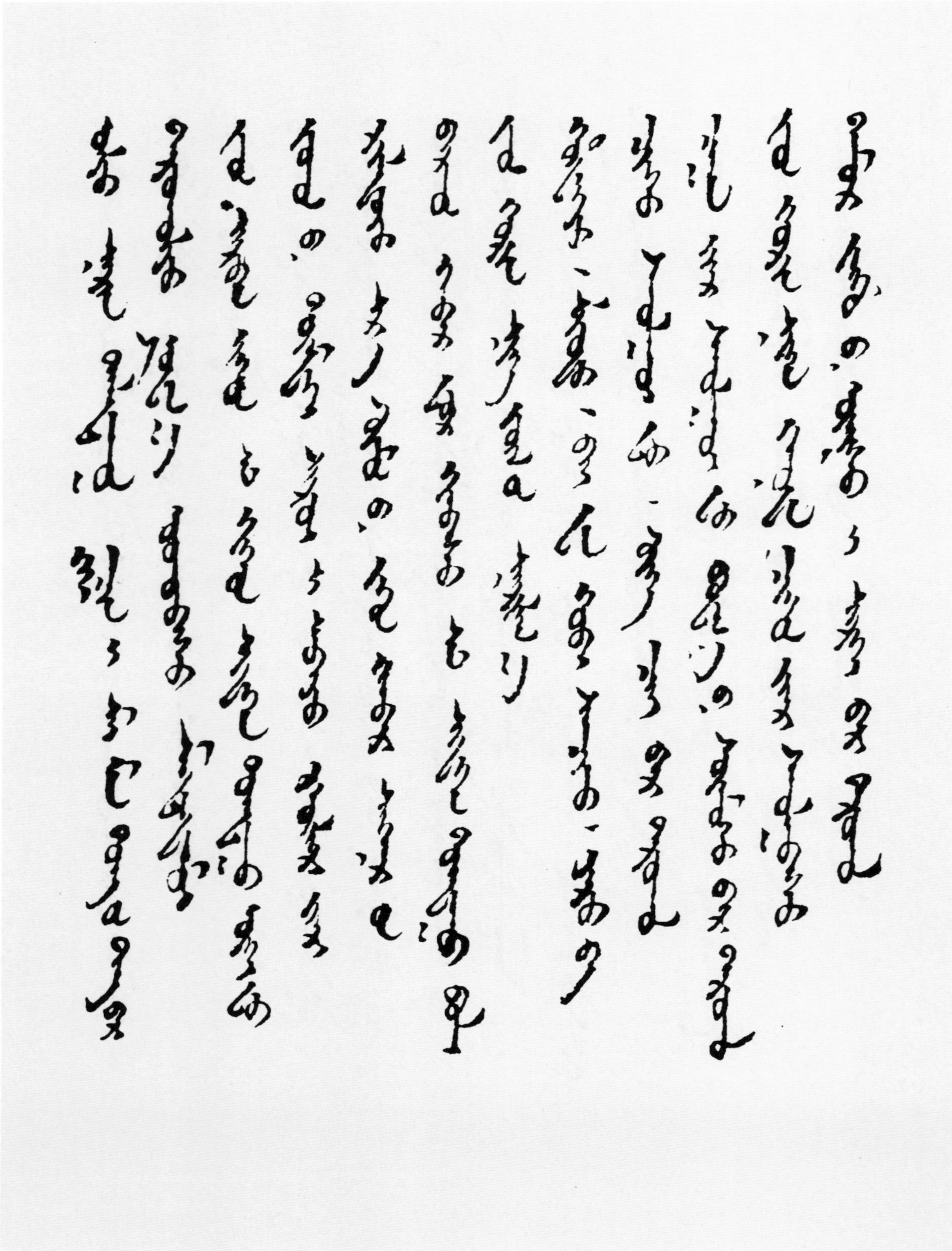

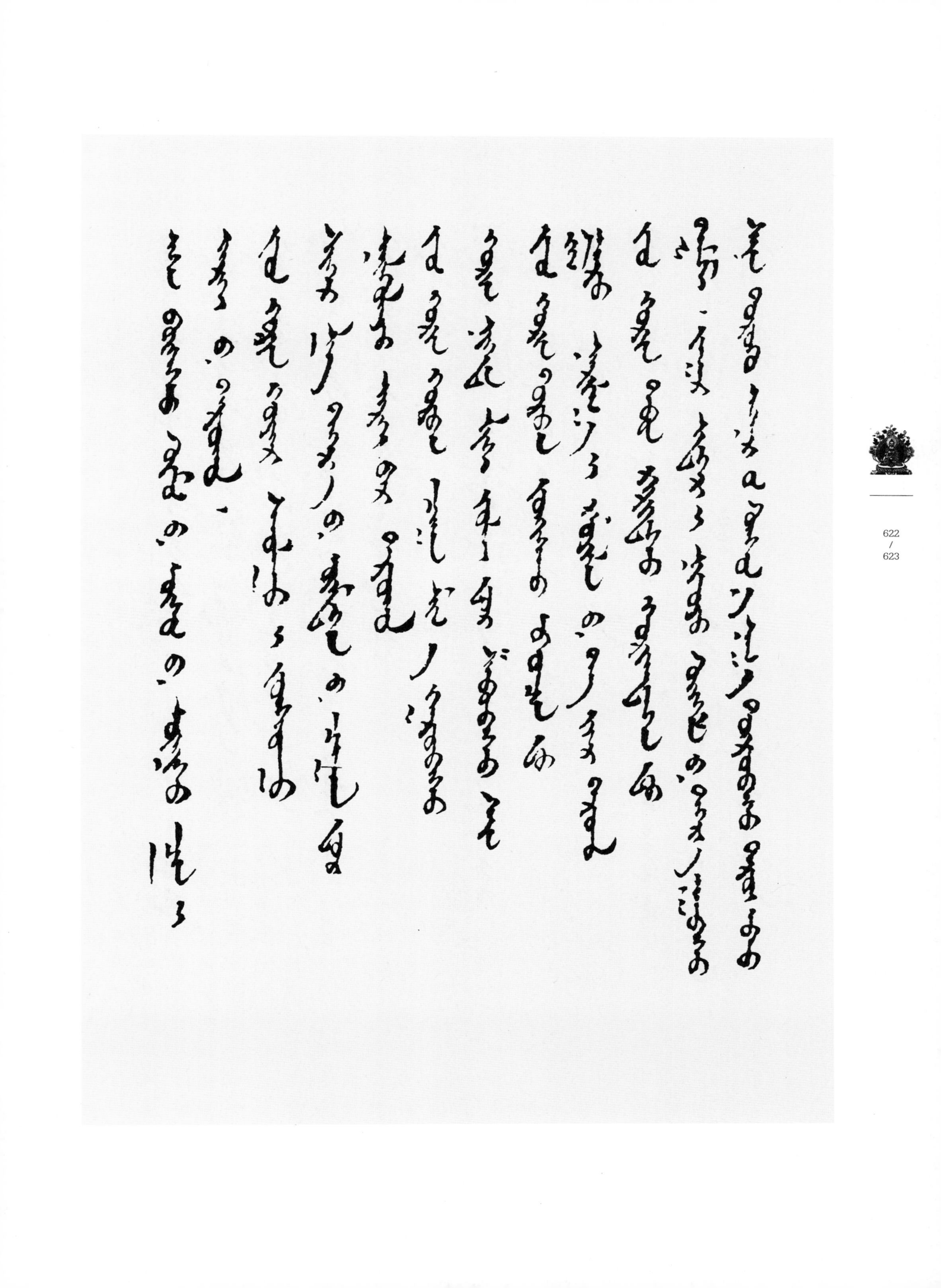

[illegible]

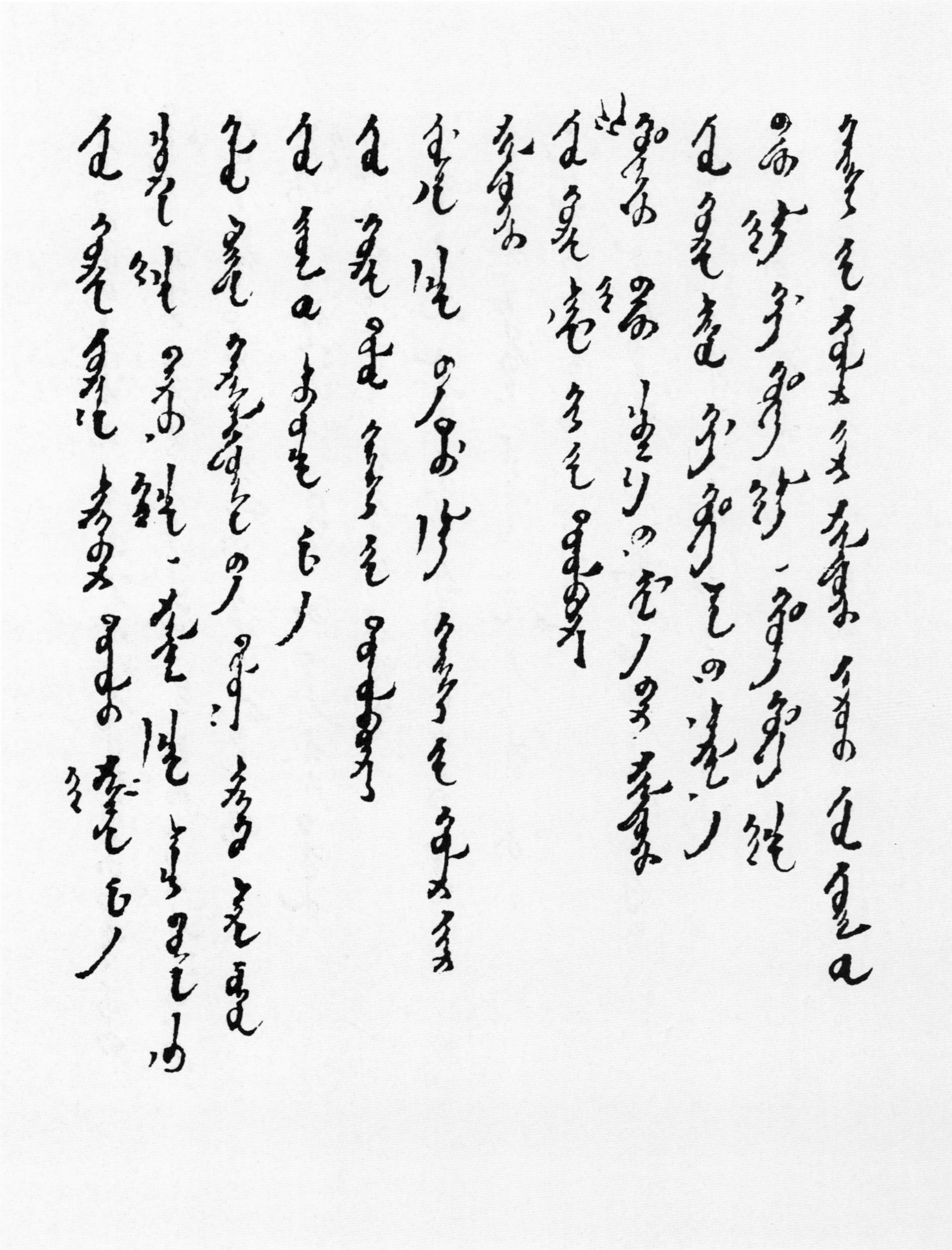

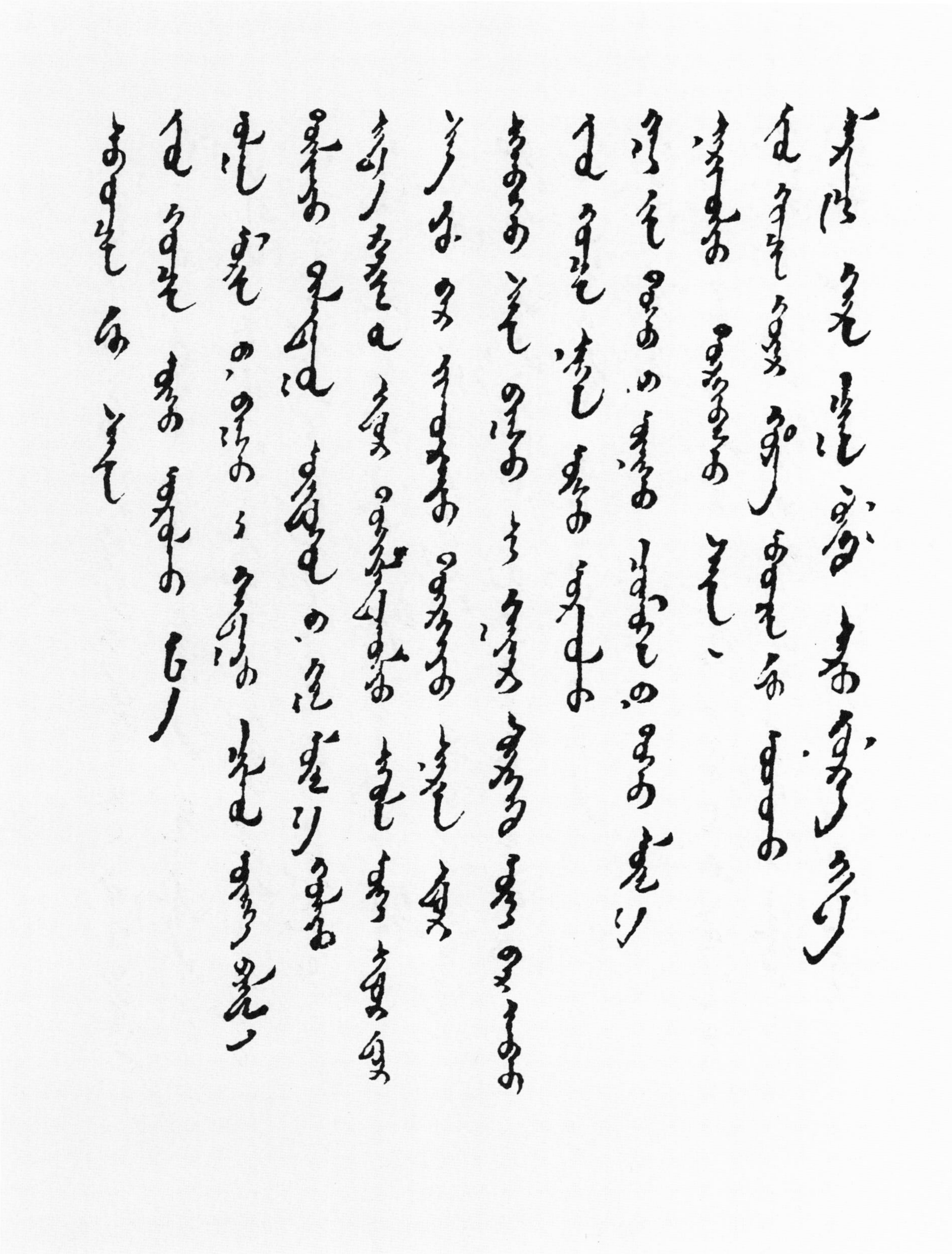

[illegible]
[illegible]
[illegible]
[illegible]
[illegible]
[illegible]
[illegible]
[illegible]
[illegible]
[illegible]
[illegible]
[illegible]
[illegible]

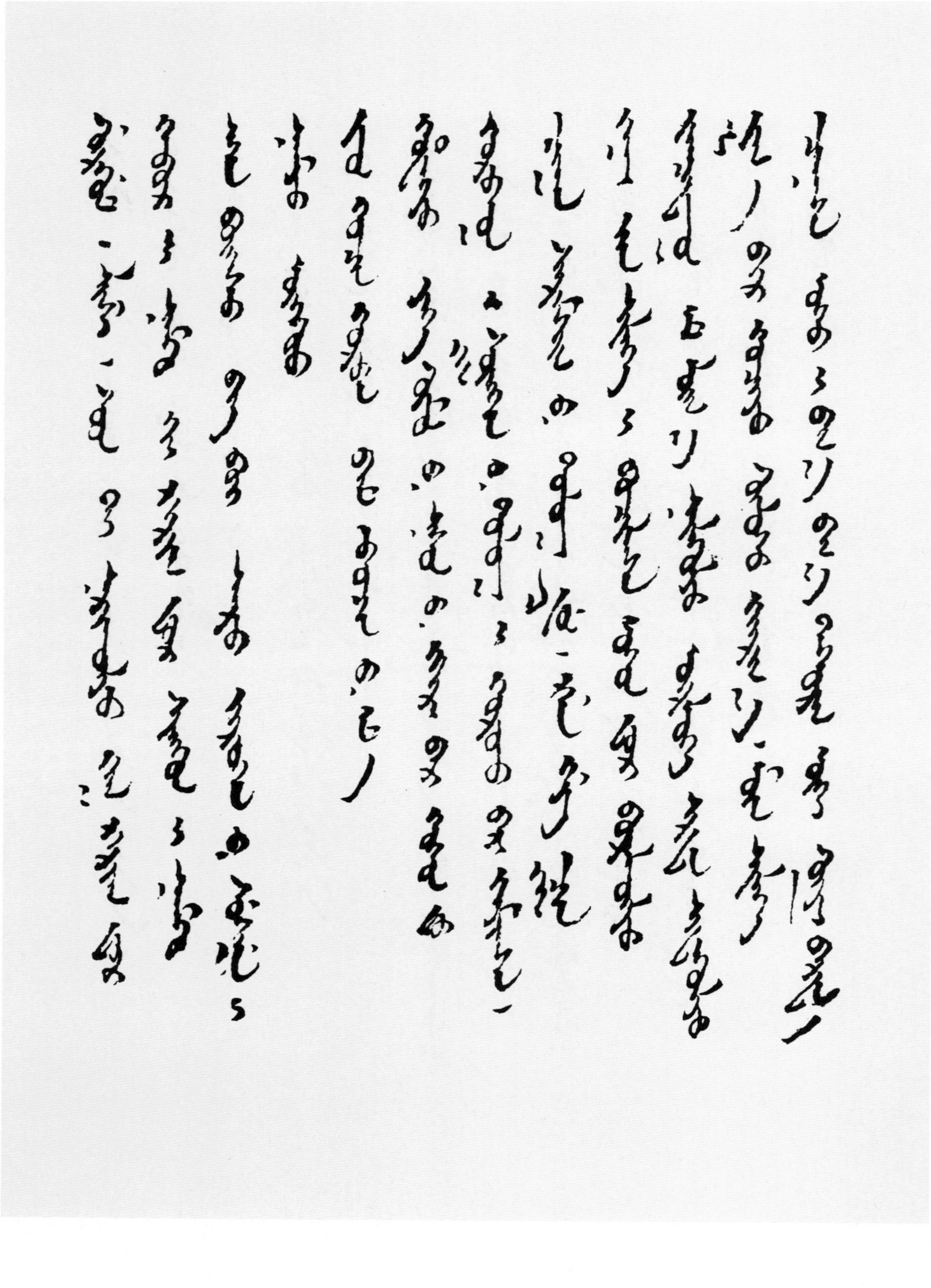

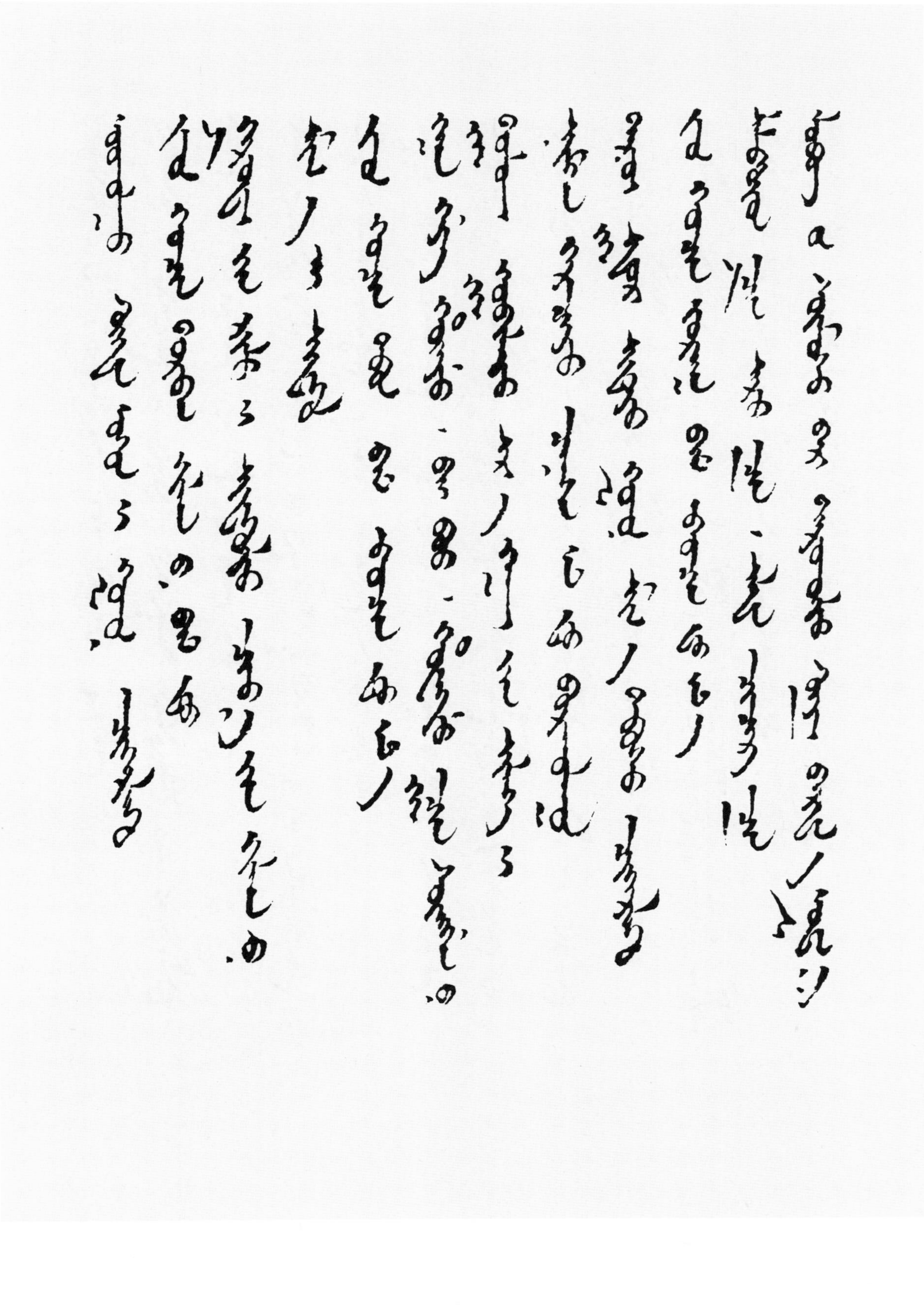

[illegible]

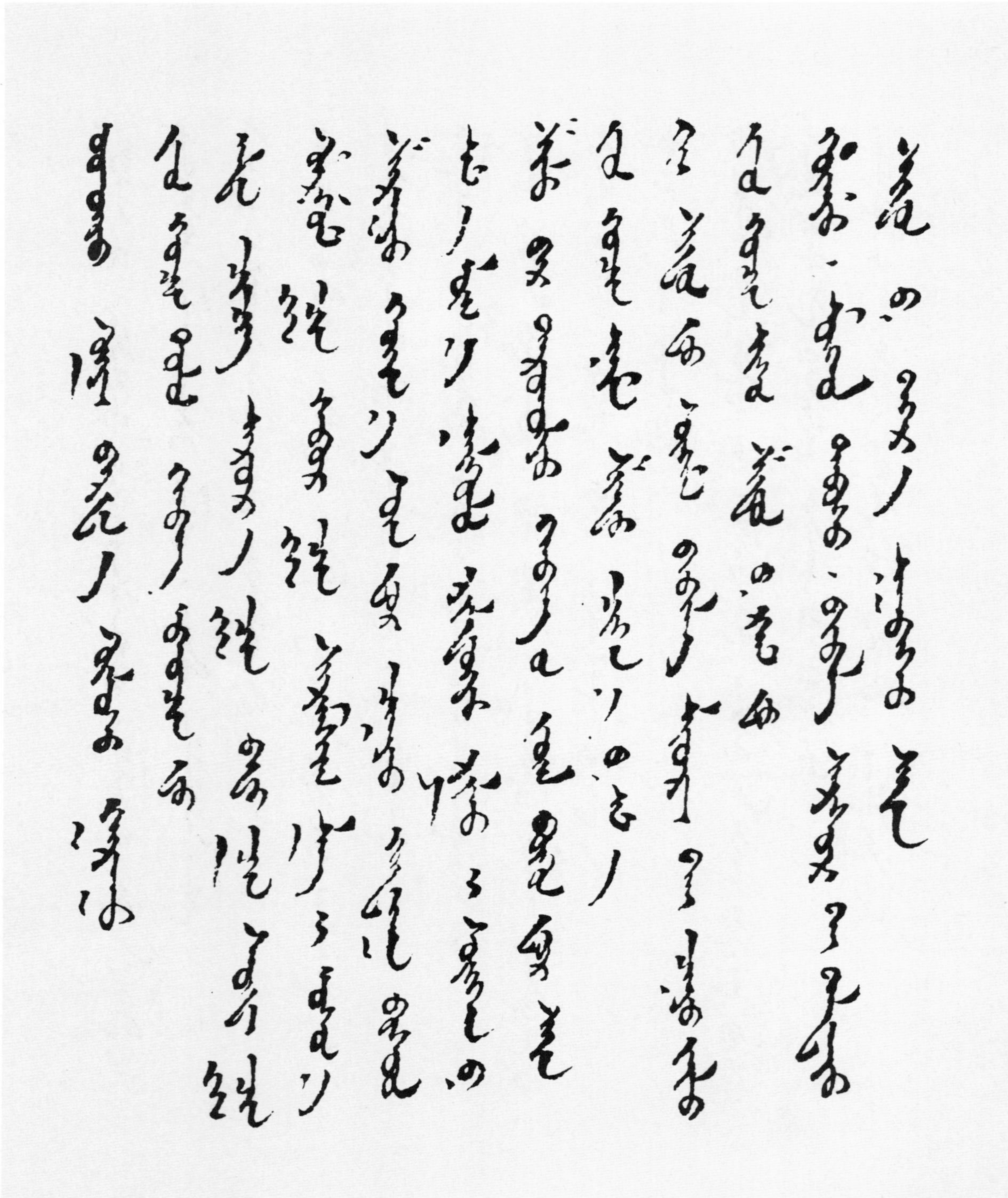

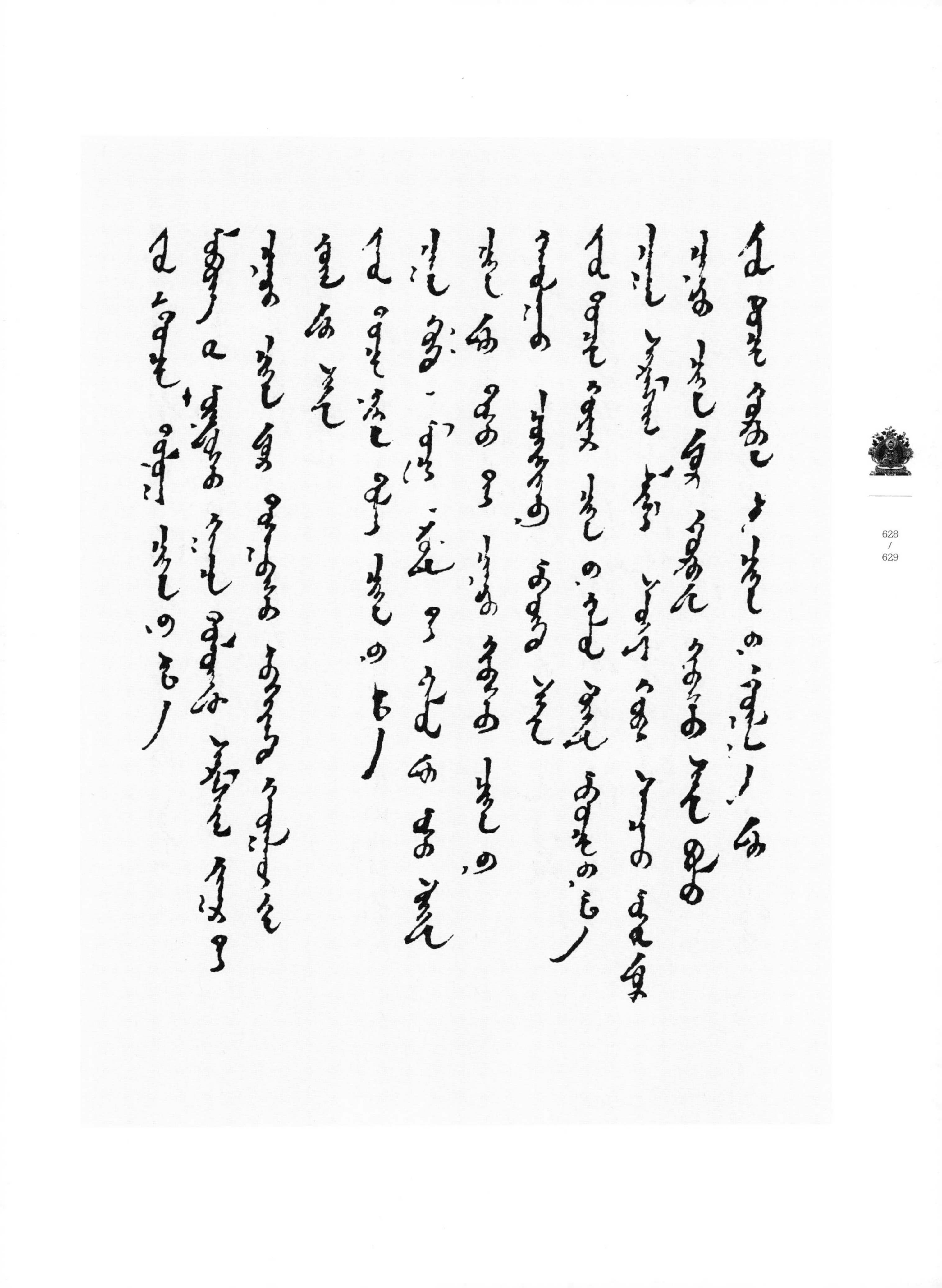

[illegible]

[illegible]

[illegible]

[illegible]

[illegible]

[illegible]

[illegible]

[illegible]

[illegible]

[illegible]

[illegible]

[illegible]

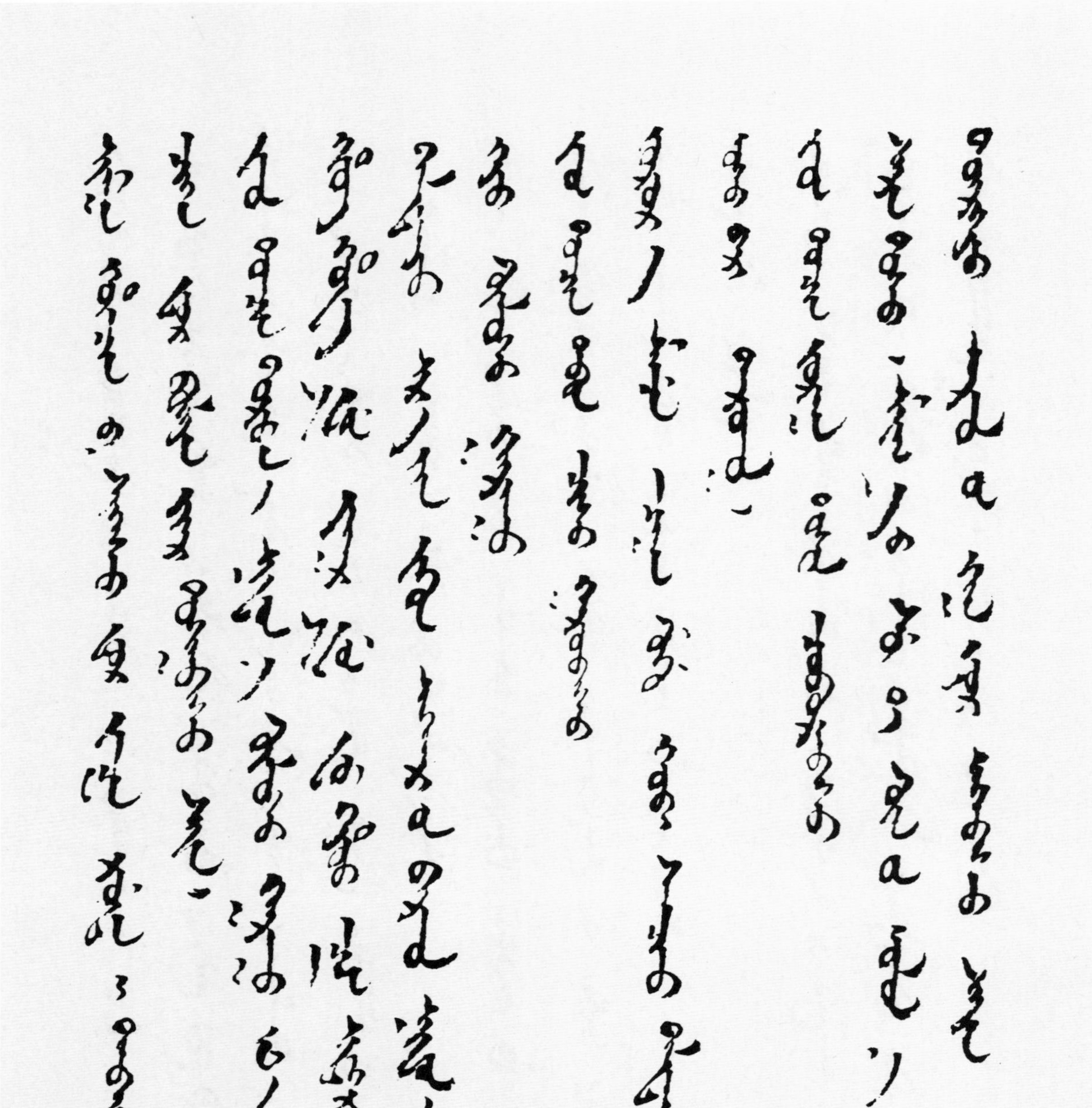

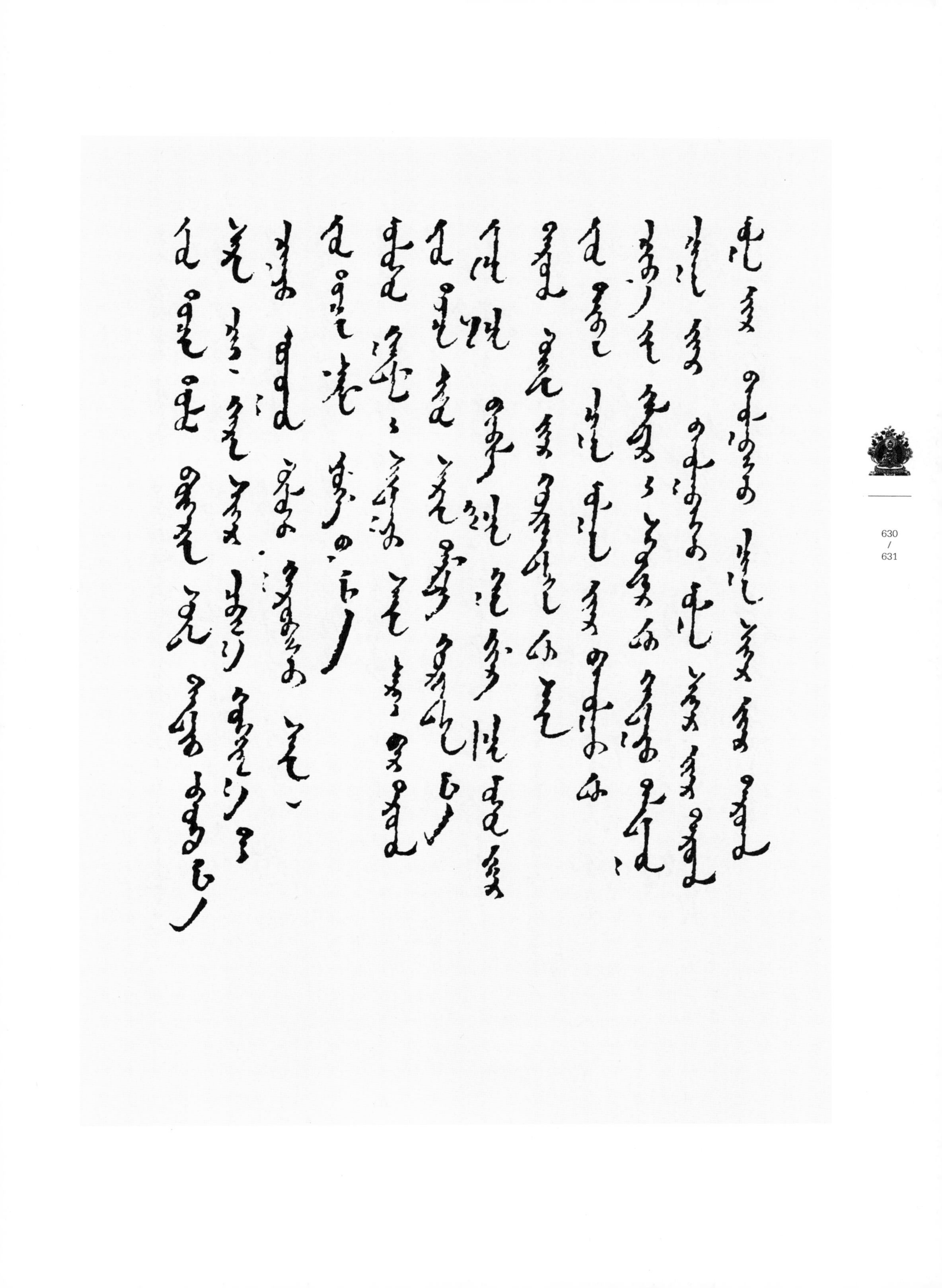

[illegible]

[illegible]

[illegible]

[illegible]

[illegible]

[illegible]

[illegible]

[illegible]

[illegible]

[illegible]

[illegible]

[illegible]

[illegible]

[illegible]

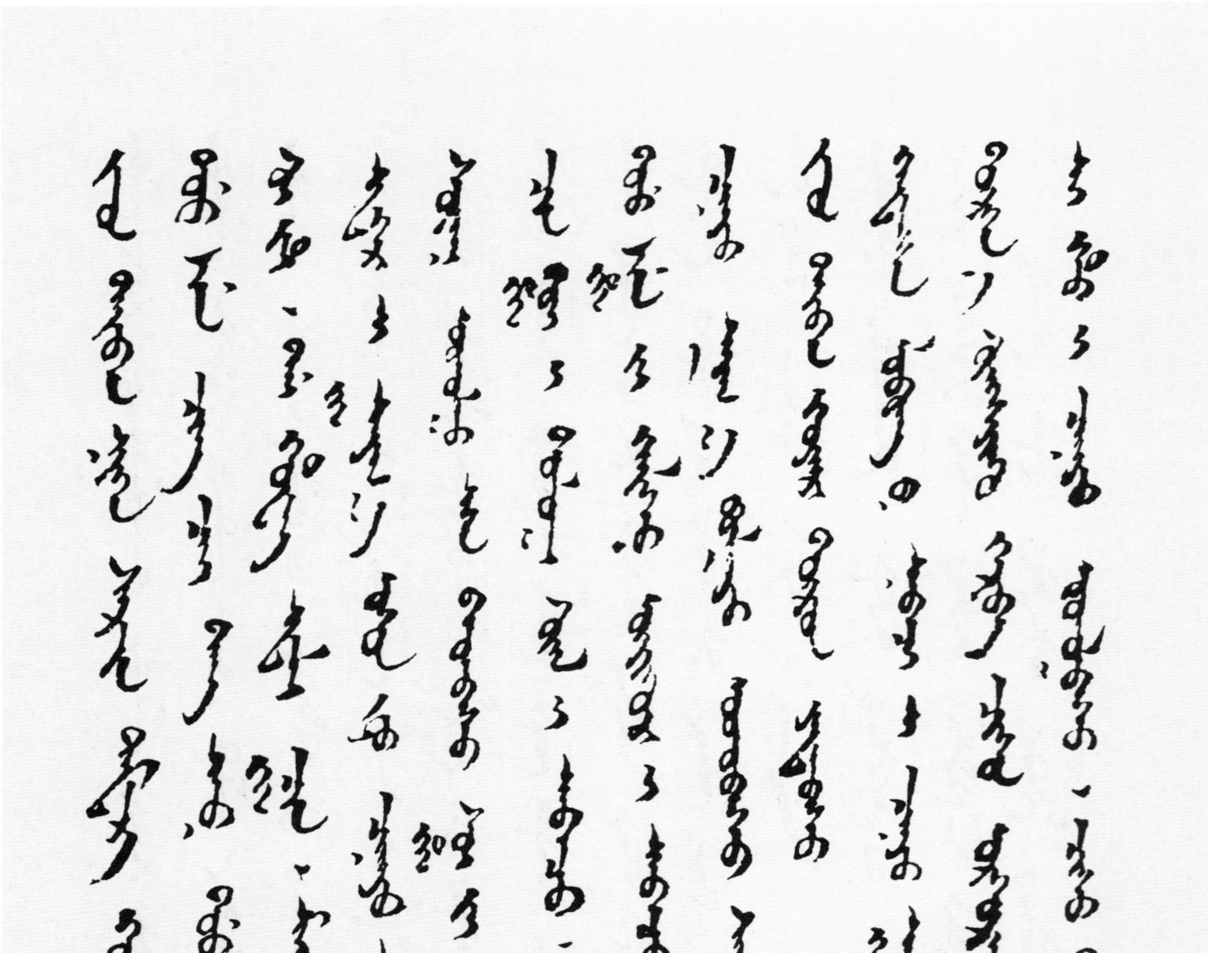

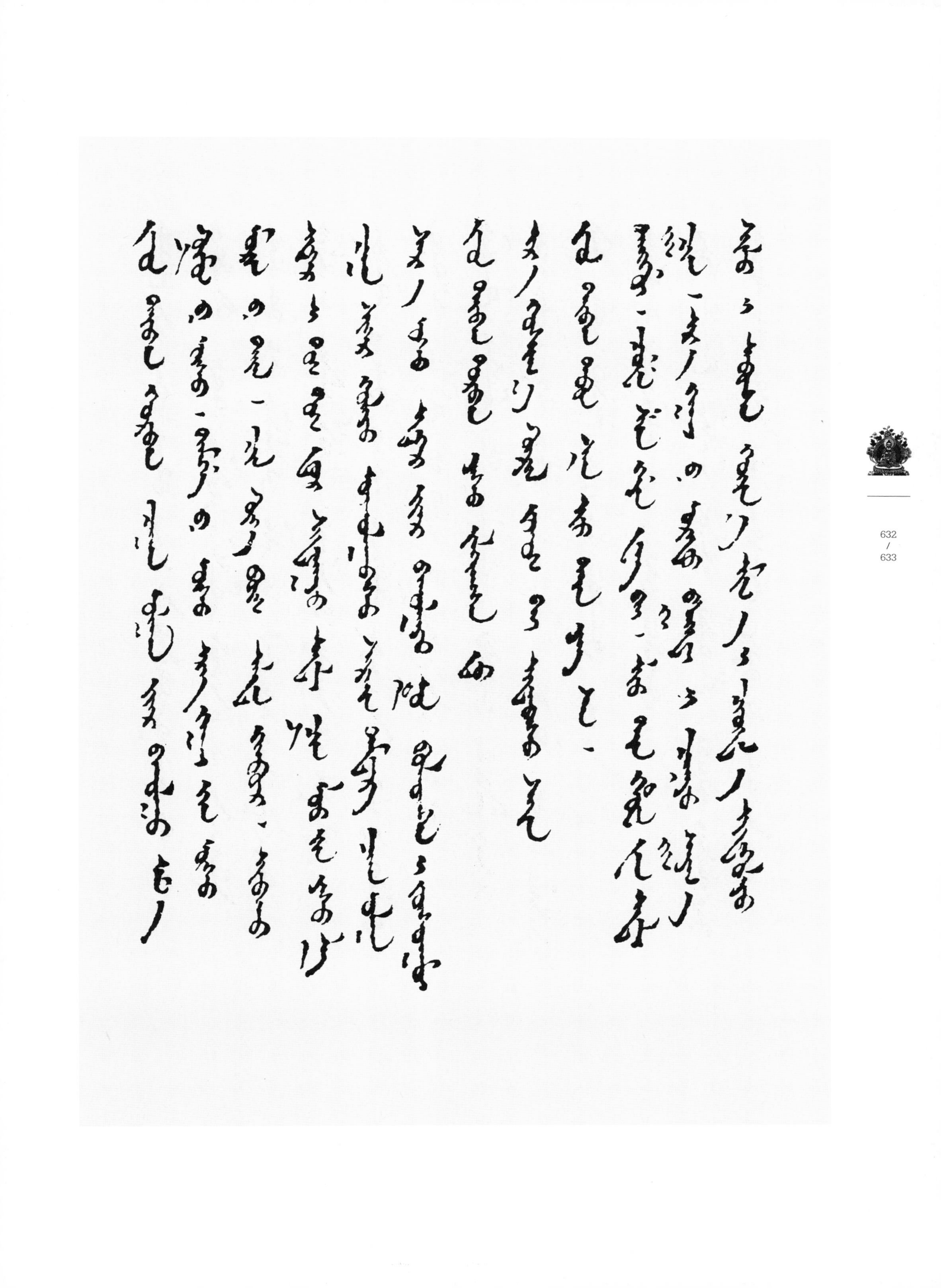

[illegible]
[illegible]
[illegible]
[illegible]
[illegible]
[illegible]
[illegible]
[illegible]
[illegible]
[illegible]
[illegible]
[illegible]
[illegible]
[illegible]

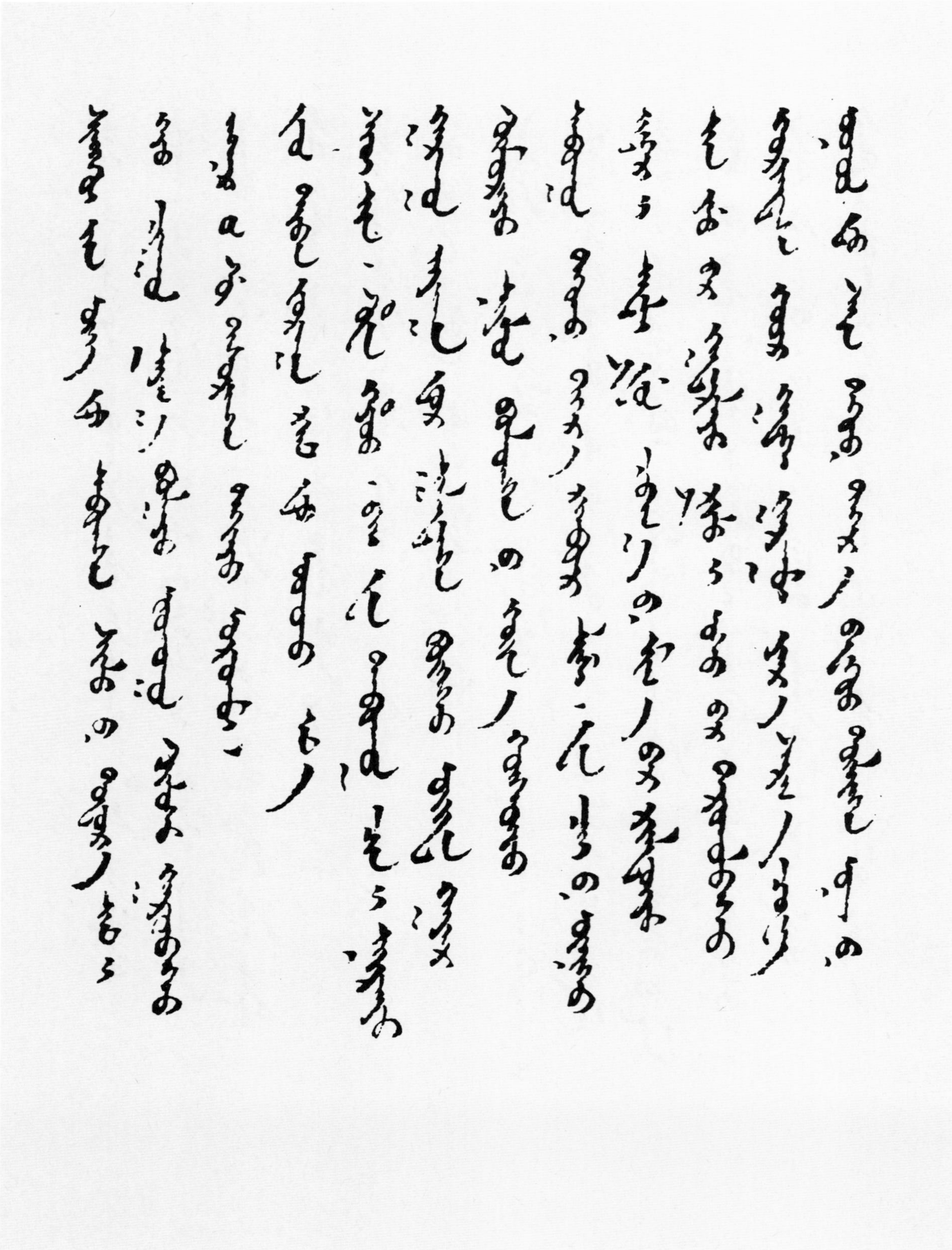

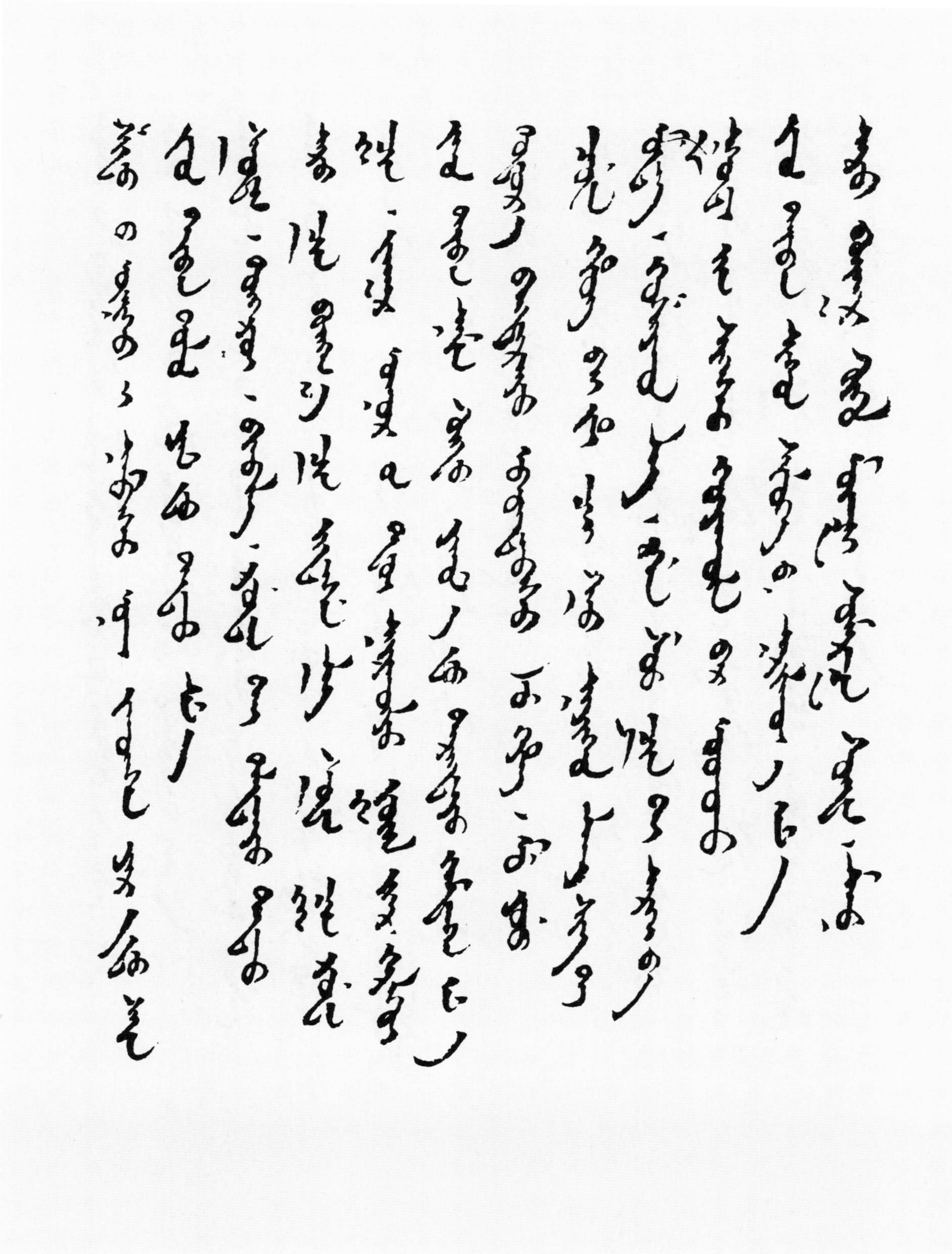

[illegible]
[illegible]
[illegible]
[illegible]
[illegible]
[illegible]
[illegible]
[illegible]
[illegible]
[illegible]
[illegible]
[illegible]

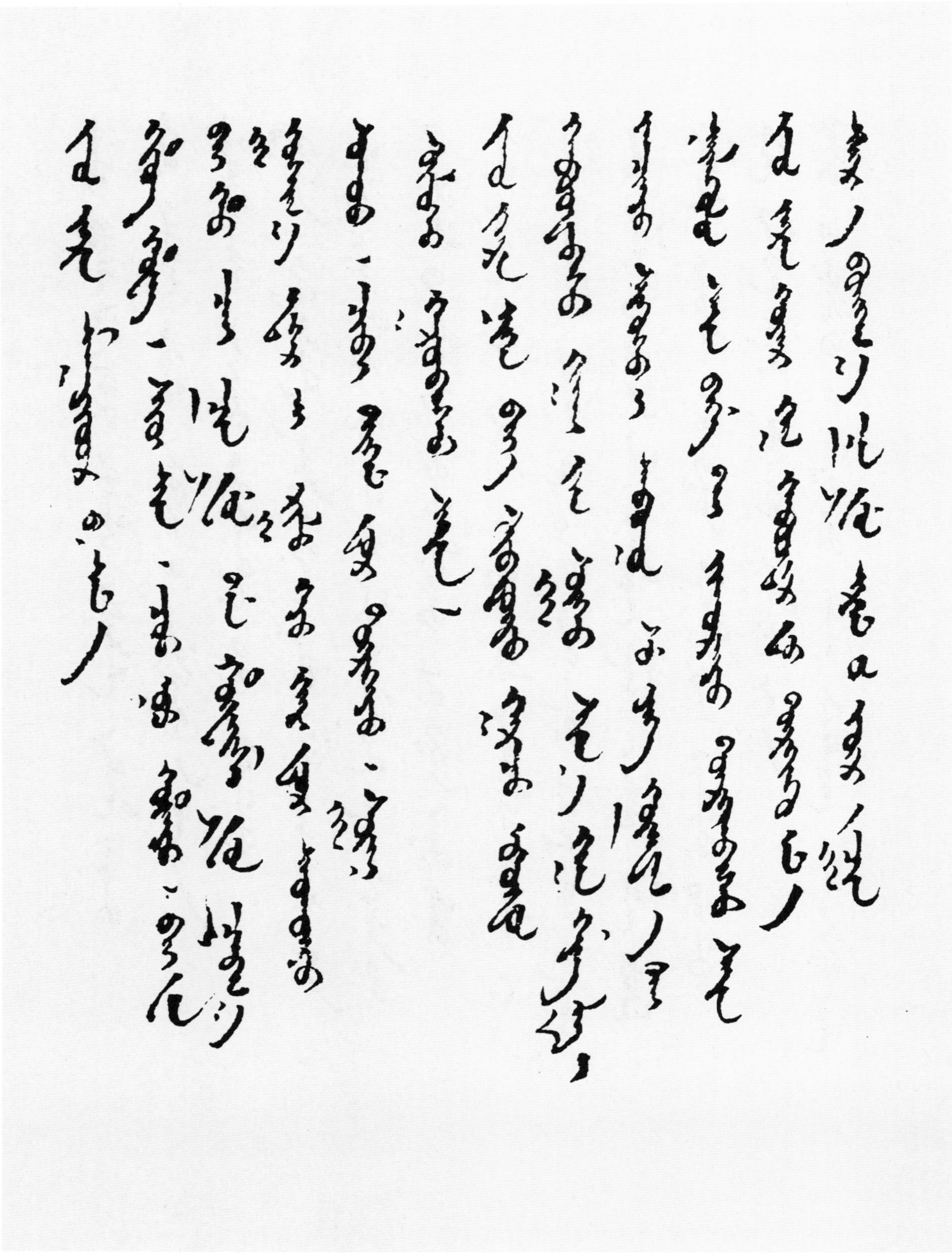

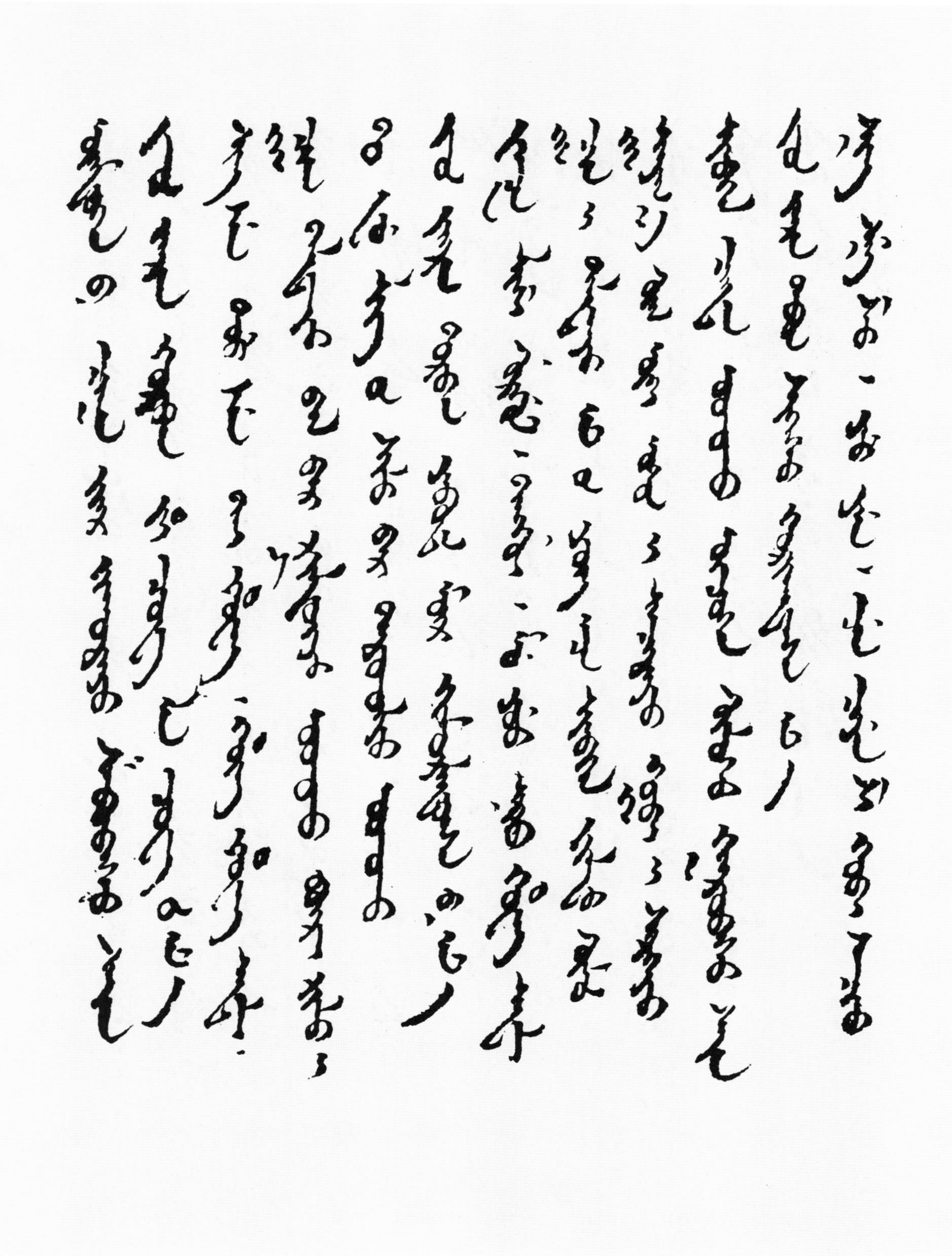

[illegible]

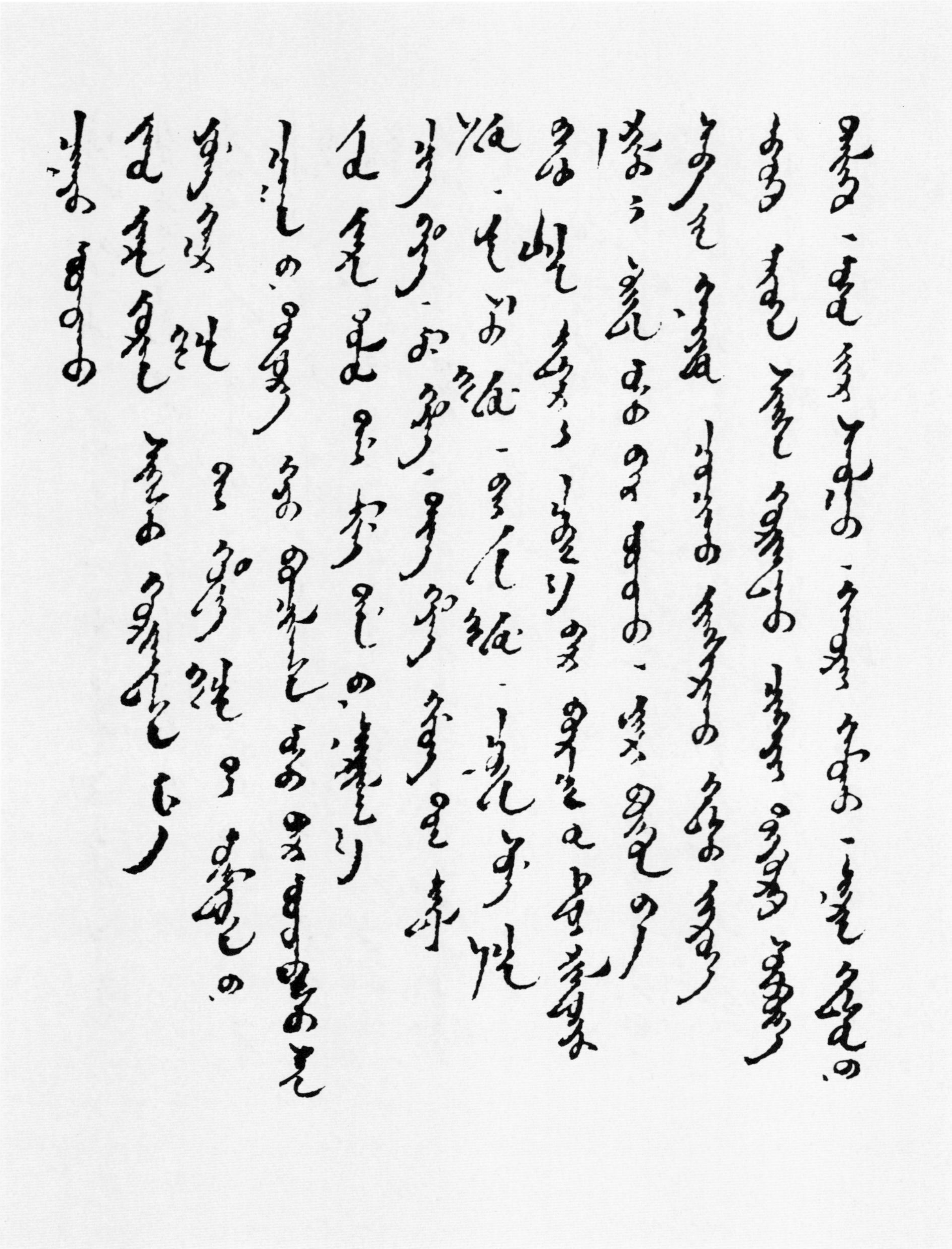

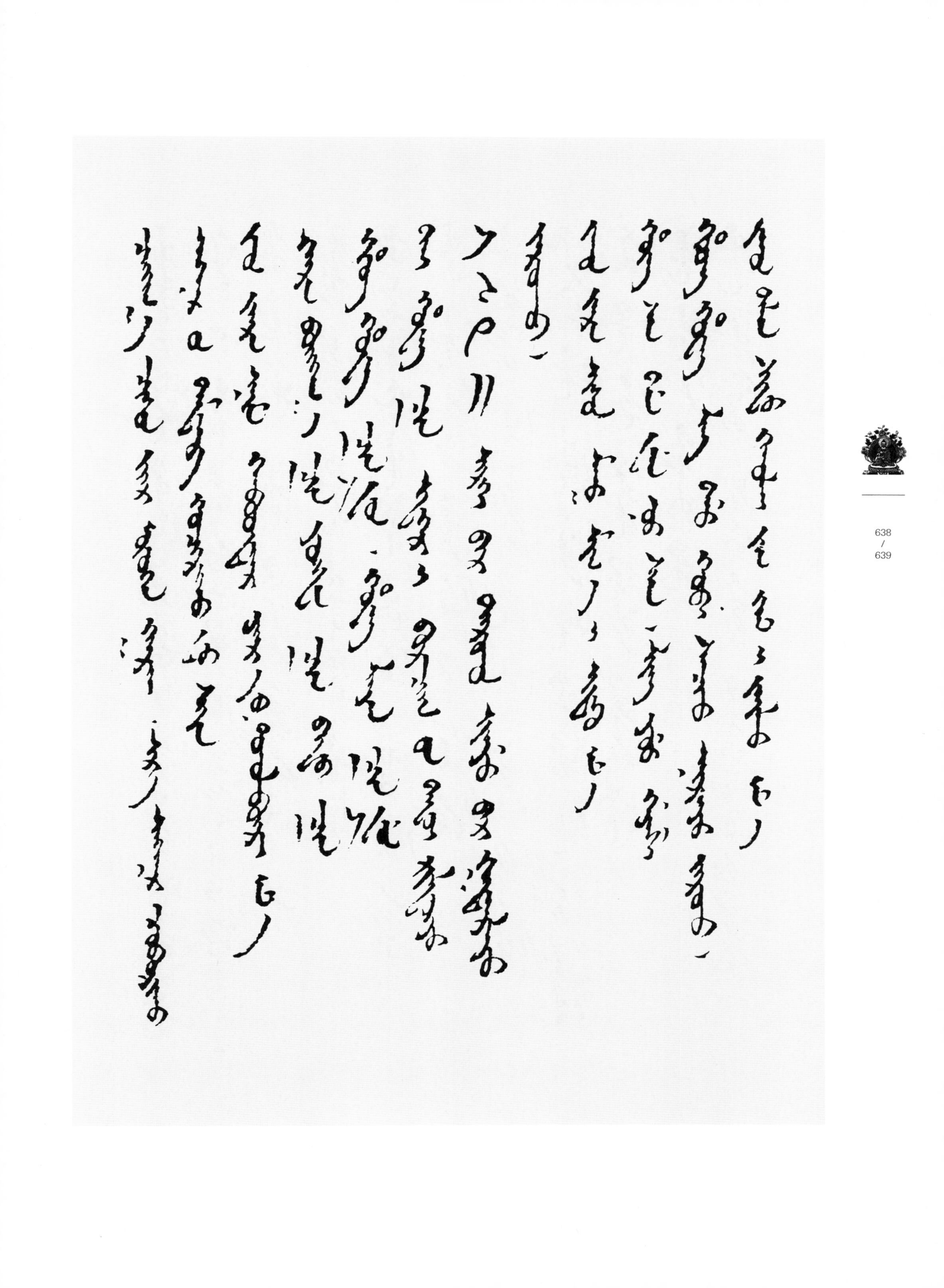

[illegible]

[illegible]

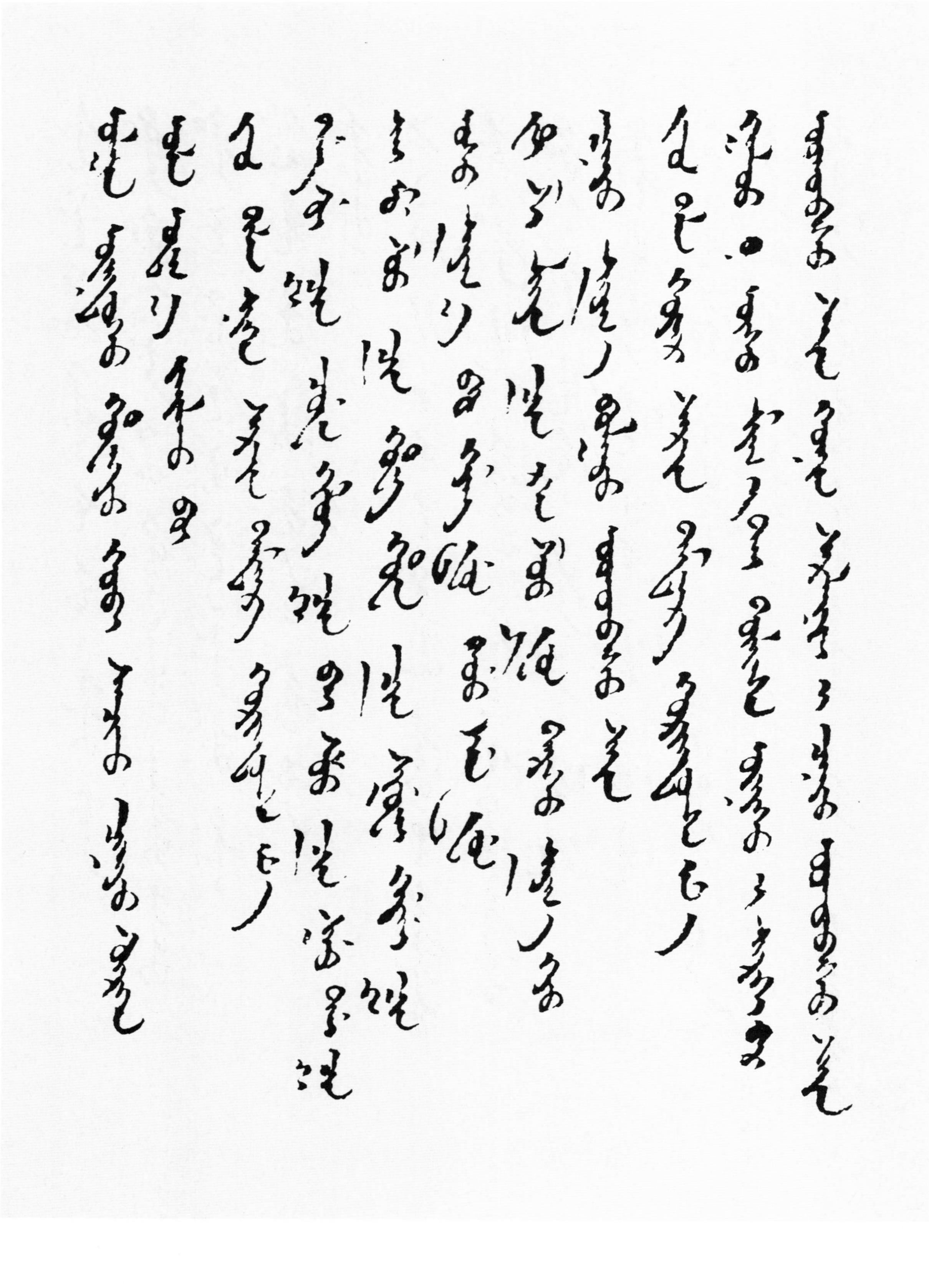

《ᠮᠣᠩᠭᠣᠯ ᠬᠡᠯᠡᠨ ᠦ ᠲᠣᠯᠢ ᠪᠢᠴᠢᠭ ᠦᠨ ᠬᠡᠪᠯᠡᠯ ᠦᠨ ᠬᠣᠷᠢᠶ᠎ᠠ ᠶᠢᠨ ᠪᠦᠲᠦᠭᠡᠯ ᠦᠨ ᠲᠣᠪᠴᠢᠶᠠᠨ》

ᠪᠢᠴᠢᠭ᠌ ᠦᠨ ᠣᠷᠴᠢᠭᠤᠯᠤᠭᠠᠳ ᠬᠡᠪᠯᠡᠭᠦᠯᠦᠨ ᠳᠤ ᠬᠣᠷᠢᠶᠠᠭᠰᠠᠨ ᠢ ᠦᠭᠡᠢᠰᠬᠡᠨ᠎ᠡ

ᠬᠡᠪᠯᠡᠯ ᠦᠨ ᠡᠷᠬᠡ ᠶᠢ ᠬᠠᠮᠠᠭᠠᠯᠠᠨ᠎ᠠ

ᠭᠠᠷᠴᠠᠭ ᠲᠠᠢ ᠪᠢᠴᠢᠭ᠌ ᠤᠨ ᠭᠠᠷᠴᠠᠭ ᠢ ᠰᠣᠯᠢᠨ᠎ᠠ ᠬᠡᠪᠯᠡᠯ ᠦᠨ ᠡᠷᠬᠡ

*

ᠦᠨᠳᠦᠰᠦᠲᠡᠨ ᠦ ᠬᠡᠪᠯᠡᠯ ᠦᠨ ᠬᠣᠷᠢᠶ᠎ᠠ ᠳᠤ ᠬᠡᠪᠯᠡᠭᠦᠯᠦᠨ ᠭᠠᠷᠭᠠᠪᠠ

ᠦᠨᠳᠦᠰᠦᠲᠡᠨ ᠦ ᠰᠣᠶᠣᠯ ᠭᠡᠭᠡᠷᠡᠯ ᠬᠡᠪᠯᠡᠯ ᠦᠨ ᠬᠣᠷᠢᠶ᠎ᠠ ᠬᠡᠪᠯᠡᠪᠡ

2018 ᠣᠨ ᠤ 7 ᠰᠠᠷ᠎ᠠ ᠳᠤ ᠨᠢᠭᠡᠳᠦᠭᠡᠷ ᠬᠡᠪᠯᠡᠯ

2021 ᠣᠨ ᠤ 1 ᠰᠠᠷ᠎ᠠ ᠳᠤ ᠬᠣᠶᠠᠳᠤᠭᠠᠷ ᠤᠳᠠᠭ᠎ᠠ ᠬᠡᠪᠯᠡᠪᠡ

ᠦᠨ᠎ᠡ : 480.00 ᠶᠤᠸᠠᠨ